# AUTISM SPECTRUM DISORDERS – FROM GENES TO ENVIRONMENT

Edited by **Tim Williams**

**Autism Spectrum Disorders – From Genes to Environment**
Edited by Tim Williams

**Published by InTech**

Janeza Trdine 9, 51000 Rijeka, Croatia



**Publishing Process Manager** Ivana Lorkovic

**Technical Editor** Teodora Smiljanic

**Cover Designe**r InTech Design Team

Additional hard copies can be obtained from orders@intechopen.com

Autism Spectrum Disorders – From Genes to Environment, Edited by Tim Williams
p. cm.
ISBN 978-953-307-558-7

For EU product safety concerns:
IN TECH d.o.o., Prolaz Marije Krucifikse Kozulić 3, 51000 Rijeka, Croatia,
info@intechopen.com or visit our website at intechopen.com.

# Meet the editor

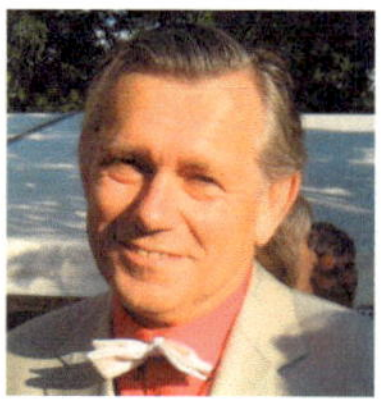

Dr. Tim Williams has known people with autism spectrum disorder since childhood. When he started his professional work as a clinical psychologist, he worked in a small residential hospital for children with autism and severe learning difficulties. His doctoral thesis was on teaching methods for children with autism, and following the closure of the hospital he was asked to set up a community based assessment and intervention service. He retired from that post in October 2010 and now works part time for a school for children with autism and learning difficulties, for the National Health Service and for the University of Reading. He has published more than forty peer reviewed papers on autism, behaviour problems and obsessive compulsive disorder.

# Contents

# Preface

DSM-V will introduce a change to the classification of autism, Asperger's syndrome and other related disorders by creating an over-arching category of Autism Spectrum Disorder (http://www.dsm5.org/ProposedRevisions/Pages/proposedrevision.aspx?rid =94#). The rationale behind this change is that autism spectrum disorder (ASD) can be diagnosed reliably, unlike the subcategories of Autism, Asperger's Syndrome and so on which cannot be reliably differentiated. Genetic studies have confirmed that the inheritance patterns are best understood as a predisposition to ASD rather than to autism or Asperger's syndrome. In this book the chapters have deliberately used a variety of terminology but with the understanding that the information contained in them can be applied to the whole autism spectrum.

The work described in this volume covers biological, psychological and environmental aspects of ASD. As editor I have organised the chapters to represent an orderly flow from genetic to environmental influences on ASD while attempting to recognise the complexities of the processes involved. Thus Millonig's group (Chapter 1) has identified one aspect of the genotype which renders people liable to the development of ASD. The genotype however does not have an inevitable outcome in terms of phenotype. One way of describing the inter-related influences is to use a diagram like that pioneered by Waddington (1956), as a series of valleys or equilibrium states into which an organism might develop depending on environmental influences. What the diagram makes clear is that with time it becomes increasingly difficult to move from one equilibrium state (valley in the diagram) to another.

The development of people with ASD can be conceptualised in a similar way. In theory, at least, early interventions are less effortful and require less environmental manipulation than later ones.

The interventions that are described in this volume can be classified as pharmacological (the use of antipsychotics (chapter 2), complementary medicine (chapters 3 and 4)), biological (direct modification of brain activity (chapter 5) and dietary (chapter 6) or psychosocial (the second section of the book).

The second section of the book is concerned with psychosocial interventions. Once again we can invoke a hierarchy to impose structure on the order of the chapters (see figure 2).

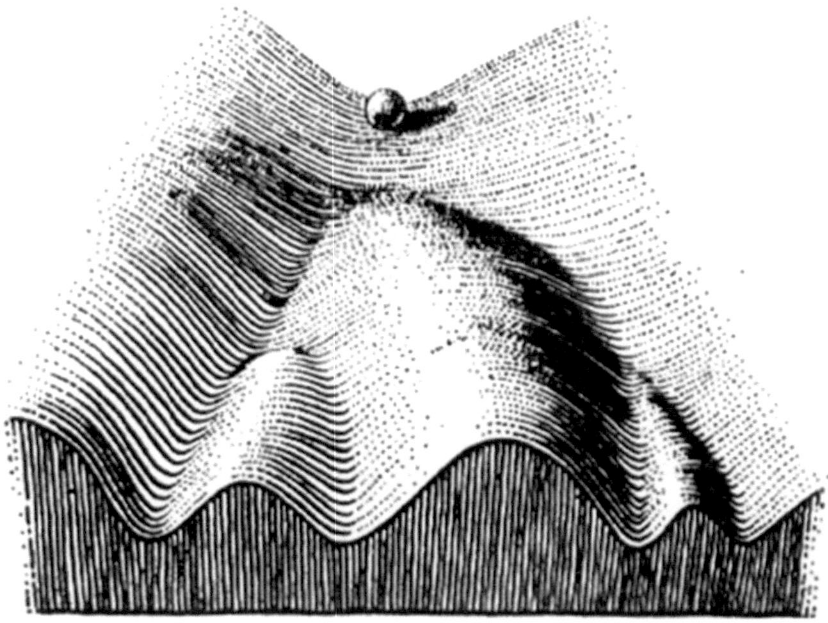

Fig. 1. Representation of the epigenetic landscape. The ball represents organism fate. The valleys are the different fates the organism might roll into. At the beginning of its journey, development is plastic, and an organism can become many fates. However, as development proceeds, certain decisions cannot be reversed easily. (From Waddington, 1956,).

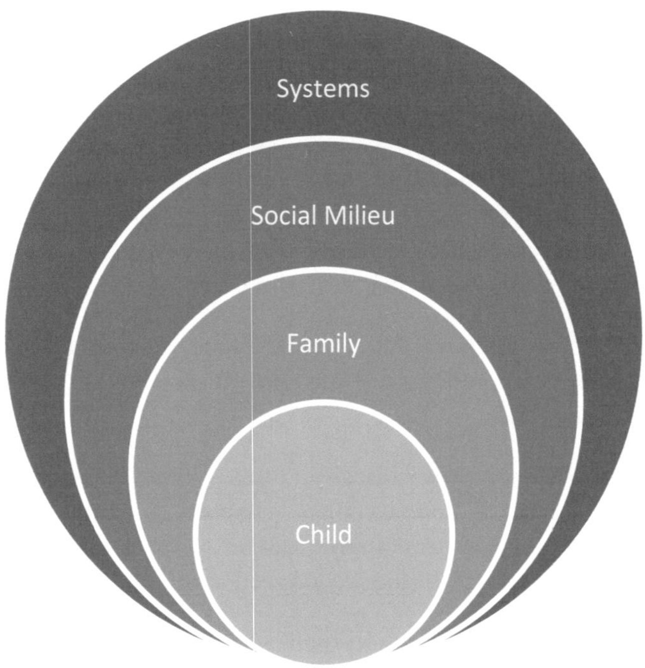


Fig. 2. Organisation of chapters

Starting from the outside chapters 7 and 8 consider how systems can be adapted to provide the most effective help for the family. Chapters 9, 10 and 11 describe adaptations to the social milieu around the child such as providing a TEACCH (chapter 9), Applied Behavior Analysis (chapter 10) or mediating literacy environment (chapter 11) or enabling a more inclusive peer system (chapter 12). Nader-Grosbois (chapter 13) then provides a useful overview of how the self-regulatory skills of the child with ASD impact on the ability of the environment to contain them and enable their development.

Chapters 14 to 17 are concerned with more targeted interventions. Field (chapter 14) has contributed a chapter on the development of imitation, Orvalho (chapter 15) has described an intervention to improve the recognition of emotions using technology and Barbro and Hansson (chapter 16) have evaluated an intervention to improve responsiveness. The use of technology recurs as a theme through chapters 17 (Thunberg), and 18 (Rodríguez-Fórtiz, Fernández-López, and Rodríguez) which are concerned with augmentative communication methods. The last intervention chapter (19) reminds us that to live a high quality life, maintenance of one's own health is a priority. The final chapter (20) stands out as a useful summary of the literature on the built environment for people with ASD, which is itself the result of an interaction of designers, the materials that they work with and people with autism spectrum disorders.

For the reader I would suggest that this book is best conceived as a series of journal articles. Like all scientific publications any one article can be critiqued, but I hope as editor that there is sufficient worth in each chapter that they can inform future work in the field of ASD studies.

**References**

Waddington, C. H., 1956, Principles of Embryology, Macmillan, New York

**Dr T. I. Williams**
Consultant Educational and Clinical Psychologist
Berkshire Healthcare NHS Trust and Priors Court Foundation
Reader in Special Education
University of Reading

# Part 1

# Biomedical Aspects

# 1

# *ENGRAILED 2* (*EN2*) Genetic and Functional Analysis

Jiyeon Choi[1], Silky Kamdar[1], Taslima Rahman[1], Paul G Matteson[1] and James H Millonig[1,2,3]
[1]*Center for Advanced Biotechnology and Medicine,*
[2]*Department of Neuroscience and Cell Biology,*
*UMDNJ-Robert Wood Johnson Medical School,*
[3]*Department of Genetics, Rutgers University, Piscataway NJ,*
*USA*

## 1. Introduction

Our autism research has focused on the homeobox transcription factor, *ENGRAILED 2* (*EN2*). Prior to the advent of genome wide association and re-sequencing analysis, we selected *EN2* as a candidate gene due to neuroanatomical similarities observed between individuals with autism and mouse *En2* mutants.

Animal studies have demonstrated that *En2* is expressed throughout CNS development and regulates numerous cell biological processes implicated in ASD including connectivity, excitatory/inhibitory (E/I) circuit balance, and neurotransmitter development. The relevance of these functions to ASD etiology is discussed.

Human genetic analysis by us determined that two intronic SNPs, *rs1861972* and *rs1861973,* are significantly associated with Autism Spectrum Disorder (ASD). We observed the common haplotype (*rs1861972-rs1861973* A-C) is over-transmitted to affected individuals while the *rs1816972-rs1861973* G-T haplotype is over-represented in unaffected siblings. Significant results were observed in 3 datasets (518 families, 2336 individuals, P=.00000035). 6 other groups have also reported association of *EN2* with ASD, suggesting that *EN2* is an ASD susceptibility gene. These results are discussed.

However if *EN2* contributes to ASD risk, we would expect the ASD-associated A-C haplotype to segregate with a polymorphism that is functional and affects either the regulation or activity of *EN2*. Linkage disequilibrium mapping, re-sequencing and additional association analysis was performed, and identified the A-C haplotype as the best candidate for functional analysis. Luciferase assays conducted in primary mouse neuronal cultures demonstrated that the A-C haplotype functions as a transcriptional activator and specifically binds a protein complex. Transgenic mouse studies have demonstrated that the A-C haplotype is also functional, increasing gene expression *in vivo*. Finally, human post-mortem studies indicate *EN2* levels are also increased in individuals with autism. Thus, the ASD-associated A-C haplotype is functional and increased *EN2* levels are consistently correlated with ASD.

Six significant CpG islands also flank human *EN2*. Preliminary studies indicate hypomethylation of these CpGs can also result in increased *EN2* levels, suggesting epigenetic alterations influenced by non-genetic environmental factors can affect *EN2* levels. To study how genetic and epigenetic changes may function together to influence *EN2* regulation and CNS development, we are creating a chromosomal engineered knock-in that will replace ~75kb of mouse *En2* with the human gene.

In summary *EN2* is consistently associated with ASD and functions in developmental pathways implicated in ASD. In addition, we have shown that the ASD-associated haplotype is functional, resulting in increased expression both in neuronal cultures *in vitro* and in transgenic mice *in vivo*. Increased levels are also observed in human post-mortem samples. Together these human genetic data along with our molecular, mouse and post-mortem studies indicate that *EN2* is an ASD susceptibility gene

## 2. Selection of *ENGRAILED 2* as a candidate gene

Before genome-wide strategies were available for identifying common and rare variants for ASD, my laboratory decided to test candidate genes based upon neuroanatomical phenotypes. When we started this work in 2003, two cerebellar neuroanatomical phenotypes were consistently observed in individuals with ASD: a decrease in cerebellar volume (hypoplasia) and fewer Purkinje neurons (Bauman and Kemper 1985; Bauman 1986; Courchesne, Yeung-Courchesne et al. 1988; Courchesne 1997; Amaral, Schumann et al. 2008). We knew of numerous mouse mutants that displayed similar morphological phenotypes so we decided to test these genes for association in the available Autism Genetic Resource Exchange (AGRE) dataset. A list of nearly 100 genes were compiled that displayed similar cerebellar phenotypes in the mouse and individuals with ASD. The list also included genes that at the time were expressed in the cerebellum in specific spatial-temporal patterns suggesting they were likely to contribute to development. These genes were then placed on the human genome to determine which ones mapped near polymorphic markers that displayed linkage to ASD.

Many of the genes mapped to possibly interesting locations so we prioritized our association analysis by the following criteria: i) distance to SSLP marker, ii) LOD score or statistical significance of marker, iii) whether segregation or linkage to the chromosomal region had been replicated in multiple studies, iv) whether the genomic region displayed linkage in the AGRE dataset which would be used for our association analysis, v) whether mouse mutants existed for the gene, vi) and the similarity between reported mouse and ASD cerebellar phenotypes

Based on these criteria we selected the homeobox transcription factor *ENGRAILED 2* (*EN2*) as a candidate gene. *EN2* belongs to a class of transcription factors that are homologous in their DNA binding domain called the homeobox. Homeobox transcription factors regulate gene expression by binding to AT-rich DNA elements, and play central roles in coordinating development. Many homeobox genes are evolutionarily conserved from Drosophila to humans. The *engrailed* gene was first identified in classical genetic screens for developmental regulators in Drosophila. Humans and mice have two *Engrailed* genes, *Engrailed 1* (*En1*) and *Engrailed 2* (*En2*). Both *En1* and *En2* regulate important aspects of CNS development (see Section 4 - *ENGRAILED 2* function)

Human *EN2* maps to distal chromosome 7 (7q36.3), near markers that display linkage to ASD in several datasets (Liu, Nyholt et al. 2001; Alarcon, Cantor et al. 2002; Auranen, Vanhala et al. 2002). Two of these studies had been performed using AGRE families. In addition two different *En2* mouse mutations existed – a traditional knock-out or deletion of

*En2*, and a transgenic misexpression mutant. In the knockout the cerebellum is reduced in size and cell counts have determined an ~30-40% reduction in all the major cerebellar cell types including Purkinje cells (Millen, Wurst et al. 1994; Kuemerle, Zanjani et al. 1997). In the trangenic *En2* is misexpressed in a subset of Purkinje cells and similar phenotypes were observed (40-50% reduction in cerebellar area; ~40% decrease in the number of adult Purkinje cells)(Baader, Sanlioglu et al. 1998).
Significant association of *EN2* with ASD was initially demonstrated by us and has now been reported by 5 additional groups (Brune, Korvatska et al. 2007; Wang, Jia et al. 2008; Yang, Lung et al. 2008; Sen, Singh et al. 2010; Yang, Shu et al. 2010). Prior to summarizing these data, we will first describe the known expression of mouse and human *EN2* as well as the cell biological processes regulated by En2 in the developing and adult brain.

## 3. *Engrailed 2* expression during development

Mouse *En2* expression has been evaluated primarily by *in situ* hybridization and lacZ knock-in mice (see Table 1 for summary). In these studies *En2* expression is initiated at E8.0 at the junction between the midbrain and hindbrain. *En2* continues to be expressed in a majority of mid-hindbrain cells from E8.5 to E12.5. These *En2* expressing cells will generate the cerebellum and midbrain colliculi dorsally, as well as parts of the serotonin (raphe nucleus) and norepinephrine (locus coeruleus) neurotransmitter systems ventrally. By E17.5 *En2* expression becomes more spatially restricted. In the chick tectum *En2* is expressed in a rostral to caudal gradient, while in the cerebellum it is stripe-like. By post-natal day 6 *En2* transcripts are restricted to the differentiating cells in the external germinal layer and developing inner granule cell layer of the cerebellum. In the adult *En2* continues to be expressed in mature cerebellar granule cells. Finally, QRTPCR studies indicate *En2* is also expressed at low levels in adult hippocampus.

| Developmental Stage | Expression | Function |
|---|---|---|
| E8.0-E12.5 | Mid-hindbrain junction | A-P patterning, Neurotransmitter development |
| E12.5-E15.5 | Developing cerebellum, colliculi, ventral mid-hindbrain nuclei including LC and RN, periaqueductal gray | Retinal-tectal mapping, Neurotransmitter development |
| E15.5-P0 | Developing cerebellum, colliculi, | Retinal-tectal mapping, cerebellar connectivity |
| P0-P12 | Cerebellum (differentiating Granule cells) | Cell cycle and differentiation |
| Adult | Mature granule cells | Unknown |

Table 1. Summary of *En2* expression and function from animal studies

A limited number of human *ENGRAILED 2* expression studies have been performed. One analysis conducted on 18-21 weeks post-conception fetuses demonstrated widespread expression for both *ENGRAILED 1* and *2* genes throughout the mid-hindbrain region including the cerebellar cortex and deep nuclei. Expression was also observed in several ventral hindbrain nuclei (inferior olive, arcuate nucleus, caudal raphe nucleus)(Zec, Rowitch et al. 1997). Western blot analysis conducted on cerebellar samples at later gestational ages (40 weeks) indicated abundant expression for both EN proteins (Logan, Hanks et al. 1992). Interestingly, recent microarray analysis performed by The Allen Institute for Brain Science demonstrates abundant expression throughout the cerebellum (cortex and deep nuclei) but also in numerous forebrain and midbrain structures (basal ganglia, amygdala, thalamus)(Figure 1). A complete developmental analysis of human *EN2* expression has not been reported. These data suggest human adult brain *EN2* expression is more widespread than mouse *En2,* and in fore- and mid-brain structures relevant to ASD phenotypes.

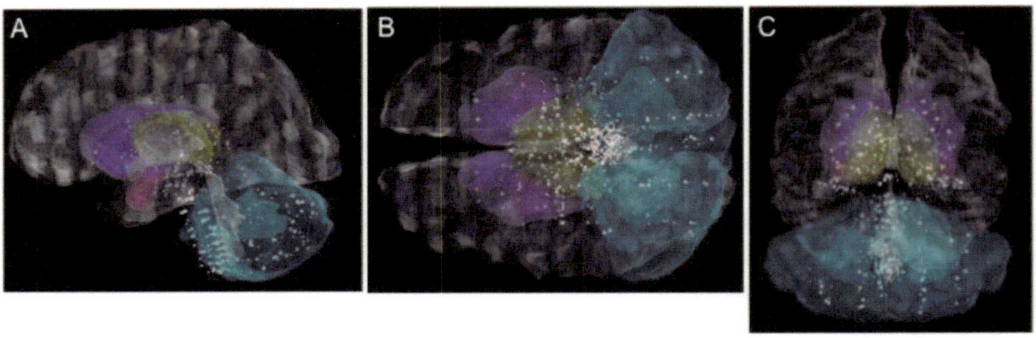


Fig. 1. Human *EN2* expression. Microarray data of microdissected brain regions performed by The Allen Institute for Brain Science indicate that *EN2* is expressed in the basal ganglia (purple), amygdala (pink), thalamus (green) as well as cerebellum and brainstem (blue). A) sagittal, B) horizontal, and C) caudal views

## 4. *ENGRAILED 2* function

Molecular studies have determined that En2 functions as a transcriptional repressor. The protein regulates numerous cell biological pathways during CNS development but has a well-characterized function in establishing connectivity maps. Emerging data also supports En2 function in E/I circuit balance as well as serotonin and norepinephrine neurotransmitter development. All of these cellular processes have been implicated in ASD etiology.

### 4.1 Transcriptional repressor function of En2

Molecular studies indicate the Engrailed 2 protein primarily functions as a transcriptional repressor, which is mediated by several different protein domains (Figure 2). DNA binding occurs through the homeodomain to a generic AT rich cis-sequence recognized by homeobox transcription factors. Two domains (engrailed homology region 1 (EH1) and EH5) contribute to Engrailed repressor activity. EH1 is located in the N-terminal portion of the protein while the EH5 domain is immediately 3′ of the homeodomain in the C terminal portion of the protein. Both domains bind the co-repressor Groucho, while EH1 is sufficient to confer repression activity when transferred to a transcriptional activator. Engrailed repressor function is mediated by two different mechanisms. The protein can actively block the trans-activation of activators by binding to nearby cis-sequences. Alternatively, the engrailed proteins compete for the binding of the basal transcriptional machinery to TATA box sequences (Ohkuma, Horikoshi et al. 1990; Jaynes and O'Farrell 1991; Tolkunova,

Fujioka et al. 1998). Finally, two other domains (EH2 and EH3) bind the Pbx family of homeodomain transcription factors, which affect DNA biding specificity (van Dijk and Murre 1994; Peltenburg and Murre 1997).

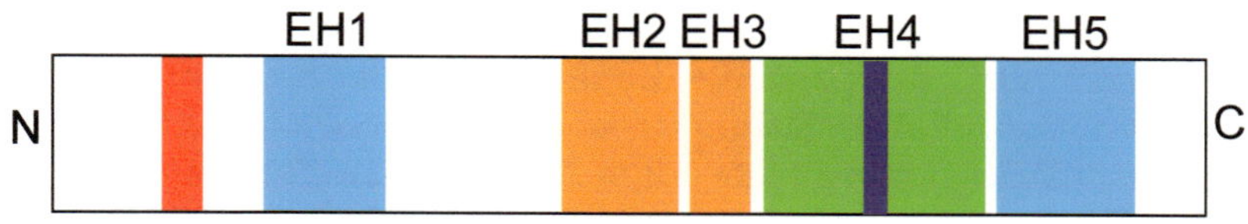


Fig. 2. En protein domains. The En protein structure is illustrated and the different En interaction domains are demarcated in following colors: translation initiation factor eIF4E binding site, transcriptional repressor domains, PBX interactions domains, homeodomain, and penetratin domain. EH1-5 indicate engrailed homology domains 1 through 5.

### 4.2 En2 regulates mid-hindbrain patterning

Mouse and chick studies have determined that En2 coordinates multiple cell biological process throughout development. From E8.0-E12.5, *En2* and *En1* are spatially overlapping at the mid-hindbrain junction and both genes function to restrict progenitors to a midbrain and hindbrain lineage (Joyner 1996). *En2* temporal expression commences a few hours after *En1* transcripts are first detected and because of this difference, the *En1* knock-out mouse displays a more severe phenotype with a deletion of mid-hindbrain structures (Wurst, Auerbach et al. 1994). Knock-in experiments where *En2* is targeted to the *En1* locus are sufficient to rescue this phenotype, demonstrating that En2 is functionally redundant to En1 at this early stage of development (Hanks, Wurst et al. 1995).

### 4.3 Engrailed genes and 5HT and NE neurotransmitter system development

Previous studies have demonstrated that the *Engrailed* genes are important in the development and maintenance of substantia nigra neurons in the dopamine neurotransmitter system. These data are reviewed elsewhere (Simon, Saueressig et al. 2001; Alberi, Sgado et al. 2004; Simon, Thuret et al. 2004; Gherbassi and Simon 2006; Sgado, Alberi et al. 2006). Instead we focus on the role of the *En* genes on serotonin (5HT) and norepinephrine (NE) development, since abnormalities in these neurotransmitter systems have been more consistently implicated in ASD.

Mutations in the Engrailed genes affect the development of ventral mid-hindbrain nuclei that synthesize NE and 5HT: the locus coeruleus (LC) and raphe nuclei (RN) respectively. The LC is generated early in development (E9-E10 in the mouse) from the dorsal mid-hindbrain junction. The LC is deleted in the double *En1*$^{-/-}$ *En2*$^{-/-}$ knockout mice but appears relatively normal in the single knockouts suggesting the genes compensate for each other during development. The RN is generated in the ventral mid-hindbrain and express 5HT by E11.5. Several transcription factors including Pet1, Lmx1b and Gata3 are important in the generation of RN. Recent analysis indicates that both *En* genes are expressed in the progenitors of RN at E11.5 and to continue to be expressed in post-mitotic rostral 5HT neurons. In addition an ~50% loss of neurons is observed in the dorsal RN by E16.5 in the double En knockouts. Like the LC phenotype the RN is relatively normal in the single knockouts suggesting the genes compensate for each other during development (Simon, Saueressig et al. 2001; Simon, Scholz et al. 2005; Sgado, Alberi et al. 2006; Fox 2010). Neurochemical data from our collaborator, Emanuel DiCicco-Bloom MD, have demonstrated abnormal levels of NE and 5HT in both the fore- and hindbrain structures of the *En2* knockout (Lin 2010). These data indicate that the development of the 5HT and NE neurotransmitter systems are regulated by the Engrailed proteins.

Numerous studies have implicated the 5HT and NE pathways in ASD. The 5HT pathway regulates mood, eating, body temperature and arousal, some of which are often perturbed in individuals with ASD. Abnormalities in the 5HT pathway have been consistently observed in individuals with ASD. Blood platelet hyperserotonemia has been reported since the 1960s in ~30% of affected individuals (Ritvo, Yuwiler et al. 1970; Campbell, Friedman et al. 1975; Takahashi, Kanai et al. 1976; Anderson 1987; Anderson, Freedman et al. 1987; McBride, Anderson et al. 1989; Cook, Rowlett et al. 1992; Lam, Aman et al. 2006). However, several studies suggest 5HT functioning is depressed in the CNS of individuals with autism. For example, serotonin reuptake inhibitors (SSRIs) can improve some of the symptoms of ASD (Cook, Rowlett et al. 1992; Gordon, State et al. 1993). In addition, the rate-limiting step of 5HT synthesis is the hydroxylation of tryptophan and acute depletion of tryptophan worsens ASD symptoms (McDougle, Naylor et al. 1996; McDougle, Naylor et al. 1996). The NE neurotransmitter system regulates attention, stress, anxiety, and memory, some of which are also affected in individuals with ASD. Unlike the 5HT system, the peripheral and central NE systems are tightly coordinated. Five studies have revealed increases in NE in the blood (Lake, Ziegler et al. 1977; Launay, Bursztejn et al. 1987; Leventhal, Cook et al. 1990; Leboyer, Bouvard et al. 1992; Minderaa, Anderson et al. 1994). However since plasma NE has a very short half-life, it remains possible that this increase is due to arousal at the time of blood drawing.

#### 4.4 En2 regulates connectivity

From E15.5-P0, *En2* is expressed in a stripe-like pattern in the cerebellum. *En2* is one of many patterning genes that are expressed in this stripe-like pattern at this age (*En1, Shh, Pax2* and *Wnt7b*)(Millen, Hui et al. 1995). Interestingly, these stripe-like expression domains are coincident with the innervation of cerebellar afferents (mossy and climbing fibers), suggesting that these patterning genes regulate the topographic mapping of axons. Consistent with this possibility, *En2* mouse mutants display connectivity phenotypes disrupting the innervation of mossy fibers (Herrup and Kuemerle 1997; Baader, Sanlioglu et al. 1998; Baader, Vogel et al. 1999; Sillitoe, Stephen et al. 2008; Sillitoe, Gopal et al. 2009; Sillitoe, Vogel et al. 2010). Thus En2 is important in establishing the cerebellar connectivity map during development.

Several studies indicate the Engrailed proteins are secreted and function as axon guidance proteins for retinal-tectal mapping. Initial EM and protein studies from the Prochiantz group indicated that a subset of the Engrailed proteins are associated with caveolae-like vesicles (Joliot, Trembleau et al. 1997). Subsequent work demonstrated that ~5% of the Engrailed protein are secreted and they are internalized by neighboring cells. A protein sequence embedded in the homeodomain called the penetratin domain is responsible for this activity (Joliot, Maizel et al. 1998). In addition, *in vitro* cultures demonstrated that exogenous En2 acts as a guidance cue for isolated retinal axons transected from the nucleus. Imaging studies indicate En2 is endocytosed by these growth cones. The protein then interacts with the eukaryotic initiation factor 4E (eIF4E), and En2 mutations that prevent eIF4E interaction fail to cause axon turning. En2 also results in the phosphorylation of eIF4E and its binding protein, 4E-BP1, in axons, which is typically associated with translation initiation (Brunet, Weinl et al. 2005). Recent antibody experiments that block exogenous

activity cause significant connectivity defects in the tectum (Wizenmann, Brunet et al. 2009). Interestingly, several other developmentally important transcription factors (Pax6, Otx2) also display non-cell autonomous phenotypes (Lesaffre, Joliot et al. 2007; Sugiyama, Di Nardo et al. 2008), suggesting this phenomenon is not specific to the Engrailed genes.
Thus, a small proportion of the Engrailed 2 protein is secreted and is important in regulating connectivity through local translation. The FMR protein, which is mutated in Fragile X Syndrome (FXS), also regulates local synaptic translation. Approximately one-third of individuals with FXS are diagnosed with ASD, suggesting synaptic translation defects could contribute to ASD etiology.
*En2* transcripts are also observed at low levels in the adult hippocampus. *En2* knock-out studies revealed a decrease in the number of inhibitory GABA interneurons in the CA3 pyramidal layer and stratum lacunosum moleculare of the adult hippocampus. The knock-out mice also display an increase in the susceptibility of kainic acid-induced seizures. These data suggest an imbalance in excitatory/inhibitory (E/I) connectivity, which has been postulated to be a contributing factor to ASD etiology (Tripathi, Sgado et al. 2009).
Post-natally, *En2* is expressed in differentiating and mature granule cells. Studies by Emanuel DiCicco-Bloom's group demonstrated that En2 functions to promote cell cycle exit and differentiation in developing granule cells (Rossman 2008). The function of En2 in mature adult granule cells has not been investigated but it is likely to regulate the expression of genes needed for synaptic plasticity and other mature neuronal functions.
In summary although *EN2* was initially selected as a candidate gene based upon similar cerebellar neuroanatomical phenotypes, En2 coordinates multiple developmental processes. In particular the protein plays an important role in regulating connectivity and neurotransmitter system during CNS development, both of which are relevant to ASD etiology.

## 5. *ENGRAILED 2* genetic analysis

### 5.1 *rs1861972-rs1861973* association in AGRE and NIMH datasets

Human *EN2* is encoded by two exons in ~8.5kb. In collaboration with Linda Brzustowicz's group at Rutgers University, association analysis was initially performed in 167 Autism Genetic Resource Exchange families (AGRE I dataset- 745 individuals). Positive association with ASD was observed for the common alleles of two intronic SNPs, *rs1861972* and *rs1816973*. Significant association was detected under a narrow (autism) and broad (ASD) diagnosis for both SNPs individually and as a haplotype (A-C *rs1861972-rs1861973*)(Table 2)(Gharani, Benayed et al. 2004). These results were then replicated in two additional datasets (AGREII -222 families, 1102 individuals; NIMH - 129 families, 566 individuals)(Table 2). When all three datasets were combined (518 families, 2413 individuals) more significant results were observed (Table 2)(Benayed, Gharani et al. 2005).
Many factors may contribute to the lack of replication in association studies of complex genetic traits. These include inadequate statistical power, the intrinsic complexity of a disease such as unknown gene-gene and gene-environment interactions as well as locus and allelic heterogeneity in different datasets. Given these limitations, replication of *rs1861972* and *rs1861973* association supports *EN2* as an ASD susceptibility gene.
Risk for the haplotype was then determined. Individual relative risk (RR) estimates the risk the haplotype confers to a given individual, and is calculated by the degree to which the haplotype is over-transmitted from heterozygous parents to affected children. Population

attributable risk (PAR) estimates the risk of the haplotype to the general population and takes into account the degree of over-transmission and frequency of the haplotype. For the 518 families individual RR was estimated as approximately 1.42 and 1.40 under the narrow and broad diagnosis respectively. Because the frequency of the *rs1861972-rs1861973* A-C haplotype is ~67% in the combined sample, this modest individual RR corresponds to a significant PAR of ~39.5% and 38% for the narrow and broad diagnosis of ASD respectively (see Benayed et al 2005 for more details). These data imply that as much as 40% of ASD cases in the population are influenced by the risk allele responsible for *rs1861972* and *rs1861973* association

| SNP | Diagnosis | AGRE I (167 families, 750 individuals) | AGRE II (222 families, 1071 individuals) | NIMH (129 families, 515 individuals) | Combined datasets (518 families, 2336 individuals) |
|---|---|---|---|---|---|
| | | *P* value | *P* value | *P* value | *P* value |
| *rs1861972* | autism | .0106 | .0834 | .0455 | .0010 |
| | ASD | .0050 | .0296 | .0500 | .0002 |
| *rs1861973* | autism | .0073 | .0268 | .0234 | .00008 |
| | ASD | .0107 | .0121 | .0181 | .000038 |
| A-C haplotype | autism | .0018 | .0168 | .0321 | .0000205 |
| | ASD | .0035 | .0061 | .0312 | .0000088 |
| All haplotypes | autism | .0009 | .0048 | .0463 | .00000065 |
| | ASD | .0024 | .0016 | .0431 | .00000035 |

Table 2. Summary of *rs1861972* and *rs1861973* association data

### 5.2 Additional *EN2* association studies

Prior to our association analysis for *EN2*, a case-control study was performed using 100 control and affected individuals from Western/central France. Significant association was observed for a PvuII RFLP that we later mapped to ~2.5kb 5′ of the promoter (*rs34808376*)(Petit, Herault et al. 1995; Benayed, Gharani et al. 2005). Since our association analysis, 5 separate studies have reported positive results for *rs1861972* or *rs1861973* either individually or as part of a haplotype (Brune, Korvatska et al. 2007; Wang, Jia et al. 2008; Yang, Lung et al. 2008; Sen, Singh et al. 2010; Yang, Shu et al. 2010). These studies were performed in datasets recruited by the authors and represent various ethnicities (Northern/Western European, Chinese, Indian). However differences have also been observed. Additional polymorphisms have been reported to be associated and the allele for *rs1861972* and *rs1861973* that is over-transmitted to affected individuals can vary. These results are summarized in Table 3. These differences could reflect variations in LD blocks for the different ethnicities. It is also possible that different risk alleles exist in various populations.

| Study | Ethnicity | n[a] | Associated polymorphisms | ASD associated allele |
|---|---|---|---|---|
| Petit et al | Western/central French | 200 | PvuII | CG |
| Brune at al | Primarily Western/ Northern European | 2476 | *rs1861972* | A<br>G |
| Wang et al | Chinese | 630 | *rs3824068* | A |
| Yang et al (2008) | Chinese | 502 | *rs1861973*<br>*rs3808331* | T<br>G |
| Yang et al (2010) | Chinese | 551 | *rs1861972*<br>*rs1861973* | A<br>C |
| Sen et al | Indian | 281 | *rs1861973* | C |

a- number of individuals recruited

Table 3. Summary of additional *EN2* association studies

In summary *EN2* association with ASD has been reported by 7 different groups. These data are consistent with *EN2* being an ASD susceptibility gene. However if *EN2* contributes to ASD risk, then we would expect these genetic associations to be due to the co-inheritance of an allele that affects either the regulation or activity of *EN2*. The identification of an associated allele that is also functional would provide additional support for *EN2* being an ASD susceptibility gene.

### 5.3 *EN2* LD mapping and re-sequencing analysis

The next step in our analysis was to identify candidate common risk alleles by performing linkage disequilibrium (LD) mapping. LD indicates the degree to which alleles in the human population segregate with each other. Two measures for LD are commonly used: D′ and $r^2$. D′ takes into account recombination rate while $r^2$ includes recombination rate and the frequency of the alleles in the population. For common risk alleles responsible for *rs1861972-rs1861973* association, we expected candidates to display the following criteria:

- Candidates must display strong LD (D′ and $r^2 > .75$) with *rs1861972* and *rs1861973*
- Candidates must be consistently associated with ASD

LD mapping was then performed for 24 additional polymorphisms that were situated throughout the *EN2* gene (Figure 3). These polymorphisms were typed in the AGRE I dataset and we found that only the intronic SNPs were in significant LD (D′ >0.72) with *rs1861972* and *rs1861973*. We then re-sequenced the intron from individuals with ASD that had inherited the A-C haplotype from at least one heterozygous parent. This identified only 1 additional polymorphism (*rs28999108*). *Rs2899108* has a minor allele frequency of 1%, indicating that additional more common polymorphisms are likely not to be identified and *ss38341503* does not fit the criteria of a common risk allele. Association analysis of all intronic SNPs demonstrated that none of them were as consistently or significantly associated as the *rs1861972-rs1861973* A-C haplotype (Benayed, Gharani et al. 2005; Benayed, Choi et al. 2009).

However, it was equally possible that *rs1861972* and *rs1861973* was in strong LD with a polymorphisms situated further 5′ or 3′ of *EN2* that was not tested for association. If this were the case, we would expect these flanking SNPs to be in strong LD with *rs1861972* or *rs1861973* and therefore display $r^2$ values similar to .767 that is observed between *rs1861972* and *rs1861973*. To identify other polymorphisms that fit these criteria, publicly available

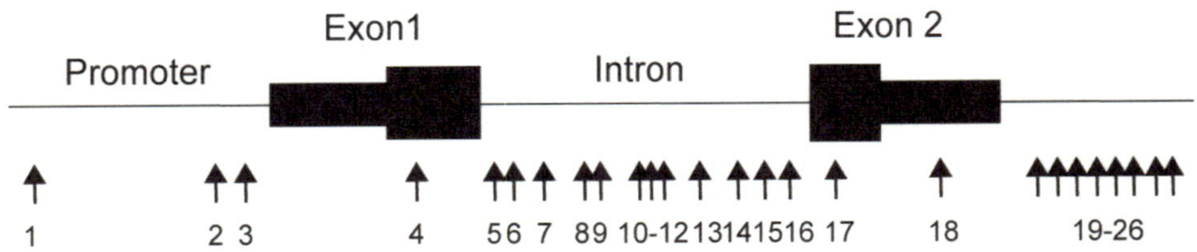


Fig. 3. **Genomic structure of *EN2*.** The exonic/intronic structure of *EN2* is illustrated. The position of 18 polymorphisms tested for association in Benayed et al 2005 is demarcated by arrows below the gene. Numbering refers to the following polymorphisms: 1-*rs6150410*, 2-PvuII (*rs3480837*), 3-*rs1345514*, 4-*rs3735653*, 5-*rs3735652*, 6-*rs6460013*, 7-*rs7794177*, 8-*rs3824068*, 9-*rs2361688*, 10-*rs3824067*, 11-*rs1861792*, 12-*rs1861973*, 13- *rs28999108*, 14-*rs3808332*, 15-*rs3808331*, 16-*rs4717034*, 17-*rs2361689*, 18-*rs3808329*, 19-*rs1895091*, 20-*rs12533271*, 21-*rs1861958*, 22-*rs3071184*, 23-*rs10259822*, 24-*rs10233570*, 25-*rs11976901*, 26-*rs10243118*. Red labeling denotes ASD association in published studies.

Hapmap data was analyzed. The Hapmap project determined the LD relationship of over 1 x $10^6$ SNPs in four human populations (CEU- Utah residents with ancestry from northern and western Europe; JPT- Tokyo, Japan; CHB- Han Chinese Beijing, China; YRI-Yoruba in Ibadan, Nigeria). $r^2$ and D′ values were first examined for 4 SNPs (*rs1861973*, *rs1861973*, *rs6460013* and *rs1861958*) typed in both the Hapmap and ASD datasets. The values were found to be nearly identical, justifying this approach to identify candidate risk allele. The inter-marker Hapmap $r^2$ values with *rs1861973* were then determined in all four Hapmap datasets for SNPs within 2 Mb of *EN2* (1Mb 5′ and 1 Mb 3′). Because 70.3% of the AGRE datasets tested for association were of Northern/Western European descent, the CEU Hapmap data were analyzed first and all SNPs within the 2 Mb region were found to be in weak $r^2$ with *rs1861973* ($r^2$<.370). Similar results were observed for the other datasets (Benayed, Choi et al. 2009). These data identified the A-C haplotype as the most appropriate common variant to test for functional differences.

It is also possible that rare variants on the A-C haplotype contribute to ASD risk and the genetic association of the haplotype with ASD. Re-sequencing over 100 individuals did not identify any non-synonymous coding polymorphisms (Benayed, Gharani et al. 2005, Rahman and Millonig, unpublished results). For all these reasons, we decided to focus our research on determining whether the ASD associated A-C haplotype was functional. Our molecular and mouse genetic studies are summarized below and demonstrate that the A-C haplotype functions as a transcriptional activator both *in vitro* and *in vivo*. These data provide molecular genetic support for *EN2* being an ASD susceptibility gene.

## 6. A-C haplotype functional studies

### 6.1 *In vitro* molecular genetic analysis

To investigate potential function of the ASD associated A-C haplotype, luciferase (luc) assays were conducted. The luc reporter system measures quanta of light, which is a sensitive and reproducible methodology for detecting transcriptional changes. Human *EN2* intron was cloned 3′ of a basal promoter and luc gene but 5′ of the polyA sequence (Figure 4). The construct also included the *EN2* splice acceptor and donor sequences. In this way the intron is transcribed and spliced like the endogenous gene. Constructs were generated for both the A-C and G-T haplotypes and are ~8kb in length. The only sequence difference between the constructs is the *rs186972-rs1861973* haplotype.

Both constructs were transfected into primary cultures of cerebellar granule cells. We chose this cell type to test the function of the A-C haplotype for the following reasons. One, cerebellar granule cells are the most abundant neuronal cell type in the brain and because of its small size they can be isolated to near homogeneity. Two, the cells can undergo various steps of development in culture including proliferation, migration, and differentiation. Three, endogenous *En2* is expressed at high levels in cerebellar granule cells.

When we transfected our constructs, the A-C haplotype resulted in significantly higher luc levels compared to the promoter control after 1 day in culture. The G-T haplotype did not display any activity compared to the promoter (Figure 4). Electrophoretic Mobility Shift Assays (EMSAs) were then performed to detect DNA-protein interactions. Granule cell nuclear extract was employed along with a 200bp fragment encompassing either the A-C or G-T haplotypes. A protein complex binds significantly better to the A-C than the G-T haplotype (data not shown). These data demonstrate that the A-C haplotype functions as a transcriptional activator *in vitro*. The A-C haplotype is one of two ASD associated alleles for which function has been ascribed.

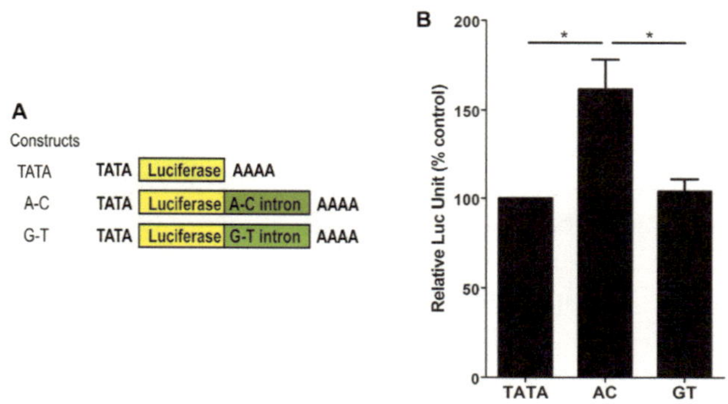


Fig. 4. **ASD-associated *rs1861972-rs1861973* A-C haplotype increases gene expression.** (A) Luciferase (luc) constructs used for transfections are diagramed: TATA - pGL3pro vector driven by SV40 minimal promoter, A-C and G-T - pGL3pro vector containing full-length human *EN2* intron with ASD-associated A-C haplotype (A-C) or unassociated G-T haplotype (G-T). The intron was cloned 3′ of luc gene and 5′ of poly A signal so it is transcribed and spliced as the endogenous gene. (B) Equimolar amount of the three constructswere transiently transfected into P6 mouse cerebellar granule neurons and cultured for 24hrs. Luciferase activities were then measured and normalized to the levels of *Renilla reniformis*. Relative luc units are expressed as percent of TATA control. Note the A-C haplotype significantly increases luc levels. N=4, *P<.05, two tailed paired Student's T test.

### 6.2 *In vivo* transgenic analysis

Because ASD is a neurodevelopmental disorder, we then generated transgenic mice to determine the developmental cell types and ages in which the A-C haplotype is functional. Our constructs include ~10kb of 5′ evolutionarily conserved sequence, the intron, and ~10kb of 3′ evolutionarily conserved sequence. Exon 1 of *EN2* was replaced with the Ds-Red fluorescent reporter and exon 2 with the polyadenylation sequence. Like our luc constructs, the intron also includes *EN2* splice acceptor and donor sequences so the intron is transcribed and spliced as the endogenous locus. Transgenes for both the A-C and G-T haplotypes were generated with the only nucleotide difference between the ~25kb transgenes being the *rs186172-rs1861973* haplotype (Figure 5).

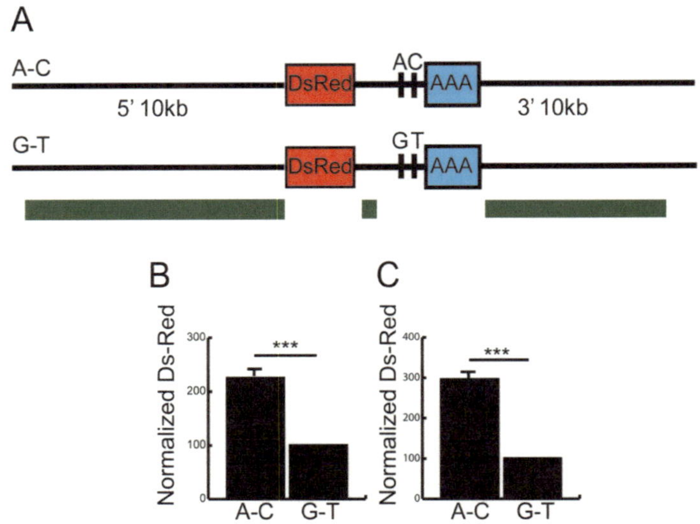


Fig. 5. **Transgenic QRTPCR results.** Top) Structure of the A-C and G-T transgenes is illustrated. Exon 1 of *EN2* is replaced with the Ds-Red reporter and exon 2 with the polyA sequence. ~20kb of flanking evolutionarily conserved sequence (green bars) drives expression of Ds-Red. The only difference between the transgenes is the two nucleotides representing the A-C and G-T haplotypes. Bottom) QRTPCR using adult cerebellar RNA was performed for Ds-Red-E5 and Gapdh in two pairs of lines with similar copy numbers: A) A-C, line F, 5 copies; G-T, line N, 6.5 copies, B) A-C, line E, 32 copies; G-T, line I, 37 copies. *** P<.001 T-test

We have begun our analysis by examining the expression of the transgenes in the adult cerebellum because *En2* is expressed specifically in granule cells. Thus we might expect to observe a similar difference in expression as observed for our *in vitro* luc analysis. Taqman QRTPCR was performed for *Ds-Red* and *Gapdh* on the adult cerebellar RNA isolated from A-C and G-T lines with similar copy numbers. These assays were performed in quadruplicate on three A-C and 3 G-T littermates. The A-C haplotype results in ~250%% increase in normalized *Ds-Red* levels compared to the G-T haplotype in the adult cerebellum (Figure 5). These results demonstrate the A-C haplotype functions as a potent activator *in vivo*. These data determined that the ASD A-C haplotype functions as a transcriptional activator both *in vitro* and *in vivo*, providing molecular genetic evidence that *EN2* contributes to ASD risk.

We are now examining levels and spatial expression at additional time points (E12.5, E17.5, P6 and adult) relevant to various described functions of *En2* (see Table 1). These studies will determine when, where, and how the A-C haplotype is functional during CNS development, providing the first *in vivo* functional analysis of any common associated allele with ASD.

### 6.3 Post-mortem and epigenetic analysis

To investigate whether *EN2* levels are also increased in individuals with ASD, post-mortem analysis has been performed. 78 age and sex matched cerebellar samples have been obtained from NICHD Brain and Tissue Bank for Developmental Disorders or Harvard Brain Tissue

Resource Center via Autism Tissue Program (49 control, 29 affected). These samples have been genotyped for *rs1861972* and *rs1861973*, and Taqman QRTPCR has been performed for *EN2* and *GAPDH*. Normalized *EN2* mRNA levels display a significant increase in affected compared to controls (Figure 6). Further examination of these data suggests that the increase is due to both the *rs1861972-rs1861973* genotype and affection status. A more detailed statistical analysis is ongoing but these results are consistent with *EN2* levels being increased in individuals with ASD. Together our *in vitro*, *in vivo*, and post-mortem studies have demonstrated that increased amounts of *EN2* are consistently associated with ASD, suggesting that elevated levels of the protein alter CNS development to increase risk for ASD.

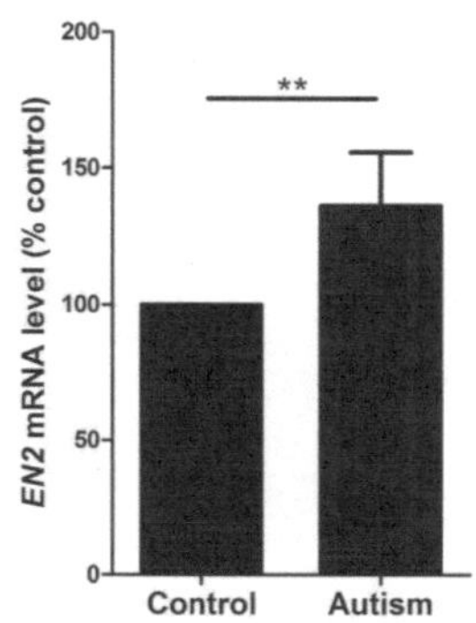


Fig. 6. ***EN2* levels are elevated in ASD individuals.** *EN2* mRNA levels were measured in 29 ASD and 49 control post-mortem cerebellum using Taqman qRT-PCR. *EN2* levels were normalized to GAPDH internal controls and average delta Ct values were obtained from triplicates of qPCR. Altered *EN2* levels of ASD individuals are presented as percent of control values. Fold difference was calculated using the formula $2^{-(EN2deltaCt-ControldeltaCt)}$. Error bars indicate standard errors. **p<.01, T-test, two-tailed, unpaired with unequal variance.

The previous data indicate the A-C haplotype results in increased gene expression. However, increased *EN2* levels could also be achieved by epigenetic mechanisms. Environmental factors can affect gene regulation through epigenetic modifications such as differential methylation. Epigenetics likely plays an important role in ASD for the following reasons. One, epigenetics provides an interface between environmental factors and genetic susceptibility. Numerous common environmental factors (e.g. bis-phenol, arsenic, certain antibiotics) affect CpG island methylation and gene expression (Villar-Garea and Esteller 2003). Thus differential environmental exposures could cause variations in epigenetic modifications and gene expression. This model provides a possible explanation for the phenotypic variability observed in ASD and other polygenic disorders (Bjornsson, Fallin et al. 2004; Feinberg 2007). In addition, the methyl-CpG binding proteins, MeCP2 and MBD2, are mutated in Rett Syndrome and ASD, pointing to the importance of epigenetic regulation in ASD (Amir, Van den Veyver et al. 1999; Li, Yamagata et al. 2005; Coutinho, Oliveira et al. 2007; Loat, Curran et al. 2008).

CG dinucleotides are clustered in regions called CpG islands that are regulated by epigenetic mechanisms. CpG dinucleotides are the substrates for cytosine methyl transferases and DNA methylation often leads to decreased expression. Six CpG islands flank human *EN2* with 3 in the gene. Interestingly, a vast majority of these CpG islands are not observed in mouse or rat, indicating they have evolved since rodent radiation to possibly regulate *EN2* expression. To investigate whether *EN2* is epigenetically regulated, we treated two human neuronal cell lines (Daoy, SH-SY5Y) that express *EN2* with the methylation inhibitor, 5-aza-2'-deoxycytidine (AZA), and a methyl group donor, S-adenosylmethionine (SAM). Preliminary bisulfite sequencing demonstrated methylation of CpGs with SAM treatment while the same dinucleotides are unmethylated in AZA treated cells (Figure 7). Importantly this difference in methylation is correlated with *EN2* mRNA levels. AZA treatment results in increased expression; SAM treatment with decreased levels (Figure 7). Thus, these data are consistent with *EN2* being epigenetically regulated

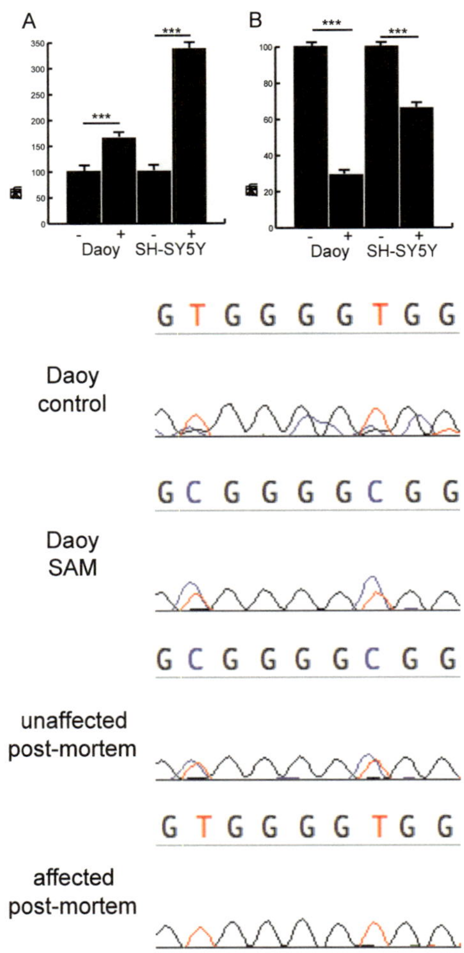


Fig. 7. ***EN2* epigenetic analysis.** A and B) Treatment of Daoy and Sh-SY5Y cells with AZA (A) resulted in increased *EN2* mRNA levels (expressed as percent difference relative to untreated). Treatment with SAM (B) resulted in decreased *EN2* mRNA levels (expressed as percent difference relative to untreated). *** P<.001 T-test. Bottom) Bisulfite sequencing of PCR products demonstrated the *EN2* promoter is hypomethylated in untreated Daoy cells but methylated upon SAM treatment. An unaffected post-mortem sample is methylated while an affected sample is methylated at the same nucleotides.

We have bisulfite sequenced the promoter in a few post-mortem samples. In affected individuals none of the CpG dinucleotides are methylated while in unaffected individuals the same CpGs were methylated. These CpGs are the same dinucleotides methylated after SAM treatment *in vitro* (Figure 7). In sum, these results are consistent with epigenetic differences contributing to the increase in *EN2* mRNA levels observed in the post-mortem samples. High-throughput epigenetic platform analysis is ongoing to investigate this hypothesis further.

## 7. Future studies

One important next step is to identify the downstream molecular and cell biological effects of increased *EN2* expression. For this analysis we are generating a humanized *EN2* knock-in

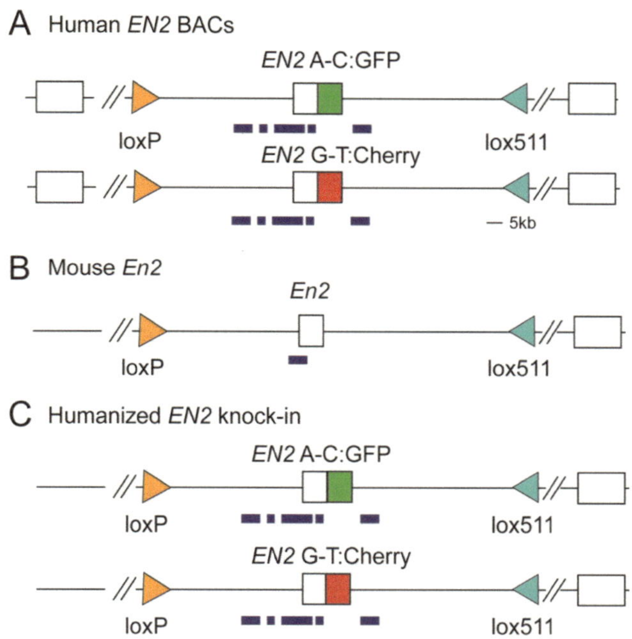


Fig. 8. **RMGR humanized *EN2* knock-in.** A) Genomic structure of the recombineered BACs is drawn to scale. Human *EN2* G-T haplotype BAC was obtained and recombineered to generate the ASD-associated A-C haplotype. IRES:GFP was then introduced downstream of the *EN2* coding region for the A-C BAC. IRES:Cherry was introduced in the same location for the G-T BAC. Heterotypic loxP (orange triangle) and lox511 (blue triangle) sites were also recombineered into both BACs, ~35kb upstream and downstream of *EN2*. This genomic region does not include any other genes. Empty boxes depict the next flanking genes. The human CpG islands are also illustrated as blue boxes. B) The mouse *En2* locus is illustrated with one small CpG island (blue box). LoxP and lox511 sites have been sequentially targeted onto the same *En2* chromosome. C) The recombineered BACs will then be transfected into our cis loxP-lox511 double-targeted ES cells. Cre recombinase will then be expressed in the ES cells. Since the heterotypic lox sites do not recombine with each other but still recognize both the cre recombinase, the mouse sequence will be replaced with the human locus via cre-mediated recombination through the flanking loxP and lox511 sites. Both A-C and G-T knock-ins will be generated, which will also contain the human CpG islands

mouse whereby we are replacing ~75kb of mouse *En2* with the human sequence. This sequence will also contain the flanking CpG islands. To accomplish this goal we are using a strategy called Recombination Mediated Genome Replacement (RMGR) developed by Andrew Smith PhD (Figure 8)(Wallace, Marques-Kranc et al. 2007). In this way we will be able to determine the molecular and cell biological effects of the A-C haplotype throughout development. Because the human sequence will include the flanking CpG islands, we will also be able to expose the mice to various non-genetic factors that affect epigenetic regulation and investigate how these environmental compounds can either improve or worsen the A-C associated phenotypes.

## 8. Summary

We have demonstrated that the *EN2 rs1861972-rs1861973* A-C haplotype is significantly associated with ASD in 3 datasets. 6 additional groups have reported *EN2* ASD association, suggesting it is an ASD susceptibility gene. If this possibility is correct, then we would expect the associated alleles to segregate with common or rare variants that functionally alter *EN2* expression or activity. To address this question, we decided to use a combinatorial approach that included human genetics, molecular biology, mouse transgenesis, and human post-mortem analysis. In the three datasets that we studied, LD mapping, re-sequencing, and additional association studies identified the A-C haplotype as the best candidate to test for function. *In vitro* luc assays demonstrated that the A-C haplotype functions as a transcriptional activator, resulting in elevated levels. Importantly transgenic mice have recapitulated these results *in vivo* and will determine when, where, and how the A-C haplotype is functional throughout CNS development. *EN2* levels are also increased in individuals with ASD. Thus elevated amounts of *EN2* seem to be correlated with increased ASD risk. Our preliminary studies indicate that *EN2* is also epigenetically regulated, suggesting exposure to environmental non-genetic factors may also increase *EN2* expression. Future experiments are directed at identifying downstream molecular and cell biological pathways affected by increased *EN2* levels. Finally, *En2* regulates developmental processes implicated in ASD, including the establishment of connectivity maps. In sum, our combinatorial approach has provided evidence that *EN2* is an ASD susceptibility gene.

## 9. Acknowledgements

We thank NICHD Brain and Tissue Bank for Developmental Disorders, the Harvard Brain Tissue Resource Center for the post-mortem samples, and all participating families for the post-mortem samples. We thank the Autism Tissue Program and especially Jane Pickett for all their help. We acknowledge the funding agencies that have supported this research: NIH (MH076624, MH080429, MH083509), Department of Defense (W81XWH-09-1-0286), NAAR/Autism Speaks, and New Jersey Governor's Council for Medical Research and Treatment of Autism

## 10. References

Alarcon, M., R. M. Cantor, et al. (2002). "Evidence for a language quantitative trait locus on chromosome 7q in multiplex autism families." Am J Hum Genet 70(1): 60-71.

Alberi, L., P. Sgado, et al. (2004). "Engrailed genes are cell-autonomously required to prevent apoptosis in mesencephalic dopaminergic neurons." Development 131(13): 3229-3236.

Amaral, D. G., C. M. Schumann, et al. (2008). "Neuroanatomy of autism." Trends in neurosciences 31(3): 137-145.

Amir, R. E., I. B. Van den Veyver, et al. (1999). "Rett syndrome is caused by mutations in X-linked MECP2, encoding methyl-CpG-binding protein 2." Nat Genet 23(2): 185-188.

Anderson, G. M. (1987). "Monoamines in autism: an update of neurochemical research on a pervasive developmental disorder." Medical biology 65(2-3): 67-74.

Anderson, G. M., D. X. Freedman, et al. (1987). "Whole blood serotonin in autistic and normal subjects." J Child Psychol Psychiatry 28(6): 885-900.

Auranen, M., R. Vanhala, et al. (2002). "A genomewide screen for autism-spectrum disorders: evidence for a major susceptibility locus on chromosome 3q25-27." Am J Hum Genet 71(4): 777-790.

Baader, S. L., S. Sanlioglu, et al. (1998). "Ectopic overexpression of engrailed-2 in cerebellar Purkinje cells causes restricted cell loss and retarded external germinal layer development at lobule junctions." J Neurosci 18(5): 1763-1773.

Baader, S. L., M. W. Vogel, et al. (1999). "Selective disruption of "late onset" sagittal banding patterns by ectopic expression of engrailed-2 in cerebellar Purkinje cells." J Neurosci 19(13): 5370-5379.

Bauman, M. (1986). "Developmental cerebellar abnormalities: A consistent finding in early infantile autism." Neurology 36(1): 190.

Bauman, M. and T. L. Kemper (1985). "Histoanatomic observations of the brain in early infantile autism." Neurology 35(6): 866-874.

Benayed, R., J. Choi, et al. (2009). "Autism-associated haplotype affects the regulation of the homeobox gene, ENGRAILED 2." Biol Psychiatry 66(10): 911-917.

Benayed, R., N. Gharani, et al. (2005). "Support for the homeobox transcription factor gene ENGRAILED 2 as an autism spectrum disorder susceptibility locus." Am J Hum Genet 77(5): 851-868.

Bjornsson, H. T., M. D. Fallin, et al. (2004). "An integrated epigenetic and genetic approach to common human disease." Trends Genet 20(8): 350-358.

Brune, C. W., E. Korvatska, et al. (2007). "Heterogeneous association between engrailed-2 and autism in the CPEA network." Am J Med Genet B Neuropsychiatr Genet.

Brunet, I., C. Weinl, et al. (2005). "The transcription factor Engrailed-2 guides retinal axons." Nature 438(7064): 94-98.

Campbell, M., E. Friedman, et al. (1975). "Blood serotonin in schizophrenic children. A preliminary study." International pharmacopsychiatry 10(4): 213-221.

Cook, E. H., Jr., R. Rowlett, et al. (1992). "Fluoxetine treatment of children and adults with autistic disorder and mental retardation." J Am Acad Child Adolesc Psychiatry 31(4): 739-745.

Courchesne, E. (1997). "Brainstem, cerebellar and limbic neuroanatomical abnormalities in autism." Curr Opin Neurobiol 7(2): 269-278.

Courchesne, E., R. Yeung-Courchesne, et al. (1988). "Hypoplasia of cerebellar vermal lobules VI and VII in autism." N Engl J Med 318(21): 1349-1354.

Coutinho, A. M., G. Oliveira, et al. (2007). "MECP2 coding sequence and 3'UTR variation in 172 unrelated autistic patients." Am J Med Genet B Neuropsychiatr Genet 144B(4): 475-483.

Feinberg, A. P. (2007). "Phenotypic plasticity and the epigenetics of human disease." Nature 447(7143): 433-440.

Fox, S. R., Deneris, E.S. (2010). Engrailed is required in the early postnatal period for maintenance of anterior 5-HT neurons. Society for Neuroscience, San Diego, CA.

Gharani, N., R. Benayed, et al. (2004). "Association of the homeobox transcription factor, ENGRAILED 2, 3, with autism spectrum disorder." Mol Psychiatry 9(5): 474-484.

Gherbassi, D. and H. H. Simon (2006). "The engrailed transcription factors and the mesencephalic dopaminergic neurons." Journal of neural transmission. Supplementum(70): 47-55.

Gordon, C. T., R. C. State, et al. (1993). "A double-blind comparison of clomipramine, desipramine, and placebo in the treatment of autistic disorder." Archives of general psychiatry 50(6): 441-447.

Hanks, M., W. Wurst, et al. (1995). "Rescue of the En-1 mutant phenotype by replacement of En-1 with En-2." Science 269(5224): 679-682.

Herrup, K. and B. Kuemerle (1997). "The compartmentalization of the cerebellum." Annual review of neuroscience 20: 61-90.

Jaynes, J. B. and P. H. O'Farrell (1991). "Active repression of transcription by the engrailed homeodomain protein." The EMBO journal 10(6): 1427-1433.

Joliot, A., A. Maizel, et al. (1998). "Identification of a signal sequence necessary for the unconventional secretion of Engrailed homeoprotein." Current biology : CB 8(15): 856-863.

Joliot, A., A. Trembleau, et al. (1997). "Association of Engrailed homeoproteins with vesicles presenting caveolae-like properties." Development 124(10): 1865-1875.

Joyner, A. L. (1996). "Engrailed, Wnt and Pax genes regulate midbrain--hindbrain development." Trends Genet 12(1): 15-20.

Kuemerle, B., H. Zanjani, et al. (1997). "Pattern deformities and cell loss in Engrailed-2 mutant mice suggest two separate patterning events during cerebellar development." J Neurosci 17(20): 7881-7889.

Lake, C. R., M. G. Ziegler, et al. (1977). "Increased norepinephrine levels and decreased dopamine-beta-hydroxylase activity in primary autism." Archives of general psychiatry 34(5): 553-556.

Lam, K. S., M. G. Aman, et al. (2006). "Neurochemical correlates of autistic disorder: a review of the literature." Res Dev Disabil 27(3): 254-289.

Launay, J. M., C. Bursztejn, et al. (1987). "Catecholamines metabolism in infantile autism: a controlled study of 22 autistic children." Journal of autism and developmental disorders 17(3): 333-347.

Leboyer, M., M. P. Bouvard, et al. (1992). "Brief report: a double-blind study of naltrexone in infantile autism." Journal of autism and developmental disorders 22(2): 309-319.

Lesaffre, B., A. Joliot, et al. (2007). "Direct non-cell autonomous Pax6 activity regulates eye development in the zebrafish." Neural development 2: 2.

Leventhal, B. L., E. H. Cook, Jr., et al. (1990). "Relationships of whole blood serotonin and plasma norepinephrine within families." Journal of autism and developmental disorders 20(4): 499-511.

Li, H., T. Yamagata, et al. (2005). "Mutation analysis of methyl-CpG binding protein family genes in autistic patients." Brain Dev 27(5): 321-325.

Lin, L., Sonsalla, P., Matteson, P.G., Silverman, J., Crawley, J.N., Millonig, J.H., DiCicco-Bloom, E. (2010). Deficiency of Engrailed 2 (En2) Produces Abnormal Development of Forebrain-Projecting, Monoamine Neurotransmitters Systems and Depression Related Behaviors. The 9th International Meeting for Autism research (IMFAR), Philadephia, PA.

Liu, J., D. R. Nyholt, et al. (2001). "A genomewide screen for autism susceptibility loci." Am J Hum Genet 69(2): 327-340.

Loat, C. S., S. Curran, et al. (2008). "Methyl-CpG-binding protein 2 polymorphisms and vulnerability to autism." Genes Brain Behav 7(7): 754-760.

Logan, C., M. C. Hanks, et al. (1992). "Cloning and sequence comparison of the mouse, human, and chicken engrailed genes reveal potential functional domains and regulatory regions." Developmental genetics 13(5): 345-358.

McBride, P. A., G. M. Anderson, et al. (1989). "Serotonergic responsivity in male young adults with autistic disorder. Results of a pilot study." Archives of general psychiatry 46(3): 213-221.

McDougle, C. J., S. T. Naylor, et al. (1996). "Effects of tryptophan depletion in drug-free adults with autistic disorder." Arch Gen Psychiatry 53(11): 993-1000.

McDougle, C. J., S. T. Naylor, et al. (1996). "A double-blind, placebo-controlled study of fluvoxamine in adults with autistic disorder." Archives of general psychiatry 53(11): 1001-1008.

Millen, K. J., C. C. Hui, et al. (1995). "A role for En-2 and other murine homologues of Drosophila segment polarity genes in regulating positional information in the developing cerebellum." Development 121(12): 3935-3945.

Millen, K. J., W. Wurst, et al. (1994). "Abnormal embryonic cerebellar development and patterning of postnatal foliation in two mouse Engrailed-2 mutants." Development 120(3): 695-706.

Minderaa, R. B., G. M. Anderson, et al. (1994). "Noradrenergic and adrenergic functioning in autism." Biol Psychiatry 36(4): 237-241.

Ohkuma, Y., M. Horikoshi, et al. (1990). "Engrailed, a homeodomain protein, can repress in vitro transcription by competition with the TATA box-binding protein transcription factor IID." Proceedings of the National Academy of Sciences of the United States of America 87(6): 2289-2293.

Peltenburg, L. T. and C. Murre (1997). "Specific residues in the Pbx homeodomain differentially modulate the DNA-binding activity of Hox and Engrailed proteins." Development 124(5): 1089-1098.

Petit, E., J. Herault, et al. (1995). "Association study with two markers of a human homeogene in infantile autism." J Med Genet 32(4): 269-274.

Ritvo, E. R., A. Yuwiler, et al. (1970). "Increased blood serotonin and platelets in early infantile autism." Archives of general psychiatry 23(6): 566-572.

Rossman, I., Lin, L., Kamdar, S., Millonig, J.H., DiCicco-Bloom, E. (2008). The Autism-Associated Gene, Engrailed 2 (En2), Has Age Dependent Effects On Cerebellar Granule Precursor Proliferation And Differentiation When Overexpressed In Vitro. Proceedings of The 7th International Meeting for Autism research (IMFAR) London, United Kingdom

Sen, B., A. S. Singh, et al. (2010). "Family-based studies indicate association of Engrailed 2 gene with autism in an Indian population." Genes Brain Behav 9(2): 248-255.

Sgado, P., L. Alberi, et al. (2006). "Slow progressive degeneration of nigral dopaminergic neurons in postnatal Engrailed mutant mice." Proceedings of the National Academy of Sciences of the United States of America 103(41): 15242-15247.

Sillitoe, R. V., N. Gopal, et al. (2009). "Embryonic origins of ZebrinII parasagittal stripes and establishment of topographic Purkinje cell projections." Neuroscience 162(3): 574-588.

Sillitoe, R. V., D. Stephen, et al. (2008). "Engrailed homeobox genes determine the organization of Purkinje cell sagittal stripe gene expression in the adult cerebellum." J Neurosci 28(47): 12150-12162.

Sillitoe, R. V., M. W. Vogel, et al. (2010). "Engrailed homeobox genes regulate establishment of the cerebellar afferent circuit map." The Journal of neuroscience : the official journal of the Society for Neuroscience 30(30): 10015-10024.

Simon, H. H., H. Saueressig, et al. (2001). "Fate of midbrain dopaminergic neurons controlled by the engrailed genes." The Journal of neuroscience : the official journal of the Society for Neuroscience 21(9): 3126-3134.

Simon, H. H., C. Scholz, et al. (2005). "Engrailed genes control developmental fate of serotonergic and noradrenergic neurons in mid- and hindbrain in a gene dose-dependent manner." Mol Cell Neurosci 28(1): 96-105.

Simon, H. H., S. Thuret, et al. (2004). "Midbrain dopaminergic neurons: control of their cell fate by the engrailed transcription factors." Cell and tissue research 318(1): 53-61.

Sugiyama, S., A. A. Di Nardo, et al. (2008). "Experience-dependent transfer of Otx2 homeoprotein into the visual cortex activates postnatal plasticity." Cell 134(3): 508-520.

Takahashi, S., H. Kanai, et al. (1976). "Reassessment of elevated serotonin levels in blood platelets in early infantile autism." Journal of autism and childhood schizophrenia 6(4): 317-326.

Tolkunova, E. N., M. Fujioka, et al. (1998). "Two distinct types of repression domain in engrailed: one interacts with the groucho corepressor and is preferentially active on integrated target genes." Molecular and cellular biology 18(5): 2804-2814.

Tripathi, P. P., P. Sgado, et al. (2009). "Increased susceptibility to kainic acid-induced seizures in Engrailed-2 knockout mice." Neuroscience 159(2): 842-849.

van Dijk, M. A. and C. Murre (1994). "extradenticle raises the DNA binding specificity of homeotic selector gene products." Cell 78(4): 617-624.

Villar-Garea, A. and M. Esteller (2003). "DNA demethylating agents and chromatin-remodelling drugs: which, how and why?" Curr Drug Metab 4(1): 11-31.

Wallace, H. A., F. Marques-Kranc, et al. (2007). "Manipulating the mouse genome to engineer precise functional syntenic replacements with human sequence." Cell 128(1): 197-209.

Wang, L., M. Jia, et al. (2008). "Association of the ENGRAILED 2 (EN2) gene with autism in Chinese Han population." American journal of medical genetics. Part B, Neuropsychiatric genetics : the official publication of the International Society of Psychiatric Genetics 147B(4): 434-438.

Wizenmann, A., I. Brunet, et al. (2009). "Extracellular Engrailed participates in the topographic guidance of retinal axons in vivo." Neuron 64(3): 355-366.

Wurst, W., A. B. Auerbach, et al. (1994). "Multiple developmental defects in Engrailed-1 mutant mice: an early mid-hindbrain deletion and patterning defects in forelimbs and sternum." Development 120(7): 2065-2075.

Yang, P., F. W. Lung, et al. (2008). "Association of the homeobox transcription factor gene ENGRAILED 2 with autistic disorder in Chinese children." Neuropsychobiology 57(1-2): 3-8.

Yang, P., B. C. Shu, et al. (2010). "Intronic single nucleotide polymorphisms of engrailed homeobox 2 modulate the disease vulnerability of autism in a han chinese population." Neuropsychobiology 62(2): 104-115.

Zec, N., D. H. Rowitch, et al. (1997). "Expression of the homeobox-containing genes EN1 and EN2 in human fetal midgestational medulla and cerebellum." J Neuropathol Exp Neurol 56(3): 236-242.

# 2

# Antipsychotics in the Treatment of Autism

Carmem Gottfried[1,2] and Rudimar Riesgo[1,2]
[1]*Neuroglial Plasticity Laboratory at Department of Biochemistry, Postgraduate Program of Biochemistry, Institute of Basic Health Sciences,*
[2]*Translational Research Group in ASD (GETEA), Child Neurology Unit, Clinical Hospital of Porto Alegre,*
[1,2]*Federal University of Rio Grande do Sul, Porto Alegre, RS, Brazil*

## 1. Introduction

The neurobehavioral syndromes are more frequent than we usually think. They are clinical challenges, because they demand knowledge from the physician as well as time for the correct approach. Such complaints are very frequent in hospital and addition to the private practice. For example, according to a survey carried out in our Hospital, the Child Neurology Unit made 10,622 evaluations in 2010, most of which were neurobehavioral syndromes including autism and other Pervasive Development Disorders.

Because of the subtlety of the boundaries between Neurology and Psychiatry, the term neurobehavioral could also be called neuropsychiatric. These boundaries have been explored both in the clinical (Nunes and Mercadante, 2004) and in the experimental area (Quincozes-Santos et al., 2010). It is important to build a bridge between the clinical and the experimental research, especially when the issue is neuropsychiatric disorders. This linkage indubitably enhances the common knowledge of neurobehavioral alterations as well as it promotes the reciprocal enthusiasm.

One of the most intriguing neurobehavioral syndromes is autism. The challenge starts with the difficulty of defining the disorder, continues with the limitations imposed by the lack of a clinical marker, and ends with the difficulties in the experimental research field.

The word autism was used for the first time by the Swiss psychiatrist Eugen Bleuler in 1911. "Autism" came from the Greek word "autos," meaning self. However, the landmark paper describing autism came from the Austrian psychiatrist Leo Kanner, who described eleven children that shared common behavior, with a peculiar inability to establish affective and interpersonal contact. He published the paper "Autistic disturbances of affective contact" in the Journal *Nervous Child* (Kanner, 1943).

In 1944, the Austrian pediatrician Hans Asperger described cases of children with some behavioral characteristics that resembled those of children with autism, but with a peculiar type of language as well as normal cognitive performance (Gadia *et al.*, 2004). He published an article in German in 1944 entitled "Die 'Autistischen Psychopathen' im Kindesalter" in *Archiv fur Psychiatrie und Nervenkrankheiten* that was translated into English only in 1989.

To date, more than half a century since Kanner´s study, the number of papers in PubMed containing the word *autism* has risen above 17,000. From this total, the percentage of published papers comprising different keywords correlated to autism (see Figure 1), reveals that the most frequent words in a set of selected targets were *developmental*, *brain* and *psychiatry*. Curiously, the word *environment* occurs in only 5% of papers. It was a surprise, considering evidence indicating that environment plays a role in the development of autism (Landrigan, 2010). In fact, the prevalence of autism is higher than previously thought and if it is rising, the rise might be associated with a shift in the environment. Further, the appearance of keywords related to glial cells (*astrocyte*, *oligodendrocytes* and *microglia*) can be noted, and, as expected, in less than 2% of papers indicating an emerging and promising field of investigation on ASD.

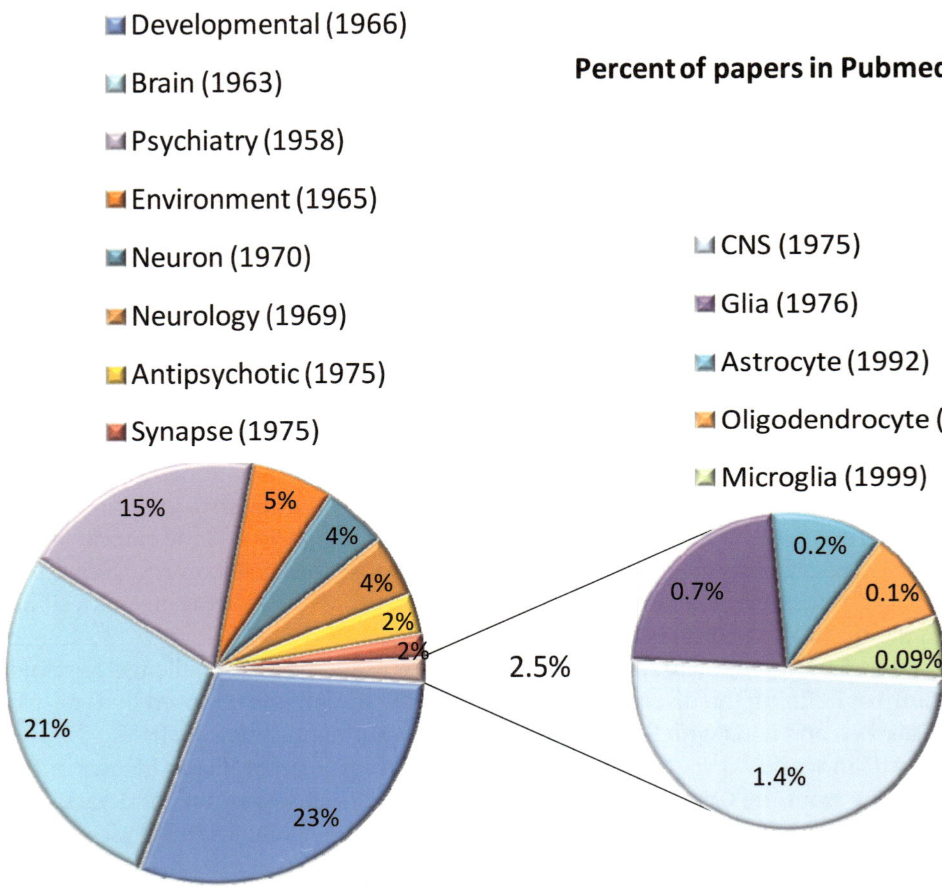


Fig. 1. **Number of papers published in PubMed.** Values were obtained combining the word "autism" with selected keywords related to ASD and neural studies. Number in parenthesis indicates the first year of publication in PubMed of each word combination. Keyword autism = 100% = 17,199 papers. E.g. autism + developmental = 23%, with the first paper with this combination having been published in 1966. Data was obtained in March 23, 2011.

According to the Diagnostic and Statistical Manual of Mental Disorders - Fourth Edition criteria, there are five clinical situations that could be encompassed by the term "PDD"

(Pervasive Developmental Disorders) or "ASD" (Autism Spectrum Disorders) with the same meaning of PDD or autism. The terms PDD or ASD are interchangeable and they are widely used in clinical practice to refer to children with autism or any other of the related disorders (Gadia *et al.*, 2004). Actually, the terms PDD and ASD are not a specific diagnosis, but a kind of umbrella with five different diagnostic categories based on clinical findings.

The five clinical ASD diagnoses admitted by DSM-IV-TR (APA, 2002) are: a) Autistic Disorder; b) Asperger Disorder; c) Rett Disorder; d) Childhood Disintegrative Disorder; e) PDD-NOS (Pervasive Developmental Disorder - Not Otherwise Specified).

In terms of frequency, our group found that the most prevalent ASD is the PDD-NOS, followed by Autistic Disorder, and then by Asperger Disorder. Rett's Disorder and Childhood Disintegrative Disorder are seen less frequently in the clinical practice (Longo *et al.*, 2009).

One of the major challenges of cognitive neuroscience is to understand how changes in the structural properties of the brain affect the plasticity exhibited whenever a person develops, ages, learns a new skill, or adapts to a neuropathology (Keller and Just, 2009). There are many hypotheses in this field attempting to explain the genetics, neurotransmitter imbalances, early childhood immunizations, xenobiotic and teratogenic agents, and maternal infection (Buehler, 2011).

With the advent of electroencephalography, the aberrant patterns observed in patients with autism have contributed to the contemporary understanding of the syndrome as a brain-based disorder. There is a positive correlation between increasing radiate white matter volume and motor skill impairment in children with autism (Mostofsky *et al.*, 2007). Moreover, macrocephaly is observed in 15-35% of patients with autism (Bailey *et al.*, 2008).

The clinical onset of autism appears to be preceded by two phases of brain growth abnormalities: a reduced head size at birth, followed by sudden and excessive increase between 1-2 months and 6–14 months of age (Pardo and Eberhart, 2007), which may reflect a disruption of multiple fundamental processes during the patterning and organization of a cortical cytoarchitecture. The effects of these disrupted processes may be manifested widely, with atypical or adaptive behaviors associated with these changes.

Considering that the etiology of autism still unknown and that there are no effective medical treatments that address the core symptoms of ASD concerning communication, inappropriate social interactions and restricted interests or behaviors, the promise of future medical treatments for ASD is through the identification of the underlying pathophysiological mechanisms, and treatment of these molecular and cellular deficits (Coury, 2010).

The psychopharmacotherapy used in autism is generally addressed to behavioral symptoms, such as: anxiety, lack of attention, irritability, hyperactivity, humor oscillations, sleep disturbances, aggressiveness and self-injury. Another clinical problem in ASD is epilepsy, reaching up to twenty times more frequency in autism. Even though, many of the above mentioned behavioral symptoms could be reduced after treatment; the antipsychotic drugs can adversely facilitate epilepsy.

Nevertheless, the antipsychotic treatment in ASD has expanded, sometimes accompanied by several clinical and metabolic side-effects of primary concern (weight gain, hyperglycemia and dyslipidemia), especially by the greater risk within the pediatric population.

In this context, the present chapter aimed to review (i) the neurotransmitter dysfunctions in ASD and the most commonly prescribed antipsychotics; (ii) the vantages and advantages regarding to the antipsychotics side effects and (iii) the non-neuronal possible targets of atypical antipsychotics in brain.

## 2. Ligand-receptor dysfunctions in autism

The wide diversity of core characteristics of ASD and the variety of comorbidities makes the diagnostic procedure and clinical management of the patient more difficult. In the immature brain, the neuronal migration and emplacement are modulated paracrinally by neurotransmitters and their receptors (Manent and Represa, 2007). The complex functions being related to neurotransmitters during brain development indicates that these molecules can play central roles in a wide variety of neurobiological alterations associated with ASD.
Likewise, the multifactorial basis of ASD is engineered by complex developmental changes in the brain that occur during the first few years of life. These changes include alterations (a) at the anatomical level, in the limbic system (hippocampus and amygdala), cerebellum, cortex, basal ganglia and brainstem (Bauman and Kemper, 2005) and (b) at the neurochemical level, in a number of key ligand-receptor systems, including serotonergic, dopaminergic, noradrenergic, cholinergic, opioid, amino acids and hormone mechanisms (Lam *et al.*, 2006). Full understanding of these systems in the brain involves different areas of knowledge such as genomics, neurochemistry, electrophysiology, and behavior.

### 2.1 Most prevalent neurotransmitter/receptor dysfunctions in ASD

#### 2.1.1 Serotonergic system

The neurotransmitter serotonin is synthesized from the essential aminoacid tryptophan. Firstly, tryptophan is hydroxylated (by tryptophan hydroxylase) into 5-hydroxytryptophan, which is then decarboxylated (by aromatic L-amino acid decarboxylase) resulting in serotonin or 5-hydroxytryptamine (5-HT).
Serotonin has been linked to a wide variety of behaviors including those having to do with feeding and body-weight regulation, social hierarchies, aggression and suicidal behavior, obsessive compulsive disorder, alcoholism, anxiety, and affective disorders. This neurotransmitter plays two important roles in the mammalian brain: it regulates serotonergic outgrowth and maturation of the target regions in the developing brain (Whitaker-Azmitia, 2005), and modulates the function and plasticity of the adult brain (Catalano, 2001).
The function of serotonin in ASD has been has been investigated by means of biomarker, neuroimaging and genetic approaches (Scott and Deneris, 2005). An important investigation by positron emission tomography (PET) shows that the normal brain developmental peak of 5-HT synthesis cannot be observed in children with autism (Chandana *et al.*, 2005; Chugani *et al.*, 1999).
5-HT has been shown to reside in platelets and is best measured in a whole blood assay. One of the most consistent biological findings related to autism is elevated whole blood 5-HT levels found in about 1/3 of cases, which may be connected to cellular immune abnormalities found in autism, as 5-HT display immunoregulatory effects primarily via 5-HT1A, 5-HT2 and 5-HT3 receptors located on lymphocytes and monocytes/macrophages (Burgess *et al.*, 2006). Besides hyperserotonemia, the binding of 5-HT2 receptors seems to be decreased in platelets or whole blood (Cook *et al.*, 1993) and in the cerebral cortex of individuals with autism (Murphy *et al.*, 2006).
Polymorphisms in the promoter region of the serotonin transporter gene SLC6A4 have also been reported to be associated with autism and cortical gray matter volume (Pardo and Eberhart, 2007). The gene ITGB3 has been suggested as a regulator of serotonin levels in autism based on genetic association studies (Weiss *et al.*, 2006).

### 2.1.2 Dopaminergic system

Dopamine (DA) is a catecholamine synthesized from the essential amino acid tyrosine. Once ingested, tyrosine is hydroxylated (by tyrosine hydroxylase) into L-dihydroxyphenylalanine (L-DOPA), which is then converted into dopamine via the enzyme DOPA decarboxylase.

Most DA-containing neurons lie in the midbrain. In particular, three important DA systems project from the *substantia nigra* and the ventral tegmental area. The dopaminergic system modulates a wide range of behaviors and functions, including cognition, motor function, brain-stimulation reward mechanisms, eating and drinking behaviors, sexual behavior, neuroendocrine regulation, and selective attention (Lam *et al.*, 2006).

The role of DA in autism begins with the observation that some DA blockers (i.e., antipsychotics), appear to be effective in treating some aspects of autism. Specifically, the antipsychotics supposedly to decrease hyperactivity, stereotypies, aggression, and self-injury (Young *et al.*, 1982). In addition, animal research has shown that stereotypies and hyperactivity can be induced by increasing dopaminergic functioning. These observations suggested that dopaminergic neurons could be overactive in autism, which led to studies of DA function. These studies have been performed using several methods, including blood and urine measurements of DA and its major metabolite, and measurements of this metabolite in CSF (Lam *et al.*, 2006).

The investigations of DA transporter binding have shown a significant and local increase of function in the medial region of the orbitofrontal cortex in patients with autism (Nakamura *et al.*, 2010). PET studies showed increased striatal dopamine $D_2$ receptor binding in children with autism confirming the over functioning in the dopaminergic system (Fernell *et al.*, 1997). Also, there are evidences pointing increased dopamine synthesis and storage in the striatum and frontal cortex of adults with Asperger syndrome (Nieminen-von Wendt *et al.*, 2004). The orbitofrontal cortex is a key structure in the network underlying emotional regulation. Dysfunction in the orbitofrontal-limbic circuit may be associated with behaviors in autism, such as impulsivity, difficulties in changing the focus of interest and aggressive behavior (Nakamura *et al.*, 2010).

### 2.1.3 Cholinergic system

Acetylcholine (ACh) is a simple molecule synthesized from choline and acetyl-CoA through the action of choline acetyltransferase and is the neurotransmitter found at the neuromuscular junction, in the autonomic nervous system ganglia and at multiple sites in the CNS (Fagerlund and Eriksson, 2009). There are two kinds of ACh receptors: nicotinic and muscarinic. Both are found in the brain, although muscarinic receptors are more prevalent.

The role of acetylcholine in ASD has been investigated due to neuropathological deficits found in cholinergic neurons located in the basal forebrain of individuals with autism (Bauman & Kemper, 1994), suggesting that a disruption in this system could be linked to the cognitive deficits that often accompany autism (e.g., problems with attention, learning) (Lam *et al.*, 2006).

### 2.1.4 Catecholaminergic system

Noradrenaline (NA) is a catecholamine that is synthesized from DA through the action of the enzyme DA beta-hydroxylase. Nearly every region of the brain receives input from noradrenergic neurons (Lam *et al.*, 2006). The neuronal projections from *locus coeruleus* are distributed widely throughout the brain, and play a critical role in attention, filtering of irrelevant stimuli, stress response, anxiety, and memory (Harris and Fitzgerald, 1991).

Since many of these functions are impaired in individuals with autism, researchers have investigated whether noradrenergic system shows alterations. Recent studies of people with autism have demonstrated variants at two polymorphic sites of the $\beta_2$-adrenergic receptor (ADRB2) leading to increased activity which could result in increased risk of autism (Cheslack-Postava *et al.*, 2007).

Noradrenergic activity has been assessed in autism via the measurement of NA and its central and/or peripheral metabolites in the blood, urine, and CSF. Noradrenergic function can be measured in the blood as NA itself, and as its principal central metabolite, 3-methoxy-4-hydroxyphenylglycol (MHPG). Unlike some of the other neurotransmitter systems, central and peripheral noradrenergic systems are tightly coupled with blood and CSF concentrations being highly correlated (Lam *et al.*, 2006).

### 2.1.5 Opioid system

Opioid receptors are G protein–coupled receptors, characterized by 7 transmembrane domains, and are located in the periphery and in all areas of the CNS. These receptors are known to be involved in integrating information about pain in the following areas: the brainstem, the medial thalamus, the spinal cord, the hypothalamus, and the limbic system. They are termed $\mu$ (mu), $\kappa$ (kappa), and $\delta$ (delta) receptors. Morphine is considered the prototypical $\mu$-agonist.

There is an "opioid hypothesis" suggesting that childhood autism may result from excessive brain opioid activity during the neonatal period which may constitutionally inhibit social motivation, yielding autistic isolation and aloofness (Sahley and Panksepp, 1987). Interestingly, some children with autism seem to feel less pain when compared with typically developed children. The hypothesis of excessive brain opioid activity is based on a similarity between autistic symptomatology and abnormal behavior induced in young animals by injections of exogenous opioids and the therapeutic effects of the long lasting opioid receptor blocking agent naltrexone in autism. Naltrexone is a Food and Drug Administration (FDA)-approved drug used as an opiate antagonist for treating opiate drug and alcohol addiction since the 1970's. It is a competitive antagonist of opioid receptors OPRM1, OPRD1 and OPRK1 and was used in children with autism in cases of hyperactivity (Desjardins *et al.*, 2009).

### 2.1.6 Aminoacid-neurotransmitter system

The activation of specific GABA and glutamate receptors during cell migration is necessary to the regulation of radial and tangential migrations (Manent and Represa, 2007) and an imbalance in this system can be involved in several brain pathologies. There is increasing evidence to suggesting a role for the opioid system in the control of pathophysiology of neurological disorders (Alzheimer's, Parkinson's, and Huntington's diseases, spinal cord injury, epilepsy, hypoxia, and autism) (Nandhu *et al.*, 2010).

Recent studies have pointed to abnormalities in glutamate and GABA neurotransmission in ASD, e.g. mutations in glutamate receptor genes *GRIN2A* and *GRIK2* and multiple GABA receptor genes (Webb, 2010). Therefore, additional studies are necessary to better understand glutamate metabolism in ASD.

From the translational point of view, the fact that ASD patients are up to twenty times more prone to have epilepsy, added to the abovementioned information, can let us suppose that the possible relationship between autism and epilepsy can be explained, at least in part, as a consequence from the imbalance between GABA and glutamate functioning.

### 2.1.7 Hormone-melatonin system

The discovery of melatonin in 1958 (Alberti, 1958) heralded a new field of research in reproductive physiology. Melatonin is produced in the dark by the pineal gland and is a key regulator of circadian and seasonal rhythms. A low melatonin level has been reported in individuals with ASD caused by a primary deficit in N-acetylserotonin O-methyltransferase (ASMT) (Melke *et al.*, 2008), an enzyme that catalyzes the final reaction in melatonin biosynthesis.

Melatonin is metabolized to 6-hydroxy-melatonine in the liver and the main metabolite excreted is 6-sulphatoxy-melatonine. Isolated measurements of melatonin are difficult to interpret given its circadian secretion. However urinary excretion of 6-sulphatoxy-melatonine may be helpful in studying pineal function.

## 3. Behavioral symptoms and psychopharmacotherapy on ASD

The qualitative deficits in the social interaction of children with autism may manifest themselves as social isolation and/or inappropriate social behavior characterized by poor eye contact, a difficulty to participate in group activities, affective indifference or inappropriate manifestation of affection or a lack of social or emotional empathy (Gadia et al., 2004). Children with Asperger disorder may also possibly not have any kind of problems in eye contact, but they may have some social inadequacy, particularly due to their difficulties with understanding the metaphors, the jokes and some social rules and behaviors. There is no available drug for improving the social abilities of ASD patients (Rotta and Riesgo, 2005).

The difficulties in communication occur in varying degrees in verbal as well as the non verbal ability to share information. Some children do not develop any kind of communication skills. Others speak an immature language characterized by abnormal prosody, inappropriate intonation, jargon, echolalia, the reversal of pronoun, etc. Those who maintain adequate capacity of expression may have the inability to initiate or continue a conversation appropriately. On the other hand, children with Asperger disorder may not have clear difficulties in communication. Their language may actually be characterized by a particularly correct speech. There is no available drug designed for improving the capacity of communication capacity in ASD patients. The best treatment for this problem is provided by speech therapy (Rotta and Riesgo, 2005).

The repetitive and stereotyped patterns of behavior, characteristic of autism include resistance to any sort of changes, the insistence on certain routines, the excessive attachment to objects and the fascination with the movement of parts, such as wheels or propellers.

Children with autism may be more interested in objects rather than people. Although some children seem to play, they may be more concerned in aligning, handle or throw away toys than use them into their symbolic purpose. The motor and verbal stereotyped pattern of behavior may also be observed in certain activities such as clapping hands repeatedly, circling, repeating certain words, phrases, jingles or even complete songs. If these stereotyped and repetitive patterns of behavior are part of an anxiety disorder, maybe they can ameliorate with anti-anxiety medications (Gadia *et al.*, 2004).

From the clinical point of view, some of these above mentioned behavioral symptoms may also occur in children with mental disability without autism, and this is a recurrent problem. Additionally, patient with autism may have varied degrees of mental disability ranging from no impact in the cognitive performance, that may occur in Asperger disorder, to the opposite side of the spectrum, characterized by of moderate mental disability that usually occur in the classic form of autism. This overlay of diagnostics, autism versus mental disability, albeit sometimes partial, can create difficulties to clinicians.

Fortunately, there are some clinical instruments that could help in distinguishing between autism and mental disability without autism, such as the Autism Screening Questionnaire (ASQ). The ASQ is useful both in the clinical practice as well as from the research point of view and its translation and validation is already available for different languages and countries (Sato *et al.*, 2009).

During routine clinical practice, the ideal situation would be to add the DSM-IV-TR (APA, 2002) criteria with the so-called "handmade diagnosis", which means the personal experience prudently combined with the officially adopted parameters. Once the diagnosis is confirmed, there is inaccuracy in measuring the autism behavior symptom's intensity. For sure, it could be easier to establish, from the clinical point of view, when compared and interconnected with the research approach.

Frequency and intensity of behavioral and psychological symptoms could be easily accessed by the physician through his making use of previous experience. However,, the same symptoms rating could be somewhat more difficult from the research perspective. One of the most useful clinical instruments for this purpose is the CARS (Childhood Autism Rating Scale), that already was translated and validated in several languages and countries (Pereira *et al.*, 2008).

In addition to the DSM-IV-TR criteria, there are other clinical findings that are frequently observed. These findings are not listed in the commonly used guidelines for autism diagnosis. For example, children with autism may have hypersensitivity to certain sounds or noises, such as a kitchen mixer, a jackhammer or fireworks. These noises can be extremely uncomfortable, leading children to covering ears with their hands and sometimes to screaming (Gomes *et al.*, 2004). Other findings not listed in the official autism criteria of autism includes: a) children with autism may keep walking on his toes for more time when compared with children with typical development; b) children with autism may have a higher pain threshold in comparison with people with typical development; c) children with autism may feel uncomfortable with the usual pediatric clinical maneuvers, such as touching or auscultation procedures; d) patients with autism may demonstrate a fear for people approaching, etc.

Sleep disorders can be identified in young children with ASD, occasionally even before the diagnosis confirmation. This symptom can be devastating to parents due its intensity. The mean age of ASD patients with sleep disorders is usually between one and three years of age, but disorders may also be identified earlier. From the research perspective, sleep disorders in these patients could be one interesting field. Sleep disorders, if not improving response to a non-medical approach, may be treated with Melatonin or with benzodiazepines.

Usually, one of the first behavioral symptoms in patients with ASD is language delay. In this case, it is mandatory to rule out hearing impairment before autism is diagnosed. In this group of patients, a normal global development it is not uncommon until about 18 or 24 months of age, followed by loss of language and social interaction. This diminution in social and communications skills may begin with poor eye contact, followed by a clear disinterest in people as opposed to objects. In this sense, it is important to monitor the development of these skills in children that show autistic symptoms, especially throughout the period when a child is between one and three years of age (Rotta and Riesgo, 2005).

When it comes to cerebral hemispheres specialization during childhood, language seems to be one of the most powerful inducers. In addition, language can also be useful in differentiating between autism and Asperger disorder. By definition, language can be unremarkable in Asperger's patients, while language is usually absent in the severe forms of autism. Actually, patients with Asperger have preserved both language and cognition, especially the latter. Sometimes, patients with Asperger present a peculiar type of pedantic and extremely correct language, leading the parents of these children to be proud of their adult-like type of expressive language (Rotta and Riesgo, 2005).

In certain cases, clinicians may have difficulties with distinguishing between these two diagnostics as the following questions arise. Is this a case of "high functioning autism" or an Asperger disease? Actually, from the clinical perspective, it is sometimes impossible to differentiate between these situations. However, it is somewhat easier to differentiate the pure form or autism from Asperger disease. In the clinical practice a simple rule exists which states that children with autism usually "live in their own world". By the other side, patients with Asperger in general "live in our world in their own way".

In terms of clinical diagnosis, to date we have no biological marker. Consequently, previous clinical experience is needed in order to assure a safe approach. Furthermore, some patients may have so many associated behavioral alterations that the core diagnosis, as for example ASD, could be delayed or may not even be taken into consideration.

For instance, some children´s behavior may show up to five alterations associated with ASD. The initial clinical diagnosis may be ADHD (Attention-Deficit/Hyperactive Disorder), and/or Bipolar Disorder, Anxiety Disorder, Depressive Disorder, Tics Disorder, etc. During the follow-up inevitably it will be clear that the principal diagnosis is actually ASD, and all the other diagnostics are just ASD associated features.

From the clinical perspective, one of the most prevalent behavioral symptoms is the pure form of hyperactivity, especially in the mentally disabled patients. It must be kept in mind that any type of environmental change can provoke this specific symptom and/or can deteriorate other associated behavioral manifestations. The approach of agitation can include both behavioral and/or psychopharmacological treatment. In these cases, when patient are extremely agitated and/or disorganized, the use of antipsychotics is one of the best choices. Unfortunately, there is a paucity of evidence-based studies of the efficacy of the antipsychotic drugs in treating autism.

The co-occurrence of ADHD and ASD is no rarity and, from the psychopharmacological perspective, it is crucial to define which one of the two is the principal cause of impairment, because the wrong choice of medication can deteriorate the patient's behavior. For example, stimulants drugs can provoke an increase in hyperactivity in ASD patients with concomitant ADHD. Long action stimulants in particular may have this effect.

In the clinical practice, at present, risperidone and aripoprazole are the better choice to ASD associated agitation. This, antipsychotic drugs are already approved by FDA for the treatment of childhood autism. Other medications related to the psychopharmacotherapy in ASD are described in Table 1. Initially, the main dosage of risperidone was considerably high, reaching up to 6mg/day. Today, clinicians are aware that, if there is no response to 3mg/day, probably no benefit will be obtained with higher doses of risperidone.

Further, in clinical practice, coincidently this specific daily dose regimen of 3mg/day of risperidone seems to be the threshold dose for inducing seizure in susceptible children. In Child Neurology, we frequently have to deal with patients with epilepsy. The mean prevalence of epilepsy in non-autistic children is about 1%. In comparison, the mean prevalence of epilepsy in children with ASD children reaches 20%, a rate that is clearly of both clinical and statistical significance. The possible relationship between ASD and epilepsy is one of the coming and intriguing challenges to be studied. This relationship is one of the "state of art" issues in autism, both from the clinical point of view as well as from the research perspective.

A further frequent symptom of behavior in clinical practice with ASD patients is the instability of the baseline mood. Children's mood normally changes faster than with adults' mood. Increasing our knowledge of mood regulation in childhood specifically, it is important to remember that mood changes in ASD patients occur more rapidly when compared with typically developed children. This kind of symptom may occur both in the mentally disabled and in the Asperger group of patients. If one ASD patient also has epilepsy, the addition of sodium divalproate can both protect against seizures and at the same time improve the mood control. Dealing with patients with a refractory humor deregulation is not unlikely. The use of lithium still is the best choice in some cases of severe mood oscillations.

Although not being an unchangeable rule, from the clinical point of view, the intensity of behavioral symptoms is clearly related to both with gender and cognition. The usual observation is that behavioral symptoms are more prominent in girls than in boys with autism. Additionally, we frequently see that the intensity of these symptoms is inversely related to cognition.

One of the principal prognostic factors in the clinical approach is cognition. In this sense, the main problem is how to evaluate the cognition in non-verbal ASD patients. Our group is now conducting a research in order to find the most useful clinical tool to evaluate cognition in non-verbal ASD patients. One of the possibilities is to attempt to use the same instruments used in another group of patients, such as those children without autism who are candidates to auditory prosthesis.

From the clinical perspective, feeding problems are frequently identified. Usually ASD patients have difficulties with changing their alimentation. For example, they are capable of repeating the same menu week after week without any complaint. Weight gain can also occur in autism, and sometimes it is difficult to identify its etiology. It can be a result of a stereotyped and exaggerated consumption and/or it can also be a consequence of the use of antipsychotic drugs. Further, children with autism may present several types of food allergy.

Additional useful clinical information could be how different behavioral symptoms change during the lifetime of ASD patients. First of all, obviously there is an ontogenetic evolution of each one of the behavioral manifestations in normally developed children. In other words, it is crucial to know how behavior can normally change during childhood neuropsychological development. For instance, hyperactivity would be a "normal" finding until children reach the age of five years because of the normal brain maturation that occurs from the occipital lobe towards to the frontal cerebral lobe.

In terms of gender versus behavior, usually hyperactivity is more prevalent in normal boys when compared with normal girls. Humor control, language skills and social competence usually improve in normally developed children as time passes. Normal girls tend to improve faster their language skills and their social competence when compared with normal boys.

| | Selected primary publications | First publication in ASD | Clinical information |
|---|---|---|---|
| Psychostimulants | | | Used in child neurology and psychiatry to treat attention deficit disorder, narcolepsy, and some forms of refractory depression, when used combined with antidepressants |
| Methylphenidate | (Barison and Massignan, 1956) | (Hoshino *et al.*, 1977) | |
| Pemoline | (Lucas and Knowles, 1963) | (King *et al.*, 1993) | |
| Buspirone | (Goldberg, 1979) | (Realmuto *et al.*, 1989) | |
| Antidepressants-tricyclic | | | Indicated to treat depression and/or associated anxiety. Imipramine may be also useful to treat nocturnal enuresis and/or associated sleep disorder |
| Imipramine | (Lehmann *et al.*, 1958) | (Campbell *et al.*, 1971) | |
| Clomipramine | (Volmat *et al.*, 1968) | (Brodkin *et al.*, 1997) | |
| Desipramine | (Olesen, 1963) | (Gordon *et al.*, 1992) | |
| Antidepressants-SSRI | | | The selective serotonin reuptake inhibitors (SSRI), are the most commonly prescribed antidepressants, relatively safe and generally cause fewer side effects than other types of antidepressants. They may be also be useful in the whole associated spectrum of anxiety symptoms |
| Paroxetine | (Lassen, 1978) | (Posey *et al.*, 1999) | |
| Fluoxetine | (Fuller *et al.*, 1974) | (Mehlinger *et al.*, 1990) | |
| Fluvoxamine | (Saletu *et al.*, 1977) | (McDougle *et al.*, 1990) | |
| Escitalopram | (Hyttel, 1977) | (Anderson *et al.*, 2002) | Antidepressant drug. |
| Antipsychotics (t, typical; a, atypical) | | | Antipsychotic drugs are used to treat psychosis and other mental and emotional conditions. In ASD they are frequently used to treat aggressiveness and/or agitation. In patients with mental disability and ADHD (Attention Deficit/Hyperactivity Disorder) risperidone may be more efficient when compared with methylphenidate |
| Haloperidol[t] | (Divry *et al.*, 1959) | (Faretra *et al.*, 1970) | |
| Risperidone[a] | (Faretra *et al.*, 1970) | (Purdon *et al.*, 1994) | |
| Olanzapine[a] | (Fuller and Snoddy, 1992) | (Malek-Ahmadi and Simonds, 1998) | |
| Quetiapine[a] | (Pullen *et al.*, 1992) | (Martin *et al.*, 1999) | |
| Ziprasidone[a] | (Bench *et al.*, 1993) | (Alessi, 2003) | |
| Aripiprazole[a] | (Kikuchi *et al.*, 1995) | (Rugino and Janvier, 2005) | |
| Clozapine[a] | (Ueki *et al.*, 1970) | (Atlas and Gerbino-Rosen, 1995) | |
| Antiepileptic (anticonvulsant) | | | There are at least two clinical reasons for their use: the frequent co-occurrence of epilepsy in ASD patients and/or the also frequent co-occurrence of affective disorders, especially mood disorders. |
| Valproic acid | (Lance and Anthony, 1975) | (Sovner, 1989) | |
| Carbamazepine | (Donner and Frisk, 1965) | (Gadow, 1992) | |
| Topiramate | (Maryanoff *et al.*, 1987) | (Pellock, 2004) | |
| Antiopioid | | | Naltrexone is an opioid |

| | | | |
|---|---|---|---|
| Naltrexone | (Martin *et al.*, 1973) | (Sahley and Panksepp, 1987) | receptor antagonist with higher affinity for mu receptors than other opioid receptor subtypes. Nowadays, this drug is not used in ASD patients. |
| Mood stabilizer | | | |
| Lithium | (Andreani, 1957) | (Campbell, 1975) | Lithium, discovered in 1817, was noticed to have mood stabilizing properties in the late 1800s. It is an extremely useful drug in ASD |
| Hormones | | | |
| Melatonin | (Alberti, 1958) | (Jan and O'Donnell, 1996) | Melatonin is a hormone that plays a key role in regulating circadian rhythms. Their use in treating sleep disorders resulted in weaker clinical responses than expected. |

Table 1. **Psychopharmacotherapy in ASD.** Pharmacotherapy options in ASD based upon the following target symptom clusters: inattention/hyperactivity, interfering repetitive and stereotypic behavior, aggression and self-injurious behavior, humor oscillations, anxiety and the core social impairment of autism.

Analyzing changes in ASD patient's symptoms during lifetime, it is clear that hyperactivity is more prevalent in boys than in girls and it is know that hyperactivity can decrease as time passes (Guan *et al.*, 2010). Although aggressiveness itself usually decreases with childhood development, we know that the consequences of aggressiveness can worsen with increasing age of patients with autism owing to the increase of muscle strength.

Anxiety can increase in stress situations and also can worsen during their lifetime in patients with ASD, especially in children with a less affected cognitive function, like patients with Asperger disorder. In this specific group of patients, the most frequent behavioral symptoms are depression and/or anxiety.

As time passes, communication tends to improve in children that are and/or became able to communicate. This improve in communication skills is clearly more prominent in the patients with Asperger disorder when comparing with other ASD patients.

The restricted repertoire of activities and interests does not change in intensity as time passes, but certainly the types of interests change. Interestingly, the social deficits do not improve significantly throughout patient's lives.

### 3.1 Historical landmarks of psychopharmacotherapy

In 1949, the Australian psychiatrist John Cade showed that lithium calmed maniac patients, and Mogens Schou in Denmark confirmed Cade's findings in a double-blind study in 1954. About 20 years later, in 1970, the FDA finally approved lithium to treat patients with manic-depressive illness. The first publications related to lithium treatment and ASD were in 1975.

The first antipsychotic drug, chlorpromazine, was discovered by the French pharmacologist Henri Laborit. In 1944, he noted the antihistamine activity of chlorpromazine, as well as other compounds and started to use these drugs in a pharmacological combination to prevent surgical shock. However, he curiously observed that chlorpromazine, besides preventing surgical shock, also induced calmness in patients before the operation. Laborit had the bright idea of trying the antipsychotic on schizophrenics and found that it stopped their symptoms. In consequence, he had unintentionally discovered the first antipsychotic drug.

In the same year, methylphenidate was synthesized by Ciba chemist Leandro Panizzon, who named the compound Ritalin™ because his wife Margherite (nicknamed Rita) used to take this drug as a stimulant before playing tennis.

The first effective pharmacologic treatment for depression was discovered by the clinician Roland Kuhn in 1956. This drug was the tricyclic antidepressant imipramine. Kuhn published the results of his observations in the *Schweizerische Medizinische Wochenschrift* (Swiss Weekly Medical Journal) in 1957. Heinz Lehmann, Clinical Director at Douglas Hospital, Montreal, Canada, treated depressed with equally good results. Lehmann and two co-workers published their results in the *Canadian Medical Association Journal* in 1958 (Lehmann *et al.*, 1958).

The typical antipsychotic drug, haloperidol, was discovered by Paul Janssen and was developed in 1957 by the Belgian company Janssen Pharmaceutica. It was approved by the by the U.S. Food and Drug Administration (FDA) in April 12, 1967.

The work which eventually led to the discovery of fluoxetine began at Eli Lilly and Company in 1970 with collaboration of Bryan Molloy and Robert Rathbun. After 20 years, the first papers related to the fluoxetine treatment of ASD patients were published.

In 1988, the American psychiatrist John Kane demonstrated that clozapine achieved a good response in schizophrenic patients refractory to treatment with other antipsychotic drugs; the FDA approves the drug in 1989.

The atypical antipsychotic risperidone was developed by Janssen-Cilag, first released in 1994, approved by the FDA in the same year to use in adult psychiatric patients and approved for treating ASD only two years later. In the brain, risperidone binds multiple neurotransmitter receptors, having a strong affinity to the serotonin 2A (5-HT2A) and dopamine D2 receptors, and a good affinity for the α-1 and α-2C adrenergic receptors and for the serotonin receptors 6 and 7 (5-HT6 and 5-HT7).

## 4. Antipsychotic side effects in ASD

The first generation of antipsychotics, today called typical antipsychotics, functions by blocking the effects of dopamine, controlling hallucinations and delusions. Because of this primary function, this medication is also named neuroleptic which means "seizing the neuron", with high efficiency to some symptoms of autism (lack in social behavior, stereotypical behavior) and in behavioral impairments that may be associated with autism (aggressive behavior, hyperactivity). However, the use of typical antipsychotics, like haloperidol, can induce extrapyramidal side effects, which often lead to persistent tardive dyskinesia, limiting the long term use of these drugs.

Atypical antipsychotics have been prescribed for ASD symptoms as they have lower frequency and intensity of side effects compared with the typical one. However, an important concern related to the use of atypical antipsychotics is the inducement of endocrine and metabolic side-effects (weight gain, obesity, and related metabolic abnormalities such as hyperglycemia and dyslipidemia). Obesity is a risk to the development of metabolic syndrome and may result in a high-risk state for future cardiovascular morbidity and mortality in adult age (Goeb *et al.*, 2010).

The atypical antipsychotics risperidone, olanzapine, quetiapine and ziprazidone are most commonly prescribed for ASD. However, only two atypical antipsychotics have been approved by the FDA for treating irritability in autistic children. Risperidone was approved in late 2006, followed by aripiprazole in 2009.

## 5. Non-neuronal targets of Risperidone

All complex nervous systems consist of two main cell types, neurons and glial cells. In the past 20 years evidence has accumulated that supports the existence of bidirectional communication between glial cells and neurons (Froes *et al.*, 1999; Gomes *et al.*, 2001). Based on this context, it is important to consider that if the functional unit of the brain is not only orchestrated by neurons but rather by the neuron-glial complex, consequently must assume that both neuronal and glial cells are involved in neural diseases.

There are three main types of glial cell populations in the CNS, termed *astrocytes* a diverse population of cells with numerous functions; *oligodendrocytes*, the myelinating cells of the CNS (McLaurin and Yong, 1995) and *microglia*, considered the immune cells of the CNS, responding to any kind of pathology with a reaction termed microglial activation (Hanisch and Kettenmann, 2007).

The idea that astrocytes, like neurons, might take up diverse roles in the development and function of the CNS has slowly been gaining recognition (Westergaard *et al.*, 1995). Nowadays, a considerable amount of evidence has revealed a more active role of astrocytes in the physiology of the CNS than previously believed (Araque *et al.*, 2001). It has been found that these cells play a crucial role in maintaining normal brain physiology during development, releasing molecules important for neuronal survival and dendrite formation. Also, astrocytes have been emerging as key modulators of neuronal excitability, synaptic transmission (Perea and Araque, 2009) and blood-brain barrier (Wang and Bordey, 2008). Common astrocytic reactions that occur in the pathological states are cellular swelling, hypertrophy-hyperplasia (astrogliosis) and proliferation (astrocytosis).

Morphology of astrocytes varies depending on regional localization and shape changes potentially may influence neuronal activity and injury via ion channels, neurotransmitter receptors and transporters on their processes (Theodosis *et al.*, 2008). In this context, we have investigated the effect of risperidone on astroglial cells, evaluating morphology, membrane integrity, viability, secretion of S100B, a neurotrophic astrocyte-derived protein and glutamate metabolism (glutamate uptake, glutamine synthetase activity and glutathione synthesis).

We demonstrate for the first time that risperidone was able to modulate cell morphology and glial adhesion (Quincozes-Santos *et al.*, 2008), contributing to the proposal that glial cells also are targets of antipsychotics. In addition, risperidone also increased S100B secretion by astroglial cells. S100B is a calcium-binding protein involved in the regulation of cytoskeleton and the proliferation of astrocytes. Beyond its intracellular role, S100B, depending on its concentration, works as a cytokine for neighboring cells (astrocytes, neurons, and microglia) and is able to protect hippocampal neurons against glutamate toxicity. Extending these findings to brain plasticity in ASD, it would be possible to conceive that risperidone stimulates S100B secretion which in turn can stimulate neuronal activity in patients.

Astrocytes respond to neuronal activity via ion channels, neurotransmitter receptors, and transporters on their processes, a plasticity that has important functional consequences since it modifies neurotransmission. We described a significant increase in glutamate uptake and in glutamine synthetase (GS) activity by astroglial cells in the presence of risperidone (Quincozes-Santos *et al.*, 2010).

Astrocytes are the only cells in the brain that have the important ability to convert glutamate into glutamine via GS. Glutamine, in turn, is taken up by neurons and used for the synthesis of glutamate (and then GABA, in GABAergic neurons). However, glutamate has another important destination in astrocytes, particularly GSH (glutathione) synthesis (Dringen *et al.*, 1999). Glutamate serves as a substrate per se for GSH synthesis and as a moiety for exchange by cysteine, another substrate for GSH synthesis. Moreover, concomitantly with the increase in glutamate uptake and GS activity, an increase in the content of GSH was seen, reinforcing the antioxidant activity of astroglial cells mediated by risperidone. In this context, astrocyte clearance of glutamate from the synaptic cleft is an important aspect to be considered in autism, from both the physiopathologic and the pharmacologic point of view.

As evidence emerging indicates that signaling between perisynaptic astrocytes and neurons at the tripartite synapse display important roles when neural circuits are formed and refined (Araque *et al.*, 1999), we propose an integrative model of the tripartite synapse modulated by this antipsychotic during treatment *in vivo* (Figure 2).

Most studies about pathological abnormalities in brains of patients with autism report differences in neuronal plasticity and migration patterns rather than alterations in glial cells (Minshew and Williams, 2007; Minshew and Keller, 2010). Also, this cells have many functions that could be relevant to abnormalities described in psychiatric disorders such as schizophrenia (Rothermundt *et al.*, 2004). However, the majority of studies about cellular mechanisms of antipsychotic drug treatment focus on neuronal effects. Therefore, a possible role of astrocytes has been largely neglected in ASD research.

## 6. Clinical recommendations of antipsychotics in ASD

The following clinical recommendations can be made after twenty years of clinical practice in Child Neurology. During this time, more than one thousand of ASD patients were seen, if children seen in private practice are added to those treated in our Child Neurology Residence Program.

First of all, it is important to remember that until now ASD encompasses five different clinical diagnostic categories. These diagnostic categories will change with the new DSM-V classification. Even the widely used expression "ASD" may disappear. Even after the changes of the new classification, what is now called ASD will remain as a heterogeneous group both in terms of behavioral symptoms as well as in terms of medical diagnosis.

In other words, before planning a psychopharmacological treatment in ASD, it is important to be sure that the diagnosis is correct. We must remember that this type of diagnosis can be catastrophic to parents and consequently an incorrect diagnosis would be even worse. This is probably one of the most important clinical recommendations. Before medications usage, make a double check in every diagnosis of this group of children.

Another important remark is that each one of the five currently adopted clinical diagnostics, considered individually, also has its own behavioral heterogeneity, when taken individually. For instance, one particular case of autism may initially present as a confused mix of different behavioral complaints that could hide the main diagnosis.

There is no single medication that can be successfully used in ASD as a whole. The guidelines recommend that monotherapy would be the best choice, but often this is difficult

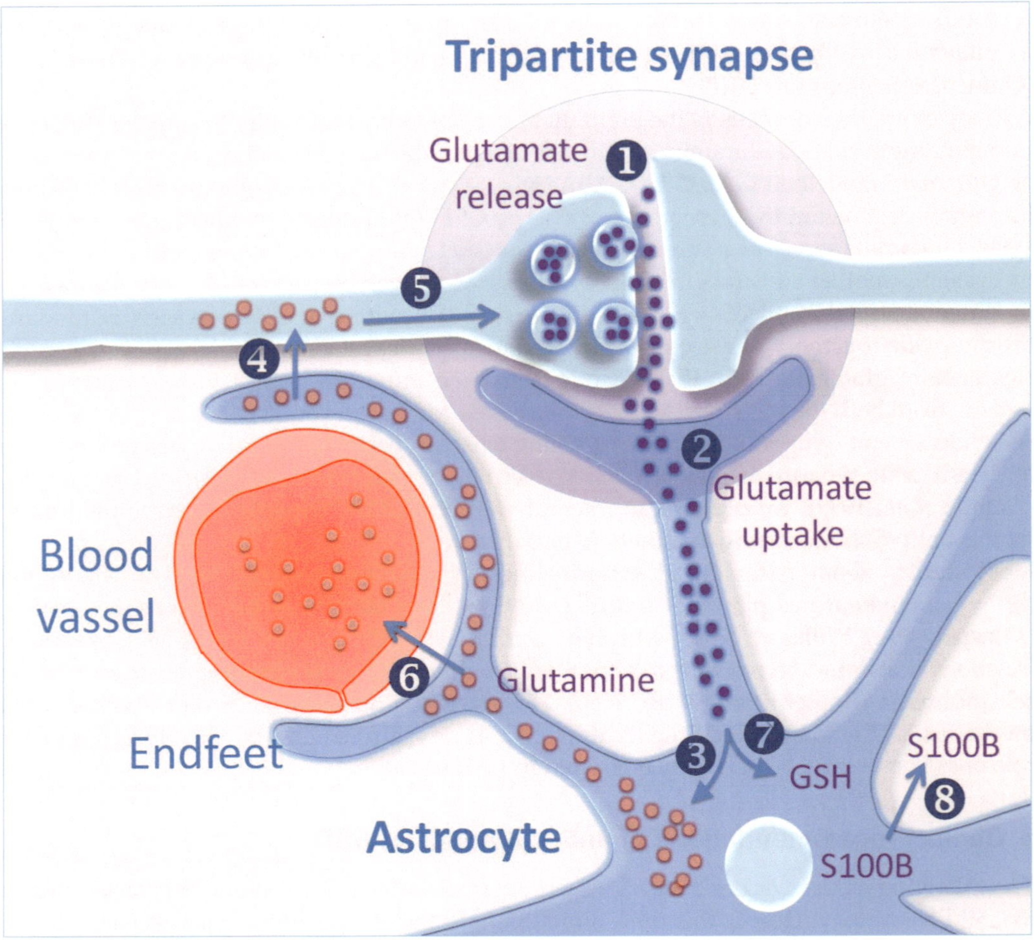


Fig. 2. **Hypothesis for the influence of Risperidone on tripartite synapse supported by its influence on astroglial cell culture and on hippocampal slices.** After the release of glutamate at the synaptic cleft (1), risperidone improves glutamate uptake by astrocytes (2); stimulates the enzyme GS to convert glutamate into glutamine (3), which in turn is taken up by neurons (4), followed by resynthesis of glutamate (5) and/or transported to the blood (6). Additionally, risperidone is able to stimulate the synthesis of another important fate of glutamate in astrocytes, the tripeptide L-glutamyl-L-cysteinyl-glycine or glutathione (GSH) (7), and to promote the secretion of the trophic factor S100B (8). This hypothesis was proposed considering the direct effect of risperidone on astroglial cells (numbers 2, 3, 7 and 8).

or even impossible to do in the real clinical world. Although there is no ASD-specific medication, the psychopharmacologic treatment can decrease the "noise" surrounding autism, as well as facilitate the non pharmacological treatments. It is important to remember that the psychopharmacological approach is only one of the available treatments for ASD patients.

The first clinical recommendation is to identify as clearly as possible each one of the behavioral symptoms. It would be extremely useful to make a list of these behavioral targets. After making the list, it is important try to put these targets into a ranking of clinical relevance, in order to choose which one of the behavioral symptoms is more prominent and/or requires prompt relief.

The second clinical recommendation is to decide if each one of the selected behavioral targets really will require psychopharmacological treatment. Obviously, this decision is somewhat more complicated and is not available in any guideline. This is the art included in clinical practice. The only safe way to make this decision is to use the previous experience. It would be helpful to discover whether a given behavioral symptom is more uncomfortable for parents or to the patient. For example, stereotyped and repetitive movements are frequently more unpleasant to parents than to the child, which can obtain a sort of relief of anxiety with these repetitive movements. In this case, no medication would be used. Instead the best recommendation would be try to find a use for the stereotyped movements.

If the given symptom really requires psychopharmacological treatment, the third clinical recommendation is to choose which would be the better medication. This appears problematic because of the paucity of good evidence based studies with regard to the efficacy of medications in the treatment of autism.

Different categories of drugs have been used to treat autism for years, despite the lack of proved efficacy of the majority of them. The following list of drugs that have been used in autism is obviously incomplete; antiepileptic drugs, mood stabilizers, antidepressants, anti-anxiety drugs, sleep inducers, stimulants, antipsychotics, etc.

Since there is no medication for autism itself, we must choose which of the undesirable behaviors could be ameliorated by antipsychotic medication. Of all of the symptoms presented by ASD patients, disrupted behavior and irritability probably are the best responders to antipsychotic drugs. It is important to mention that many of the drugs used in the psychopharmacological treatment in autism, including antipsychotics, can decrease the seizure threshold (Tuchman, 2009). Because of ASD children are almost twenty times more prone to have epilepsy when compared with a child who had a normal neurodevelopment, probably it would be safer to consider the usefulness of an electroencephalogram examination before prescribing psychoactive drugs. Also, before prescribing antipsychotic drugs, it is useful to obtain a baseline laboratory profile, which includes a complete blood count, evaluation of blood lipids and glucose, liver function as well as prolactin levels. It is also important to measure the weight and height as well as the blood pressure. It is also prudent to make a complete physical and neurological examination.

After prescribing antipsychotic drugs, it is necessary to monitor both the above mentioned measures, such as laboratorial findings as well as the clinical examination findings. In clinical practice, different antipsychotic drugs have been used, but only few of them still continue in the medical arsenal. To date, atypical antipsychotic drugs are preferred when compared with the typical antipsychotic drugs because of their relative safety in terms of side effects, especially neurologic impregnation.

In the past, haloperidol was the typical antipsychotic more frequently used in the treatment of children. The daily dose usually ranges between 1 to 2 mg. The most problematic side effect of haloperidol seems to be neurological side effects manifested by Parkinson-like symptoms, extrapiramidal signs and/or tardive dyskinesia.

Many of the available atypical antipsychotic drugs used in adult patients have also been used in children. The most frequently prescribed antipsychotics for ASD patients are risperidone, olanzapine, quetiapine, clozapina, ziprazidone and aripiprazole, however only two of them have been approved by the FDA for use in childhood autism. Risperidone was the first atypical antipsychotic drug to be approved by the FDA, in 2006. The second drug of this group of medications was aripiprazole, which was approved in 2009. The usual daily dose of risperidone varies from 1 to 3 mg, and the usual daily dose of aripiprazole is up to 15 mg in children and adolescents. Aripiprazole seems to be better when compared with risperidone in terms of side effects, because as there is a relatively lower risk of metabolic side effects and/or weigh gain.

## 7. Conclusions and future remarks

The first generation of antipsychotics (now called typical) has been used since the 1950s, and is dopamine-2 (D2) receptor antagonist. Nevertheless, the second generation, or atypical, has many clinical applications in neuropsychiatric practice (Schwartz and Stahl, 2011). Since the mid-1990's, it is clear that atypical antipsychotics are safer in regard to inducing fewer extrapyramidal symptoms and tardive dyskinesia.

At first sight, the bulk of neurochemical research in autism has been inconclusive. In addition, the high levels of use of many different psychotropic agents, often in combination, is concerning and is necessary to study the results of interactions of different types of medical and educational treatment for children with ASD.

As a result of our translational research in autism, we became enthusiasts of changing the traditional "neuronal neuropsychiatry" approach into the modern "neuroglial neuropsychiatry" concept. In our opinion, the first one is somewhat simplistic because is totally based only on the neurons activity, and the last one is indubitably the more comprehensive, because there is no way to deny the importance of glial cells working together with neurons in the neurobiology of development and behavior, coincidentally two of the most altered areas in ASD patients.

## 8. References


Alberti, C., 1958. [Melatonin: the first hormone isolated from the pineal body]. Farmaco Sci. 13, 604-5.

Alessi, N.E., 2003. Ziprasidone in autism. J Am Acad Child Adolesc Psychiatry. 42, 622-3.

Anderson, G.M., Gutknecht, L., Cohen, D.J., Brailly-Tabard, S., Cohen, J.H., Ferrari, P., Roubertoux, P.L., Tordjman, S., 2002. Serotonin transporter promoter variants in autism: functional effects and relationship to platelet hyperserotonemia. Mol Psychiatry. 7, 831-6.

Andreani, G., 1957. [Electrocardiographic findings during treatment of mental patients with lithium salts]. G Clin Med. 38, 1759-75.

APA, 2002. Diagnostic and Statistical Manual of Mental Disorders: DSM-IV-TR., Vol., Artes Medicas, Porto Alegre.

Araque, A., Parpura, V., Sanzgiri, R.P., Haydon, P.G., 1999. Tripartite synapses: glia, the unacknowledged partner. Trends Neurosci. 22, 208-15.

Araque, A., Carmignoto, G., Haydon, P.G., 2001. Dynamic signaling between astrocytes and neurons. Annu Rev Physiol. 63, 795-813.

Atlas, J.A., Gerbino-Rosen, G., 1995. Differential diagnostics and treatment of an inpatient adolescent showing pervasive developmental disorder and mania. Psychol Rep. 77, 207-10.

Bailey, A.R., Giunta, B.N., Obregon, D., Nikolic, W.V., Tian, J., Sanberg, C.D., Sutton, D.T., Tan, J., 2008. Peripheral biomarkers in Autism: secreted amyloid precursor protein-alpha as a probable key player in early diagnosis. Int J Clin Exp Med. 1, 338-44.

Barison, F., Massignan, L., 1956. [Observations on neurotic depressions with reference to a combined serpasil-ritalin treatment]. Rass Neuropsichiatr. 10, 198-209.

Bauman, M.L., Kemper, T.L., 2005. Neuroanatomic observations of the brain in autism: a review and future directions. Int J Dev Neurosci. 23, 183-7.

Bench, C.J., Lammertsma, A.A., Dolan, R.J., Grasby, P.M., Warrington, S.J., Gunn, K., Cuddigan, M., Turton, D.J., Osman, S., Frackowiak, R.S., 1993. Dose dependent occupancy of central dopamine D2 receptors by the novel neuroleptic CP-88,059-01: a study using positron emission tomography and 11C-raclopride. Psychopharmacology (Berl). 112, 308-14.

Brodkin, E.S., McDougle, C.J., Naylor, S.T., Cohen, D.J., Price, L.H., 1997. Clomipramine in adults with pervasive developmental disorders: a prospective open-label investigation. J Child Adolesc Psychopharmacol. 7, 109-21.

Buehler, M.R., 2011. A proposed mechanism for autism: an aberrant neuroimmune response manifested as a psychiatric disorder. Med Hypotheses.

Burgess, N.K., Sweeten, T.L., McMahon, W.M., Fujinami, R.S., 2006. Hyperserotoninemia and altered immunity in autism. J Autism Dev Disord. 36, 697-704.

Campbell, M., Fish, B., Shapiro, T., Floyd, A., Jr., 1971. Imipramine in preschool autistic and schizophrenic children. J Autism Child Schizophr. 1, 267-82.

Campbell, M., 1975. Pharmacotherapy in early infantile autism. Biol Psychiatry. 10, 399-423.

Catalano, M., 2001. Functionally gene-linked polymorphic regions and genetically controlled neurotransmitters metabolism. Eur Neuropsychopharmacol. 11, 431-9.

Chandana, S.R., Behen, M.E., Juhasz, C., Muzik, O., Rothermel, R.D., Mangner, T.J., Chakraborty, P.K., Chugani, H.T., Chugani, D.C., 2005. Significance of abnormalities in developmental trajectory and asymmetry of cortical serotonin synthesis in autism. Int J Dev Neurosci. 23, 171-82.

Cheslack-Postava, K., Fallin, M.D., Avramopoulos, D., Connors, S.L., Zimmerman, A.W., Eberhart, C.G., Newschaffer, C.J., 2007. beta2-Adrenergic receptor gene variants and risk for autism in the AGRE cohort. Mol Psychiatry. 12, 283-91.

Chugani, D.C., Muzik, O., Behen, M., Rothermel, R., Janisse, J.J., Lee, J., Chugani, H.T., 1999. Developmental changes in brain serotonin synthesis capacity in autistic and nonautistic children. Ann Neurol. 45, 287-95.

Cook, E.H., Jr., Arora, R.C., Anderson, G.M., Berry-Kravis, E.M., Yan, S.Y., Yeoh, H.C., Sklena, P.J., Charak, D.A., Leventhal, B.L., 1993. Platelet serotonin studies in hyperserotonemic relatives of children with autistic disorder. Life Sci. 52, 2005-15.

Coury, D., 2010. Medical treatment of autism spectrum disorders. Current Opinion in Neurology. 23, 131-136.

Desjardins, S., Doyen, C., Contejean, Y., Kaye, K., Paubel, P., 2009. [Treatment of a serious autistic disorder in a child with Naltrexone in an oral suspension form]. Encephale. 35, 168-72.

Divry, P., Bobon, J., Collard, J., Pinchard, A., Nols, E., 1959. [Study & clinical trial of R 1625 or haloperidol, a new neuroleptic & so-called neurodysleptic agent]. Acta Neurol Psychiatr Belg. 59, 337-66.

Donner, M., Frisk, M., 1965. Carbamazepine treatment of epileptic and psychic symptoms in children and adolescents. Ann Paediatr Fenn. 11, 91-7.

Dringen, R., Pfeiffer, B., Hamprecht, B., 1999. Synthesis of the antioxidant glutathione in neurons: supply by astrocytes of CysGly as precursor for neuronal glutathione. J Neurosci. 19, 562-9.

Fagerlund, M.J., Eriksson, L.I., 2009. Current concepts in neuromuscular transmission. Br J Anaesth. 103, 108-14.

Faretra, G., Dooher, L., Dowling, J., 1970. Comparison of haloperidol and fluphenazine in disturbed children. Am J Psychiatry. 126, 1670-3.

Fernell, E., Watanabe, Y., Adolfsson, I., Tani, Y., Bergstrom, M., Hartvig, P., Lilja, A., von Knorring, A.L., Gillberg, C., Langstrom, B., 1997. Possible effects of tetrahydrobiopterin treatment in six children with autism--clinical and positron emission tomography data: a pilot study. Dev Med Child Neurol. 39, 313-8.

Froes, M.M., Correia, A.H., Garcia-Abreu, J., Spray, D.C., Campos de Carvalho, A.C., Neto, M.V., 1999. Gap-junctional coupling between neurons and astrocytes in primary central nervous system cultures. Proc Natl Acad Sci U S A. 96, 7541-6.

Fuller, R.W., Perry, K.W., Molloy, B.B., 1974. Effect of an uptake inhibitor on serotonin metabolism in rat brain: studies with 3-(p-trifluoromethylphenoxy)-N-methyl-3-phenylpropylamine (Lilly 110140). Life Sci. 15, 1161-71.

Fuller, R.W., Snoddy, H.D., 1992. Neuroendocrine evidence for antagonism of serotonin and dopamine receptors by olanzapine (LY170053), an antipsychotic drug candidate. Res Commun Chem Pathol Pharmacol. 77, 87-93.

Gadia, C.A., Tuchman, R., Rotta, N.T., 2004. [Autism and pervasive developmental disorders]. J Pediatr (Rio J). 80, S83-94.

Gadow, K.D., 1992. Pediatric psychopharmacotherapy: a review of recent research. J Child Psychol Psychiatry. 33, 153-95.

Goeb, J.L., Marco, S., Duhamel, A., Kechid, G., Bordet, R., Thomas, P., Delion, P., Jardri, R., 2010. [Metabolic side effects of risperidone in early onset schizophrenia]. Encephale. 36, 242-52.

Goldberg, H.L., 1979. Buspirone--a new antianxiety agent not chemically related to any presently marketed drugs [proceedings]. Psychopharmacol Bull. 15, 90-2.

Gomes, E., Rotta, N.T., Pedroso, F.S., Sleifer, P., Danesi, M.C., 2004. Auditory hypersensitivity in children and teenagers with autistic spectrum disorder. Arq Neuropsiquiatr. 62, 797-801.

Gomes, F.C., Spohr, T.C., Martinez, R., Moura Neto, V., 2001. Cross-talk between neurons and glia: highlights on soluble factors. Braz J Med Biol Res. 34, 611-20.

Gordon, C.T., Rapoport, J.L., Hamburger, S.D., State, R.C., Mannheim, G.B., 1992. Differential response of seven subjects with autistic disorder to clomipramine and desipramine. Am J Psychiatry. 149, 363-6.

Guan, B.Q., Luo, X.R., Deng, Y.L., Wei, Z., Ye, H.S., Yuan, X.H., Ning, Z.J., Yang, W., Ding, J., 2010. [Prevalence of psychiatric disorders in primary and middle school students in Hunan Province]. Zhongguo Dang Dai Er Ke Za Zhi. 12, 123-7.

Hanisch, U.K., Kettenmann, H., 2007. Microglia: active sensor and versatile effector cells in the normal and pathologic brain. Nat Neurosci. 10, 1387-94.

Harris, G.C., Fitzgerald, R.D., 1991. Locus coeruleus involvement in the learning of classically conditioned bradycardia. J Neurosci. 11, 2314-20.

Hoshino, Y., Kumashiro, H., Kaneko, M., Takahashi, Y., 1977. The effects of methylphenidate on early infantile autism and its relation to serum serotonin levels. Folia Psychiatr Neurol Jpn. 31, 605-14.
Hyttel, J., 1977. Neurochemical characterization of a new potent and selective serotonin uptake inhibitor: Lu 10-171. Psychopharmacology (Berl). 51, 225-33.
Jan, J.E., O'Donnell, M.E., 1996. Use of melatonin in the treatment of paediatric sleep disorders. J Pineal Res. 21, 193-9.
Kanner, L., 1943. Autistic Disturbances of Affective Contact. Nervous Child. 217-250.
Keller, T.A., Just, M.A., 2009. Altering cortical connectivity: remediation-induced changes in the white matter of poor readers. Neuron. 64, 624-31.
Kikuchi, T., Tottori, K., Uwahodo, Y., Hirose, T., Miwa, T., Oshiro, Y., Morita, S., 1995. 7-(4-[4-(2,3-Dichlorophenyl)-1-piperazinyl]butyloxy)-3,4-dihydro-2(1H)-qui nolinone (OPC-14597), a new putative antipsychotic drug with both presynaptic dopamine autoreceptor agonistic activity and postsynaptic D2 receptor antagonistic activity. J Pharmacol Exp Ther. 274, 329-36.
King, B.H., Au, D., Poland, R.E., 1993. Low-dose naltrexone inhibits pemoline-induced self-biting behavior in prepubertal rats. J Child Adolesc Psychopharmacol. 3, 71-9.
Lam, K.S., Aman, M.G., Arnold, L.E., 2006. Neurochemical correlates of autistic disorder: a review of the literature. Res Dev Disabil. 27, 254-89.
Lance, J.W., Anthony, M., 1975. Sodium valproate in the management of intractable epilepsy: comparison with clonazepam. Proc Aust Assoc Neurol. 12, 55-60.
Landrigan, P.J., 2010. What causes autism? Exploring the environmental contribution. Current Opinion in Pediatrics. 22, 219-225.
Lassen, J.B., 1978. Influence of the new 5-HT-uptake inhibitor paroxetine on hypermotility in rats produced by p-chloroamphetamine (PCA) and 4,alpha-dimethyl-7-tyramine (H 77/77). Psychopharmacology (Berl). 57, 151-3.
Lehmann, H.E., Cahn, C.H., De Verteuil, R.L., 1958. The treatment of depressive conditions with imipramine (G 22355). Can Psychiatr Assoc J. 3, 155-64.
Longo, D., Schuler-Faccini, L., Brandalize, A.P., dos Santos Riesgo, R., Bau, C.H., 2009. Influence of the 5-HTTLPR polymorphism and environmental risk factors in a Brazilian sample of patients with autism spectrum disorders. Brain Res. 1267, 9-17.
Lucas, C.J., Knowles, J.B., 1963. The Trial of a New Stimulant, Pemoline, in the Treatment of Fatigue in Students. J Am Coll Health Assoc. 12, 187-94.
Malek-Ahmadi, P., Simonds, J.F., 1998. Olanzapine for autistic disorder with hyperactivity. J Am Acad Child Adolesc Psychiatry. 37, 902.
Manent, J.B., Represa, A., 2007. Neurotransmitters and brain maturation: early paracrine actions of GABA and glutamate modulate neuronal migration. Neuroscientist. 13, 268-79.
Martin, A., Koenig, K., Scahill, L., Bregman, J., 1999. Open-label quetiapine in the treatment of children and adolescents with autistic disorder. J Child Adolesc Psychopharmacol. 9, 99-107.
Martin, W.R., Jasinski, D.R., Mansky, P.A., 1973. Naltrexone, an antagonist for the treatment of heroin dependence. Effects in man. Arch Gen Psychiatry. 28, 784-91.
Maryanoff, B.E., Nortey, S.O., Gardocki, J.F., Shank, R.P., Dodgson, S.P., 1987. Anticonvulsant O-alkyl sulfamates. 2,3:4,5-Bis-O-(1-methylethylidene)-beta-D-fructopyranose sulfamate and related compounds. J Med Chem. 30, 880-7.

McDougle, C.J., Price, L.H., Goodman, W.K., 1990. Fluvoxamine treatment of coincident autistic disorder and obsessive-compulsive disorder: a case report. J Autism Dev Disord. 20, 537-43.
McLaurin, J.A., Yong, V.W., 1995. Oligodendrocytes and myelin. Neurol Clin. 13, 23-49.
Mehlinger, R., Scheftner, W.A., Poznanski, E., 1990. Fluoxetine and autism. J Am Acad Child Adolesc Psychiatry. 29, 985.
Melke, J., Goubran Botros, H., Chaste, P., Betancur, C., Nygren, G., Anckarsater, H., Rastam, M., Stahlberg, O., Gillberg, I.C., Delorme, R., Chabane, N., Mouren-Simeoni, M.C., Fauchereau, F., Durand, C.M., Chevalier, F., Drouot, X., Collet, C., Launay, J.M., Leboyer, M., Gillberg, C., Bourgeron, T., 2008. Abnormal melatonin synthesis in autism spectrum disorders. Mol Psychiatry. 13, 90-8.
Minshew, N.J., Williams, D.L., 2007. The new neurobiology of autism: cortex, connectivity, and neuronal organization. Arch Neurol. 64, 945-50.
Minshew, N.J., Keller, T.A., 2010. The nature of brain dysfunction in autism: functional brain imaging studies. Current Opinion in Neurology. 23, 124-130.
Mostofsky, S.H., Burgess, M.P., Gidley Larson, J.C., 2007. Increased motor cortex white matter volume predicts motor impairment in autism. Brain. 130, 2117-22.
Murphy, D.G., Daly, E., Schmitz, N., Toal, F., Murphy, K., Curran, S., Erlandsson, K., Eersels, J., Kerwin, R., Ell, P., Travis, M., 2006. Cortical serotonin 5-HT2A receptor binding and social communication in adults with Asperger's syndrome: an in vivo SPECT study. Am J Psychiatry. 163, 934-6.
Nakamura, K., Sekine, Y., Ouchi, Y., Tsujii, M., Yoshikawa, E., Futatsubashi, M., Tsuchiya, K.J., Sugihara, G., Iwata, Y., Suzuki, K., Matsuzaki, H., Suda, S., Sugiyama, T., Takei, N., Mori, N., 2010. Brain serotonin and dopamine transporter bindings in adults with high-functioning autism. Arch Gen Psychiatry. 67, 59-68.
Nandhu, M.S., Naijil, G., Smijin, S., Jayanarayanan, S., Paulose, C.S., 2010. Opioid system functional regulation in neurological disease management. J Neurosci Res. 88, 3215-21.
Nieminen-von Wendt, T.S., Metsahonkala, L., Kulomaki, T.A., Aalto, S., Autti, T.H., Vanhala, R., Eskola, O., Bergman, J., Hietala, J.A., von Wendt, L.O., 2004. Increased presynaptic dopamine function in Asperger syndrome. Neuroreport. 15, 757-60.
Nunes, M.L., Mercadante, M.T., 2004. [Neurobiology of behavior: exploring the frontier between the mind and the brain]. J Pediatr (Rio J). 80, S1-2.
Olesen, K.M., 1963. [Endogenous Depressions Treated with Pertofrane]. Nord Psykiatr Tidsskr. 17, 183-6.
Pardo, C.A., Eberhart, C.G., 2007. The neurobiology of autism. Brain Pathol. 17, 434-47.
Pellock, J.M., 2004. Understanding co-morbidities affecting children with epilepsy. Neurology. 62, S17-23.
Perea, G., Araque, A., 2009. GLIA modulates synaptic transmission. Brain Res Rev.
Pereira, A., Riesgo, R.S., Wagner, M.B., 2008. Childhood autism: translation and validation of the Childhood Autism Rating Scale for use in Brazil. J Pediatr (Rio J). 84, 487-94.
Posey, D.I., Litwiller, M., Koburn, A., McDougle, C.J., 1999. Paroxetine in autism. J Am Acad Child Adolesc Psychiatry. 38, 111-2.
Pullen, R.H., Palermo, K.M., Curtis, M.A., 1992. Determination of an antipsychotic agent (ICI 204,636) and its 7-hydroxy metabolite in human plasma by high-performance

liquid chromatography and gas chromatography-mass spectrometry. J Chromatogr. 573, 49-57.
Purdon, S.E., Lit, W., Labelle, A., Jones, B.D., 1994. Risperidone in the treatment of pervasive developmental disorder. Can J Psychiatry. 39, 400-5.
Quincozes-Santos, A., Abib, R.T., Leite, M.C., Bobermin, D., Bambini-Junior, V., Goncalves, C.A., Riesgo, R., Gottfried, C., 2008. Effect of the atypical neuroleptic risperidone on morphology and S100B secretion in C6 astroglial lineage cells. Mol Cell Biochem. 314, 59-63.
Quincozes-Santos, A., Bobermin, L.D., Tonial, R.P., Bambini-Junior, V., Riesgo, R., Gottfried, C., 2010. Effects of atypical (risperidone) and typical (haloperidol) antipsychotic agents on astroglial functions. Eur Arch Psychiatry Clin Neurosci. 260, 475-81.
Realmuto, G.M., August, G.J., Garfinkel, B.D., 1989. Clinical effect of buspirone in autistic children. J Clin Psychopharmacol. 9, 122-5.
Rothermundt, M., Ponath, G., Arolt, V., 2004. S100B in schizophrenic psychosis. Int Rev Neurobiol. 59, 445-70.
Rotta, N.T., Riesgo, R.S., 2005. Rotinas em Neuropediatria. In: Autismo Infantil. Vol., N.T. Rotta, L. Ohlweiler, R.S. Riesgo, ed.^eds. Artes Medicas, Porto Alegre, pp. 161-172.
Rugino, T.A., Janvier, Y.M., 2005. Aripiprazole in children and adolescents: clinical experience. J Child Neurol. 20, 603-10.
Sahley, T.L., Panksepp, J., 1987. Brain opioids and autism: an updated analysis of possible linkages. J Autism Dev Disord. 17, 201-16.
Saletu, B., Schjerve, M., Grunberger, J., Schanda, H., Arnold, O.H., 1977. Fluvoxamine-a new serotonin re-uptake inhibitor: first clinical and psychometric experiences in depressed patients. J Neural Transm. 41, 17-36.
Sato, F.P., Paula, C.S., Lowenthal, R., Nakano, E.Y., Brunoni, D., Schwartzman, J.S., Mercadante, M.T., 2009. Instrument to screen cases of pervasive developmental disorder: a preliminary indication of validity. Rev Bras Psiquiatr. 31, 30-3.
Schwartz, T.L., Stahl, S.M., 2011. Treatment strategies for dosing the second generation antipsychotics. CNS Neurosci Ther. 17, 110-7.
Scott, M.M., Deneris, E.S., 2005. Making and breaking serotonin neurons and autism. Int J Dev Neurosci. 23, 277-85.
Sovner, R., 1989. The use of valproate in the treatment of mentally retarded persons with typical and atypical bipolar disorders. J Clin Psychiatry. 50 Suppl, 40-3.
Theodosis, D.T., Poulain, D.A., Oliet, S.H., 2008. Activity-dependent structural and functional plasticity of astrocyte-neuron interactions. Physiol Rev. 88, 983-1008.
Tuchman, R., 2009. CSWS-related autistic regression versus autistic regression without CSWS. Epilepsia. 50 Suppl 7, 18-20.
Ueki, A., Tada, H., Seno, S., 1970. Antigenicity of chlorpromazine and clozapine to rabbits. Acta Med Okayama. 24, 323-32.
Volmat, R., Allers, G., Vittouris, N., 1968. [Clomipramine or anafranil. Apropos of treatment of 100 depressive states]. Encephale. 57, 116-42.
Wang, D.D., Bordey, A., 2008. The astrocyte odyssey. Prog Neurobiol. 86, 342-67.
Webb, S., 2010. Drugmakers dance with autism. Nat Biotechnol. 28, 772-4.
Weiss, L.A., Ober, C., Cook, E.H., Jr., 2006. ITGB3 shows genetic and expression interaction with SLC6A4. Hum Genet. 120, 93-100.

Westergaard, N., Sonnewald, U., Schousboe, A., 1995. Metabolic trafficking between neurons and astrocytes: the glutamate/glutamine cycle revisited. Dev Neurosci. 17, 203-11.

Whitaker-Azmitia, P.M., 2005. Behavioral and cellular consequences of increasing serotonergic activity during brain development: a role in autism? Int J Dev Neurosci. 23, 75-83.

Young, J.G., Kavanagh, M.E., Anderson, G.M., Shaywitz, B.A., Cohen, D.J., 1982. Clinical neurochemistry of autism and associated disorders. J Autism Dev Disord. 12, 147-65.

3

# Complementary Medicine Products Used in Autism - Evidence for Rationale

Susan Semple, Cassie Hewton, Fiona Paterson and Manya Angley
*Quality Use of Medicines and Pharmacy Research Centre,*
*Sansom Institute for Health Research,*
*School of Pharmacy and Medical Sciences,*
*University of South Australia,*
*Australia*

## 1. Introduction

The use of complementary and alternative medicine (CAM) is increasing in children with chronic illness or disability (Mamtani&Cimino 2002; Ernst 2005; Hyman&Levy 2005; Sinha&Efron 2005). Generally, the term CAM includes complementary therapies, such as behavioural/physical therapies, in addition to products such as herbals and vitamins that are administered systemically. This study specifically considers CAM products and supplements. Prevalence of biologically-based CAM product use in children with autism spectrum disorder (ASD) is among the highest of any population, with reported lifetime use of between 35% and 70% (Hanson et al. 2007; Christon et al. 2010; Green et al. 2006; Senel 2010). High CAM usage in autism has been attributed to the availability of few conventional pharmacological treatments that have a limited evidence base and are often associated with significant adverse effects.

Recent well-designed studies using whole-genome scanning methods, cytogenetics and genetic linkage/association analyses indicate genetic factors play a key role in the aetiology of autism (Eapen, 2011). Environmental and epigenetic factors have also been shown to impact on susceptibility to autism (Persico&Bourgeron 2006). Evidence is building that autism represents a cluster of syndromes that have distinct aetiologies involving inflammation, increased oxidative stress, impaired gastrointestinal (GI) health, mitochondrial dysfunction, autoimmune processes, and impaired ability to neutralise toxins (London 2007).

There is a belief that CAM products may ameliorate biological abnormalities that are reported to occur in autism. Reasons cited by parents for using CAM products for their children with autism include general health maintenance as well as specific symptoms such as moodiness, aggression, irritability, hyperactivity, inattention, GI symptoms, and sleep difficulties (Wong&Smith 2006). Another reason commonly cited by caregivers for implementing CAM products is that sensory processing difficulties and aberrant behaviour that can occur in children with autism may lead to poor feeding patterns and the possibility of nutritional deficiencies (Geraghty et al. 2010).

A study by Golnik and Ireland (2009) surveyed 539 medical practitioners (19% response rate using email and regular post) regarding CAM use in children with autism. The study revealed physicians encouraged use of multi-vitamins (49%), PUFAs (25%), melatonin (25%) and probiotics (19%) in children with autism and discouraged use of chelation (61%) and secretin (43%). In the same study medical practitioners responded positively when asked if they desired more complementary alternative medicine training for these patients (Golnik&Ireland 2009).

Despite this widespread use of CAM products in children with autism, it is of concern that there is a distinct lack of accurate, unbiased and evidence-based information about CAMs available for health professionals and caregivers of children with autism. Ready access to information through the Internet has contributed to the general increased frequency of caregivers implementing CAMs (Hyman&Levy 2005). Families perceive CAMs as a risk-free approach that may improve their child's outcome (Hyman&Levy 2005). However, all treatments used in children should be judged on standards of scientific research (Levy&Hyman 2003). Studies supporting CAM usage in autism need to be evaluated for scientific study design, clinical safety and scientific validity (Levy&Hyman 2003). There have been few published reviews examining the evidence for rationale, safety and efficacy of CAM products in autism (Angley et al. 2007; Weber&Newmark 2007; Levy&Hyman 2008; Atkins et al. 2010), and none were conducted systematically. To address this gap, we have endeavoured to address this area systematically in this chapter.

This chapter presents the first part of a two-part review. The rationale for a range of CAM products that are used in the management of autism is examined in this chapter. It is hoped this information will inform researchers and health care professionals about the theoretical or proven basis for a range of CAM products used in autism.

Chapter 4 which is the second part of the two-part review includes an examination of the evidence for efficacy and safety of a range of CAM products in autism. Each CAM product for which randomised controlled trials have been conducted has been assigned to a category of the Natural Standard Research Collaboration grading rationale for efficacy (Natural Standard Research Collaboration 2010). To determine safety of the range of CAM products investigated, all types of trials where a specific CAM product has been investigated in autism have been examined.

## 2. Aim

To systematically review the literature to determine the rationale of a range of CAM products used in ASD. Specifically, the following interventions were investigated: vitamins A, B, C and E, dimethylglycine (DMG), calcium, iron, magnesium, selenium, zinc, probiotics, digestive enzymes, colostrum, secretin, olive leaf extract, polyunsaturated fatty acids (PUFAs), melatonin, chelating agents (dimercaptosuccinic acid and thiamine tetrahydrofuryl disulphide), metallothionein promotion, glutathione and glutamine.

## 3. Method

For part 1 of this 2-part review (i.e. Chapter 3), a generalised review of the literature was performed to examine the possible rationale behind the use of these CAMs in ASD which included locating articles describing and investigating the biological basis of autism. Cross-sectional studies investigating biochemical abnormalities that occur in autism were also retrieved. For part 2, (i.e. Chapter 4) randomised controlled trials or randomised cross-over

| Topic | Search Terms |
|---|---|
| *Calcium* | Calcium/, calcium.mp, bone meal.mp |
| *Chelation/Allithiamine/TTFD/DMSA* | chelating agent$.mp, ttfd.mp, tetrahydrofurfuryl disulfide.mp, allithiamine.mp, Chelating Agents/, Chelation Therapy/, Thiamine/, Garlic/ dimercaptosuccinic acid.mp, dmsa.mp |
| *Colostrum* | colostrum.mp, Colostrum/ |
| *Dimethylglycine* | dimethylglycine.mp, DMG.mp |
| *Enzyme therapy* | Enzymes/, Peptide hydrolases/, Pancrelipase/, Lipase/, Amylases/, gastrointestinal agents/, proteolytic enzyme$.mp., enzyme$.mp., pancreatic enzyme$.mp., enzyme therapy.mp., carboxyl peptidase.mp., |
| *Fatty acids* | Fatty Acids, Essential/, Fish Oils/, Docosahexaenoic Acids/, Fatty Acids, Omega-3/, Cod Liver Oil/, Fatty Acids, Unsaturated/, Eicosapentaenoic Acid/ Fatty Acids, Omega-6/, gamma-Linolenic Acid/, Linoleic Acid/, Evening Primrose/, Onagraceae/, Oenothera/, essential fatty acid.mp, fish oil.mp, docosahexaenoic acid.mp, omega 3.mp, w-3 fatty acid.mp, cod liver oil.mp, marine oil.mp, menhaden oil.mp, highly unsaturated fatty acid.mp, eicosapentaenoic acid.mp, evening primrose oil.mp, fever plant.mp, gamma linolenic acid.mp, linoleic acid.mp, night willow herb.mp, primrose.mp, sun drop.mp, onagraceae.mp, oenothera$.mp |
| *Iron* | Iron/, Ferrous Compounds/, iron.mp, ferrous$.mp. |
| *L-glutamine* | Glutamine/, l-glutamine.mp, glutamine.mp |
| *Magnesium* | Magnesium/, Magnesium Compounds, magnesium.mp. |
| *Melatonin* | Melatonin/, melatonin.mp |
| *Metallothionein* | metallothionein.mp, mt promoter.mp, metallothionein promoter.mp, Metallothionein/ |
| *Olive leaf extract* | Olea/, Olive/, olive lea$.mp., olea.mp., oleuropein.mp., olea europaea.mp. |

| Topic | Search Terms |
|---|---|
| *Probiotics* | Probiotics/, Probiotic/, Yogurt/, Lactobacillus/, Bifidobacterium/, probiotic$.mp., yeast.mp., microbes.mp., yogurt.mp., yoghurt.mp. flora.mp.,lactobacillus.mp.,candidiasis.mp., saccharomyces.mp., bifidobacteria.mp., acidophilus. |
| *Reduced l-glutathione* | reduced glutathione.mp, glutathione.mp, Glutathione/ |
| *Selenium* | Selenium.mp, Selenium/, Selenium Compounds |
| *Secretin* | Secretin/, secretin.mp |
| *Vitamins* | Vitamin A/, Retinoids/, vitamin A.mp, retino$.mp, Fat-soluble vitamin$.mp, water soluble vitamin$.mp., Ascorbic Acid/, vitamin B6.mp, pyridoxine.mp, Vitamin B 6/, Pyridoxine/, Vitamin B 6 deficiency/, folic acid.mp, folinic acid.mp, folate.mp, vitamin B9.mp, Folic Acid/, Leucovorin/, Folic Acid Deficiency/, Vitamin B Complex/, vitamin B12.mp, cyanocobalamin.mp, methylcobalamin.mp, Vitamin B 12/, vitamin C.mp, ascorbic acid.mp, ascorbate.mp, ascorbyl$.mp. Vitamin E/, Tocopherols/, Tocotrienols/, vitamin E.mp, tocopherol.mp, tocotrienol.mp. |
| *Zinc* | zinc.mp, Zn.mp, Zinc/ |

/ at the end of a term denotes a subject heading in MEDLINE, AMED or CINAHL. Some subject headings differ between these databases.
In some databases the symbol $ is used to truncate a word, in some databases the symbol * is used instead

Table 1. Search terms used in database searches.

trials in which participants served as their own controls, were used to assess effectiveness of specific CAMs in individuals with ASD. Clinical trials of all designs were used to examine reported adverse effects of the CAMs in this population.

For the purposes of this review, the term CAM was used only in reference to non-conventional medications, sometimes termed 'biological treatments' or 'dietary supplements' (Levy&Hyman 2005) used in ASD, but not other forms of complementary or alternative therapy (e.g. touch therapies, manipulation therapies). Off-label use of prescription medications was not considered in this review.

The list of CAM products selected for review was developed using previous literature reporting CAM products being implemented by caregivers in their children with autism (Green et al. 2006; Wong&Smith 2006; Hanson et al. 2007; Christon et al. 2010) and consensus amongst authors based on our own research experiences.

Computerised literature searches were performed to locate articles reporting clinical trials of CAMs in children or adults with ASD. The databases searched were Medline (via Ovid), EMBASE, International Pharmaceutical Abstracts (IPA), Allied and Complementary Medicine (AMED), CINAHL, the Natural Medicines Comprehensive Database (Therapeutic Research Faculty) and The Cochrane Library.

To search for articles relevant to ASD standardised search terms were used including: autis$.mp, Asperger$.mp, developmental disabilit$.mp, pervasive developmental disorder$.mp (as key words); and Autistic Disorder/, Asperger Syndrome/, Child Development Disorders/, Developmental Disabilities/, Speech Disorders/, Child Psychiatry/ Communication Disorders/, Language Disorders (as subject headings).

These terms were combined with other terms to identify articles on specific CAMs as indicated in Table 1. Studies were restricted to English language. Searches were restricted to the years 1970 to December 2010. The reference lists of published studies and systematic reviews were also checked for relevant articles.

For the Natural Medicines Comprehensive Database the Product Effectiveness Checker was used to search for articles examining effectiveness for autism or Asperger Syndrome.

## 4. Results

### 4.1 Rationale

CAM product usage in autism generally has a theoretical basis rather than a proven rationale. However, there are some instances where biochemical abnormalities have been demonstrated in studies which can be normalised with administration of CAM products. For example James et al. (2004) showed biomarkers of oxidative stress in children with autism could be normalised following supplementation with betaine, folinic acid and vitamin B12. Some studies have also examined how the effects of biochemical normalisation translate into quantifiable outcome measures of behaviour in autism.

The rationale for the use of the CAM products investigated was found to fall into one or more of the following categories: promote GI health, reduce oxidative stress, enhance detoxification of heavy metals, modulate the immune system, normalise neurotransmitter abnormalities, promote sleep and prevent or treat nutritional deficiencies. The theoretical or proven abnormality occurring in autism, rationale for the CAM products investigated and behaviour targeted where known are summarised in Table 2.

#### 4.1.1 Promotion of gastrointestinal health

A high frequency of GI disturbance occurring in individuals with autism was first reported almost 40 years ago (Goodwin et al. 1971), but data regarding prevalence are conflicting. High rates of functional gastrointestinal disorders (FGIDs) in individuals with ASD have been reported in several studies including abdominal pain, constipation, diarrhoea, diarrhoea and alternating constipation and GI inflammation (Horvath et al. 1999; Molloy&Manning-Courtney 2003; Levy et al. 2007). A prospective study by Valicenti-McDermott et al. reported an increased prevalence of GI conditions in children with ASD (n=50, 70%) compared with matched controls that included both neurotypical children (n=50, 28%) and those with non-ASD developmental disorders (n=50, 42%) (2006). However, a recent well-designed population-based study by Ibrahim et al. found that the overall incidence of GI symptoms did not differ between cases of autism and controls (2009).

Recently Campbell et al. have provided genetic evidence supporting the link between GI dysfunction and autism and reported an association between a single nucleotide polymorphism in the promoter of the mesenchymal epithelial transition (MET) factor gene and autism (2009). Evidence is also emerging that intestinal permeability (D'Eufemia et al. 1996; Horvath et al. 1999; de Magistris et al. 2010), GI mucosal inflammation (de Magistris et al. 2010), fermentation products (Yap et al. 2010) and GI microbiota profiles (Finegold et al. 2002; Song et al. 2004; Parracho et al. 2005; Finegold et al. 2010) in individuals with autism are different from those of the general population.

#### 4.1.1.1 Intestinal hyper-permeability in autism

Functional changes have been reported in the GI tracts of children with autism including increased intestinal permeability (Horvath&Perman 2002). Intestinal permeability, as measured by the urinary excretion of metabolically inert sugars, is a surrogate marker of mucosal integrity and gut barrier function (de Magistris et al. 2010). It has been hypothesised that impaired GI function may not only be a symptom of autism but may also contribute to the phenotypic presentation by increasing absorption of chemicals from the GI tract. There is a body of thought that increased absorption of opioid-like peptides that are derived from gluten and casein (i.e. the 'opioid excess theory') may disturb neurological function, as may GI overgrowth of neurotoxin-producing bacteria (Shattock&Whiteley 2002).

#### 4.1.1.2 Altered gut fermentation products in autism

A growing appreciation for the role of intestinal microflora in health and disease has emerged over the last few years, however the beneficial and potentially adverse contributions of bacterial fermentation by-products have not been well established and are largely uncharacterised in children with ASD. A recent metabonomic study revealed metabolic phenotype (metabotype) differences were observed between autistic and control children, which were associated with perturbations in the relative patterns of urinary mammalian microbial co-metabolites including dimethylamine, hippurate, and phenyacetylglutamine (Yap et al. 2010). Another study by Altieri et al. (2011) found higher levels of p-cresol in urine of young children with autism than controls and also reported a positive correlation between urinary p-cresol and autism severity. P-cresol is a toxic metabolite of tyrosine catabolism by gut bacteria such as clostridial species and *Pseudomonas stutzeri* (Altieri et al. 2011). Whether the observed differences in urinary metabolites observed contribute to, or reflect, GI dysfunction in individuals with ASD requires further investigation.

#### 4.1.1.3 Altered GI microbiota profiles in autism

Several studies have found some bacterial species, particularly some *Clostridium* species, are present in higher numbers in children with autism experiencing GI disturbance (Finegold et al. 2002; Song et al. 2004; Parracho et al. 2005; Finegold et al. 2010). Some workers have speculated that the differences in the GI microbiotica could be contributing to the pathophysiology of ASD (Bolte 1998; Finegold 2008).

#### 4.1.1.4 Altered digestive enzyme capacity in autism

It has been hypothesised that digestion of dietary gluten and casein in the small intestine by pancreatic and intestinal peptidases releases short chain peptide molecules (exorphins) which are structurally similar to endogenous opioid substances (White 2003). Other hypotheses suggest that excessive opioid activity linked with dietary peptides from gluten and casein have an aetiological role in the pathogenesis of autism (Reichelt&Knivsberg 2003). The 'opioid excess' theory of autism proposes that many of the behaviours found in individuals with ASD mimic the influence of opioids on human brain function (White 2003). In addition Horvath & Perman (2002) demonstrated that 44 of 90 (49%) of children with autism showed at least one deficient disaccharidase enzyme activity. Lactase and maltase were the enzymes most commonly measured to have deficient activity, followed by sucrase, palatinase and glucoamylase. They found that all of the children with reduced enzyme activity had flatulence and/or loose stools. It is hypothesised that disaccharide malabsorption may cause chronic diarrhoea and flatulence in children with ASD and may contribute to abnormal behaviour (Patel et al. 2002). Hence, supplementation with these enzymes may cause a reduction in autism related symptoms. For example supplementation with lactase may resolve the symptoms related to lactose malabsorption (Horvath&Perman 2002).

It is speculated that GI symptoms exacerbate the behavioural manifestations of autism contributing to the severity of the disorder (Buie et al. 2010). Abdominal pain, constipation, and/or diarrhoea are unpleasant and can be painful and likely to produce frustration, behavioural problems, and possibly sleep disturbance, aggression and self abuse, especially in children unable to communicate their discomfort.

Various CAMs are used to ameliorate the GI symptoms in children with autism as outlined in Table 2. Probiotics and prebiotics are used to promote gut health. Dietary interventions include the exclusion of gluten and casein containing foods together with dietary supplementation with peptidase enzymes. Peptidase enzymes are implemented in children with autism in an attempt to remove the opioid-like peptides that may exert a neurotoxic effect on the brain (Brudnak et al. 2002). Less obvious candidates are PUFAs which are used with the rationale that they can decrease GI inflammation and improve a 'leaky gut'.

### 4.1.2 Oxidative stress

A leading theory implicated in the aetiology of autism is oxidative stress, which results from a complex interplay of genetic and environmental factors. Oxidative stress occurs when reactive oxygen species (ROS) levels exceed the antioxidant capacity of a cell leading to damage and functional impairment (McGinnis 2004). "It is thought that autism could result from an interaction between genetic and environmental factors with oxidative stress as a potential mechanism linking the two" (Ming et al. 2005, p.379). These ROS target lipids, proteins and nucleic acids (Chauhan&Chauhan 2006) resulting in a risk of neurologic deficits, especially during early life (Zecavati&Spence 2009). A range of evidence has emerged in recent years supporting the role of oxidative stress in the aetiology of autism.

#### 4.1.2.1 Lipid peroxidation

It has also been found that lipid peroxidation (an oxidative biomarker) in plasma is significantly increased in children with autism when compared to their non-autistic siblings reflecting increased oxidative stress in autism (Chauhan et al. 2004).

#### 4.1.2.2 Antioxidants

Reduced endogenous antioxidant capacity i.e. low levels of the plasma antioxidant enzymes glutathione peroxidase and superoxide dismutase have been found in autistic individuals (Sogut et al. 2003). Furthermore, Yorbik et al. (2002) found that the activities of erythrocyte superoxide dismutase and erythrocyte and plasma glutathione peroxidase were significantly lower in 45 autistic children compared with 41 controls. Chauhan et al. (2004) also found a significant reduction of the major endogenous antioxidants transferrin and ceroplasmin in the serum of children with autism as compared to their typically developing siblings. An excess of toxic free radicals e.g. nitric oxide has also been reported in children with autism as compared to age and sex matched controls (Sogut et al. 2003). Ming et al. (2005) also describe increased nitrite concentrations, thiobarbituric acid reactive substances and xanthine oxidase activity in red blood cells in children with autism compared to controls. Notably, decreased plasma levels of the antioxidant vitamins A, C and E were reported in the same autistic cohort (Ming et al. 2005).

#### 4.1.2.3 Mitochondrial disease

Mitochondria serve a primary role in energy production during normal physiological function and generate high levels of ROS which are normally neutralised by free radical scavengers. In the event there is excess ROS relative to the antioxidant defence, mitochondrial dysfunction occurs exacerbating oxidative stress. Mitochondrial disease is associated with impaired neurodevelopment. Two recent studies have reported mitochondrial dysfunction in autism. Post-mortem samples showed increased mitochondrial metabolism and oxidised mitochondrial proteins in the brains of six people with autism compared with controls (Palmieri et al. 2010). Another study showed that 11/21 patients with ASD had definite mitochondrial disease while the rest had probable mitochondrial disease (Weissman et al. 2008).

#### 4.1.2.4 Abnormalities in the trans-methylation and trans-sulphuration pathways

There is emerging evidence that a deficient trans-methylation (i.e. folate/methionine) pathway has a role in the aetiology of autism (Boris et al. 2004; James et al. 2004; James et al. 2006). The folate/methionine pathway (Figure 1) is responsible for the synthesis of the deoxynucleotide triphosphate (dNTP) pools required for DNA synthesis and repair, the establishment and maintenance of stable DNA methylation patterns for tissue-specific gene expression and chromatin conformation and maintenance of the redox balance within each cell.

As shown in Figure 1, the methionine cycle involves the re-methylation of homocysteine to methionine either by methionine synthase (MS) which is folate and vitamin B12 dependent or by the betaine homocysteine methyltransferase (BHMT) reaction. The methyl group is donated by 5-methyl tetrahydrofolate synthesised by methylene tetrahydrofolate (MTHFR) from 5,10 methyl tetrahydrofolate.

Methionine is activated by methionine adenosyl transferase (MAT) to S-adenosyl-methinine (SAM), the major methyl donor for cellular methyltransferase reactions (MTases). Following methyl transfer, SAM is converted to S-adenosylhomocysteine (SAH). This is further metabolised in a reversible reaction to homocysteine and adenosine. Adenosine is either phosphorylated to adenosine nucleotides by adenosine kinase (AK) or catabolised to inosine by adenosine deaminase (ADA). Homocysteine may be permanently removed from the methionine cycle by irreversible conversion to cystathionine by cystathione-β-synthase (CßS). Cystathionine is converted to cysteine which is the rate-limiting amino acid for the synthesis of glutathione.

A decrease in turnover of the folate/methionine pathway will lead to decreased synthesis of SAM which is vital for normal methylation activity and decreased synthesis of cysteine and glutathione required for normal antioxidant activity.

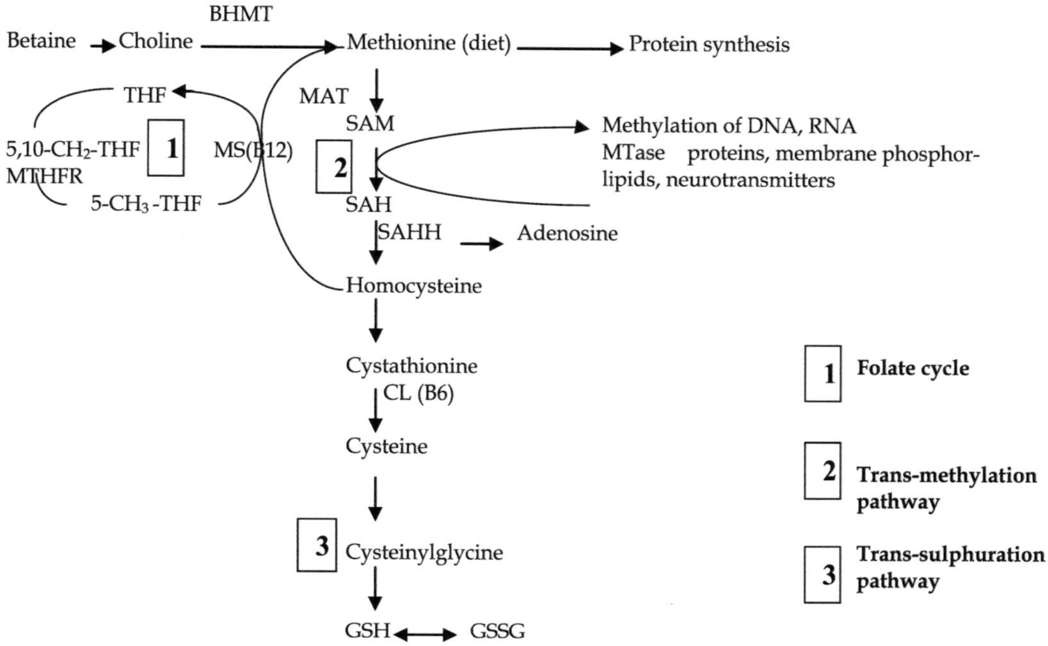


Source: Ms P.A.E. Main, 2011. Used with permission

**Metabolites** THF: tetrahydrofolate; SAM: S-adenosyl-methionine; SAH: S-adenosyl-homocysteine; GSH: reduced active glutathione; GSSG: oxidised disulfide form of glutathione

**Enzymes** MS: methionine synthase; BHMT : Betaine homocysteine methyltransferase; MAT: methionine adenosyl transferase; SAHH: SAH hydroxylase; CßS: Cystathione-β-synthase; CL: Cystathione lyase; MTHFR: methylene-tetra-hydrofolate reductase; MTRR: methionine synthase reductase

Fig. 1. Folate cycle and the trans-methylation and trans-sulphuration pathways

A systematic literature review identifying studies reporting metabolites, co-factors or genes of the folate/methionine pathway in autism found there are significant differences in the levels of various metabolites of the methionine/folate cycle in individuals with autism compared with controls although there are some inconsistencies between studies which may be due to different methodologies (Main et al. 2010).

Elevated levels of oxidised GSH and subsequent reduction in GSH:GSSG ratio together with a decrease in cysteine (a rate limiting amino acid for glutathione synthesis) and increased lipid peroxidation suggests that oxidative stress may play a significant role in the aetiology of autism (James et al. 2004; Wu et al. 2004). The conclusion of a review of oxidative pathways as potential drug targets in autism by Villagonzalo et al. (2010) was that although there is significant evidence demonstrating that oxidative pathways are disturbed in autism, there is insufficient evidence to decide whether oxidative stress is the cause of autism, or contributes to the illness, or is simply a consequence of the illness. They stated that further research is required to determine if children will benefit from antioxidant treatment and that longitudinal studies exploring oxidative biomarkers and autism symptomatology over time may be a methodology for investigation.

Thus as outlined in Table 2, oxidative stress in autism provides a rationale for the use of CAM products that are antioxidants in their own right, metabolites or co-factors of the trans-methylation or trans-sulphuration pathways, co-factors of plasma antioxidant enzymes and include: vitamins A, C & E, vitamin B12, DMG, magnesium, selenium, zinc, melatonin and glutathione.

### 4.1.3 Heavy metal toxicity

Heavy metals, such as arsenic, lead, and mercury have been associated with a variety of neurologic deficits and disorders, including lower IQ, Alzheimer's disease, and Parkinson's disease (Zecavati&Spence 2009). It has been suggested that some children with autism have an increased body-burden of mercury which may result from biochemical and genomic susceptibilities within detoxification pathways (Mutter et al. 2005).

As mentioned above James et al. (2004) found a significantly reduced GSH: GSSG ratio in children with autism compared with controls. An impaired glutathione redox ratio is thought to play a role in the aetiology of autism by delaying the clearance of heavy metals from the body (Deth et al. 2008). The association between heavy metal exposure and autism, in particular mercury, has attracted considerable interest (Counter et al. 2002; Holmes et al. 2003; Palmer et al. 2006; Geier&Geier 2007). Mercury has been implicated in immune, sensory, neurological, motor, and behavioural dysfunction resulting in clinical manifestations similar to those defining or associated with autism. Some studies have suggested that mercury can disrupt neurotransmitter levels and biochemistry (Faustman et al. 2000; Redwood et al. 2001; Bernard et al. 2002) and impact on normal child development. A suspected source of mercury is thiomersal, a preservative used in vaccines. Notably, although thiomersal has not been included in US vaccines since 2000, autism prevalence rates have continued to rise (Fombonne 2008).

As shown in Table 2, CAM products that are implemented based on the rationale that autism is associated with heavy metal toxicity include probiotics, allithiamine/TTFD, DMSA, metallothionein promoter, glutathione and glutamine.

### 4.1.4 Immune dysregulation in autism

There is evidence to suggest the immune system plays a role in the aetiology of autism (Kidd 2002a). It is hypothesised that some cases of autism are associated with immune factors and that autism related symptoms may be associated with immune deficiencies or autoimmunity (Levy&Hyman 2005). Immunological anomalies involving cytokines, immunoglobulins, inflammation, and cellular activation have been reported in individuals with autism (Goines&Van de Water 2010).

#### 4.1.4.1 Immune deficiencies and autism

Immune deficiencies in children with ASD have been reported due to frequently encountered medical problems including recurrent ear infection/rhinosinusitis/upper respiratory tract infection, adverse reactions to multiple medications, allergies, GI problems and prolonged courses of illness as compared to typically developing siblings (Jyonouchi et al. 2005; Levy&Hyman 2005). Various immune system deficits including abnormalities in cell-mediated immunity have been reported in autism. Abnormalities of macrophages, B cells, T cells and natural killer cells have been reported in individuals with ASD which may compromise defence against infection (Gupta 2000).

#### 4.1.4.2 Autoimmune disease and autism

A survey administered to families of 61 children with autism and 46 control families with typically developing children discovered that the mean number of autoimmune disorders was greater in families who had children with autism (Comi et al. 1999). In this study, Comi et al. (1999) found that 46% of the families of children with autism had two or more family members with autoimmune disorders (e.g. type 1 diabetes, adult rheumatoid arthritis and hypothyroidism). In addition, this finding may further suggest that genetic predisposition plays an important role in autism. However, Micali, Chakrabarti & Fombonne (2004) did not have the same findings following administration of a semi-structured questionnaire to 79 parents of children with pervasive developmental disorders (PDDs) and 61 controls (parents with typically developing children). They found the rates for any autoimmune disorder for both mothers and fathers combined was 22.4% for parents of controls and 30.9% for parents of children with PDDs which was not significantly different.

It is hypothesised that autoimmune disease in autism may lead to neurodevelopmental damage. Autoantibodies against proteins associated with the central nervous system (CNS) has been reported in some children with autism (Singh et al. 1988; Plioplys et al. 1994; Vojdani et al. 2004). In recent studies, antibodies against the fetal brain have been detected in some mothers of children with autism; these antibodies have the ability to alter behavioural outcomes in the offspring of animal models (Enstrom et al. 2009).

A review by Theoharides et al (2008) proposes a relationship between GI factors, oxidative stress and immune dysregulation and proposes potential drug targets in autism.

#### 4.1.4.3 Vaccination and autism

Although an array of epidemiological studies do not support causality (DeStefano 2007; Baker 2008), the alleged link between autism and vaccination has been debated extensively and many parents and parent advocacy groups continue to suspect that vaccines cause autism. Putative mechanisms for vaccine associated autism include: "1) immune response directed towards a vaccine that cross reacts with host antigens, 2) host response to a vaccine that would result in the production of cytokines and a subsequent autoimmune reaction and 3) toxic components of a vaccine that directly impact on the immune or nervous system" (Levy&Hyman 2005, p.134).

Therefore as outlined in Table 2, immune dysfunction in autism provides a rationale for the use of CAM products that are claimed to be immunomodulators/immunoadjuvants and include: vitamin A, DMG, vitamin C, zinc, colostrum and glutamine.

### 4.1.5 Normalise neurotransmitters and neurotransmitter metabolites

Many studies (Young et al. 1978; Garnier et al. 1986; Launay et al. 1987; Minderaa et al. 1987; Barthelemy et al. 1988; Garreau et al. 1988; Barthelemy et al. 1989; Minderaa et al. 1989; Martineau et al. 1991; Martineau et al. 1992; Herault et al. 1993; Martineau et al. 1994; Minderaa et al. 1994; Herault et al. 1996; Croonenberghs et al. 2000; Mulder et al. 2005; Mulder et al. 2005; Mulder et al. 2009) have focused on neurotransmitter abnormalities in individuals with autism. Abnormalities in various neurotransmitters have been implicated in the development of autism, including serotonin (5-hydroxytryptamine, 5-HT), dopamine (DA), noradrenaline (NA), gamma-aminobutryic acid, glutamate and neuropeptides.

#### 4.1.5.1 Serotonin and metabolites

5-HT is a monoamine neurotransmitter that plays an important role in the developing brain by directing both neuronal proliferation and maturation (McDougle et al. 2005). CNS 5-HT activity has been involved in a range of physiological functions, such as sleep, sensory perception and appetite, which are often disrupted in autism (Young et al. 1982). High levels of 5-HT during early development may cause a loss of 5-HT receptors and therefore impact on subsequent neuronal development (Whitaker-Azmitia 2001). Neuroimaging studies suggest altered developmental regulation of 5-HT synthesis may be associated with the pathogenesis of autism (Chugani et al. 1999). Hyperserotonemia has been consistently reported in people with autism in more than 25 published studies (Lam et al. 2006).

#### 4.1.5.2 Dopamine and metabolites

Dopamine (DA) is a catecholamine which acts as a major neurotransmitter in the brain. Generally, the dopaminergic system is thought to affect a wide range of functions, including cognition and attention (Nieoullon 2002), motor function (Niimi et al. 2009), predictive reward signal mechanisms (Schultz 1998) and immunity (Basu&Dasgupta 2000). Some animal research has shown that stereotypies and hyperactivity can be induced by increasing dopaminergic functioning suggesting dopaminergic neurons may be overactive in autism (Miller et al. 2010).

#### 4.1.5.3 Noradrenaline

Noradrenaline (NA) is synthesized from DA by dopamine β-hydroxylase and released from noradrenergic neurons as well as from the adrenal medulla into the bloodstream. NA plays a critical role in attention, the stress response (i.e. the "fight or flight" response), anxiety, and memory (Amaral&Sinnamon 1977; Fitzgerald 2009), which are frequently observed to be impaired in individuals with autism. Previous studies have shown that measurements of NA (i.e. in plasma and urine) are generally well correlated with measurements in the CNS (Roy et al. 1988). A range of neurochemical studies have attempted to examine excretion of urinary NA and / or adrenaline (A) in individuals with autism compared with controls and have yielded inconsistent findings. Three studies found higher levels of NA and/or A in autism compared to controls (Barthelemy et al. 1988; Herault et al. 1993; Martineau et al. 1994), while four studies found no differences (Launay et al. 1987; Martineau et al. 1992; Minderaa et al. 1994; Croonenberghs et al. 2000).
Therefore as outlined in Table 2, the range of neurotransmitter abnormalities that have been shown to occur in autism provide a rationale for the use of CAM products that are claim to normalise neurotransmitter levels and function such as: high dose pyridoxine and magnesium, metabolites and co-factors of the transmethylation and trans-sulphuration cycles (see Figure 1), vitamin C, zinc and secretin.

### 4.1.6 Sleep

Sleep problems in children with ASD are common with a prevalence of 44-83% in comparison to 10-20% of typically developing young children (Wright et al. 2011). Sleep difficulties contribute to significant morbidity in children and to family stress. Melatonin is a hormone that is synthesised in the pineal gland from the precursor tryptophan. Its production is light-sensitive, beginning in the early evening and reaching peak levels at approximately 3am. Daytime secretion of melatonin is generally insignificant (Jan et al.

1999). The main functions of melatonin within the body are the synchronisation of circadian rhythm and control of sleep patterns and endocrine secretions (Natural Medicines Comprehensive Database 2011). The suprachiasmatic nucleus of the anterior hypothalamus is responsible for the generation of circadian rhythm. Transmission of light through the retina activates this tissue, causing either inhibition or stimulation of melatonin synthesis in the pineal gland. Sleep induction is thought to occur as a result of direct inhibition of the 'wakefulness generating system' by melatonin (Jan et al. 1999).
Two studies have suggested a tendency for autistic children to be deficient in the essential amino acid tryptophan, a precursor in the biosynthesis of melatonin (D'Eufemia et al. 1995; Arnold et al. 2003). Additionally, Tordjman et al. (2005) found a significantly lower excretion rate of 6-sulphatoxymelatonin, the prominent metabolite of melatonin, in children with autistic disorder compared to sex and age-matched controls. These results support the above hypothesis that children with autism may have impaired synthesis of melatonin. Therefore, in theory, supplementation with melatonin could potentially improve their quality of sleep and hence also their daytime behaviour.

### 4.1.7 Nutritional deficiencies

Factors that contribute to nutritional concerns and deficiencies in children with autism are summarised by Geraghty et al. (2010) and include sensory processing difficulties, rituals and routines and non-compliance behaviours at meal times. Significantly lower levels of nutrients in blood, hair, and other tissues have been seen in autistic children including low levels of magnesium (Strambi et al. 2006), iron (Latif et al. 2002), zinc (Yorbik et al. 2004), vitamins A, C and E, (Ming et al. 2005) and polyunsaturated fatty acids (PUFAs) (Vancassel et al. 2001; Bell et al. 2004; Meguid et al. 2008). Further, medications prescribed for children with autism may have nutrition related adverse effects and restrictive diets that are frequently implemented in autism may compromise nutritional intake. As a result, caregivers may elect to implement CAM interventions to treat or prevent nutritional deficiencies.

| CAM product used in autism | Abnormality theorised/reported to occur in autism | Rationale for use | Specific symptom/behaviour targeted |
|---|---|---|---|
| Vitamin A | Hippocampal retinoid receptor dysfunction<br><br>Immune system dysfunction (Goines&Van de Water 2010)<br><br>Oxidative stress (Villagonzalo et al. 2010)<br><br>Deficiency (Clark et al. 1993; Steinemann &Christiansen 1998; Ming et al. 2005) | Reconnect retinoid receptor pathways (Megson 2000)<br><br>Immunomodulation (Megson 2000)<br><br>Antioxidant (Natural Medicines Comprehensive Database 2011)<br><br>Prevent or treat deficiency | General autistic behaviours |

| CAM product used in autism | Abnormality theorised/reported to occur in autism | Rationale for use | Specific symptom/behaviour targeted |
|---|---|---|---|
| Pyridoxine (vitamin B6) and magnesium | Dysfunctional pyridoxine metabolism (Adams&Holloway 2004; Adams et al. 2006) | Normalise neurotransmitter synthesis (Kidd 2002b; Levy&Hyman 2005)<br><br>Magnesium is synergistic with pyridoxine (Abraham et al. 1981) | Repetitive behaviour |
| | Oxidative stress (Villagonzalo et al. 2010) | Magnesium protects against oxidative damage via activation of CNS copper-zinc superoxide dismutase (CuZnSOD) (Johnson 2001) | General autistic behaviours |
| | Magnesium deficiency (Strambi et al. 2006) | Magnesium is necessary for many cellular metabolic processes and transmission of nerve and muscle potentials (Natural Medicines Comprehensive Database 2011) | |
| Cyanocobalamin (vitamin B12) | Gut dysbiosis and inflammation results in decreased GI synthesis of B12 and/or absorption (Kidd 2002b; Erickson et al. 2005) | Normalise B12 levels (Bertoglio et al. 2010) | |
| | Trans-methylation and trans-sulphation pathway abnormalities (James et al. 2004; Bertoglio et al. 2010) causing oxidative stress (Villagonzalo et al. 2010) | Correct folate/methionine metabolite profile and other indexes of oxidative stress (James et al. 2004; James et al. 2009; Bertoglio et al. 2010) | |

| CAM product used in autism | Abnormality theorised/reported to occur in autism | Rationale for use | Specific symptom/behaviour targeted |
|---|---|---|---|
| Folate/folinic acid (vitamin B9) | Trans-methylation pathway abnormalities (James et al. 2004; Bertoglio et al. 2010) causing oxidative stress (Villagonzalo et al. 2010)<br><br>Neurotransmitter level abnormalities (Lam et al. 2006) | Correct folate/methionine metabolite profile and other indexes of oxidative stress (James et al. 2004; James et al. 2009)<br><br>Modulate neurotransmitters (Fernstrom 2000) | |
| Dimethylglycine (DMG) | Immune system dysfunction (Goines&Van de Water 2010)<br><br>Neurotransmitter level abnormalities (Lam et al. 2006)<br><br>Folate/methionine pathway abnormalities (James et al. 2004; Bertoglio et al. 2010)<br><br>Oxidative stress (Villagonzalo, et al. 2010) | Immunoadjuvant (Graber et al. 1981)<br><br>Modulate neurotransmitters (Kern et al. 2001)<br><br>Methyl donor (Kern et al. 2001)<br><br>Antioxidant(Kern et al. 2001) | General autistic behaviours |
| Vitamin C | Neurotransmitter level abnormalities (Lam et al. 2006)<br><br>Oxidative stress (Villagonzalo et al. 2010)<br><br>Immune system dysfunction (Goines&Van de Water 2010)<br><br>Deficiency (Ming et al. 2005) | Cofactor for neurotransmitter synthesis (Kidd 2003)<br><br>Antioxidant (Natural Medicines Comprehensive Database 2011)<br><br>Immune function regulation (Natural Medicines Comprehensive Database 2011)<br><br>Prevent or treat deficiency | General autistic behaviours |

| **CAM product used in autism** | **Abnormality theorised/reported to occur in autism** | **Rationale for use** | **Specific symptom/behaviour targeted** |
|---|---|---|---|
| Vitamin E | Oxidative stress (Villagonzalo et al. 2010)<br>Low erythrocyte levels (Jory & McGinnis 2007)<br><br>Deficiency (Ming et al. 2005) | Antioxidant (Natural Medicines Comprehensive Database 2011)<br><br>Prevent or treat deficiency | General autistic behaviours |
| Selenium | Oxidative stress (Villagonzalo et al. 2010) | Antioxidant (glutathione peroxidase is selenium dependent) (Thorne Research Inc. 2003) | General autistic behaviours |
| Calcium | | Prevent or treat deficiency | Treat deficiency |
| Iron | Neurotransmitter level abnormalities (Lam et al. 2006)<br><br>Deficiency (Latif et al. 2002) | Cofactor for neurotransmitter synthesis (Natural Medicines Comprehensive Database 2011)<br><br>Optimise neural development<br><br>Prevent or treat deficiency | Treat deficiency |
| Zinc (Zn) | Immune system dysfunction (Goines& Van de Water 2010)<br><br>GI disturbance<br><br>Neurotransmitter level abnormalities (Lam et al. 2006)<br><br>Oxidative stress (Villagonzalo et al. 2010)<br><br>Deficiency (Yorbik et al. 2004) | Immunomodulation<br><br>Correct GI disturbance<br><br>Modulate neurotransmitter synthesis<br><br>Zn is a component of CuZnSOD<br><br>Prevent or treat deficiency | |

| CAM product used in autism | Abnormality theorised/reported to occur in autism | Rationale for use | Specific symptom/behaviour targeted |
|---|---|---|---|
| Probiotics | GI dysbiosis (Finegold et al. 2002; Parracho et al. 2005; Finegold et al. 2010)<br><br>Heavy metal toxicity (Al-Ayadhi 2005; Fido &Al-Saad 2005) | Correct dysbioisis by promoting gut health (Parracho et al. 2010)<br><br>Detoxify heavy metals (Brudnak 2002) | Normalise gut pathology |
| Digestive enzymes | Leaky gut (Horvath&Perman 2002) | Used in conjunction with the casein-/ gluten-free diet to prevent absorption of potentially neurotoxic opioid-like peptides (Munasinghe et al. 2010) | Aid digestion/GI disturbance<br><br>General autistic behaviours |
| Olive leaf extract | GI dysbiosis (Finegold et al. 2002; Parracho et al. 2005; Finegold et al. 2010) | Correct dysbioisis due to antimicrobial action (Markin et al. 2003) | GI abnormalities |
| Colostrum | Immune system dysfunction (Goines&Van de Water 2010)<br><br>Lower levels of cerebrospinal fluid (CSF) insulin-like growth factor 1(IGF-I) (Vanhala et al. 2001)<br><br>Leaky gut (Horvath& Perman 2002) | Immunomodulation<br><br>Rich source of IGF-I (Mero et al. 2002)<br><br>GI protective (Natural Medicines Comprehensive Database 2011) | General autistic behaviours<br><br>Ameliorate GI disturbance |
| Secretin | GI disturbance i.e. gastroesophageal reflux disease (GORD) (Patel et al. 2002)<br><br>Neurotransmitter level abnormalities (Lam et | Correct GI disturbance (Patel et al. 2002)<br><br>Increase GI elimination of neurotoxic substances (Patel et al. 2002)<br><br>Acts as CNS neuropeptide (Levy&Hyman 2005)<br><br>Increase brain neurotransmitters | Ameliorate GI disturbance<br><br>General autistic behaviours |

| CAM product used in autism | Abnormality theorised/reported to occur in autism | Rationale for use | Specific symptom/behaviour targeted |
|---|---|---|---|
| | al. 2006) | synthesis (Patel et al. 2002)<br>Increase cerebral blood flow (Patel et al. 2002) | |
| Polyunsaturated fatty acids (PUFAs) | Functional deficiencies/imbalances of PUFAs (Vancassel et al. 2001; Bell et al. 2004; Meguid et al. 2008)<br>Leaky gut (Horvath&Perman 2002) | Optimise neural development (Freeman et al. 2006)<br>Prevent or treat deficiency (Meguid, Atta et al. 2008; Bent et al. 2010)<br>Reduce GI inflammation (Garvey 2002) | Cognition<br>Attention/ hyperactivity<br>GI abnormalities |
| Melatonin | Tryptophan deficiency (melatonin precursor) (D'Eufemia et al. 1995; Arnold et al. 2003)<br>Lower excretion rate of 6-sulphatoxymelatonin (melatonin metabolite) (Tordjman et al. 2005)<br>Oxidative stress (Villagonzalo et al. 2010) | Normalise melatonin levels to reduce sleep latency<br>Antioxidant (Natural Medicines Comprehensive Database 2011) | Improve sleep quality |
| Allithiamine/ thiamine tetrahydrofuryl disulphide (TTFD) | Heavy metal toxicity (Al-Ayadhi 2005; Fido &Al-Saad 2005)<br>Impaired sulphation capacity (Waring&Klovrza 2000)<br>Reduced excretion of cyanide i.e. lower urinary thiocyanate (Waring&Klovrza 2000) | Chelate and reduce heavy metal levels (Lonsdale 2004)<br>Enhance sulphation capacity by acting as a sulphate donor (Waring&Klovrza 2000)<br>Enhance excretion of neurotoxic cyanide (Lonsdale 2004) | General autistic behaviours |
| Dimercaptosuccinic acid (DMSA) | Heavy metal toxicity (Al-Ayadhi 2005; Fido &Al-Saad 2005) | Chelate and reduce heavy metal levels (Lonsdale 2004; Adams et al. 2009) | General autistic behaviours |

| CAM product used in autism | Abnormality theorised/reported to occur in autism | Rationale for use | Specific symptom/behaviour targeted |
|---|---|---|---|
| Metallothionein promotion | Elevated blood copper-to-zinc ratios (Faber et al. 2009) | Regulate levels of redox-active metals (Copper (Cu) and Zn) (Faber et al. 2009)<br><br>Defense against toxic heavy metals (Faber et al. 2009) | General autistic behaviours |
| Glutathione | Abnormal trans-sulphuration pathway leading to low GSH:GSSG (James et al. 2004; James et al. 2006), an index of oxidative stress (Villagonzalo et al. 2010) | Antioxidant (Thorne Research Inc. 2001)<br><br>Augments chelation therapy (Thorne Research Inc. 2001)<br><br>Regulates metallothionein expression (Thorne Research Inc. 2001) | General autistic behaviours |
| Glutamine | Abnormal glutamine levels (Shinohe et al. 2006) | Enhance immunity (Natural Medicines Comprehensive Database 2011)<br><br>Is a pre-cursor to glutathione (see above)<br><br>GI protective (van der Hulst&van Kreel 1993) | General autistic behaviours<br><br>GI abnormalities |

Table 2. CAM products used in autism, theoretical or proven abnormality in autism, rationale for use and symptom/behaviour targeted

## 5. Conclusion

Available evidence for the theoretical or proven rationale of a range of CAM products has been compiled to give researchers and health professionals insight into why such agents are recommended and implemented in autism. This information forms the basis for the second part of this 2-part review which follows examining the efficacy and safety of a range of CAM products used in autism.

## 6. References

Abraham, G., Schwartz, U. &Lubran, M. (1981). Effect of vitamin B-6 on plasma and red blood cell magnesium levels in premenopausal women. *Annals of Clinical and Laboratory Science* Vol. 11 No. 4: pp. 333-336

Adams, J. B., Baral, M., Geis, E., Mitchell, J., Ingram, J., Hensley, A., et al. (2009). Safety and efficacy of oral DMSA therapy for children with autism spectrum disorders: Part A--medical results. *BMC Clinical Pharmacology* Vol. 9 No. 16: pp. 16.1472-6904 (Electronic) 1472-6904 (Linking)

Adams, J. B., George, F. &Audhya, T. (2006). Abnormally High Plasma Levels of Vitamin B6 in Children with Autism Not Taking Supplements Compared to Controls Not Taking Supplements. *The Journal of Alternative and Complementary Medicine* Vol. 12 No. 1: pp. 59-63

Adams, J. B. &Holloway, C. (2004). Pilot Study of a Moderate Dose Multivitamin/Mineral Supplement for Children with Autistic Spectrum Disorder. *The Journal of Alternative and Complementary Medicine* Vol. 10 No. 6: pp. 1033-1039

Al-Ayadhi, L. (2005). Heavy metals and trace elements in hair samples of autistic children in central Saudi Arabia. *Neurosciences* Vol. 10 No. 3: pp. 213-218

Altieri, L., Neri, C., Sacco, R., Curatolo, P., Benvenuto, A., Muratori, F., et al. (2011). Urinary p-cresol is elevated in small children with severe autism spectrum disorder. *Biomarkers* Vol.: pp.1366-5804 (Electronic) 1354-750X (Linking)

Amaral, D. G. &Sinnamon, H. M. (1977). The locus coeruleus: Neurobiology of a central noradrenergic nucleus. *Progress in Neurobiology* Vol. 9 No. 3: pp. 147-196

Angley, M., Semple, S., Hewton, C. &Paterson, F. (2007). Children and autism--Part 2--management with complementary medicines and dietary interventions. *Australian Family Physician* Vol. 36 No. 10: pp. 827-830.0300-8495 (Print) 0300-8495 (Linking)

Arnold, G. L., Hyman, S. L., Mooney, R. A. &Kirby, R. S. (2003). Plasma Amino Acid Profiles in Children with Autism: Potential Risk of Nutritional Deficiencies. *Journal of Autism and Developmental Disorders* Vol. 33 No. 4: pp. 449-454

Atkins, R. S., Angkustsiri, K. &Hansen, R. L. (2010). Complementary and Alternative Medicine in Autism: An Evidence-Based Approach to Negotiating Safe and Efficacious Interventions with Families. *The Journal of the American Society for Experimental NeuroTherapeutics* Vol. 7 No. 7: pp. 307-319

Baker, J. P. (2008). Mercury, vaccines, and autism: one controversy, three histories. *American Journal of Public Health* Vol. 98 No. 2: pp. 244-253.1541-0048 (Electronic) 0090-0036 (Linking)

Barthelemy, C., Bruneau, N., Cottet-Eymard, J. M., Domenech-Jouve, J., Garreau, B., Lelord, G., et al. (1988). Urinary free and conjugated catecholamines and metabolites in autistic children. *Journal of Autism and Developmental Disorders* Vol. 18 No. 4: pp. 583-591

Barthelemy, C., Bruneau, N., Jouve, J., Martineau, J., Muh, J. P. &Lelord, G. (1989). Urinary dopamine metabolites as indicators of the responsiveness to fenfluramine treatment in children with autistic behavior. *Journal of Autism and Developmental Disorders* Vol. 19 No. 2: pp. 241-254.0162-3257 (Print) 0162-3257 (Linking)

Basu, S. &Dasgupta, P. S. (2000). Dopamine, a neurotransmitter, influences the immune system. *Journal of Neuroimmunology* Vol. 102 No. 2: pp. 113-124.0165-5728

Bell, J. G., MacKinlay, E. E., Dick, J. R., MacDonald, D. J., Boyle, R. M. &Glen, A. C. (2004). Essential fatty acids and phospholipase A2 in autistic spectrum disorders. *Prostaglandins Leukotrienes and Essential Fatty Acids* Vol. 71 No. 4: pp. 201-204

Bent, S., Bertoglio, K., Ashwood, P., Bostrom, A. &Hendren, R. L. (2010). A Pilot Randomized Controlled Trial of Omega-3 Fatty Acids for Autism Spectrum

Disorder. *Journal of Autism and Developmental Disorders* Vol. 41 No. 5: pp. 545 - 554 (Electronic) 0162-3257 (Linking)

Bernard, S., Enayati, A., Roger, H., Binstock, T. &Redwood, L. (2002). The role of mercury in the pathogenesis of autism. *Molecular Psychiatry* Vol. 7 No. SUPPL. 2: pp. S42 - S43

Bertoglio, K., James, S.J, Deprey, L., Brule, N. &Hendren, R. L. (2010). Pilot study of the effect of methyl B12 treatment on behavioral and biomarker measures in children with autism. *The Journal of Alternative and Complementary Medicine* Vol. 16 No. 5: pp. 555-560.1557-7708 (Electronic) 1075-5535 (Linking)

Bolte, E. R. (1998). Autism and Clostridium tetani. *Medical Hypotheses* Vol. 51 No. 2: pp. 133-144.0306-9877 (Print) 0306-9877 (Linking)

Boris, M., Goldblatt, A., Goalanko, J. &James, S. (2004). Association of MTHFR gene variants with autism. *Journal of American Physicians and Surgeons* Vol. 9 No. 4: pp. 106-108

Brudnak, M. A. (2002). Probiotics as an adjuvant to detoxification protocols. *Medical Hypotheses* Vol. 58 No. 5: pp. 382-385.0306-9877

Brudnak, M. A., Rimland, B., Kerry, R. E., Dailey, M., Taylor, R., Stayton, B., et al. (2002). Enzyme-based therapy for autism spectrum disorders--is it worth another look? *Medical Hypotheses* Vol. 58 No. 5: pp. 422-428

Buie, T., Fuchs, G. J., 3rd, Furuta, G. T., Kooros, K., Levy, J., Lewis, J. D., et al. (2010). Recommendations for evaluation and treatment of common gastrointestinal problems in children with ASDs. *Pediatrics* Vol. 125 Suppl 1: pp. S19-29.1098-4275 (Electronic) 0031-4005 (Linking)

Campbell, D. B., Buie, T. M., Winter, H., Bauman, M., Sutcliffe, J. S., Perrin, J. M., et al. (2009). Distinct genetic risk based on association of MET in families with co-occurring autism and gastrointestinal conditions. *Pediatrics* Vol. 123 No. 3: pp. 1018-1024.1098-4275 (Electronic) 0031-4005 (Linking)

Chauhan, A. &Chauhan, V. (2006). Oxidative stress in autism. *Pathophysiology* Vol. 13 No. 3: pp. 171-181

Chauhan, A., Chauhan, V., Brown, W. T. &Cohen, I. (2004). Oxidative stress in autism: increased lipid peroxidation and reduced serum levels of ceruloplasmin and transferrin--the antioxidant proteins. *Life Sciences* Vol. 75 No. 21: pp. 2539-2549.0024-3205

Christon, L. M., Mackintosh, V. H. &Myers, B. J. (2010). Use of complementary and alternative medicine (CAM) treatments by parents of children with autism spectrum disorders. *Research in Autism Spectrum Disorders* Vol. 4 No.: pp. 249-259

Chugani, D. C., Muzik, O., Behen, M., Rothermel, R., Janisse, J. J., Lee, J., et al. (1999). Developmental changes in brain serotonin synthesis capacity in autistic and nonautistic children. *Annals of Neurology* Vol. 45 No. 3: pp. 287-295.0364-5134 (Print) 0364-5134 (Linking)

Clark, J. H., Rhoden, D. K. &Turner, D. S. (1993). Symptomatic vitamin A and D deficiencies in an eight-year-old with autism. *Journal of Parenteral and Enteral Nutrition* Vol. 17 No. 3: pp. 284-286

Comi, A. M., Zimmerman, A. W., Frye, V. H., Law, P. A. &Peeden, J. N. (1999). Familial clustering of autoimmune disorders and evaluation of medical risk factors in autism. *Journal of Child Neurology* Vol. 14 No. 6: pp. 388-394

Counter, S. A., Buchanan, L. H., Ortega, F. &Laurell, G. (2002). Elevated blood mercury and neuro-otological observations in children of the Ecuadorian gold mines. *Journal of*

*Toxicology and Environmental Health* Vol. 65 No. 2: pp. 149-163.1528-7394 (Print) 0098-4108 (Linking)

Croonenberghs, J., Delmeire, L., Verkerk, R., Lin, A. H., Meskal, A., Neels, H., et al. (2000). Peripheral markers of serotonergic and noradrenergic function in post-pubertal, caucasian males with autistic disorder. *Neuropsychopharmacology* Vol. 22 No. 3: pp. 275-283.0893-133X (Print)

D'Eufemia, P., Celli, M., Finocchiaro, R., Pacifico, L., Viozzi, L., Zaccagnini, M., et al. (1996). Abnormal intestinal permeability in children with autism. *Acta Paediatrica* Vol. 85 No. 9: pp. 1076-1079.0803-5253 (Print) 0803-5253 (Linking)

D'Eufemia, P., Finocchiaro, R., Celli, M., Viozzi, L., Monteleone, D. &Giardini, O. (1995). Low serum tryptophan to large neutral amino acids ratio in idiopathic infantile autism. *Biomedicine and Pharmacotherapy* Vol. 49 No. 6: pp. 288-292

de Magistris, L., Familiari, V., Pascotto, A., Sapone, A., Frolli, A., Iardino, P., et al. (2010). Alterations of the intestinal barrier in patients with autism spectrum disorders and in their first-degree relatives. *Journal of Pediatric Gastroenterology and Nutrition* Vol. 51 No. 4: pp. 7

DeStefano, F. (2007). Vaccines and autism: evidence does not support a causal association. *Clinical Pharmacology and Therapeutics* Vol. 82 No. 6: pp. 756-759.1532-6535 (Electronic) 0009-9236 (Linking)

Deth, R., Muratore, C., Benzecry, J., Power-Charnitsky, V. A. &Waly, M. (2008). How environmental and genetic factors combine to cause autism: A redox/methylation hypothesis. *NeuroToxicology* Vol. 29 No. 1: pp. 190-201

Enstrom, A. M., Van de Water, J. A. &Ashwood, P. (2009). Autoimmunity in autism. *Current Opinion in Investigational Drugs* Vol. 10 No. 5: pp. 463-473.2040-3429 (Electronic) 1472-4472 (Linking)

Eapen, V. (2011). Genetic basis of autism: is there a way forward? *Current Opinion in Psychiatry* Vol. 24 No. 3: pp. 226-236.1473-6578 (Electronic) 0951-7367 (Linking)

Erickson, C. A., Stigler, K. A., Corkins, M. R., Posey, D. J., Fitzgerald, J. F. &McDougle, C. J. (2005). Gastrointestinal factors in autistic disorder: a critical review. *Journal of Autism and Developmental Disorders* Vol. 35 No. 6: pp. 713-727.0162-3257 (Print) 0162-3257 (Linking)

Ernst, E. (2005). Why alternative medicines are used. *The Pharmaceutical Journal* Vol. 275: pp. 55

Faber, S., Zinn, G. M., Kern, J. C., 2nd &Kingston, H. M. (2009). The plasma zinc/serum copper ratio as a biomarker in children with autism spectrum disorders. *Biomarkers* Vol. 14 No. 3: pp. 171-180.1366-5804 (Electronic) 1354-750X (Linking)

Faustman, E. M., Silbernagel, S. M., Fenske, R. A., Burbacher, T. M. &Ponce, R. A. (2000). Mechanisms underlying children's susceptibility to environmental toxicants. *Environmental Health Perspectives* Vol. 108 No. SUPPL. 1: pp. 13-21

Fernstrom, J. D. (2000). Can nutrient supplements modify brain function? *American Journal of Clinical Nutrition* Vol. 71(suppl) No. 6: pp. 1669S-1673S

Fido A &Al-Saad S (2005). Toxic trace elements in the hair of children with autism. *Autism* Vol. 9 No. 3: pp. 290-298

Finegold, S. M. (2008). Therapy and epidemiology of autism-clostridial spores as key elements. *Medical Hypotheses* Vol. 70 No. 3: pp. 508-511

Finegold, S. M., Dowd, S. E., Gontcharova, V., Liu, C., Henley, K. E., Wolcott, R. D., et al. (2010). Pyrosequencing study of fecal microflora of autistic and control children. *Anaerobe* Vol. 16 No. 4: pp. 444-453

Finegold, S. M., Molitoris, D., Song, Y., Liu, C., Vaisanen, M.-L., Bolte, E., et al. (2002). Gastrointestinal microflora studies in late-onset autism. *Clinical Infectious Diseases* Vol. 35 No. 1: pp. S6-16

Fitzgerald, P. J. (2009). Is elevated noradrenaline an aetiological factor in a number of diseases? *Autonomic and Autacoid Pharmacology* Vol. 29 No. 4: pp. 143-156.1474-8673 (Electronic) 1474-8665 (Linking)

Fombonne, E. (2008). Thimerosal disappears but autism remains. *Archives of General Psychiatry* Vol. 65 No. 1: pp. 15-16.1538-3636 (Electronic) 0003-990X (Linking)

Freeman, M. P., Hibbeln, J. R., Wisner, K. L., Davis, J. M., Mischoulon, D., Peet, M., et al. (2006). Omega-3 fatty acids: evidence basis for treatment and future research in psychiatry. The *Journal of Clinical Psychiatry* Vol. 67 No. 12: pp. 1954-1967.1555-2101 (Electronic) 0160-6689 (Linking)

Garnier, C., Barthelemy, C. &Leddet, I. (1986). Dopamine-beta-hydroxylase (DBH) and homovanicillic acid (HVA) in autistic children. *Journal of Autism and Developmental Disorders* Vol. 16 No. 1: pp. 23-29

Garreau, B., Barthelemy, C., Jouve, J., Bruneau, N., Muh, J. P. &Lelord, G. (1988). Urinary homovanillic acid levels of autistic children. *Developmental Medicine and Child Neurology* Vol. 30 No. 1: pp. 93-98

Garvey, J. (2002). Diet in autism and associated disorders. *Journal of Family Health Care* Vol. 12 No. 2: pp. 34-38.1474-9114

Geier, D. A. &Geier, M. R. (2007). A prospective study of mercury toxicity biomarkers in autistic spectrum disorders. *Journal of Toxicology and Environmental Health A* Vol. 70 No. 20: pp. 1723-1730

Geraghty, M. E., Depasquale, G. M. &Lane, A. E. (2010). Nutritional Intake and Therapies in Autism : A Spectrum of What We Know: Part 1. *ICAN: Infant, Child, and Adolescent Nutrition* Vol. 2: pp. 62-69

Goines, P. &Van de Water, J. (2010). The immune system's role in the biology of autism. *Current Opinion in Neurology* Vol. 23 No. 2: pp. 111-117.1473-6551 (Electronic) 1080-8248 (Linking)

Golnik, A. E. &Ireland, M. (2009). Complementary alternative medicine for children with autism: a physician survey. *Journal of Autism and Developmental Disorders* Vol. 39 No. 7: pp. 996-1005.1573-3432 (Electronic) 0162-3257 (Linking)

Goodwin, M. S., Goodwin, T. C. &Cowen, M. A. (1971). Malabsorption and cerebral dysfunction: A multivariate and comparative study of autistic children. *Journal of Autism and Childhood Schizophrenia* Vol. 1 No. 1: pp. 48-62

Graber, C. D., Goust, J. M., Glassman, A. D., Kendall, R. &Loadholt, C. B. (1981). Immunomodulating Properties of Dimethylglycine in Humans. *The Journal of Infectious Diseases* Vol. 143 No. 1: pp. 101-105

Green, V. A., Pituch, K. A., Itchon, J., Choi, A., O'Reilly, M. &Sigafoos, J. (2006). Internet survey of treatments used by parents of children with autism. *Research in Developmental Disabilities* Vol. 27 No. 1: pp. 70-84

Gupta, S. (2000). Immunological treatments for autism. *Journal of Autism and Developmental Disorders* Vol. 30 No. 5: pp. 475-479

Hanson, E., Kalish, L. A., Bunce, E., Curtis, C., McDaniel, S., Ware, J., et al. (2007). Use of complementary and alternative medicine among children diagnosed with autism spectrum disorder. *Journal of Autism and Developmental Disorders* Vol. 37 No. 4: pp. 628-636.0162-3257 (Print) 0162-3257 (Linking)

Herault, J., Martineau, J., Perrot-Beaugerie, A., Jouve, J., Tournade, H., Barthelemy, C., et al. (1993). Investigation of whole blood and urine monoamines in autism. *European Child and Adolescent Psychaitry* Vol. 2 No. 4: pp. 211-220

Herault, J., Petit, E., Martineau, J., Cherpi, C., Perrot, A., Barthelemy, C., et al. (1996). Serotonin and autism: biochemical and molecular biology features. *Psychiatry Research* Vol. 65 No. 1: pp. 33-43.0165-1781 (Print) 0165-1781 (Linking)

Holmes, A. S., Blaxill, M. F. &Haley, B. E. (2003). Reduced levels of mercury in first baby haircuts of autistic children. *International Journal of Toxicology* Vol. 22 No. 4: pp. 277-285

Horvath, K., Papadimitriou, J. C., Rabsztyn, A., Drachenberg, C. &Tyson Tildon, J. (1999). Gastrointestinal abnormalities in children with autistic disorder. *Journal of Pediatrics* Vol. 135 No. 5: pp. 559-563

Horvath, K. &Perman, J. A. (2002). Autism and gastrointestinal symptoms. *Current Gastroenterology Reports* Vol. 4 No. 3: pp. 251-258.1522-8037

Hyman, S. L. &Levy, S. E. (2005). Introduction: novel therapies in developmental disabilities--hope, reason, and evidence. *Mental Retardation and Developmental Disabilities Research Reviews* Vol. 11 No. 2: pp. 107-109.1080-4013

Ibrahim, S. H., Voigt, R. G., Katusic, S. K., Weaver, A. L. &Barbaresi, W. J. (2009). Incidence of gastrointestinal symptoms in children with autism: a population-based study. *Pediatrics* Vol. 124 No. 2: pp. 680-686.1098-4275 (Electronic) 0031-4005 (Linking)

James, S.J, Cutler, P., Melnyk, S., Jernigan, S., Janak, L., Gaylor, D., et al. (2004). Metabolic biomarkers of increased oxidative stress and impaired methylation capacity in children with autism *American Journal of Clinical Nutrition* Vol. 80 No. 6: pp. 1611-1617

James, S. J., Melnyk, S., Jernigan, S., Cleves, M. A., Halsted, C. H., Wong, D. H., et al. (2006). Metabolic endophenotype and related genotypes are associated with oxidative stress in children with autism. *American Journal of Medical Genetics Part B: Neuropsychiatric Genetics* Vol. 141B No. 8: pp. 947-956.1552-4841 (Print) 1552-4841 (Linking)

James, S. J., Melnyk, S., Fuchs, G., Reid, T., Jernigan, S., Pavliv, O., et al. (2009). Efficacy of methylcobalamin and folinic acid treatment on glutathione redox status in children with autism. *American Journal of Clinical Nutrition* Vol. 89 No. 1: pp. 425-430.1938-3207 (Electronic) 0002-9165 (Linking)

Jan, J. E., Freeman, R. D. &Fast, D. K. (1999). Melatonin treatment of sleep-wake cycle disorders in children and adolescents. *Developmental Medicine and Child Neurology* Vol. 41: pp. 491-500

Johnson, S. (2001). Micronutrient accumulation and depletion in schizophrenia, epilepsy, autism and Parkinson's disease? *Medical Hypotheses* Vol. 56 No. 5: pp. 641-645.0306-9877

Jory, J. &McGinnis, W. L. (2007). Red-cell trace minerals in children with autism. *American Journal of Biotechnology and Biochemistry* Vol. 3 No. 2: pp. 60-63

Jyonouchi, H., Geng, L., Ruby, H. &Zimmerman-Bier, B. (2005). Dysregulated Innate Immune Responses in Young Children with Autism Spectrum Disorders: Their Relationship to Gastrointestinal Symptoms and Dietary Intervention. *Neuropsychobiology* Vol. 51 No. 2: pp. 77-85

Kern, J. K., Miller, V. S., Cauller, L., Kendall, R., Mehta, J. &Dodd, M. (2001). Effectiveness of N,N-Dimethylglycine in Autism and Pervasive Developmental Disorder. *Journal of Child Neurology* Vol. 16 No. 3: pp. 169-173

Kidd, P. M. (2002a). Autism, an extreme challenge to integrative medicine. Part: 1: the knowledge base. *Alternative Medicine Review* Vol. 7 No. 4: pp. 292-316.1089-5159

Kidd, P. M. (2002b). Autism, an extreme challenge to integrative medicine. Part 2: medical management. *Alternative Medicine Review* Vol. 7 No. 6: pp. 472-499.1089-5159

Kidd, P. M. (2003). An approach to the nutritional management of autism. *Alternative Therapies in Health and Medicine* Vol. 9 No. 5: pp. 22-32

Lam, K. S., Aman, M. G. &Arnold, L. E. (2006). Neurochemical correlates of autistic disorder: a review of the literature. *Research in Developmental Disabilities* Vol. 27 No. 3: pp. 254-289.0891-4222 (Print) 0891-4222 (Linking)

Latif, A., Heinz, P. &Cook, R. (2002). Iron deficiency in autism and Asperger syndrome. *Autism* Vol. 6 No. 1: pp. 103-114.1362-3613

Launay, J. M., Bursztejn, C., Ferrari, P., Dreux, C., Braconnier, A., Zarifian, E., et al. (1987). Catecholamines metabolism in infantile autism: A controlled study of 22 autistic children. *Journal of Autism and Developmental Disorders* Vol. 17 No. 3: pp. 333-347

Levy, S. E. &Hyman, S. L. (2003). Use of complementary and alternative treatments for children with autistic spectrum disorders is increasing. *Pediatric Annals* Vol. 32 No. 10: pp. 685-691

Levy, S. E. &Hyman, S. L. (2005). Novel Treatments for Autism Spectrum Disorders. *Mental Retardation and Developmental Disabilities Research Reviews* Vol. 11 No. 2: pp. 131-142.1080-4013 (Print) 1080-4013 (Linking)

Levy, S. E. &Hyman, S. L. (2008). Complementary and alternative medicine treatments for children with autism spectrum disorders. *Child and Adolescent Psychiatric Clinics of North America* Vol. 17 No. 4: pp. 803-820, ix.1056-4993 (Print) 1056-4993 (Linking)

Levy, S. E., Souders, M. C., Ittenbach, R. F., Giarelli, E., Mulberg, A. E. &Pinto-Martin, J. A. (2007). Relationship of dietary intake to gastrointestinal symptoms in children with autistic spectrum disorders. *Biological Psychiatry* Vol. 61 No. 4: pp. 492-497.0006-3223 (Print) 0006-3223 (Linking)

London, E. (2007). The role of the neurobiologist in redefining the diagnosis of autism. *Brain Pathology* Vol. 17 No. 4: pp. 408-411.1015-6305 (Print) 1015-6305 (Linking)

Lonsdale, D. (2004). Thiamine tetrahydrofurfuryl disulfide: a little known therapeutic agent. *Medical Science Monitor* Vol. 10 No. 9: pp. 199-203

Main, P. A., Angley, M. T., Thomas, P., O'Doherty, C. E. &Fenech, M. (2010). Folate and methionine metabolism in autism: a systematic review. *American Journal of Clinical Nutrition* Vol. 91 No. 6: pp. 1598-1620.1938-3207 (Electronic) 0002-9165 (Linking)

Mamtani, R. &Cimino, A. (2002). A primer of complementary and alternative medicine and its relevance in the treatment of mental health problems. *Psychiatric Quarterly* Vol. 73 No. 4: pp. 367-381.0033-2720

Markin, D., Duek, L. &Berdicevsky, I. (2003). In vitro antimicrobial activity of olive leaves. *Mycoses* Vol. 46 No. 3-4: pp. 132-136.0933-7407

Martineau, J., Barthelemy, C., Herault, J., Jouve, J. &Muh, J. P. (1991). Monoamines in autistic children: A study of age-related changes. *Brain Dysfunction* Vol. 4 No. 4: pp. 141-146

Martineau, J., Barthelemy, C., Jouve, J., Muh, J. P. &Lelord, G. (1992). Monoamines (serotonin and catecholamines) and their derivatives in infantile autism: Age-related changes and drug effects. *Developmental Medicine and Child Neurology* Vol. 34 No. 7: pp. 593-603

Martineau, J., Herault, J., Petit, E., Guerin, P., Hameury, L., Perrot, A., et al. (1994). Catecholaminergic metabolism and autism. *Developmental Medicine and Child Neurology* Vol. 36 No. 8: pp. 688-697.0012-1622 (Print) 0012-1622 (Linking)

McDougle, C. J., Erickson, C. A., Stigler, K. A. &Posey, D. J. (2005). Neurochemistry in the pathophysiology of autism. *Journal of Clinical Psychiatry* Vol. 66 Suppl 10: pp. 9-18.0160-6689 (Print) 0160-6689 (Linking)

McGinnis, W. R. (2004). Oxidative stress in autism. *Alternative Therapies in Health and Medicine* Vol. 10 No. 6: pp. 22-36.1078-6791

Megson, M. N. (2000). Is autism a G-alpha protein defect reversible with natural vitamin A? *Medical Hypotheses* Vol. 54 No. 6: pp. 979-983.0306-9877

Meguid, N. A., Atta, H. M., Gouda, A. S. &Khalil, R. O. (2008). Role of polyunsaturated fatty acids in the management of Egyptian children with autism. *Clinical Biochemistry* Vol. 41 No. 13: pp. 1044-1048.1873-2933 (Electronic) 0009-9120 (Linking)

Mero, A., Kahkonen, J., Nykanen, T., Parvianen, T., Jokinen, I., Takala, T., et al. (2002). IGF-1, IgA, and IgG responses to bovine colostrum supplementation during training. *Journal of Applied Physiology* Vol. 93 No. 2: pp. 732-739

Micali, N., Chakrabarti, S. &Fombonne, E. (2004). The broad autism phenotype. *Autism* Vol. 8 No. 1: pp. 21-37

Miller, J. S., Tallarida, R. J. &Unterwald, E. M. (2010). Inhibition of GSK3 attenuates dopamine D1 receptor agonist-induced hyperactivity in mice. *Brain Research Bulletin* Vol. 82 No. 3-4: pp. 184-187.1873-2747 (Electronic) 0361-9230 (Linking)

Minderaa, R. B., Anderson, G. M. &Volkmar :R, F. (1987). Urinary 5-hydroxyindoleacetic acid and whole blood serotonin and tryptophan in autistic and normal subjects. *Biological Psychiatry* Vol. 22 No. 8: pp. 933-940

Minderaa, R. B., Anderson, G. M., Volkmar, F. R., Akkerhuis, G. W. &Cohen, D. J. (1989). Neurochemical study of dopamine functioning in autistic and normal subjects. *Journal of the American Academy of Child and Adolescent Psychiatry* Vol. 28 No. 2: pp. 190-194.0890-8567 (Print) 0890-8567 (Linking)

Minderaa, R. B., Anderson, G. M., Volkmar, F. R., Akkerhuis, G. W. &Cohen, D. J. (1994). Noradrenergic and adrenergic functioning in autism. *Biological Psychiatry* Vol. 36 No. 4: pp. 237-241

Ming, X., Stein, T. P., Brimacombe, M., Johnson, W. G., Lambert, G. H. &Wagner, G. C. (2005). Increased excretion of a lipid peroxidation biomarker in autism. *Prostaglandins Leukotrienes and Essential Fatty Acids* Vol. 73 No. 5: pp. 379-384.0952-3278

Molloy, C. A. &Manning-Courtney, P. (2003). Prevalence of chronic gastrointestinal symptoms in children with autism and autistic spectrum disorders. *Autism* Vol. 7 No. 2: pp. 165-171.1362-3613

Mulder, E. J., Anderson, G. M., Kema, I. P., Brugman, A. M., Ketelaars, C. E., de Bildt, A., et al. (2005). Serotonin transporter intron 2 polymorphism associated with rigid-compulsive behaviors in Dutch individuals with pervasive developmental disorder. *American Journal of Medical Genetics Part B: Neuropsychiatric Genetics* Vol. 133B No. 1: pp. 93-96.1552-4841 (Print) 1552-4841 (Linking)

Mulder, E. J., Anderson, G. M., Kemperman, R. F. J., Oosterloo-Duinkerken, A., Minderaa, R. B. &Kema, I. P. (2009). Urinary excretion of 5-hydroxyindoleacetic acid, serotonin and 6-sulphatoxymelatonin in normoserotonemic and hyperserotonemic autistic individuals. *Neuropsychobiology* Vol. 61 No. 1: pp. 27-32

Mulder, E. J., Oosterloo-Duinkerken, A., Anderson, G. M., De Vries, E. G. E., Minderaa, R. B. &Kema, I. P. (2005). Automated on-line solid-phase extraction coupled with HPLC for measurement of 5-hydroxyindole-3-acetic acid in urine. *Clinical Chemistry* Vol. 51 No. 9: pp. 1698-1703

Munasinghe, S. A., Oliff, C., Finn, J. &Wray, J. A. (2010). Digestive enzyme supplementation for autism spectrum disorders: a double-blind randomized controlled trial. *Journal of Autism and Developmental Disorders* Vol. 40 No. 9: pp. 1131-1138.1573-3432 (Electronic) 0162-3257 (Linking)

Mutter, J., Naumann, J., Schneider, R., Walach, H. &Haley, B. (2005). Mercury and autism: accelerating evidence? *Neuroendocrinology Letters* Vol. 26 No. 5: pp. 439-446.0172-780X (Print) 0172-780X (Linking)

Natural Medicines Comprehensive Database (2011). Monographs. In. Retrieved 3 March 2011, Available from: http://www.naturaldatabase.com/(S(i2p051ajm3jul455nejtyui1))/home.aspx?li=0 &st=0&cs=&s=ND

Natural Standard Research Collaboration (2010). Natural Standard evidence-based validated grading rationale ™. In. Retrieved November 16, 2010, Available from: http://www.naturalstandard.com/grading.asp

Nieoullon, A. (2002). Dopamine and the regulation of cognition and attention. *Progress in Neurobiology* Vol. 67 No. 1: pp. 53-83.0301-0082 (Print) 0301-0082 (Linking)

Niimi, K., Takahashi, E. &Itakura, C. (2009). Analysis of motor function and dopamine systems of SAMP6 mouse. *Physiology and Behavior* Vol. 96 No. 3: pp. 464-469.0031-9384 (Print) 0031-9384 (Linking)

Palmer, R. F., Blanchard, S., Stein, Z., Mandell, D. &Miller, C. (2006). Environmental mercury release, special education rates, and autism disorder: an ecological study of Texas. *Health and Place* Vol. 12 No. 2: pp. 203-209.1353-8292 (Print) 1353-8292 (Linking)

Palmieri, L., Papaleo, V., Porcelli, V., Scarcia, P., Gaita, L., Sacco, R., et al. (2010). Altered calcium homeostasis in autism-spectrum disorders: evidence from biochemical and genetic studies of the mitochondrial aspartate/glutamate carrier AGC1. *Molecular Psychiatry* Vol. 15 No. 1: pp. 38-52.1476-5578 (Electronic) 1359-4184 (Linking)

Parracho, H. M., Bingham, M. O., Gibson, G. R. &McCartney, A. L. (2005). Differences between the gut microflora of children with autistic spectrum disorders and that of healthy children. *Journal of Medical Microbiology* Vol. 54 pp. 987-991.0022-2615 (Print) 0022-2615 (Linking)

Parracho, H. M. R. T., Gibson, G. R., Knott, F., Bosscher, D., Kleerebezem, M. &McCartney, A. L. (2010). A double-blind, placebo-controlled, crossover-designed probiotic feeding study in children diagnosed with autistic spectrum disorders. *International Journal of Probiotics and Prebiotics* Vol. 5 No. 2: pp. 69-74

Patel, N. C., Yeh, J. Y., Shepherd, M. D. &Crismon, M. L. (2002). Secretin treatment for autistic disorder: a critical analysis. *Pharmacotherapy* Vol. 22 No. 7: pp. 905-914.0277-0008

Persico, A. M. &Bourgeron, T. (2006). Searching for ways out of the autism maze: genetic, epigenetic and environmental clues. *Trends in Neurosciences* Vol. 29 No. 7: pp. 349-358.0166-2236 (Print) 0166-2236 (Linking)

Plioplys, A. V., Greaves, A., Kazemi, K. &Silverman, E. (1994). Lymphocyte function in autism and Rett syndrome. *Neuropsychobiology* Vol. 29 No. 1: pp. 12-16

Redwood, L., Bernard, S. &Brown, D. (2001). Predicted mercury concentrations in hair from infant immunizations: Cause for concern. *NeuroToxicology* Vol. 22 No. 5: pp. 691-697

Reichelt, K. L. &Knivsberg, A. M. (2003). Can the pathophysiology of autism be explained by the nature of the discovered urine peptides? *Nutritional Neuroscience* Vol. 6 No. 1: pp. 19-28.1028-415X

Roy, A., Pickar, D., De Jong, J., Karoum, F. &Linnoila, M. (1988). Norepinephrine and its metabolites in cerebrospinal fluid, plasma, and urine. Relationship to hypothalamic-pituitary-adrenal axis function in depression. *Archives of General Psychiatry* Vol. 45 No. 9: pp. 849-857.0003-990X (Print) 0003-990X (Linking)

Schultz, W. (1998). Predictive reward signal of dopamine neurons. *Journal of Neurophysiology* Vol. 80 No. 1: pp. 1-27

Senel, H. G. (2010). Parents' views and experiences about complementary and alternative medicine treatments for their children with autistic spectrum disorder. *Journal of Autism and Developmental Disorders* Vol. 40 No. 4: pp. 494-503.1573-3432 (Electronic) 0162-3257 (Linking)

Shattock, P. &Whiteley, P. (2002). Biochemical aspects in autism spectrum disorders: updating the opioid-excess theory and presenting new opportunities for biomedical intervention. *Expert Opinion on Therapeutic Targets* Vol. 6 No. 2: pp. 175-183

Shinohe, A., Hashimoto, K., Nakamura, K., Tsujii, M., Iwata, Y., Tsuchiya, K. J., et al. (2006). Increased serum levels of glutamate in adult patients with autism. *Progress in Neuropsychopharmacology & Biological Psychiatry* Vol. 30 No. 8: pp. 1472-1477.0278-5846 (Print) 0278-5846 (Linking)

Singh, V. K., Fudenberg, H. H., Emerson, D. &Coleman, M. (1988). Immunodiagnosis and immunotherapy in autistic children. *Annals of New York Academy of Science* Vol. 540 No. 11: pp. 602-604

Sinha, D. &Efron, D. (2005). Complementary and alternative medicine use in children with attention deficit hyperactivity disorder. *Journal of Paediatrics and Child Health* Vol. 41 No. 1-2: pp. 23-26

Sogut, S., Zoroglu, S. S., Ozyurt, H., Yilmaz, H. R., Ozugurlu, F., Sivasli, E., et al. (2003). Changes in nitric oxide levels and antioxidant enzyme activities may have a role in the pathophysiological mechanisms involved in autism. *Clinica Chimica Acta* Vol. 331 No. 1-2: pp. 111-117.0009-8981

Song, Y., Liu, C. &Finegold, S. M. (2004). Real-time PCR quantitation of clostridia in feces of autistic children. *Applied and Environmental Microbiology* Vol. 70 No. 11: pp. 6459-6465.0099-2240 (Print) 0099-2240 (Linking)

Steinemann, T. L. &Christiansen, S. P. (1998). Vitamin A deficiency and xerophthalmia in an autistic child. *Archives of Ophthalmology* Vol. 116 No. 3: pp. 392-393.0003-9950

Strambi, M., Longini, M., Hayek, J., Berni, S., Macucci, F., Scalacci, E., et al. (2006). Magnesium profile in autism. *Biological Trace Element Research* Vol. 109 No. 2: pp. 97-104.0163-4984 (Print) 0163-4984 (Linking)

Theoharides, T. C., Doyle, R., Francis, K., Conti, P. &Kalogeromitros, D. (2008). Novel therapeutic targets for autism. *Trends in Pharmacological Sciences* Vol. 29 No. 8: pp. 375-382.0165-6147 (Print) 0165-6147 (Linking)

Thorne Research Inc. (2001). Glutathione, Reduced (Monograph). *Alternative Medicine Review* Vol. 6 No. 6: pp. 601-607

Thorne Research Inc. (2003). Selenium (Monograph). *Alternative Medicine Review* Vol. 8 No. 1: pp. 63-71

Tordjman, S., Anderson, G. M., Pichard, N., Charbuy, H. &Touitou, Y. (2005). Nocturnal Excretion of 6-Sulphatoxymelatonin in Children and Adolescents with Autistic Disorder. *Biological Psychiatry* Vol. 57: pp. 134-138

Valicenti-McDermott, M., McVicar, K., Rapin, I., Wershil, B. K., Cohen, H. &Shinnar, S. (2006). Frequency of gastrointestinal symptoms in children with autistic spectrum disorders and association with family history of autoimmune disease. *Journal of Developmental and Behavioral Pediatrics* Vol. 27 No. 2 Suppl: pp. S128-136.0196-206X (Print) 0196-206X (Linking)

van der Hulst, R. M. W. J. &van Kreel, B. K. (1993). Glutamine and the preservation of gut integrity. *The Lancet* Vol. 341 No. 8857: pp. 1363-1365

Vancassel, S., Durand, G., Barthelemy, C., Lejeune, B., Martineau, J., Guilloteau, D., et al. (2001). Plasma fatty acid levels in autistic children. *Prostaglandins Leukotrienes and Essential Fatty Acids* Vol. 65 No. 1: pp. 1-7

Vanhala, R., Turpeinen, U. &Riikonen, R. (2001). Low levels of insulin-like growth factor-I in cerebrospinal fluid in children with autism. *Developmental Medicine and Child Neurology* Vol. 43 No. 9: pp. 614-616

Villagonzalo, K. A., Dodd, S., Dean, O., Gray, K., Tonge, B. &Berk, M. (2010). Oxidative pathways as a drug target for the treatment of autism. *Expert Opinion on Therapeutic Targets* Vol. 14 No. 12: pp. 1301-1310.1744-7631 (Electronic) 1472-8222 (Linking)

Vojdani, A., O'Bryan, T., Green, J. A., McCandless, J., Woeller, K. N., Vojdani, E., et al. (2004). Immune response to dietary proteins, gliadin and cerebellar peptides in children with autism. *Nutritional Neuroscience* Vol. 7 No. 3: pp. 151-161

Waring, R. H. &Klovrza, L. V. (2000). Sulphur Metabolism in Autism. *Journal of Nutritional and Environmental Medicine* Vol. 10 No. 1: pp. 25-32

Weber, W. &Newmark, S. (2007). Complementary and alternative medical therapies for attention-deficit/hyperactivity disorder and autism. *Pediatric Clinics of North America* Vol. 54 No. 6: pp. 983-1006; xii.0031-3955 (Print) 0031-3955 (Linking)

Weissman, J. R., Kelley, R. I., Bauman, M. L., Cohen, B. H., Murray, K. F., Mitchell, R. L., et al. (2008). Mitochondrial disease in autism spectrum disorder patients: a cohort analysis. *PLoS One* Vol. 3 No. 11: pp. e3815.1932-6203 (Electronic) 1932-6203 (Linking)

Whitaker-Azmitia, P. M. (2001). Serotonin and brain development: role in human developmental diseases. *Brain Research Bulletin* Vol. 56 No. 5: pp. 479-485.0361-9230 (Print) 0361-9230 (Linking)

White, J. F. (2003). Intestinal pathophysiology in autism. *Experimental Biology and Medicine* Vol. 228 No. 6: pp. 639-649

Wong, H. H. &Smith, R. G. (2006). Patterns of complementary and alternative medical therapy use in children diagnosed with autism spectrum disorders. *Journal of Autism and Developmental Disorders* Vol. 36 No. 7: pp. 901-909.0162-3257 (Print) 0162-3257 (Linking)

Wright, B., Sims, D., Smart, S., Alwazeer, A., Alderson-Day, B., Allgar, V., et al. (2011). Melatonin versus placebo in children with autism spectrum conditions and severe sleep problems not amenable to behaviour management strategies: a randomised controlled crossover trial. *Journal of Autism and Developmental Disorders* Vol. 41 No. 2: pp. 175-184.1573-3432 (Electronic) 0162-3257 (Linking)

Wu, G., Fang, Y. Z., Yang, S., Lupton, J. R. &Turner, N. D. (2004). Glutathione metabolism and its implications for health. *Journal of Nutrition* Vol. 134 No. 3: pp. 489-492

Yap, I. K., Angley, M., Veselkov, K. A., Holmes, E., Lindon, J. C. &Nicholson, J. K. (2010). Urinary metabolic phenotyping differentiates children with autism from their unaffected siblings and age-matched controls. *Journal of Proteome Research* Vol. 9 No. 6: pp. 2996-3004.1535-3907 (Electronic) 1535-3893 (Linking)

Yorbik O, Akay C, Sayal A, Cansever A, Sohmen T &Cavdar AO (2004). Zinc Status in Autistic Children. *The Journal of Trace Elements in Experimental Medicine* Vol. 17 No. 2: pp. 101-107

Yorbik, O., Sayal, A., Akay, C., Akbiyik, D. I. &Sohmen, T. (2002). Investigation of antioxidant enzymes in children with autistic disorder. *Prostaglandins Leukotrienes and Essential Fatty Acids* Vol. 67 No. 5: pp. 341-343.0952-3278

Young, J. G., Cohen, D. J. &Roth, J. A. (1978). Association between platelet monoamine oxidase activity and hematocrit in childhood autism. *Life Sciences* Vol. 23 No. 8: pp. 797-806.0024-3205 (Print) 0024-3205 (Linking)

Young, J. G., Kavanagh, M. E., Anderson, G. M., Shaywitz, B. A. &Cohen, D. J. (1982). Clinical neurochemistry of autism and associated disorders. *Journal of Autism and Developmental Disorders* Vol. 12 No. 2: pp. 147-165.0162-3257 (Print) 0162-3257 (Linking)

Zecavati, N. &Spence, S. J. (2009). Neurometabolic disorders and dysfunction in autism spectrum disorders. *Current Neurology and Neuroscience Reports* Vol. 9 No. 2: pp. 129-136.1534-6293 (Electronic) 1528-4042 (Linking)

4

# Complementary Medicine Products Used in Autism - Evidence for Efficacy and Safety

Susan Semple, Cassie Hewton, Fiona Paterson and Manya Angley
*Quality Use of Medicines and Pharmacy Research Centre,*
*Sansom Institute for Health Research,*
*School of Pharmacy and Medical Sciences,*
*University of South Australia*
*Australia*

## 1. Introduction

In Chapter 3 the rationale for a range of CAM products that are used in the management of autism was presented with the view to inform researchers and health care professionals about the theoretical or proven basis for a range of CAM products in autism.
This Chapter is the second part of the two-part review and examines the evidence for efficacy and safety of a range of CAM products in autism. Each CAM product for which randomised controlled trials have been conducted has been assigned to a category of the Natural Standard Research Collaboration grading rationale for efficacy (Natural Standard Research Collaboration 2010). To determine safety of the range of CAM products investigated, all types of trials where specific a CAM product has been investigated in autism were examined.

## 2. Aim

To systematically review the literature to determine the efficacy and safety of a range of CAM products used in autism. Specifically, the following interventions were investigated: vitamins A, B, C and E, dimethylglycine (DMG), calcium, iron, magnesium, selenium, zinc, probiotics, digestive enzymes, colostrum, secretin, olive leaf extract, polyunsaturated fatty acids (PUFAs), melatonin, chelating agents (dimercaptosuccinic acid, DMSA & thiamine tetrahydrofuryl disulphide, TTFD), glutathione and glutamine.

## 3. Method

The method used to retrieve articles for the purposes of the review of efficacy and safety of CAM products used in autism was as described in Chapter 3.
Randomised controlled trials or randomised cross-over trials that were retrieved via the method described in Chapter 3, were used to assess effectiveness of specific CAM products in individuals with autism spectrum disorder (ASD). The grading system used by the Natural Standard Research Collaboration (Natural Standard Research Collaboration 2010) was used to assign a rating (A to F) signifying the level of evidence that exists for the use of

each complementary medicine in treating autism. A rating A is assigned to strong positive evidence and a rating of F indicates strong negative evidence.
Relevant articles were read in full by two independent reviewers and data extracted using a pre-defined protocol including study design, number and characteristics of subjects, interventions and comparisons, length of follow-up, outcome measures, and results. Randomised controlled trials, used to examine evidence for efficacy, were assessed for study quality and given a rating from 0 to 5 on the Jadad scale (Jadad et al. 1996). This scale awards points for description of randomisation, blinding and drop-outs with a score of 5 indicating the highest study quality. Any discrepancies between reviewers were resolved by discussion. Studies published only in abstract form were excluded from the analysis of efficacy. Adverse effects reported in all relevant studies were summarised and assessed. Clinical trials of all designs were used to examine reported adverse effects of the CAMs products in the autism population.

## 4. Results

### 4.1 Efficacy

Overall there is a distinct lack of good quality clinical evidence to support the efficacy of the wide variety of CAM products that are used in autism. There were no published studies of any kind conducted specifically examining efficacy for the following CAM products in autism: vitamin A or E, selenium, calcium, zinc, olive leaf extract, colostrum, Metallothionein promoter or glutamine. For the remainder of the CAM products investigated, various types of trials were retrieved. Evidence for efficacy was assessed based on findings from randomised controlled trials. For those CAM products where randomised controlled trials have been published, evidence for efficacy in autism was rated as being either unclear or conflicting for the majority of agents i.e. a Natural Standard Research Collaboration Efficacy Rating C as shown in Table 1.

#### 4.1.1 High dose pyridoxine and magnesium (HDPM)

A total of 15 studies describing the administration of vitamin B6 and/or magnesium to children with autism were identified through the literature search (Lelord et al. 1978; Rimland et al. 1978; Barthelemy et al. 1980; Martineau et al. 1981; Lelord et al. 1982; Barthelemy et al. 1983; Jonas et al. 1984; Martineau et al. 1985; Martineau et al. 1986; Martineau et al. 1988; Martineau et al. 1989; Ménage et al. 1992; Tolbert et al. 1993; Findling et al. 1997; Kuriyama et al. 2002;). As shown in Table 2, there were three randomised controlled trials that examined the effects of pyridoxine and magnesium in autism that had a Jadad score of 3 or above and therefore were of sufficient quality to use to determine evidence for efficacy. A study by Kuriyama et al. (2002) comparing pyridoxine versus placebo found that verbal IQ improved in the treatment group while two other studies by Findling et al (1997) and Tolbert et al. (1993) found no significant differences in response between HDPM and placebo. The sample sizes of all studies were small i.e. n = 8, 10 & 15 respectively. Notably, a study by Mousain-Bosc et al. (2006) found children with PDD had significantly lower magnesium prior to supplementation with HDPM which normalised following treatment with an improvement in PDD symptoms. According to the Natural Standard Research Collaboration grading rationale (Natural Standard Research Collaboration 2010), vitamin B6 plus or minus magnesium for the treatment of autism as shown in Table 1 would be assigned to category C. This corresponds to unclear or conflicting scientific evidence

| Complementary Medicine | Natural Standard Research Collaboration Rating | Trials used to determine the Natural Standard Research Collaboration Rating |
|---|---|---|
| Vitamin B6 + magnesium | C | Kuriyama et al. 2002; Findling et al. 1997; Tolbert et al. 1993 |
| Vitamin B12 | C | Bertoglio et al. 2010 |
| Multivitamins/minerals (Spectrum Support) | C | Adams&Holloway 2004 |
| Dimethylglycine (DMG) | C | Bolman &Richmond 1999; Kern et al. 2001 |
| Vitamin C | C | Dolske et al. 1993 |
| Probiotics | C | Parracho et al. 2010 |
| Digestive enzymes | D | Munasinghe et al. 2010 |
| Secretin | F | Williams et al. 2009 (Cochrane review that examined 14 randomised controlled trials) |
| Polyunsaturated fatty acids (PUFAs) | C | Amminger et al. 2007; Bent et al. 2010 |
| Melatonin | B | Garstang&Wallis 2006; Wright et al. 2011 |
| All others | Lack of scientific evidence | |

Level of Evidence Grade A: Strong Scientific Evidence; B: Good Scientific Evidence; C: Unclear or conflicting scientific evidence; D: Fair Negative Scientific Evidence; F: Strong Negative Scientific Evidence.

Table 1. Evidence for the efficacy of selected complementary medicines in treating autism

on the basis that there is no apparent majority of the properly-conducted trials indicating evidence of benefit or ineffectiveness. In conclusion, the long-term administration of high-dose vitamin B6 to autistic children should not be recommended, pending further research. There is a need for randomised, controlled clinical trials with adequate power to be performed in this population before efficacy can be confirmed.

### 4.1.2 Vitamin B12, folinic acid and betaine

A small case control study by James et al (2004) showed that the metabolic profile within the folate/methionine pathway was normalised in children with autistic disorder (AD) when they received supplementation with folinic acid and betaine for three months (n=8), particularly the ratio of S-adenosyl-methionine: S-adenosylhomocysteine (SAM:SAH), comparable to the profile in individuals without autism. The addition of vitamin B12 to this regimen for a further one month acted mainly on the trans-sulphuration pathway, increasing the ratio of reduced glutathione: oxidised glutathione (GSH:GSSG), although it also led to further normalisation of methionine metabolites. Clinical improvements in both speech and cognition were observed but these were not quantitatively measured. The same researchers conducted a larger intervention in 40 children with AD and reduced methylation capacity or GSH:GSSG in which they were supplemented with folinic acid and methylcobalamin for 3 months (James et al. 2009). The new regimen, which used half the dose of folinic acid than their earlier study (James et al. 2004), improved the mean metabolite concentrations significantly after intervention, although they remained below those in unaffected control children. In the earlier 2004 study, objective behavioural measures were not reported. As these studies were not randomised controlled trials and behavioural measures were not quantitatively measured and reported, vitamin B12 and folinic acid plus or minus betaine for the management of autism would be assigned to the 'lack of evidence' category of the Natural Standard Research Collaboration grading rationale

#### 4.1.3 Folinic acid

Studies have reported the effect of treatment with folinic acid on low cerebrospinal fluid (CSF) levels of 5-methyltetrahydrofolate (5-MTHF) in a subgroup of children with autism and at least one symptom of cerebral folate deficiency (CFD) (Moretti et al. 2005; Ramaekers et al. 2007; Moretti et al. 2008). One of these studies showed that treatment with folinic acid resulted in improved autistic, motor and other neurological symptoms in young children (<3.5 years) and improvements in motor and neurological symptoms in older children, although there was no change in autistic symptoms in the older age group (Ramaekers et al. 2007). It remains to be determined whether gains can be achieved with folinic acid supplementation in children with AD without CFD. As these studies were not randomised controlled trials, folinic acid for the management of autism would be assigned to the 'lack of evidence' category of the Natural Standard Research Collaboration grading rationale.

#### 4.1.4 Vitamin B12

As summarised in Table 2, a double-blinded randomised placebo-controlled trial was recently published where participants (n=30) were administered either methyl-cobalamin or placebo for 6 weeks and then switched without washout for a further 6 weeks (Bertoglio et al. 2010). Overall, there was no significant change in GSH, GSH:GSSH or behaviour, however, 30% of participants showed a significant improvement against objective behavioural measures which correlated with improved plasma GSH and GSH:GSSH. Therefore, given there was no overall benefit but a benefit shown in a subgroup of children with autism, vitamin B12 for the treatment of autism would be assigned to category C of the Natural Standard Research Collaboration grading rationale as shown in Table 1. Further studies in the subgroup which show improvements in plasma GSH and GSH:GSSH with B12 treatment are warranted.

#### 4.1.5 Multivitamin/mineral supplement

Multivitamins are widely implemented by caregivers of children with autism and one physician survey found 49% of respondents recommended their use in children with autism (Golnik&Ireland 2009). Adams & Hollloway (2004) conducted a 3-month pilot randomised controlled trial of a moderate dose multivitamin/mineral supplement (Spectrum Support II transitioning to III) in children with autism (n=20). Mothers completed a Global Impressions survey and results showed statistically significant improvements in sleep and gastrointestinal (GI) symptoms in those children taking the supplement versus placebo. Therefore this study shows Spectrum Support multivitamin/mineral supplement holds promise for the treatment of sleep and GI disturbance in autism . However, due to the small sample size it would be assigned to category C of the Natural Standard Research Collaboration grading rationale as shown in Table 1 and indicates a larger study is warranted.

#### 4.1.6 Dimethylglycine (DMG)

Although there are numerous anecdotal reports that DMG reduces autistic behaviours and improves speech, as summarised in Table 2, administration of low dose DMG demonstrated no statistically significant effect on autistic behaviours in two double-blind, placebo-controlled trials (n = 8 & 37) (Bolman &Richmond 1999; Kern et al. 2001). Therefore, DMG for the treatment of autism would be assigned to category C of the Natural Standard Research Collaboration grading rationale, i.e. unclear or conflicting scientific evidence as shown in Table 1. This is on the basis that although there is an indication that DMG is ineffective in two randomised controlled trials, the sample sizes are too small to provide conclusive evidence.

#### 4.1.7 Vitamin C

One small randomised double-blind, crossover study (n=18) reported decreased stereotypic behaviours in children who received ascorbic acid (Dolske et al. 1993). This study had a number of methodological flaws including a small sample size, heterogeneity of subjects, lack of ascorbate-free baseline and a lack of different, multiple dependent variables. In addition this study has not been replicated (Levy&Hyman 2003). As the study was of poor quality (i.e. a Jadad rating of 2) vitamin C as a treatment for autism is assigned to category C of the Natural Standard Research Collaboration grading rationale i.e. unclear or conflicting scientific evidence on the basis that there is no apparent majority of the properly-conducted trials indicating evidence of benefit or ineffectiveness. It is important to note that the use of vitamin C to prevent/treat deficiency (scurvy) in any individual would gain a Natural Standard Research Collaboration rating of A (strong scientific evidence), however the focus of this study is to examine the efficacy of vitamin C as a treatment for the disorder of autism.

#### 4.1.8 Iron

An open-label uncontrolled study was undertaken as a pilot study to examine the effects of iron supplementation in children with autism (n=33, 2-10 years of age) (Dosman et al. 2007). The study examined effects on ferritin levels and sleep. An oral iron supplement at a dose of 6 mg elemental iron/kg/day was administered for 8 weeks. Parents completed two sleep questionnaires, a three-day food record, and a Clinical Global Impression Scale questionnaire at baseline and after 8 weeks of iron supplementation. Blood samples were taken at baseline and post-treatment to determine serum ferritin and transferrin receptor and other blood chemistry. There was a significant increase ($p < 0.001$) in blood ferritin levels from 15.72 microgram/L at baseline to 28.8 microgram/L post-treatment. The Restless Sleep score improved significantly post-treatment ($p< 0.04$), however no statistically significant relationship was found between Restless Sleep score and ferritin concentration. One study has shown that iron levels may be problematic in children with ASD (Latif et al. 2002), and clearly there are obvious benefits in treating iron deficiency. However, in terms of actually improving sleep and behaviour, the study conducted by Dosman et al. (2007) provides insufficient evidence for efficacy and is assigned to the 'lack of evidence' category of the Natural Standard Research Collaboration grading rationale.

#### 4.1.9 Probiotics

Probiotics are widely used in autism, with one survey reporting 19% of medical practitioners recommend probiotics as a treatment in autism (Golnik&Ireland 2009).

Probiotics are live bacteria that, when administered, can provide health benefits to the host. As summarised in Table 2, a randomised double-blind, placebo-controlled, crossover-designed probiotic feeding study was undertaken in children diagnosed with ASD. Children (n=17, 4-16 years of age) received either *Lactobacillus plantarum* WCFS1 for 3 weeks with a 3 week wash out period. The overall indicator of behavioural/emotional disturbances was not significantly different between the two feeding periods. The observed benefit of the probiotic was a higher percentage of 'formed' stool samples compared to the placebo feeding, whilst the percentage of 'hard' stool samples was lower during probiotic feeding. No significant differences were observed between probiotic and placebo for GI disturbance (Parracho et al. 2010). Although probiotics hold promise as a treatment in autism they are currently assigned to category C of the Natural Standard Research Collaboration grading rationale as shown in Table 1. Notably Parracho et al.'s study (2010) only examined one type of probiotic feeding i.e. with *Lactobacillus plantarum* WCFS1 and thus even the benefits on stool consistency are not be generalisable to all probiotic interventions.

#### 4.1.10 Digestive enzymes

One randomised double-blind, placebo-controlled, crossover-designed study (Munasinghe et al. 2010) examined the efficacy of 3 months treatment (with a 1 week washout) with a digestive enzyme (Peptizyde ™) in autism (n=27, mean age 69.4 months). As summarised in Table 2, this study found treatment with enzyme compared with placebo was not associated with clinically significant improvement in behaviour, food variety, GI symptoms, sleep quality, engagement with therapist, or the Language Development Survey Vocabulary or Sentence Complexity Scores (Munasinghe et al. 2010). As this study was of high quality (i.e. Jadad score of 5) and showed no benefit on a range of outcome measures it is assigned to category D of the Natural Standard Research Collaboration grading rationale. Notably, only one type of enzyme product was tested and results may not be generalisable to other digestive enzyme products that are used for this purpose.

Although only randomised controlled trials were used to assess efficacy in this study, it is noteworthy that Brudnak et al. (2002) reported a case series with post-test outcomes following supplementation with a formulated combination of enzymes in children with ASD. Twenty-nine of the 46 subjects completed the trial, with personal issues, lack of palatability, and behavioural or medical side effects given as reasons for withdrawal from the study. The results of this study are limited due to its open, uncontrolled design, however Brudnak et al. (2002) reported a significant positive trend for each of the 13 parameters measured on the Symptom Outcome Survey.

#### 4.1.11 Secretin

A systematic review of intravenous secretin for ASD was undertaken through the Cochrane Collaboration and published in 2005. An editorial update to this review in 2009 made no changes to the conclusions of the review (Williams et al. 2009). The objectives of the review were to examine whether intravenous secretin: a) improved the core features of autism; b) improved the non-core aspects of behaviour or function ; c) improved the quality of life of individuals with ASD and their carers; d) had a short term and long term effects on outcomes; e) caused harm. The review included literature covered by major health and biomedical databases and unpublished studies that could be located from 1998 to March 2005. Studies were included if they were randomised controlled trials of intravenous secretin comparing it with a placebo treatment in children or adults diagnosed with ASD, where at least one standardised outcome measure (such as a standardised checklist) was reported. Studies under consideration were evaluated for methodological quality and relevance by two independent reviewers using standardised Cochrane methods for assessing study quality.

Fourteen studies met the inclusion criteria for the review. These studies represented data for 618 children aged under 18 years. Nine studies used a cross-over design and five were a parallel design. The analysis of cross-over trials in the review was limited to the first phase to prevent biased underestimation of treatment effectiveness due to potentially inadequate wash-out periods. Different types of secretin were used in different studies including porcine, synthetic porcine and synthetic human secretin. Some studies used single doses of secretin while others used two or three doses of secretin 4 - 6 weeks apart.

It was found that 25 established standardised outcome measures were reported in the included studies with no more than four studies reporting the same outcome measure. Outcomes were reported at between three and six weeks with no outcomes beyond six weeks post-intervention reported in the included studies. It was only possible to perform a meta-analysis on the outcome measure of the Childhood Autism Rating Scale (CARS).

Ten studies presented information about core features of autism as an outcome measure. Analyses of outcome measures including subscales of the Autism Behavior Checklist (ABC), the Autism Diagnostic Observation Scale (ADOS), the Childhood Autism Rating Scale (CARS), Gilliam Autism Rating Scale: Autism Quotient and Autism Behavior Checklist found no significant differences between secretin and placebo. Overall it was concluded that the "RCTs of efficacy of secretin in autism have not shown improvements for core features of autism". Overall, analysis of individual areas such as communication, behaviour, affect, visio-spatial skills and quality of life found no conclusive evidence in favour of secretin.

The authors concluded that there was no evidence that secretin was effective in ASD and should not be recommended as a treatment. While no conclusions could be drawn about the effectiveness of secretin for certain subgroups of people with autism, it was suggested that further explorations of effectiveness in such subgroups should only be undertaken if there is a biologically plausible explanation for effectiveness in these groups. Secretin is therefore assigned to category F of the Natural Standard Research Collaboration grading rationale i.e. strong negative evidence for efficacy as shown in Table 1.

#### 4.1.12 Polyunsaturated fatty acids (PUFAs)

PUFAs (also called omega -3 and -6 fatty acids), are recognised as vital building blocks for developing neurological systems. These essential fatty acids (EFAs) are present in fish oils, evening primrose oil and linseed (flaxseed) oil (Bell et al. 2004). A study by Green et al. (2006) revealed that 27.8% of caregivers of children with autism implemented PUFAs in their affected child. One survey reported PUFAs are recommended by 25% of medical practitioners for the management of autism (Golnik&Ireland 2009).

As summarised in Table 2, one small randomised controlled trial (n = 13) investigating the efficacy of PUFAs (1.5g/day) in autism noted non-significant improvements in hyperactivity and stereotypy after 6 weeks treatment (Amminger et al. 2007). Another randomised controlled trial by Bent et al. (2010) examined PUFAs (1.3 g/day) for the treatment of hyperactivity in 27 children with ASD. They also found there were non-significant improvements after 12 weeks in hyperactivity, as measured by the ABC. The remaining five studies, four uncontrolled trials in children and one case report were small (n = 30, 22, 19, 9, and 1) with four (Johnson&Hollander 2003; Bell et al. 2004; Patrick&Salik 2006; Meguid et al. 2008) reporting improvements in a wide range of outcomes including language and learning skills, parental observations of general health and behaviour, a clinician administered symptom scale, and clinical observations of anxiety. In contrast one uncontrolled trial in young adults with severe autism did not show a benefit (Politi et al. 2008).

In summary, the small sample size for both PUFA randomised controlled trials limits the conclusions that can be drawn. Although both studies were of high quality, and showed a lack of significant effect overall (but with a trend towards improvements in hyperactivity), the sample sizes are too small to give a conclusion of negative evidence. Therefore, the evidence for the efficacy of PUFAs in autism is currently inconclusive and PUFAs are assigned to category C of the Natural Standard Research Collaboration grading rationale.

#### 4.1.13 Melatonin

Melatonin is another complementary medicine that is currently receiving attention in the management of sleep problems in autism. One survey found 25%of medical practitioners reported they recommend melatonin as a treatment in autism (Golnik&Ireland 2009) As summarised in Table 2, two randomised controlled trials (n=7 & 17) have been performed in autism that suggest melatonin is effective at reducing sleep latency, or time taken for initiation of sleep, and total sleep time in children with sleep problems and autism (Garstang&Wallis 2006; Wright et al. 2011). Further, one of the trials also showed melatonin improved the number of wakings per night (Garstang&Wallis 2006) and the other showed it improved daytime behaviour (Wright et al. 2011). Therefore on the basis of the findings in the two randomised controlled trials, melatonin is assigned to category B of the Natural Standard Research Collaboration grading rationale as shown in Table 1.

Other types of trials also support the benefits of melatonin in the treatment of sleep disturbance in autism. There have also been two open trials conducted in a population of subjects with ASD (Paavonen et al. 2003; Giannotti et al. 2006). Paavonen et al. (2003) found a statistically significant reduction in sleep latency with melatonin administration to 15 children with Asperger's Syndrome (AS) and Giannotti et al. (2006) found sleep patterns of all children with autism (n=20) improved during treatment. There were significant reductions in bedtime resistance and number and duration of night awakenings, and a significant increase in sleep duration. Andersen et al. (2008) and Galli-Carminati et al. (2009) have conducted observational retrospective trials in autistic populations (n= 107 children & 6 adults respectively). Andersen et al.'s (2008) melatonin study found parents of 27/107 (25%) children no longer reported sleep concerns after initiation of melatonin. Parents of 64/107 (60%) of children reported improved sleep but with ongoing concerns. Parents of 14 children (13%) continued to report sleep problems as an ongoing concern with only 1 child (1%) having worse sleep after starting melatonin, and 1 child having undetermined response (1%). Melatonin resulted in improvements in adults including length of sleep, time to fall asleep, nocturnal awakenings and early morning awakenings (Galli-Carminati et al. 2006).

#### 4.1.14 Chelating agents

Approved uses for chelation therapy include heavy metal poisoning and digitalis toxicity, although it used in an off-label manner in autism. Practitioners are using a variety of chelating agents and routes of administration for children with ASD, with oral dimercaptosuccinic acid (DMSA), also known as succimer, probably the most common. Several of the agents are not approved for use or are given through unlicensed routes of administration such as rectally or transdermally. A 5-year old child with autism died after being administered intravenous edetate disodium (Atwood&Woeckner 2009). The survey conducted by Golnik and Ireland (Golnik&Ireland 2009) reported that 61% of medical practitioners surveyed discouraged caregivers' use of chelation in the management of autism.

A study conducted by Adams et al. (2009a; 2009b) examined the effects of oral DMSA as a chelating agent in children with a diagnosis of ASD. While the study was designed as a randomised double-blind study, the complex study design and carry-over effects from the first round of DMSA administered to all participants in the first phase of the study meant that the study lacked a true placebo control group. Essentially the study compared the effects of one round of DMSA therapy (and 6 rounds of placebo) with 7 rounds of DMSA. A round of DMSA therapy consisted of oral DMSA 10mg/kg administered three times a day for three days. This was followed by 11 days of no DMSA. Patients randomised to receive a topical reduced glutathione lotion (180 mg reduced l-glutathione/day) in the initial phase of the study received the DMSA therapy (up to 7 rounds in total) in the second study phase, while those receiving a placebo lotion received placebo in the second phase. A total of 82 children were enrolled with 65 completing phase one and 41 completing phase two. Effects on urinary excretion of toxic metals and blood chemistry were examined, with a single round of DMSA found to cause a significant increase urinary excretion of lead, tin and bismuth and normalisation of red blood cell glutathione levels. Effects on behaviour were also assessed using a variety of measures including the Autism Diagnostic Observation Schedule (ADOS); Severity of Autism Scale (SAS); Pervasive Developmental Disorders - Behaviour Inventory (PDD-BI), Autism Treatment Evaluation Checklist (ATEC), and Parental Global Impressions questionnaire. Both the groups receiving one round and seven rounds of DMSA therapy were found to have significant improvements compared to baseline using most of these measures. However the differences in improvement between the groups were not significant.

Another uncontrolled study assessed a combination of DMSA (administered orally at 10mg/kg three times a day) with the anti-androgen leuprolide acetate (administered intramuscularly and subcutaneously) in 11 children with ASD (Geier and Geier, 2006). DMSA was to be administered transdermally if oral dosing caused severe GI disturbance. However, the number of participants, if any, experiencing GI disturbances was not reported. It was reported that the treatment had no adverse effect on kidney, thyroid or liver function tests. Children in the study received vitamin and mineral supplementation during the study and no effects on serum potassium, calcium, iron, magnesium, copper or zinc were observed.

On the basis that these chelation trials were not properly conducted randomised controlled trials chelation for the management of autism would be assigned to the 'lack of evidence' category of the Natural Standard Research Collaboration grading rationale.

#### 4.1.15 Others

No studies of any description investigating use in children with autism were located for the remainder of the interventions under investigation i.e. calcium, selenium, colostrum, glutamine, magnesium, metallotheionein, olive leaf extract, vitamin A or vitamin E. Hence, the remaining interventions are assigned to the 'lack of evidence' category of the Natural Standard Research Collaboration grading rationale with respect to their use in the management of autism. It is important to remember that, as with vitamin C, supplementation with vitamin A, vitamin E, calcium and magnesium to treat or prevent deficiency in any individual would gain a Natural Standard Research Collaboration rating of A (strong scientific evidence). The focus of this study, however, was to examine their efficacy when used to specifically reducing the symptoms of autism, where they all lacked evidence for use.

| Reference | No. of Subjects | Patient Characteristics | Intervention | Comparison | Length of Follow-up | Outcome Measure(s) | Results | Funding Source | Comments |
|---|---|---|---|---|---|---|---|---|---|
| Trials of pyridoxine/magnesium | | | | | | | | | |
| Findling et al. (1997) | 12 patients enrolled, 10 completed the study (2 patients withdrew during two week lead-in period due to refusal to take study medicine). | Aged 3-17, met Diagnostic and Statistical Manual of Mental Disorders (DSM-III-R) criteria for autistic disorder, all living at home with a parent/guardian. Exclusion criteria: Significant past or current medical or neurological disorder, use of a psychotropic agent within 3 months prior to start of study. | Pyridoxine 30mg/kg/day (max. 1g) + Mg. oxide 10mg/kg/day (max. 350mg) Doses given twice daily at 8am and 12pm. All subject s received placebo for the first two weeks (baseline period), after which they were randomised and received either treatment or placebo for four weeks, and then the opposite for the next four weeks. | Placebo (identical appearance, efforts made to match taste) At baseline, all subjects received placebo for 2 weeks in a single-blind fashion before randomisation. | Subjects were evaluated every other week for a 10-week period. | Childhood Autism Rating Scale (CARS), Clinical Global Impression scale (CGI scale), Children's Psychiatric Rating Scale(CPRS), Obsessive Compulsive Scale (OCS). | ANOVA revealed no statistically significant effects of vit.B6 + Mg. on any of the outcome measures. 50% of patients had a $\geq$ 30% reduction in CPRS score during the placebo lead-in phase of the study. | Not specified | Jadad score = 4 |
| Kuriyama et al. (2002) | 15 patients were recruited, but four met the exclusion criteria. 11 completed the baseline study, 3 were then excluded based on immeasurable IQs. Therefore 8 patients were randomised (4 in treatment group, 4 in placebo). | Met DSM-IV criteria for PDDs, had expressive verbal disorders, developmental motor coordination disorders and hypersensitivity to sound, aged 6-17. Exclusion criteria: History of epilepsy or an epileptiform EEG, use of a psychotropic agent within 3 mths of starting the study, inability to measure IQ, brain image abnormalities on MRI, history of homocystinuria or fragile-x syndrome. In both groups, one child had AS and three PDD-NOS. | Pyridoxine 100mg in powder form once daily for the first 2 weeks, 100mg twice daily for the second 2 weeks (after breakfast and after dinner). | Placebo (powder form, identical in appearance and taste). | Subjects were evaluated at baseline and after 4 weeks of treatment. | Changes in IQ scores (both verbal IQ and performance IQ) using the Wechsler Intelligence Scale for Children-III (WISC-III), social quotient (SQ) scores measured with the Social Maturity Scale (SM) test assessed by the subjects' parents. | There was a statistically significant increase in verbal IQ in the vit.B6 group relative to the placebo group, although verbal IQ did increase in both groups (by 11.2 in the treatment group and by 6.0 in the placebo group). The difference was still significant after controlling for sex, age, body weight, interval between tests and baseline verbal IQ using ANOVA. No significant difference in performance IQ and SQ scores was found. | Not specified | Jadad score = 5 Limited by small sample size and short-term nature Mg was not given |
| Tolbert et al. (1993) | 15 patients were randomised. A further 5 subjects not receiving any treatment served as controls. | Ages 6-18, all diagnosed with autism according to the DSM-III-R criteria, all residential students and receiving a standardised diet. No subjects had lactose intolerance, no pyridoxine deficiencies were | Pyridoxine 200mg/70kg/day in 50mg tablets in divided doses. Magnesium 100mg/70kg/day in 27mg tablets in divided doses. | Placebo (matching tablets) and control. Group 1: treatment for 20 weeks then placebo for 10 weeks Group 2: treatment for 10 weeks, placebo for 10 weeks, | Subjects were evaluated after baseline and after each of three 10-week blocks (i.e. 30 weeks) | Ritvo-Freeman Real Life Rating Scale for Autism (R-F) - quantitates 47 specific behaviours grouped into 5 subscales: sensory-motor, social, affective, sensory responses language. | No significant differences among the three groups at any of the time points. There was a statistically significant reduction in scores across the time period for each group, possible due to other non-pharmacological therapy that patients | Not specified | Jadad score = 3 This study specifically used much lower doses of pyridoxine than previous studies in an attempt to reduce the risk of |

| | | | | | | | | | |
|---|---|---|---|---|---|---|---|---|---|
| | | identified. | | treatment for 10 weeks. (after 5-week baseline period) | | Raters observed subjects involved in classroom activities from a room equipped with one-way mirrors and sound amplification. | were receiving throughout the trial. | | peripheral neuropathies. |
| Trials of dimethylglycine (DMG) | | | | | | | | | |
| Bolman and Richmond (1999) | 10 were recruited, 8 completed full testing. | Ages 4-30, diagnosed according to DSM-III-R criteria, not taking other medication within one month prior to the study. | DMG tablets, doses varied with weight (from 125mg/day for under 70lbs to 375mg/day for over 120lbs) | Look-alike placebos 2-week baseline period, 4 weeks of either DMG or placebo, 2-week washout period, 4 weeks of placebo or DMG, 2-week baseline period. | 14 weeks (3 ½ months) | Campbell-NIMH 14-point Autism Rating Scale (ARS)(patients were videotaped weekly following a semi-structured set of guidelines in a playroom) An experimental 10-item checklist developed by Rimland Individualised scales developed with help of parents (3 scales) | Videotaping (ARS): no significant changes in behaviour observed. Experimental checklist: no significant differences between any of the study periods Individualised scales: From a group total of 55 scale items, 5 showed improvement with DMG vs. placebo, 14 worsened and 36 showed no difference. | Not specified | Jadad score = 3 Only 3 out of 8 parents could correctly guess during which period their child had taken DMG or placebo (less than chance). |
| Kern et al. (2001) | 39 began the study, 37 completed it | Ages 3-11, diagnosis of autism or pervasive developmental disorder (DSM-IV) 7 children were on psychoactive medications (held constant throughout the study). | Foil-wrapped 125mg DMG tablets (no. of tablets taken varied with weight, from 125mg/day for under 40lbs to 625mg/day for over 130lbs). | Identical placebo tablets (mannitol 125mg) | 4 weeks | Behavioural Assessments (Vineland Maladaptive Behaviour Domain, Aberrant Behaviour Checklist) Neurologic assessments | Combined analysis of behavioural assessments revealed a significant improvement over the 4 weeks across all subjects (both placebo and treatment). There was no difference in improvement between the DMG group and the placebo group. No effect of DMG on any of the behavioural measures was observed. DMG treatment did not affect the neurological status. | Not specified | Jadad score = 4 Parents reported improvement in 58% of the DMG group and 53% of the placebo group. Parents reported worsening in 16% of the DMG group and 32% of the placebo group |
| Trials of ascorbic acid | | | | | | | | | |
| Dolske et al. (1993) | 18 (13 male and 5 female). | Inclusion: subjects diagnosed under the DMS-III-R criteria by two independent child psychiatrists, no lactose intolerance and plasma ascorbate levels >30µg/ml i.e. within normal range. Prior to the initiation of the study, subjects ascorbic acid supplementation ranged from 0-4g/70kg/day. Participants were aged between 6 and 19 years (mental age ranged from 2.0-6.7, IQs ranged from <20-65). Subjects received a standardised diet throughout the duration of the study | Ascorbic acid was administered at 8g/70kg/day in 500mg tablets, divided into two or three separate doses. Phase 1: Initially all subjects received ascorbic acid for a ten-week block. Phase 2: After the first ten-week block, half the subjects were randomly assigned to continue to receive the ascorbic acid (Group 1) and the other half to receive a placebo (Group 2) for an additional ten weeks. Phase 3: For the final ten weeks the treatments were reversed. | Matching placebo tablet (film coated and identical in appearance). | Each treatment phase lasted 10 weeks and behaviours were rated weekly using the R-F scale. The weekly R-F scores (total and each subscale) in each 10-week block were averaged for each subject. 30-week trial overall. | R-F was used as an instrument to determine drug treatment evaluation. Raters observed subjects participating in routine classroom activities from an observation room equipped with one-way mirrors and sound amplification. | Comparison of total scores revealed a significant interaction when comparing Phase 2 and Phase 3 (p=0.02). Behaviour worsened in group 1 when going from ascorbate (Phase 2) to placebo (Phase 3), where as behaviour improved in group 2 when going from placebo (Phase 2) to ascorbate (Phase 3). On the sensory motor scale (subscale 1), a significant interaction was found (group x phase 2 and 3) p=0.01. No other subscales revealed significant findings for main effects of group and phase interaction. | Not stated | Jaded score= 2 Article did not report any adverse effects. Small sample size, hetero-geneous population, lack of ascorbate-free baseline, confound-ing neuroleptic variable, lack of different multiple dependent measures. |

| | | | | | | | | | |
|---|---|---|---|---|---|---|---|---|---|
| | | Nine of the children were on neuroleptics concurrent with the study. Prior to the study, the neuroleptic doses had been stabilised and were maintained throughout the study. | | | | | There were no significant differences (p>0.05) between R-F total scores and subscales of children receiving vs not receiving neuroleptic medication during the initial 10-week phase of the trial. Therefore this medication variable was not included in the subsequent analyses. | | |
| Trials of vitamin B12 | | | | | | | | | |
| Bertoglio et al. 2010 | 30 cases | Children aged 3-8 diagnosed with autism with DSM-IV-TR and Autism Diagnostic Observation Schedule (ADOS) plus non-verbal IQ ≥49 measured by Wechsler Preschool and Primary Scale of Intelligence, Mullen Scales of Early learning or Wechsler Intelligence Scale for Children. | Methyl-cobalamin 64.5 µg/kg sc for 6 wks followed by cross-over for 6 wks (no washout period). | Placebo | 12 week trial was followed by 6 month open label for 22 cases | Plasma GSH and GSH:GSSH linked to Global Clinical Impressions Score and other objective behavioural measures | Overall, no significant difference in GSH, GSH: GSSH or behavioural outcomes. No serious adverse events were reported, only hyperactivity and increased mouthing of objects. | Institute of the Univer-sity of California, Davis Medical Centre | Jadad score = 4 Increased GSH, & GSH:GSSH and improved behavioural outcomes in 9/30 children which were identified as a "responder group". |
| Trials of multivitamin supplements | | | | | | | | | |
| Adams et al. (2004) | 25 subjects were enrolled, 5 dropped out for varying reasons (20 completed - 9 in placebo group, 11 in supplement group) | Ages 3-8 yrs, diagnosis of ASD by a psychiatrist, no changes in any treatment therapies within 2 months prior to the start of the study, no prior use of a multivitamin/mineral supplement other than a standard children's multivitamin/mineral. | Spectrum Support II -dosage was increased to maximum over 24 days and then held constant until day 34. Gradual transition during days 35-50 to Spectrum Support III which was continued until day 90. Full dosage: 1ml/5lbs bodyweight three times daily with food. | Placebo, matched to colour and consistency. | 3 months | Global Impressions survey filled out by mothers | Mothers reported statistically significant improvements in sleep and GI symptoms in those children taking the supplement versus placebo. | Not specified | Jadad score = 4 Spectrum support is a liquid multi-vitamin prepara-tion with a moderate level of vit.B6 and no copper |
| Trials of probiotics | | | | | | | | | |
| Parracho et al. (2010) | 39 subjects, Group I (n=19), Group II (n=20) commenced the study. 17 participants withdrew before end of first arm, 8 from group I and 9 from group II. 3 subjects withdrew due to adverse effects, 1 with rash, 1 with diarrhoea and 1 with weight loss in feeding period. A further 2 subjects withdrew after first feeding arm and 3 after first | Children with ASD aged 4-16y | Lactobacillus plantarum WCFS1 ($4.5x10^{10}$ colony-forming units per capsule). Probiotic feeding for 3 wks followed by cross-over for 3 wks (3 week washout period). | Placebo | 12 weeks | DBC administered immediately prior to commencing the feeding period i.e. baseline (B1), at the end of each feeding (F1 & F2) and washout period (W1 & W2). Two faecal samples were taken in the week prior to the study (commencing B1 & B2) and at F1, F2, W1 and W2 and bacterial populations examined. Bowel function and GI symptoms were also determined. | The overall indicator of behavioural/emotional disturbances i.e. Total Behaviour Problem Score (TBPS) was not significantly different between the two feeding periods. Probiotic feeding resulted in a higher percentage of 'formed' stool samples (73.3 %) compared to the placebo feeding (64.8 %), whilst the percentage of 'hard' stool samples was lower during probiotic feeding. No significant differences were observed between probiotic and | Not stated | Jadad score = 5 Encapsulation of both placebo and probiotic, and blind coding of the capsules, was performed by Orafti (Belgium). Adverse effects monitored for. *Lactobacillus plantarum* WCFS1 and the placebo were supplied by Nizo Food Research, The Nether-lands. High drop-out rate from study affected statistical power |

| | | | | | | | | | |
|---|---|---|---|---|---|---|---|---|---|
| | washout. 17 subjects completed study (9 from group I and 8 from group II). | | | | | | placebo for GI symptoms (abdominal pain, intestinal bloating and flatulence) | | |
| Trials of digestive enzymes | | | | | | | | | |
| Munasingh et al. (2010) | 43 subjects, 27 completed intervention. 3 were lost to follow up; 2 from Sequence 1 (S1) & 1 from Sequence (S2). 1 subject withdrew due to family issues (S1), 4 because of perceived behaviour deterioration (3 from S1 & 1 from S2), 5 due to difficulties with capsule administration (4 from S1 & 1 from S2) and 3 gave no reason (S2). | Children diagnosed with AD or PDD-NOS with the DSM-IV. Mean age was 69.4 months. | Digestive Enzyme S1 received Peptizyde ™ for 3 months, then crossed over and received placebo. S2 received placebo for 3 months, then crossed over and received Peptizyde™ for 3 months. (1 week washout period between treatment sequences) | Placebo | 6 months and 1 week | Global Behaviour Rating Scale (GBRS), Additional Rating scale (ARS), Language Development Survey (LDS) | No significant difference on the GBRS, ARS and LDS questionnaires. A small statistically significant improvement on enzyme therapy was seen for the food variety scores that was not deemed clinically significant. | Not stated | Jadad score = 5 Enzyme and placebo provided by Houston Nutraceuticals |
| Trials of polyunsaturated fatty acids (PUFAs) | | | | | | | | | |
| Amminger et al. (2007) | 13 subjects, PUFA (n =7) or placebo (n =6). One individual from the placebo group withdrew from the trial after 2 weeks because of GI complaints and lack of symptom improvement. | Children with average age 10.4, (5-17y) diagnosed with autism with DSM-IV-TR and ADOS | 7X 1g capsules of Menhaden fish oil containing 840 mg eicosa-pentaenoic acid (EPA), 700 mg docosa-hexaenoic acid (DHA) & 7 mg Vitamin E (i.e. 1.54g of PUFA/day) for 6 weeks | Placebo i.e. coconut oil with 1 mg fish oil and 1 mg vitamin E | 6 weeks | Aberrant Behavior Checklist (ABC) | Non-significant trends towards improvement. Mild adverse events reported included fever in the experimental group and headache and insomnia in the placebo group. | Not stated | Jadad score = 4 Small sample size Trends for improve-ment in hyper-activity, but not statisticallysignificant. Omega Protein Co-operation, provided medication |
| Bent et a. (2010) | 25 subjects included in analysis, PUFA (n=13) or placebo (n=12). PUFA group, lost to follow-up (n=1, disliked taste), discontinued intervention (n=4, 2 disliked taste, 1 rash, 1 GI symptoms). Placebo group, lost to follow-up (n=1, blood draw anxiety), discontinued intervention (n=2, 1 disliked taste, 1 increased self-stimulatory behaviour) | Children ages 3-8 diagnosedwith ASD (with the ADOS, social communication questionnaire (SCQ) & DSM-IV-TR) and hyperactivity (with the ABC) | PUFAs were provided as orange-flavoured pudding packets (Coromega_, Vista, CA) containing 650 mg of omega-3 fatty acids, including 350 mg of EPA and 230 mg of DHA, given twice daily for a daily dose of 1.3 g of PUFAs (and 1.1 g of DHA/EPA) for 12 weeks. | Placebo packets had the same orange-flavoured pudding with an identical appearance and taste, but included safflower oil instead of the PUFAs. | 12 weeks | ABC (hyperactivity was primary outcome measure) Peabody Picture Vocabulary Test Expressive Vocabulary Test Social Responsiveness Scale Behavioral Assessment System for Children Clinical Global Impression-Improvement (CGI-I) scale. | Overall there were no statistically significant changes in any of the outcome measures. Hyperactivity as measured on the ABC improved 2.7 (+/-4.8) points in the PUFA group compared to 0.3 (+/-7.2) points in the placebo group (p = 0.40; effect size = 0.38) but was not statistically significant. | Autism Speaks, the Higgins Family Found-ation, The Emch Found-ation, The Taube Foundation ,NIH/NCRR UCSF-CTSI Grant Number UL1 RR024131 (Dr. Bent) and the MIND Institute. | Jadad score = 5 Small sample size (pilot study) Correl-ations were found between decreases in five fatty acid levels and decreases in hyperactivity. Treatment was well tolerated. |
| Trials of melatonin | | | | | | | | | |
| Garstang & Wallis (2006) | 7 children completed the study. | Children with a diagnosis of ASD (by a | Melatonin 5mg, given at bedtime for 4 weeks | Placebo | No follow-up | Parents kept daily sleep logs from which the | Mean and 95% confidence interval (CI) reported. There | Coventry primary care trust | Jadad score = 4 Possible |

| | | | | | | | | | |
|---|---|---|---|---|---|---|---|---|---|
| | 11 children were initially enrolled (2 discontinued the study after the trial was suspended as placebo capsules were empty, 1 dropped out because of a house move and 1 dropped out because she was involved in a child protection enquiry. | paediatrician or psychiatrist) aged 4-16, with significant difficulties sleeping at night | | | | primary outcome measures were sleep latency, total hours of sleep, and number of night awakenings. | was a decrease in mean sleep latency, wakings per night and increased total sleep time with melatonin compared to baseline & placebo Sleep latency : Baseline 2.60 h [95% CI 2.28-2.93]; Placebo 1.91 h [1.78-2.03]; melatonin 1.06h [0.98-1.13] Wakings per night: Baseline 0.35 [0.18-0.53]; Placebo 0.26 [0.20-0.34]; melatonin 0.08 [0.04-0.12] Total sleep : Baseline 8.05 h [7.65 - 8.44]; Placebo 8.75 h [8.56-8.98]; melatonin 9.84 h [9.68-9.99] | The melatonin and placebo were supplied free of charge by Penn Pharmaceuticals Ltd. | unblinding due to problems with placebo capsules. Statistical methods were not clearly described Adverse effects not described Small sample size |
| Wright et al. (2011) | 20 subjects were enrolled, 17 included in analysis. | Children diagnosed with ASD based on ICD-10 and confirmed by Autism Diagnostic Interview – Revised (ADI) or ADOS if necessary. Included 14 with autism, 4 atypical autism and 2 with AS. Children had all been referred for serious sleep problems. Children were aged 4-16 years and not taking psychotropic medication. | 2 mg and titrated up to 10mg standard release melatonin, 1 hour prior to bedtime for 3 months | Placebo | | Parents completed sleep diaries daily which were collected monthly for 9 months. Primary outcome measures were sleep latency, total sleep time, and number of wakenings Sleep Difficulties Questionnaire, Developmental Behaviour Checklist (DBC) and General Health Questionnaire collected at the start and end of each 3-month period of medication/ placebo and on completion. A Side Effects Questionnaire was completed at start, end and at end of each 3-month period of medication/ placebo | Melatonin significantly improved sleep latency (by an average of 47 minutes, p=0.004) and total sleep (by an average of 52 minutes, p = 0.002) compared to placebo, but not number of night awakenings p = 0.209. There was a statistically significant difference in the total score of the DBC of 6.0 between melatonin and placebo (p=0.05). There was a significant difference in favour of melatonin for the dysomnias subscale of the Sleep Difficulties questionnaire p=0.041) but not other subscales. Adverse effect profile low and similar between arms. | York Innov-ations Fund and the London law Trust | Jadad score = 5 Placebo was manufactured to be identical in appearance and constitution as the active form. |

Table 2. Published randomised, double-blind, controlled trials of CAM products for the treatment of autism.

### 4.2 Safety

Most interventions were associated with only mild adverse effects, although there is a lack of long-term safety data available (Table 3).

#### 4.2.1 High dose pyridoxine and magnesium (HDPM)

Each of the 15 original studies that investigated the effects of pyridoxine plus or minus magnesium was analysed in order to determine adverse effects seen with administration of vitamin B6 and/or magnesium to an autistic population. In two studies (Martineau et al. 1988; Kuriyama et al. 2002), no subjects reported adverse effects. Loose stools and symptoms

| Complementary medicine | Most prevalent adverse effects |
|---|---|
| Vitamin B6 + magnesium | Loose stools, URTI symptoms, nausea, excitability |
| Vitamin B12 | Hyperactivity and increased mouthing of objects |
| Dimethylglycine (DMG) | Agitation, hyperactivity |
| Vitamin C | None mentioned |
| Iron | GI irritation, stained teeth |
| Probiotics | Rash, diarrhoea, weight loss |
| Digestive enzymes | Hyperactivity, aggression, diarrhoea, increased self-stimulatory behaviours, loose stools, provocation or red ears and cheeks, increased hunger and cessation of eating. |
| Secretin | Rash, hyperactivity, fever, tachycardia, vomiting, photosensitivity, increased irritability and generalised flushing. |
| Polyunsaturated fatty acids | GI irritation, hyperactivity, behavioural worsening, increase the risk of bleeding |
| Melatonin | Tiredness, headache, dizziness, diarrhoea, agitation |
| Thiamine tetrahydrofuryl disulphide (TTFD) | Unpleasant odour |
| DMSA | Sleep problems, increased tantrums |

Table 3. Major adverse effects observed during trials of selected CAM products in people with autism

of an upper respiratory tract infection (URTI) were each experienced by five subjects in the study by Findling et al. (1997), with emesis and fatigue experienced by a single subject. The authors hypothesised that the loose stools could have been caused by the cathartic effect of magnesium oxide. Lelord et al. (1981) reported nausea in 3 subjects, increased excitability in 3 subjects and an increase in autistic symptoms in 4 subjects. No other studies mentioned monitoring for adverse effects, which does not necessarily indicate that they did not occur.

Safety reviews of pyridoxine based on data from human and animal studies in wider populations were conducted in the 1980s and 1990s (Cohen&Bendich 1986; Bendich&Cohen 1990). It was found that pyridoxine doses of less than 500mg/day appeared to be safe in adults, based on durations of administration ranging from 6 months to 6 years, but that daily doses of greater than 500mg for extended periods can cause sensory neuropathy. Since April 2006, the Therapeutic Goods Administration in Australia (Therapeutic Goods Administration 2006) has required products containing pyridoxine, pyridoxal or pyridoxamine to carry a label stating 'this medicine may be dangerous when used in large amounts or for a large period of time', indicating that these findings are still relevant.

### 4.2.2 Vitamin B12

In the B12 randomised controlled trial by Bertoglio et al. (2010) reported side effects were increased hyperactivity and increased mouthing of objects. No serious adverse events were reported. The authors concluded that the mild nature, and limited number of side-effects observed, supports that subcutaneous administration of methyl B12 appears safe to use in autism.

### 4.2.3 Dimethylglycine (DMG)

In the DMG study by Kern et al. (2001), a greater number of adverse effects occurred in the placebo group than in the group receiving DMG. In the DMG group, 1 subject experienced difficulty sleeping, another experienced increased aggressiveness and 2 were reported to have hyperactivity. These same effects were observed in the placebo group, but in greater numbers. Bolman and Richmond (1999) reported that 1 subject became more 'edgy' during their DMG trial. The average scores on Rimland's checklist were lower with DMG than placebo for the areas of speech, cooperation, understanding, attention, bizarre behaviour, tantrums, and activity level, indicating an overall worsening of behaviour with DMG.

### 4.2.4 Vitamin C

The single publication located examining the use of high dose vitamin C in children with autism did not mention adverse effects (Dolske et al. 1993). The Natural Medicines Comprehensive Database (Natural Medicines Comprehensive Database 2011) and the Mayo Clinic (Mayo Clinic 2011) state that Vitamin C supplements are generally regarded as safe if used within recommended doses in the general population. Adverse effects are rarely reported and are dose-related. Such adverse effects can include nausea, vomiting, heartburn, abdominal cramps and headaches. Doses of vitamin C greater than the tolerable upper limit of intake have been associated with significant adverse effects such as kidney stones, severe diarrhoea, nausea and gastritis. In addition, large doses may precipitate haemolysis in patients with glucose-6-phosphate dehydrogenase deficiency (Mayo Clinic 2011). Rare reports of flushing, dizziness, faintness and fatigue have also been noted. There are also rare reports of scurvy due to tolerance or resistance following cessation after long-term use of vitamin C (Mayo Clinic 2011; Natural Medicines Comprehensive Database 2011).

### 4.2.5 Iron

In the iron study conducted by Dosman et al (2007), nine of the 33 (27%) children who completed the study experienced GI effects including constipation, loose stools abdominal pain and decreased appetite. However, there was a high rate of baseline GI symptoms in 76% (25/33) of participants. While it was reported that there was exacerbation of GI symptoms in some of the children (possibly related to the high dose of elemental iron administered) it was stated this was not a common reason for withdrawal from the study. Stained teeth were reported for two children (6%).

### 4.2.6 Probiotics

In the probiotic study conducted by Parracho et al. (2010), three subjects withdrew from the study because of adverse events. One experienced a skin rash three days after starting the first feeding period (probiotic) and withdrew from the study. Two further subjects withdrew from the study after the first washout period, one experienced diarrhoea during the probiotic feeding period and the other lost 1.2 kg during the probiotic feeding period.

The Mayo Clinic (Mayo Clinic 2011) and The Natural Medicines Comprehensive Database (Natural Medicines Comprehensive Database 2011) agree that the common probiotics *Lactobacillus acidophilus*, *Bifidobacteria* and *Saccharomyces boulardii* (taken orally) are well tolerated in the general population and few side effects are reported when used at recommended doses. Orally, probiotics can cause GI upset including: abdominal discomfort and flatulence. It is reported that this effect is usually transient and mild and subsides with continued use (Mayo Clinic 2011; Natural Medicines Comprehensive Database 2011). In addition, *Bifidobacteria* can cause diarrhoea in children (Natural Medicines Comprehensive Database 2011).

Since probiotic preparations contain live and active microorganisms there is concern that they might cause pathological infection in some patients. There have been rare reports of septicaemia (*Lactobacillus acidophilus* and *Bifidobacteria*) and fungaemia (*Saccharomyces boulardii*) in severely ill and/or immunocompromised patients. This effect would not be expected to occur from taking oral probiotics in most healthy patients (Mayo Clinic 2011; Natural Medicines Comprehensive Database 2011).

#### 4.2.7 Digestive enzymes

An open and uncontrolled trial that investigated the efficacy of a dietary enzyme supplement (ENZYMAID) in autism also investigated adverse effects (Brudnak et al. 2002). Six of the children (13%) enrolled in the study experienced adverse effects including: hyperactivity, increased aggression, increased self-stimulatory behaviours, diarrhoea, loose stools, provocation or red ears and cheeks, increased hunger and cessation of eating. In addition behavioural or medical side affects were listed as reasons for leaving the study.

In the randomised controlled trial investigating the efficacy of Peptizyde™, no serious adverse effects were noted during the study period (Munasinghe et al. 2010). Two children were observed by their parents to have transient behavioural deterioration which they initially attributed to commencement on capsules. The behaviours described included increased irritability and aggression and inattentiveness. Both families opted to discontinue the study, however, follow-up in subsequent weeks showed that the behavioural difficulties persisted despite cessation. A further two children were observed by their parents to have negative changes in behaviour again initially attributed to capsule use. The behaviours included irritability, and difficulties engaging in the classroom. Both opted to withdraw from the study, however, on follow-up felt that changing family and school environmental factors were probably the significant precipitants.

#### 4.2.8 Secretin

No serious adverse events, such as anaphylaxis, were reported in the 14 trials included in the systematic review of intravenous secretin use in autism (Williams et al. 2009). Some adverse effects possibly attributable to secretin were reported in some studies including rash, hyperactivity, fever, tachycardia, vomiting, photosensitivity, increased irritability and generalised flushing.

#### 4.2.9 Polyunsaturated fatty acids (PUFAs)

GI side effects are reported in the general population following treatment with PUFAs and include: nausea, diarrhoea, increased belching, acid/reflux/heartburn/ indigestion, abdominal bloating, and abdominal pain. Fishy after-taste is commonly experienced and rare reports of skin rash have occurred (Mayo Clinic 2011).

In the PUFA randomised controlled trial conducted by Amminger et al. (2007) where children with autism received a 6 week course of PUFAs or placebo, 1/13 children withdrew due to GI complaints and lack of perceived benefit. In another randomised controlled trial conducted by

Bent et al. (2010), no serious adverse events were reported during the study in the 27 participants, and there was no difference in the number of reported non-serious adverse events in the two treatment groups. 5/14 patients reported adverse events in the PUFA group (2 rashes, 1 upper respiratory infection, 1 nose bleed, 1 increased GI symptoms); 4/13 patients reported adverse events in the placebo group (3 increased hyperactivity, 1 increased self-stimulatory behaviour). In an uncontrolled study by Patrick and Salik (Patrick&Salik 2006), 2/22 children withdrew due to reports of increased physical activity, but no other adverse effects were noted. In another uncontrolled study, a "few parents" reported "increased hyperactivity and behavioral problems" (Bell et al. 2004). Two uncontrolled studies (Meguid et al. 2008; Politi et al. 2008) and a case report (Johnson&Hollander 2003) did not discuss whether adverse events were assessed. Meiri et al. (2009) conducted an open study where 9 children with autism received a 12 week course of PUFAs and no adverse effects were reported. A systematic review by Bent et al. (2009) that examined safety and efficacy of PUFAs in autism highlighted that most studies indicate that omega-3 fatty acids are relatively safe, although there are some concerns that it may increase the risk of bleeding (and therefore should be avoided in persons at increased risk for bleeding).

#### 4.2.10 Melatonin

In the randomised controlled trial of melatonin conducted by Garstang and Wallis (2006), adverse effects were not described. In the randomised controlled trial in 17 children with autism by Wright et al. (2011) adverse effects were low and similar between the two arms. The side effects that occurred more frequently in the melatonin arm were as follows: daytime drowsiness, reduced appetite, reduced alertness and diarrhoea however, differences in the frequency of these adverse effects were not statistically significant. The observational retrospective study in 107 children with autism conducted by Andersen et al. (2008) reported 3 children experienced mild adverse effects including increased enuresis, morning sleepiness and "fogginess". In Paavonen et al.'s study (2003) in a cohort of 15 children with AS one subject reported extreme tiredness, diarrhoea, headache and dizziness; one reported mild tiredness and headache on days 1 and 2 of the study and another reported prolonged wakeful periods at the beginning of the treatment. In the open prospective study in 20 young children with autism conducted by Gianotti et al. (2006) and the observational retrospective study in six adults with autism by Galli-Carminati (2009) no adverse effects were reported but were monitored for. A recent case series reported melatonin induced agitation in three patients with intellectual disability (Richings&Feroz-Nainar 2010).

In a recent review of the safety and efficacy of exogenous melatonin used for secondary sleep disorder in a more generalised population (Buscemi et al. 2006), it was reported that the most frequently-occurring adverse effects were headache, dizziness, nausea and drowsiness. However, the incidence of these effects was found to be similar during both the placebo and melatonin phases of trials. The safety review encompassed a total of 17 studies, both controlled and uncontrolled, with 651 participants overall. No mention of an increase in seizure frequency being caused by melatonin administration was made.

#### 4.2.11 Chelating therapies

Lonsdale et al. (2002) examined the efficacy of the chelating agent TTFD in autism in an open pilot study in children with autism aged 3 to 8 (n=10) The only adverse effect documented by Lonsdale et al. (2002) was parental reports of a 'skunk-like odour' in 9/10 subjects. There was also a worsening of autistic symptoms in 1 subject. According to the Mayo Clinic, long-term doses of thiamine up to 200mg daily are considered non-toxic, although doses greater than 100mg may result in drowsiness or muscle relaxation (Mayo Clinic 2011).

Adverse effects were monitored for in the study by Adams et al (2009a; 2009b) examining the chelating agent DMSA in autism. In phase one of the study: one "mild adverse reaction" (lethargy and decreased appetite) was reported. In Phase two, four participants dropped out due to adverse effects including sleep problems (one on DMSA); behaviour and some skills worsened (one on DMSA); worsened behaviour (two on placebo). Additionally, two participants on DMSA who ended the study early had moderate sleep problems (both children) and increased tantrums (one child) that resolved on stopping treatment.

Despite the availability of the studies of the chelating agent DMSA in autism that showed some benefits, and acceptable levels of tolerability in a limited number of children, there are significant concerns about the safety of chelation therapy in the management of autism. It is notable that a randomised controlled trial designed to examine the safety and efficacy of DMSA for mercury chelation in autism was halted by the US National Institute for Mental Health after an assessment that the study treatment presented more than minimal risk (Mitka 2008). This was partly due to a study in rats designed to assess the effects of chelation with DMSA following lead exposure. This study had the unexpected finding that a single 3-week course of succimer treatment in rats not exposed to lead during their early development produced lasting cognitive dysfunction when assessed over a 7-month period (Stangle et al. 2007).

Furthermore the US Food and Drug Administration (FDA) issued a warning in 2010 to manufacturers of a number of different chelation products available without prescription and readily obtained over the internet (FDA, 2011). The FDA has indicated that the companies have not provided evidence to substantiate their claims that their products are safe and effective in treating conditions such as ASD. The FDA has threatened legal action if companies continue to make unsubstantiated claims.

#### 4.2.12 Others

No studies of any description involving children with autism were located for the remainder of the interventions under investigation. Hence, safety of the remaining CAM products in autism could not be elucidated. The authors refer the reader to the monographs available through the Mayo Clinic website (Mayo Clinic 2011) and the Natural Medicines Comprehensive Database (Natural Medicines Comprehensive Database 2011) that both report side effects associated with taking a range of supplements in the general population.

## 5. Conclusion

Available evidence for efficacy and safety for a range of CAM products has been compiled that will equip health professionals with information so they can sensitively disclose and discuss CAM product usage with patients and their families. Therefore, health professionals can ethically and responsibly assist patients and caregivers with their decision making regarding CAM product usage. Pleasingly, when medical practitioners were surveyed regarding which CAMs they recommended to caregivers for their children with autism it was revealed it was the agents for which there is emerging evidence for benefit and reasonable safety profiles i.e. multivitamins (49%), PUFAs (25%), melatonin (25%) and probiotics (19%) (Golnik&Ireland 2009). On the other hand, 61% of medical practitioners surveyed reported they discourage use of chelation therapy which does not have evidence of benefit in the management of autism and potential safety risks (Golnik&Ireland 2009). The information compiled can also be accessed by researchers. This study highlights there is an urgent need for more well-designed clinical trials to improve the evidence base on which people with autism, caregivers and health care professionals can make decisions about treatment options. Health care professionals and caregivers need to be informed that for many CAM products, the rationale for use is only theoretical and not biologically proven. Further, the use of CAM products in autism is not risk-free and often lacks sound clinical evidence for efficacy.

## 6. References

Adams, J. B., Baral, M., Geis, E., Mitchell, J., Ingram, J., Hensley, A., et al. (2009a). Safety and efficacy of oral DMSA therapy for children with autism spectrum disorders: Part A--medical results. *BMC Clinical Pharmacology* Vol. 9 pp. 16.1472-6904 (Electronic)1472-6904 (Linking)

Adams, J. B., Baral, M., Geis, E., Mitchell, J., Ingram, J., Hensley, A., et al. (2009b). Safety and efficacy of oral DMSA therapy for children with autism spectrum disorders: part B - behavioral results. *BMC Clinical Pharmacology* Vol. 9 pp. 17.1472-6904 (Electronic)1472-6904 (Linking)

Adams, J. B. & Holloway, C. (2004). Pilot Study of a Moderate Dose Multivitamin/Mineral Supplement for Children with Autistic Spectrum Disorder. *The Journal of Alternative and Complementary Medicine* Vol. 10 No. 6: pp. 1033-1039

Amminger, G. P., Berger, G. E., Schafer, M. R., Klier, C., Friedrich, M. H. &Feucht, M. (2007). Omega-3 fatty acids supplementation in children with autism: a double-blind randomized, placebo-controlled pilot study. *Biological Psychiatry* Vol. 61 No. 4: pp. 551-553.0006-3223 (Print)0006-3223 (Linking)

Andersen, I. M., Kaczmarska, J., McGrew, S. G. &Malow, B. A. (2008). Melatonin for insomnia in children with autism spectrum disorders. *Journal of Child Neurology* Vol. 23 No. 5: pp. 482-485.0883-0738 (Print)0883-0738 (Linking)

Atwood, K. C. &Woeckner, E. (2009). In pediatric fatality, edetate disodium was no accident. *Clinical Toxicology (Philadelphia PA)* Vol. 47 No. 3: pp. 256; author reply 256-257.1556-9519 (Electronic)1556-3650 (Linking)

Barthelemy, C., Garreau, B., Leddet, I., Sauvage, D., Domenech, J., Muh, J. P., et al. (1980). Effets cliniques et biologiques de l'administration orale du magnésium seul ou du magnésium associé à la vitamine B6 sur certains troubles observés dans l'autisme infantile. *Thérapie* Vol. 35 No. 5: pp. 627-632

Barthelemy, C., Garreau, B., Leddet, I., Sauvage, D., Muh, J. P., Lelord, G., et al. (1983). Intérêt des échelles de comportement et des dosages de l'acide homovanilique urinaire pour le côntrole des effets d'un traitement associant vitamine B6 et magnésium chez des enfants ayant un comportement autistique. *Neuropsychiatrie de l'Enfance* Vol. 31 No. 5-6: pp. 289-301

Bell, J. G., MacKinlay, E. E., Dick, J. R., MacDonald, D. J., Boyle, R. M. &Glen, A. C. (2004). Essential fatty acids and phospholipase A2 in autistic spectrum disorders. *Prostaglandins Leukotrienes and Essential Fatty Acids* Vol. 71 No. 4: pp. 201-204

Bendich, A. &Cohen, M. (1990). Vitamin B6 safety issues. *Annals of the New York Academy of Sciences* Vol. 585 pp. 321-330

Bent, S., Bertoglio, K., Ashwood, P., Bostrom, A. &Hendren, R. L. (2010). A Pilot Randomized Controlled Trial of Omega-3 Fatty Acids for Autism Spectrum Disorder. *Journal of Autism & Developmental Disorders* DOI 10.1007/s10803-010-1078-8 (Electronic)0162-3257 (Linking)

Bent, S., Bertoglio, K. &Hendren, R. L. (2009). Omega-3 fatty acids for autistic spectrum disorder: a systematic review. *Journal of Autism & Developmental Disorders* Vol. 39 No. 8: pp. 1145-1154.1573-3432 (Electronic)0162-3257 (Linking)

Bertoglio, K., James, S. J., Deprey, L., Brule, N. &Hendren, R. (2010). Pilot study of the effect of methyl B12 treatment on behavioural and biomarker measures in children with autism. *The Journal of Alternative and Complementary Medicine* Vol. 16 No. 5: pp. 555-560

Bolman WM &Richmond JA (1999). A double-blind, placebo-controlled, cross-over pilot trial of low dose dimethylglycine in patients with autistic disorder. *Journal of Autism & Developmental Disorders* Vol. 29 No.: pp. 191-194

Brudnak, M. A., Rimland, B., Kerry, R. E., Dailey, M., Taylor, R., Stayton, B., et al. (2002). Enzyme-based therapy for autism spectrum disorders--is it worth another look? *Medical Hypotheses* Vol. 58 No. 5: pp. 422-428

Buscemi, N., Vandermeer, B., Hooton, N., Pandya, R., Tjosvold, L., Hartling, L., et al. (2006). Efficacy and safety of exogenous melatonin for secondary sleep disorders and sleep disorders accompanying sleep restriction: meta-analysis. *British Medical Journal* Vol. 332 No. 7538: pp. 385-393.1468-5833 (Electronic)0959-535X (Linking)

Cohen, M. &Bendich, A. (1986). Safety of Pyridoxine - a review of human and animal studies. *Toxicology Letters* Vol. 34 No. 2-3: pp. 129-139

Dolske, M. C., Spollen, J., McKay, S., Lancashire, E. &Tolbert, L. (1993). A preliminary trial of ascorbic acid as supplemental therapy for autism. *Progress in Neuro-Psychopharmacology & Biological Psychiatry* Vol. 17 No. 5: pp. 765-774.0278-5846

Dosman, C. F., Brian, J. A., Drmic, I. E., Senthilselvan, A., Harford, M. M., Smith, R. W., et al. (2007). Children with autism: effect of iron supplementation on sleep and ferritin. *Pediatric Neurology* Vol. 36 No. 3: pp. 152-158.0887-8994 (Print)0887-8994 (Linking)

FDA. FDA Warns Marketers of Unapproved 'Chelation' Drugs. In. Retrieved March 23, Available from: http://www.fda.gov/ForConsumers/ConsumerUpdates/ucm229358.htm

Findling RL, Maxwell K, Scotese WL, Huang J, Yamashita T &Wiznitzer M (1997). High-dose pyridoxine and magnesium administration in children with autistic disorder: An absence of salutary effects in a double blind, placebo-controlled study. *Journal of Autism & Developmental Disorders* Vol. 27 pp. 467-478

Galli-Carminati, G., Chauvet, I. &Deriaz, N. (2006). Prevalence of gastrointestinal disorders in adult clients with pervasive developmental disorders. *Journal of Intellectual Disability Research* Vol. 50 No. 10: pp. 711-718.0964-2633 (Print)0964-2633 (Linking)

Galli-Carminati, G., Deriaz, N. &Bertschy, G. (2009). Melatonin in treatment of chronic sleep disorders in adults with autism: a retrospective study. *Swiss Medical Weekly* Vol. 139 No. 19-20: pp. 293-296.1424-7860 (Print)0036-7672 (Linking)

Garstang, J. &Wallis, M. (2006). Randomized controlled trial of melatonin for children with autistic spectrum disorders and sleep problems. *Child: Care, Health & Development* Vol. 32 No. 5: pp. 585-589.0305-1862 (Print)0305-1862 (Linking)

Giannotti, F., Cortesi, F., Cerquiglini, A. &Bernabei, P. (2006). An open-label study of controlled-release melatonin in treatment of sleep disorders in children with autism. *Journal of Autism & Developmental Disorders* Vol. 36 No. 6: pp. 741-752.0162-3257 (Print)0162-3257 (Linking)

Golnik, A. E. &Ireland, M. (2009). Complementary alternative medicine for children with autism: a physician survey. *Journal of Autism & Developmental Disorders* Vol. 39 No. 7: pp. 996-1005.1573-3432 (Electronic)0162-3257 (Linking)

Green, V. A., Pituch, K. A., Itchon, J., Choi, A., O'Reilly, M. &Sigafoos, J. (2006). Internet survey of treatments used by parents of children with autism. *Research in Developmental Disabilities* Vol. 27 No. 1: pp. 70-84.0891-4222 (Print)Jadad, A. R., Moore, R. A., Carroll, D., Jenkinson, C., Reynolds, D. J., Gavaghan, D. J., et al. (1996). Assessing the quality of reports of randomized clinical trials: is blinding necessary? *Controlled Clinical Trials* Vol. 17 No. 1: pp. 1-12.0197-2456

James, S. J., Cutler, P., Melnyk, S., Jernigan, S., Janak, L., Gaylor, D. W., et al. (2004). Metabolic biomarkers of increased oxidative stress and impaired methylation capacity in children with autism. *American Journal of Clinical Nutrition* Vol. 80 No. 6: pp. 1611-1617

James, S. J., Melnyk, S., Fuchs, G., Reid, T., Jernigan, S., Pavliv, O., et al. (2009). Efficacy of methylcobalamin and folinic acid treatment on glutathione redox status in children with autism. *American Journal of Clinical Nutrition* Vol. 89 pp. 425-430

Johnson, S. M. &Hollander, E. (2003). Evidence that eicosapentaenoic acid is effective in treating autism. *Journal of Clinical Psychiatry* Vol. 64 No. 7: pp. 848-849

Jonas, C., Etienne, T., Barthelemy, C., Jouve, J. &Mariotte, N. (1984). Intérêt clinique et biochimique de l'association vitamine B6 + magnésium dans le traitement de l'autisme résiduel à l'âge adulte. *Thérapie* Vol. 39 No. 6: pp. 661-669

Kern JK, Miller VS, Cauller L, Kendall R, Mehta J &Dodd M (2001). Effectiveness of N,N-Dimethylglycine in Autism and Pervasive Developmental Disorder. *Journal of Child Neurology* Vol. 16 No. 3: pp. 169-173

Kuriyama S, Kamiyama M, Watanabe M, Tamahashi S, Muraguchi I, Watanabe T, et al. (2002). Pyridoxine treatment in a subgroup of children with pervasive developmental disorders. *Developmental Medicine and Child Neurology* Vol. 44 pp. 284-286

Latif, A., Heinz, P. &Cook, R. (2002). Iron deficiency in autism and Asperger syndrome. *Autism* Vol. 6 No. 1: pp. 103-114.1362-3613

Lelord, G., Callaway, E. &Muh, J. P. (1982). Clinical and Biological Effects of High Doses of Vitamin B6 and Magnesium on Autistic Children. *Acta Vitaminologica et Enzymologica* Vol. 4 No. 1-2: pp. 27-44

Lelord, G., Callaway, E., Muh, J. P., Arlot, J. C., Sauvage, D., Garreau, B., et al. (1978). L'acide homovanilique urinaire et ses modifications par ingestion de vitamine B6: exploration fonctionelle dans l'autisme de l'enfant? *Rev. Neurol. (Paris)* Vol. 134 No. 12: pp. 797-801

Lelord, G., Muh, J. P., Barthelemy, C., Martineau, J. &Garreau, B. (1981). Effects of Pyridoxine and Magnesium on Autistic Symptoms - Initial Observations. *Journal of Autism & Developmental Disorders* Vol. 11 No. 2: pp. 219-230

Levy, S. E. &Hyman, S. L. (2003). Use of complementary and alternative treatments for children with autistic spectrum disorders is increasing. *Pediatric Annals* Vol. 32 No. 10: pp. 685-691

Lonsdale D, Shamberger RJ &Audhya T (2002). Treatment of autism spectrum children with thiamine tetrahydrofurfuryl disulfide: A pilot study. *Neuroendocrinology Letters* Vol. 23 pp. 303-308

Martineau, J., Barthelemy, C., Cheliakine, C. &Lelord, G. (1988). Brief Report: An Open Middle-Term Study of Combined Vitamin B6-Magnesium in a Subgroup of Autistic

Children Selected on Their Sensitivity to This Treatment. *Journal of Autism & Developmental Disorders* Vol. 18 No. 3: pp. 435-447

Martineau, J., Barthelemy, C., Garreau, B. &Lelord, G. (1985). Vitamin B6, Magnesium, and Combined B6-Mg: Therapeutic Effects in Childhood Autism. *Biological Psychiatry* Vol. 20 pp. 467-478

Martineau, J., Barthelemy, C. &Lelord, G. (1986). Long-Term Effects of Combined Vitamin B6-Magnesium Administration in an Autistic Child. *Biological Psychiatry* Vol. 21 pp. 511-518

Martineau, J., Barthelemy, C., Roux, S., Garreau, B. &Lelord, G. (1989). Electrophysiological effects of fenfluramine or combined vitamin B6 and magnesium on children with autistic behaviour. *Developmental Medicine and Child Neurology* Vol. 31 pp. 721-727

Martineau, J., Garreau, B., Barthelemy, C., Callaway, E. &Lelord, G. (1981). Effects of Vitamin B6 on Average Evoked Potentials in Infantile Autism. *Biological Psychiatry* Vol. 16 No. 7: pp. 627-641

Mayo Clinic (2011). MayoClinic.com: tools for healthier lives. In. Retrieved 8 September 2010 - 1 April 2011, Available from: http://www.mayoclinic.com

Meguid, N. A., Atta, H. M., Gouda, A. S. &Khalil, R. O. (2008). Role of polyunsaturated fatty acids in the management of Egyptian children with autism. *Clinical Biochemistry* Vol. 41 No. 13: pp. 1044-1048.1873-2933 (Electronic)0009-9120 (Linking)

Meiri, G., Bichovsky, Y. &Belmaker, R. H. (2009). Omega 3 fatty acid treatment in autism. *Journal of Child & Adolescent Psychopharmacology* Vol. 19 No. 4: pp. 449-451.1557-8992 (Electronic)1044-5463 (Linking)

Ménage, P., Thibault, G., Barthelemy, C., Lelord, G. &Bardos, P. (1992). CD4+CD45RA+T Lymphocyte Deficiency in Autistic Children: Effect of a Pyridoxine-Magnesium Treatment. *Brain Dysfunction* Vol. 5 pp. 326-333

Mitka, M. (2008). Chelation therapy trials halted. *Journal of the American Medical Association* Vol. 300 No. 19: pp. 2236.1538-3598 (Electronic)0098-7484 (Linking)

Moretti, P., Peters, S. U., Del Gaudio, D., Sahoo, T., Hyland, K., Bottiglieri, T., et al. (2008). Brief report: autistic symptoms, developmental regression, mental retardation, epilepsy, and dyskinesias in CNS folate deficiency. *Journal of Autism & Developmental Disorders* Vol. 38 No. 6: pp. 1170-1177.0162-3257 (Print)0162-3257 (Linking)

Moretti, P., Sahoo, T., Hyland, K., Bottiglieri, T., Peters, S., del Gaudio, D., et al. (2005). Cerebral folate deficiency with developmental delay, autism, and response to folinic acid. *Neurology* Vol. 64 No. 6: pp. 1088-1090.1526-632X (Electronic)0028-3878 (Linking)

Mousain-Bosc, M., Roche, M., Polge, A., Pradal-Prat, D., Rapin, J. &Bali, J. P. (2006). Improvement of neurobehavioral disorders in children supplemented with magnesium-vitamin B6. II. Pervasive developmental disorder-autism. *Magnesium Research* Vol. 19 No. 1: pp. 53-62.0953-1424 (Print)0953-1424 (Linking)

Munasinghe, S. A., Oliff, C., Finn, J. &Wray, J. A. (2010). Digestive enzyme supplementation for autism spectrum disorders: a double-blind randomized controlled trial. *Journal of Autism & Developmental Disorders* Vol. 40 No. 9: pp. 1131-1138.1573-3432 (Electronic)0162-3257 (Linking)

Natural Medicines Comprehensive Database (2011). Monographs. In. Retrieved 3 March 2011, Available from: http://www.naturaldatabase.com/(S(i2p051ajm3jul455nejtyui1))/home.aspx?li=0&st=0&cs=&s=ND

Natural Standard Research Collaboration (2010). Natural Standard evidence-based validated grading rationale ™. In. Retrieved November 16, 2010, Available from: http://www.naturalstandard.com/grading.asp

Paavonen EJ, Nieminen-von Wendt T, Vanhala R, Aronen ET &von Wendt L (2003). Effectiveness of Melatonin in the Treatment of Sleep Disturbances in Children with Asperger Disorder. *Journal of Child and Adolescent Psycopharmacology* Vol. 13 No. 1: pp. 83-95

Parracho, H. M. R. T., Gibson, G. R., Knott, F., Bosscher, D., Kleerebezem, M. &McCartney, A. L. (2010). A double-blind, placebo-controlled, crossover-designed probiotic feeding study in children diagnosed with autistic spectrum disorders. *International Journal of Probiotics and Prebiotics* Vol. 5 No. 2: pp. 69-74

Patrick, L. &Salik, R. (2005). Autism; Study shows benefits for autism, Asperger syndrome with fatty acid supplements. *Science Letter* Vol. pp. 95.1538-9111

Politi, P., Cena, H., Comelli, M., Marrone, G., Allegri, C., Emanuele, E., et al. (2008). Behavioral effects of omega-3 fatty acid supplementation in young adults with severe autism: an open label study. *Archives of Medical Research* Vol. 39 No. 7: pp. 682-685.0188-4409 (Print)0188-4409 (Linking)

Ramaekers, V. T., Blau, N., Sequeira, J. M., Nassogne, M. C. &Quadros, E. V. (2007). Folate receptor autoimmunity and cerebral folate deficiency in low-functioning autism with neurological deficits. *Neuropediatrics* Vol. 38 No. 6: pp. 276-281.0174-304X (Print)0174-304X (Linking)

Richings, C. &Feroz-Nainar, C. (2010). Case series: melatonin induced agitation in three patients with intellectual disability. *The British Journal of Developmental Disabilities* Vol. 56 No. 110: pp. 77-82

Rimland, B., Callaway, E. &Dreyfus, P. (1978). The Effect of High Doses of Vitamin B6 on Autistic Children: A Double-Blind Crossover Study. *American Journal of Psychiatry* Vol. 135 No. 4: pp. 472-475

Stangle, D. E., Smith, D. R., Beaudin, S. A., Strawderman, M. S., Levitsky, D. A. &Strupp, B. J. (2007). Succimer chelation improves learning, attention, and arousal regulation in lead-exposed rats but produces lasting cognitive impairment in the absence of lead exposure. *Environmental Health Perspectives* Vol. 115 No. 2: pp. 201-209.0091-6765 (Print)0091-6765 (Linking)

Therapeutic Goods Administration (2006). Required Advisory Statements for Medicine Labels. In. Retrieved 5-7-10, Available from: http://www.tga.gov.au/meds/rasml.pdf

Tolbert L, Haigler T, Waits MM &Dennis T (1993). Brief Report: Lack of Response in an Autistic Population to a Low Dose Clinical Trial of Pyridoxine Plus Magnesium. *Journal of Autism & Developmental Disorders* Vol. 23 No. 1: pp. 193-199

Williams, K. W., Wray, J. J. &Wheeler, D. M. (2009). Intravenous secretin for autism spectrum disorder. *Cochrane Database of Systematic Reviews* No. 3: pp. CD003495.1469-493X (Electronic)1361-6137 (Linking)

Wright, B., Sims, D., Smart, S., Alwazeer, A., Alderson-Day, B., Allgar, V., et al. (2011). Melatonin versus placebo in children with autism spectrum conditions and severe sleep problems not amenable to behaviour management strategies: a randomised controlled crossover trial. *Journal of Autism & Developmental Disorders* Vol. 41 No. 2: pp. 175-184.

5

# Neurofeedback Treatment for Autism Spectrum Disorders – Scientific Foundations and Clinical Practice

Mirjam E.J. Kouijzer, Hein T. van Schie,
Berrie J.L. Gerrits, and Jan M.H. de Moor
*Behavioural Science Institute, Radboud University Nijmegen*
*The Netherlands*

## 1. Introduction

Neurofeedback is a technique to enable individuals to change their brain activity by using an instrument that provides information on the activity of the brain. The goal of neurofeedback is to improve behavioral or cognitive processes related to brain activity. The technique of neurofeedback, although available for some time, is rapidly gaining interest as a treatment of various disorders (Yucha & Montgomery, 2008). Recent evidence indicates that the technique may also be used beneficially for the treatment of autism spectrum disorders.

Currently, the most frequent application of neurofeedback lies in the treatment of epilepsy and attention deficit hyperactivity disorder (ADHD). Epilepsy has been treated with neurofeedback since the 70s of the previous century. Epilepsy is a chronic neurological disorder characterized by abnormal, excessive or synchronous neuronal activity in the brain resulting in seizures. The main focus of neurofeedback in epilepsy is to enhance the sensorimotor rhythm (SMR) originating from the sensorimotor cortex of the brain. This 12 to 15 Hz activity is involved in the inhibition and control of movement. Increased SMR is found to be related to improved movement inhibition and consequently offers protection to seizures in individuals with epilepsy (Sterman & Egner, 2006). Scientific studies that investigated the efficacy of neurofeedback in individuals with epilepsy were recently evaluated by Tan and colleagues (2009). They found that in a total of nine studies, neurofeedback was effective in reducing the number of seizures in 79% of participants with severe epilepsy who did not respond to medication. The number of sessions that was used in these studies varied from 24 to more than 200 sessions. It was concluded that neurofeedback is a promising treatment for individuals with severe epilepsy, but that future randomized, sham controlled studies are required to confirm the efficacy of neurofeedback (Tan et al., 2009).

Most research on neurofeedback has been conducted in individuals with ADHD. ADHD is a developmental disorder characterized by inattention, hyperactivity and impulsivity (American Psychiatric Association, 2000). The EEG profiles of 85 to 90% of the individuals with ADHD show elevated theta power and reduced beta power over frontal and central, midline cortical brain areas (Monastra et al., 2005). Neurofeedback in ADHD aims to inhibit theta power and to elevate beta power in these cases. A recent meta-analysis on the efficacy of EEG-biofeedback in ADHD (Arns, de Ridder, Strehl, Breteler, & Coenen, 2009) demonstrated large effects on clinical symptoms of inattention and impulsivity and a medium effect on symptoms of hyperactivity. These conclusions, however, are mainly based on studies that were non-randomized and used no blinding of participants. Therefore, a conclusion on the efficacy of neurofeedback in ADHD is still preliminary at this point.

Neurofeedback has recently also been applied to individuals with autism. The term autism in this chapter refers to disorders of the entire autistic spectrum. The present chapter first provides an overview of the history of neurofeedback, followed by a detailed explanation of the practice of the technique as it is used in clinical practices. We furthermore describe what is known about working mechanisms that are involved in neurofeedback and provide an overview of the benefits of neurofeedback for individuals with autism. Finally, we review the existing literature on neurofeedback and autism and discuss several options for future research.

## 2. The origin of neurofeedback

The origin of neurofeedback goes back to the 1960s when Joseph Kamiya successfully trained human individuals to control alpha waves. Alpha waves are oscillations in the 8 to 12 Hz frequency range that are predominantly generated in occipital and parietal lobes and can be recorded during wakeful relaxation with eyes closed. In the experiment by Kamiya, participants were instructed to indicate whether they thought they were 'in alpha', i.e. whether their brain produced alpha as the dominant frequency, or not each time a tone sounded. They received feedback on whether the answer was correct or not. Initially the participants answered correct in about fifty percent of the trials. After alpha training was provided, some participants developed the ability to recognize the alpha state and to answer correctly in most of the trials. In a second experiment, the same participants were asked to go into the alpha state when a tone sounded once and not to go into the alpha state when the tone sounded twice. Interestingly, Kamiya found that some participants were able to enter the alpha state on command, whereas others were not (Kamiya, 1968).

Around the same time, Barry Sterman accidentally discovered the curative power of neurofeedback for patients with epilepsy. Sterman set up an experiment where he taught cats to produce 12 to 15 Hz oscillations along the sensorimotor cortex of the brain. He rewarded the cats with milk each time they produced 12 to 15 Hz oscillations and concluded that cats could learn to increase the sensorimotor rhythm (SMR). Increased SMR brought the motor suppression response under experimental control and helped to reduce muscle tone, reflex amplitudes, and cellular discharge in motor pathways. After this experiment ended, the cats were used for another experiment investigating the toxic symptoms of exposure to rocket fuel. Sterman's cats turned out to be more seizure resistant than cats that had not received SMR training (Wyricka & Sterman, 1968). It took only a few years before Sterman treated the first human patients with epilepsy. These patients showed a reduction of electroencephalographic and clinical epileptic manifestations after three months of SMR training (Sterman, Macdonald, & Stone, 1974).

Joel Lubar continued Sterman's work and used SMR training in patients with ADHD to reduce hyperactivity. Lubar and Shouse (1976) reported the results of 142 neurofeedback sessions in an 11-year old boy with ADHD who was trained to enhance SMR and to reduce theta power. After several months, the boy showed less undirected activities, less out-of-seat behavior, and less oppositional behaviors. In addition, there was increased cooperation and improvement in school work. In the reversal phase of the study, the boy's behavior and school work were found to worsen and to improve again when the initial training was recommenced.

Margaret Ayers, fascinated by the outcomes of these experimental studies, opened the first neurofeedback practice in 1975. One of her patients was Brian, a boy with severe epilepsy whose severe epilepsy significantly reduced after neurofeedback treatment. The parents of Brian, Siegfried and Sue Othmer, were impressed by the results of neurofeedback in their son. They started to promote neurofeedback in the United States of America. In 1987 they introduced a computerized neurofeedback tool and subsequently started a clinical practice for neurofeedback.

After these initial cases, the application of neurofeedback in patients with epilepsy and ADHD further extended in the 90s of the previous century. Subsequently, neurofeedback has also been applied in healthy individuals and in patients with various other disorders like depression, learning disability, post traumatic stress disorder, traumatic brain injury, and autism spectrum disorders (see review in: Yucha & Montgommery, 2008).

## 3. The practice of neurofeedback

In a typical neurofeedback session, a client sits in front of a computer screen while his or her electroencephalographic (EEG) activity is recorded by one or more electrodes. Figure 1 shows an example of the set up of a neurofeedback session in which a Nexus-4 device (MindMedia, the Netherlands) was used.

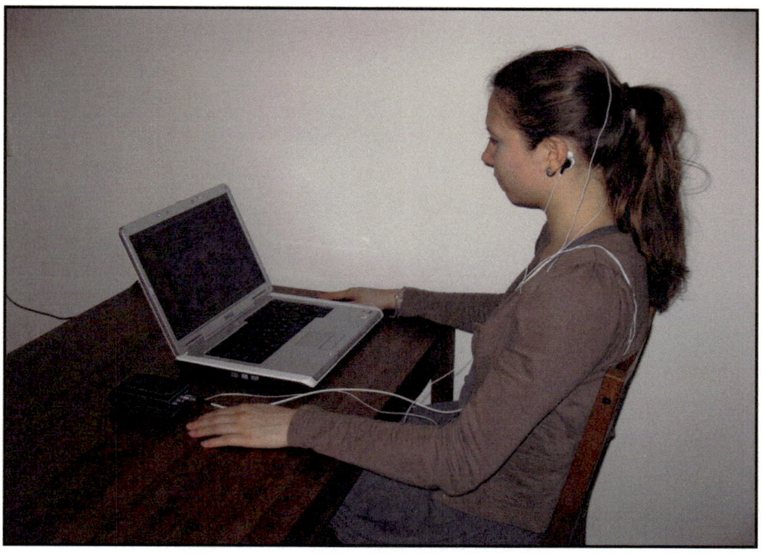

Fig. 1. An example of the set up of a neurofeedback session.

Before a client can commence with neurofeedback treatment, a treatment plan needs to be determined specifying the frequency component (or components) that is to be altered and the exact locations on the scalp at which training will take place. In the field of neurofeedback, such a treatment plan is often referred to as a treatment protocol. The

components and locations for training of such a treatment protocol are typically determined by comparing a 19-channel EEG recording of the client with a normative database containing the EEG spectra of typically developing individuals of the same age.
Typically, an EEG recording is collected using a stretchable electrode cap that contains multiple electrodes to map the distribution of brain waves over multiple sites on the scalp. Each of the electrodes is connected to the client's scalp using a conductive electro gel. Figure 2 shows an example of the experimental setup of an EEG assessment using the Mitsar EEG 201 System (Mitsar Medical Diagnostic Equipment, Russia). Following the correct preparation of all electrodes in the cap, a client's EEG is recorded for several minutes in one or more conditions. The conditions eyes opened and eyes closed are usually included in the EEG assessment. In these conditions, the client is instructed to sit still on a comfortable chair while keeping the eyes opened or closed. Next to the recording of EEG in these rest conditions, the EEG may be recorded in task conditions like reading or math.

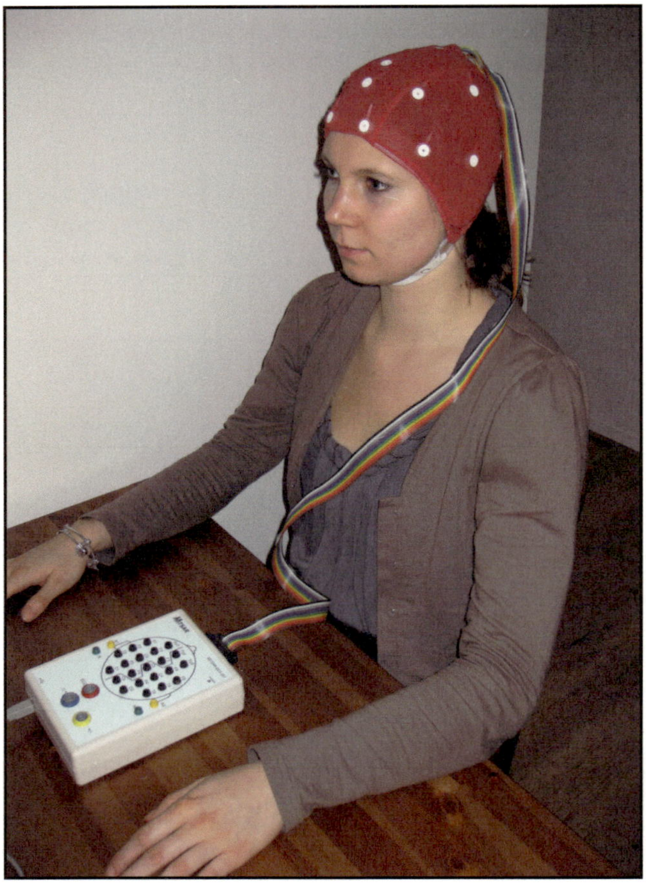

Fig. 2. An example of the set up of a 19-channel EEG assessment using the Mitsar EEG 201 System.

Raw EEG recordings are analyzed to construct a quantitative EEG (QEEG) containing the absolute and relative power spectra of the client's EEG per electrode. Relative power expresses the ratio of power in a particular frequency band relative to the total power across frequencies. The client's absolute and relative QEEG data may be subsequently compared with a normative database containing EEG data of healthy individuals of the same age to estimate possible deviations from normality. Two databases that are often used are NxLink designed by John, Prischep, & Easton (NxLink, Ltd.) and NeuroGuide, designed by Thatcher (Applied Neuroscience, Inc.). These databases produce color-coded maps and data in digital format, providing information on a client's deviations from the norm group. The output of such a database comparison may be used to guide the selection of the frequency components and the location for the subsequent neurofeedback treatment.

Figure 3 shows part of the output of the NeuroGuide database revealed by comparing the QEEG of a 15-year old girl with Asperger disorder to this database. The maps indicate that, relative to the database, power in the theta range over central and frontal electrodes exceeds the population mean, i.e. a population of girls of the same age without an autism spectrum disorder, by more than one and a half standard deviations. As a consequence, neurofeedback might, in this case, target the inhibition of 3 to 7 Hz power over fronto-central scalp regions.

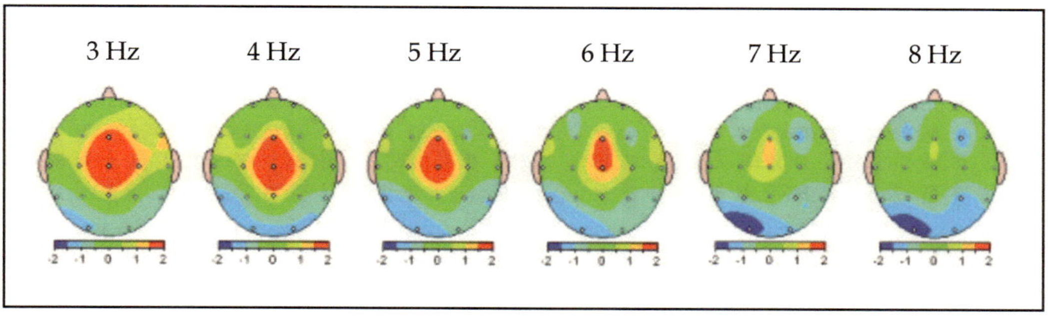


Fig. 3. An example of the output of a comparison between the QEEG of a 15-year old girl with Asperger disorder and the NeuroGuide database. Across fronto-central scalp sites a deviation of one and a half standard deviation is seen (color coded in red) of low frequency power in the 3-7 Hz frequency range compared to a norm group of girls with same age, without autism.

In addition to the method of using a database to determine possible frequency components and locations for training, a neurofeedback protocol may also be specified by visual inspection of the raw 19-channel EEG recording of the client. This procedure requires extensive knowledge of the raw EEG. A raw EEG signal is composed of separate brain waves with different frequencies and amplitudes, often arranged in separate frequency bands, i.e. delta (1-3 Hz) theta (4-7 Hz), alpha (8-12 Hz), beta (13-30 Hz), and gamma (above 30 Hz). These frequency bands can be identified in the raw EEG on the basis of the unique waveform patterns of each frequency band. Figure 4 shows an example of raw EEG data of a 10-year old boy with PDD-NOS in WinEEG software (Mitsar Medical Diagnostic Equipment, Russia). This example includes raw EEG activity measured by electrodes across several frontal sites. Visual inspection of this EEG fragment reveals clear theta activity at electrode Fz, which is indicated by the black arrow.

Instead of using individualized treatment plans wherein the frequency component and treatment location are determined on the basis of an individual's EEG characteristics, neurofeedback treatment may also be guided by predefined treatment protocols. Probably

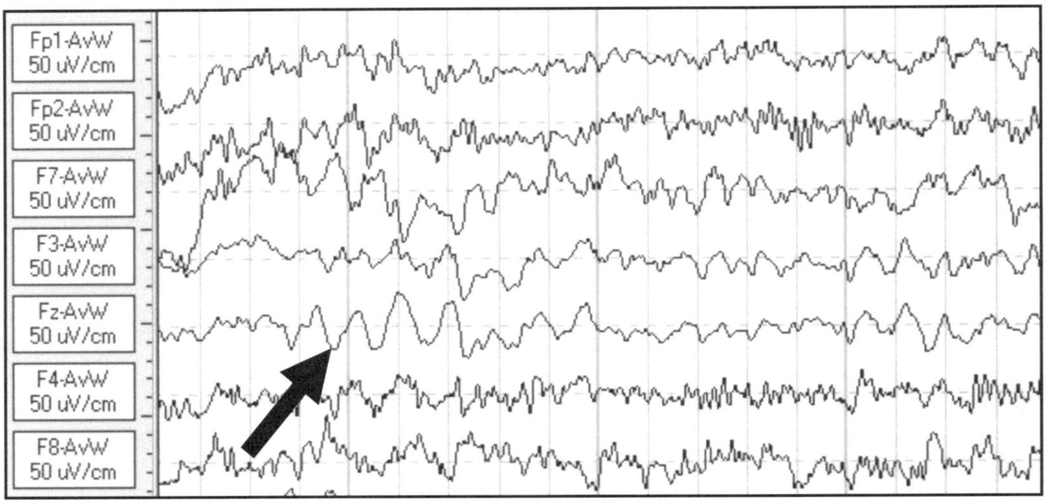


Fig. 4. Raw EEG data of a 10-year old boy with PDD-NOS in WinEEG software. The black arrow indicates the theta activity that is observed at electrode Fz.

the best known protocol is the theta/beta protocol that is used often in the treatment of ADHD. This protocol prescribes the decrease of theta power while beta power is increased at frontal or central, midline regions (Monastra et al., 2005). This protocol was developed after the finding that 85 to 90% of the individuals with ADHD have elevated theta power and reduced beta power over frontal and central, midline cortical regions of the brain (Monastra et al., 2005). Although the theta/beta protocol was originally applied to individuals with ADHD, this neurofeedback protocol has also been applied successfully to individuals with autism (Jarusiewicz, 2002; Kouijzer et al., 2009b; Scolnick, 2005; Sichel, Fehmi, & Goldstein, 1995; Thompson, Thompson, & Reid, 2010).

After a treatment plan has been established, the actual neurofeedback treatment may commence. In each neurofeedback session, an electrode needs to be attached to the selected treatment location by using conductive electrode paste. In addition, reference and ground electrodes are to be attached. Often the reference electrode is located somewhere on the head at a location where little or no of the frequency component that is selected for treatment is found, e.g. at an earlobe or at the bone behind one of the ears, i.e. the mastoid. The ground electrode is typically placed somewhere on the body, e.g. at the mastoid. Figure 5 provides an example of electrode configuration during a typical neurofeedback session, showing an EEG electrode that is used for feedback attached to the scalp (in red) and a reference electrode (in black) attached to the left mastoid.

During a neurofeedback session, information about the level of EEG activity in the frequency component that was selected for training is fed back to the client. Although in principle feedback may take any form or modality, most neurofeedback therapists use a bar graph on the computer screen to reflect the ongoing changes in EEG power over time. Figure 6 shows an example of such a computer screen created with BioTrace software (MindMedia, the Netherlands). The larger the amplitude of the recorded EEG activity is, the higher the orange bar graph on the computer screen will be presented. In this way, the bar graph informs the client about the amplitude of his or her EEG activity, almost immediately after it occurs. A criterion line is drawn together with the bar graph representing a concrete

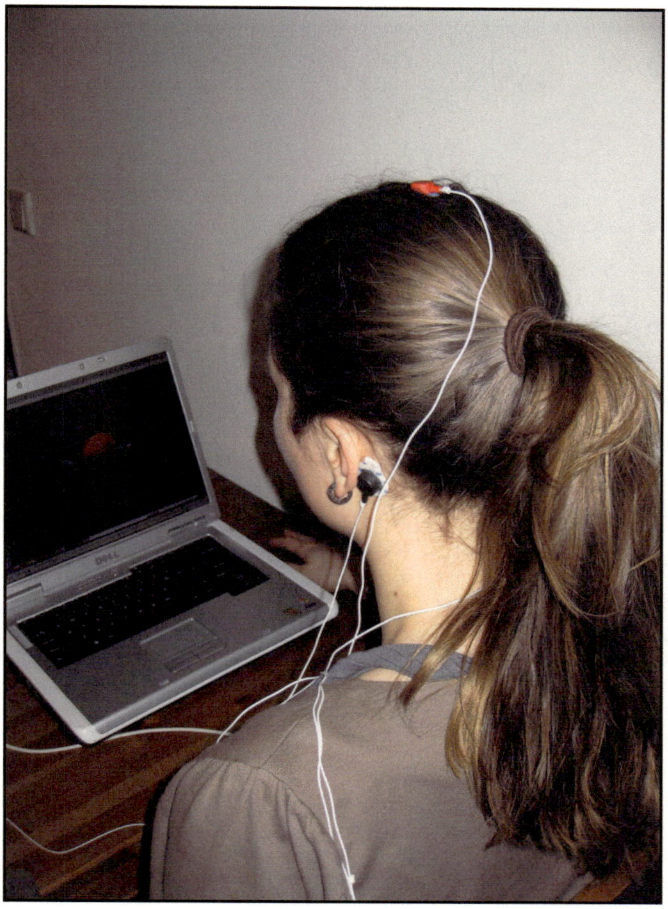

Fig. 5. Electrodes attached to the scalp and the mastoid during neurofeedback.

goal for the trainee. That is, depending on the treatment plan (i.e. increase or decrease activation in a particular frequency range), the client may be directed at keeping the bar graph amplitude beneath or above the criterion line. At first, meeting the criterion is accidental, but over time participants may learn to maintain the bar graph below or above the indicated criterion.

Whenever the client manages to keep the bar graph below or above the criterion line for a minimal amount of time, visual and auditory rewards may be provided, often in the form of a film clip presented next to the bar graph. Film clips are usually presented with corresponding music or sound and are chosen according to to the age and interests of the client. Clients can also be rewarded by a counter that counts the number of seconds the criterion is met. If desired, the bar graph can change color when the EEG activity is not within the desired range, or the film clip can shrink to remove the reward. Some clients with autism show resistance to the combination of many different rewards, such as a shrinking film clip, music, a counter, and a color changing bar graph. Therefore, the exact form in which the reward is presented should reflect the preferences of the client.

A typical neurofeedback session consists of training and rest intervals. During training intervals, the client's goal is to move the bar graph below or above a criterion line. These

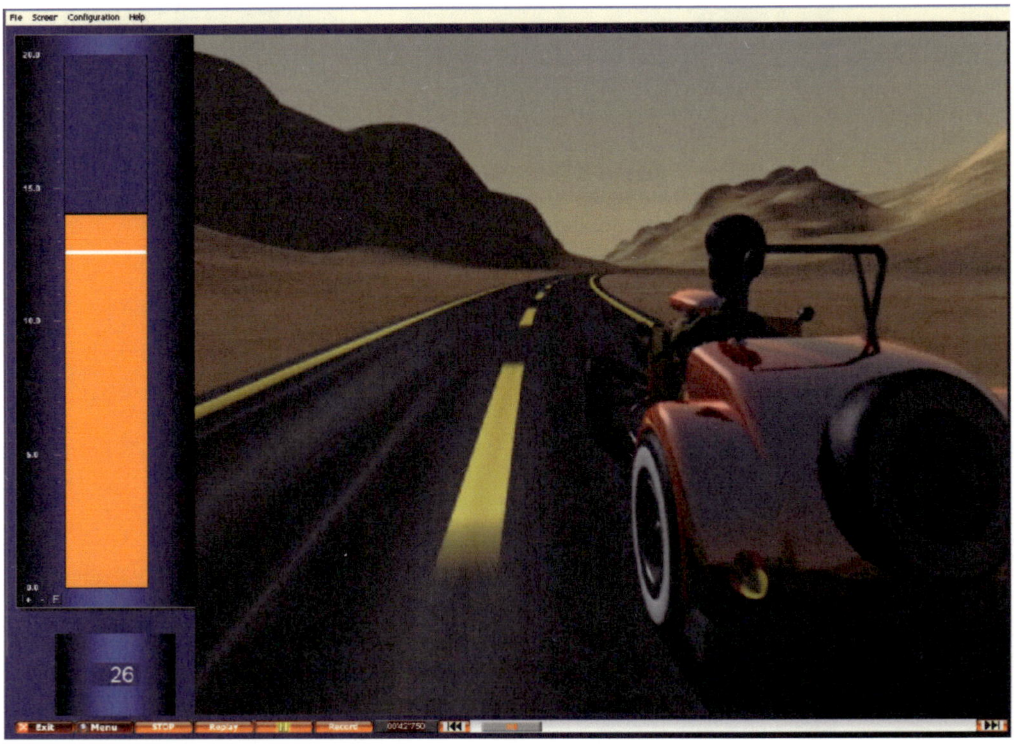


Fig. 6. An example of a computer screen where the mean amplitude of the EEG frequency of interest is fed back to the client via an orange bar graph with a white criterion line. In addition, a film clip and a counter are shown as rewards for the client.

training intervals are alternated with rest intervals, in which the client can relax for a short time. The length of the training intervals depends largely on the attention span of the client. Clients with a larger attention span may be presented with longer training intervals. A training interval of three minutes was chosen in several studies where neurofeedback was applied in children and adolescents with autism (e.g. Kouijzer et al., under review). If necessary, the length of training intervals may be adapted during the course of the training. Training and rest intervals are alternated manually or by predefined scripts. Clients with a high need for structure, like many clients within the autistic spectrum, might benefit from the accuracy that is provided by such a script.

Neurofeedback training is usually provided in psychological practices and typically takes place twice or thrice per week. Some neurofeedback therapists provide home training programs. The number of sessions is determined by the specific complaints of the client and on the progression of the client during the training. Neurofeedback for individuals with autism generally includes at least 40 sessions.

## 4. Cognitive and neuronal mechanisms underlying neurofeedback

Although the number of publications on the effects of neurofeedback is growing, little has been written about the actual functional and neuronal mechanisms that may be involved in its application and its resulting effects. In this paragraph we present an overview of several functional and neuronal mechanisms that may play a role in changing brain activation via neurofeedback and discuss why some individuals are responsive to the application of neurofeedback whereas others are not. We end with a discussion on possible neural mechanisms in autism that may be targeted by neurofeedback.

### 4.1 Functional mechanisms underlying neurofeedback

Operant conditioning involves a process of behavior modification whereby the consequences of an action determine the likelihood that the same action will be expressed in the future. Positively reinforced actions will be performed more frequently, whereas negatively reinforced behavior will fade out (Gazzaniga & Heatherton, 2003). Closely related to operant conditioning is Thorndike's law of effect, stating that any behavior that leads to a satisfying state of affairs is more likely to occur again, and behavior that leads to an annoying state of affairs is less likely to occur again (Thorndike, 1933). The principles of operant conditioning are considered to be a major factor in the capacity of neurofeedback to effectuate changes in EEG. During a neurofeedback session, a client is rewarded each time he or she manages to move the bar graph on the computer screen below or above the criterion line. That is, a film clip turns on, music starts playing, or a counter starts running. Assuming that these rewards are satisfying to the client, chances increase that the patterns of EEG activity that preceded the reward are generated in the future. Vice-versa, brain activity that produces no rewarding effects will tend to fade away.

Following the principles of operant conditioning, the EEG activity of most clients who take part in neurofeedback is found to change during consecutive neurofeedback sessions. Notwithstanding the success of neurofeedback training in some clients, often however, there is also a second group of clients whose EEG activity is not found to change over time, and for whom neurofeedback does not seem to work. These two groups of clients are referred to as responders to neurofeedback and non-responders to neurofeedback, respectively. Responders to neurofeedback are clients whose EEG activity successfully changes during neurofeedback sessions. In non-responders there is no significant change in EEG activity observed during the course of the neurofeedback sessions. Figure 7 shows examples of EEG activity of a responder and a non-responder to neurofeedback. Both clients were trained to reduce theta power in 40 consecutive neurofeedback sessions. The responder to neurofeedback shows a clear decrease of average theta power, whereas the non-responder does not show such a decrease.

Response rates of neurofeedback in individuals with autism have been reported to vary between 54 and 76% (Coben & Padolsky, 2007; Kouijzer et al., 2009b; Kouijzer et al., 2010; Kouijzer et al., under review). This means that in more than half of the clients with autism who participated in a scientific study, EEG activity was successfully changed over the course of the neurofeedback treatment. At the same time, there is also a substantial group of clients that was unable to respond to neurofeedback over time. As such it may be interesting to speculate about the reasons why some individuals may turn out to be responsive to treatment with neurofeedback, whereas others may not.

Although the reason why some participants respond to neurofeedback whereas others do not is unclear at this time, it may be that responders and non-responders differ on certain psychological dimensions such as differences in attention span, cognitive flexibility or sensitivity to reward. Alternatively, there might be physiological differences between

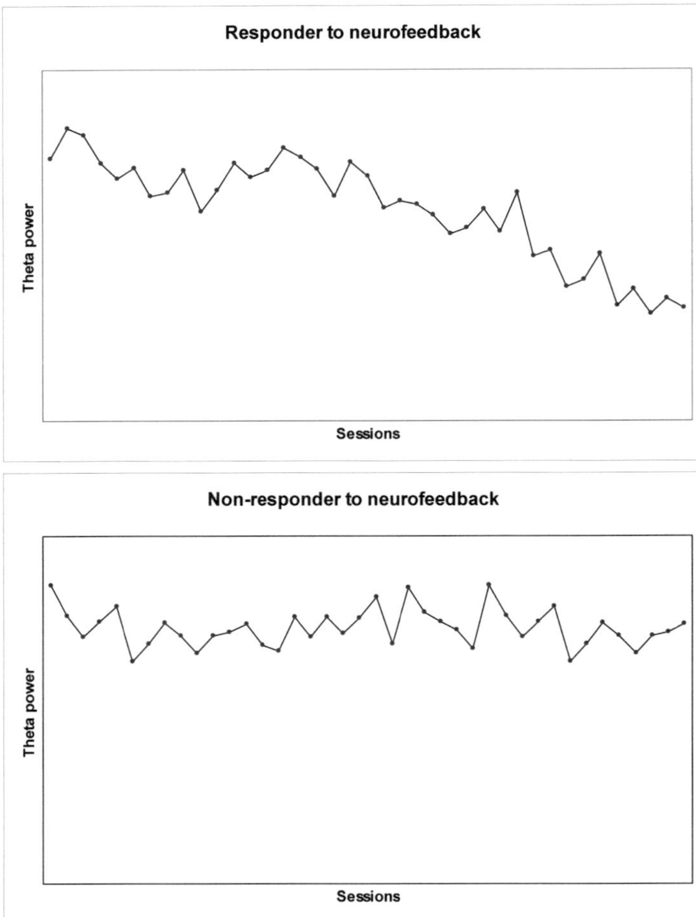


Fig. 7. Mean values of theta power of two clients who were trained to decrease theta power in 40 consecutive neurofeedback sessions. The upper part of the figure shows the mean values of theta power per session of a responder to neurofeedback; the lower part of the figure displays the mean values of theta power per session of a non-responder to neurofeedback.

responders and non-responders, for instance with regard to individual differences in QEEG profiles. Another possibility is that there may be differences between responders and non-responders in terms of the amount and the quality of the rewards they received during the neurofeedback treatment. That is, most therapists adapt the rewards to what they think works best for the individual client, which might introduce differences in both the quantity and quality of rewards between clients. For example, it may be that some clients respond best if they receive rewards in 80% of the time, whereas other clients may need more challenge and only respond to conditions in which rewards are provided in 50% of the time, or less. Similarly, some clients may be more responsive to exciting film clips, whereas others may benefit more from quiet and highly structured film clips. Inadequate choices of the therapist might influence a client's responsiveness to the treatment. A further understanding of individual preferences in both the amount and the type of rewards that are provided during neurofeedback is required to optimize the response rates of clients to neurofeedback training. In addition, the application of neurofeedback as a treatment may benefit strongly from developing predictors, i.e. specific psychological or physiological differences between individuals that allow an early distinction between responders and non-responders, and thus to save time, effort, and money on treatment of non-responders.

Whereas operant conditioning is generally considered to be a relatively passive process on which the trainee has little or no direct influence, learning processes during neurofeedback sessions might also be influenced by active processes. It is often reported that clients manage to develop deliberate control over their EEG activity, allowing them increase or decrease the height of the bar graph in a voluntary manner. There are also clients, however, who never gain deliberate control over their EEG activity. These clients might be responders to neurofeedback, but they can not intentionally act upon the EEG signal. Kamiya (1968) was to first to provide evidence for deliberate control over EEG activity. In his study, participants were first trained to produce alpha waves and some of them subsequently managed to recognize the state of these alpha waves on instruction. Nowadays, the deliberate control over EEG activity is used frequently in clinical settings where patients with neuromuscular impairments or locked-in syndrome use brain computer interfaces (BCI) to control external devices. Birbaumer and colleagues (1999), for example, showed that paralyzed patients who completely lack muscular control can learn to communicate with their environment by using an electronic spelling device that is controlled by EEG activity. By intentionally activating EEG activity in a specific frequency range, a computer cursor is controlled to point out and select different letters of the alphabet to construct a message.

The functional mechanisms that are used to control electrical activity of the brain in a deliberate way may not be so different from functional mechanisms that we use for controlling our body. A dominant theory in motor control is the Ideomotor Theory (Greenwald, 1970), which states that our actions are primarily controlled at the level of their sensory effects. For instance, when learning how to ride a bike, the motor system is attempting to match the anticipated visual and tactile consequences of the actions with an appropriate motor command. Development of new movement repertoire, e.g. in case children are learning how to drink from a cup without spilling its content, requires internal models that map the relation between sensory consequences and action output that need to be formed through experience. The ability to control one's own brain waves may well operate on similar principles, whereby the trainee's brain, over time, establishes the relationship between motor intentions and their sensory consequences, allowing an internal model to form and control the sensory effects that are provided by the neurofeedback. A simple experiment provides a convincing demonstration of this idea. Most people are unable to wiggle their ears but may easily learn to do so when the signal of the muscles controlling their ears is made explicit to them (Bair, 1901). You can try this yourself by putting your fingers behind your ears on the tendons that are controlling their movement. The direct sensory effect will make it much easier to establish control. In a sense, neurofeedback is no different from this example. All it does is make unconscious biological signals explicit to the client so that he or she may learn to control these signals in a deliberate manner.

### 4.2 Neuronal mechanisms behind neurofeedback

The exact cortical and subcortical mechanisms of the brain supporting neurofeedback training have received little or no attention so far, as have its neural effects. There is one fMRI study that investigated the effects of neurofeedback on neural substrates in children with ADHD (Beauregard & Levesque, 2006). Fifteen children were trained to reduce 4 to 7 Hz power at Cz while enhancing power in the 12 to 15 Hz and 15 to 18 Hz frequency ranges. After neurofeedback training participants in the neurofeedback group showed significant loci of activation in brain systems mediating selective attention and response inhibition compared to the control group that had no neurofeedback training. The results of this study suggest that neurofeedback has the capacity to functionally normalize brain systems in children with ADHD.

Sterman theorized on possible neuronal mechanisms underlying the effects of neurofeedback targeting SMR (Sterman, 1996; Sterman & Egner, 2006). SMR is a 12 to 15 Hz rhythm that is found maximal over the sensorimotor cortex of the brain. SMR was found positively associated with control over excitation in the thalamocortical somatosensory and somatomotor pathways of the brain (Sterman, 1996; Sterman & Egner, 2006). By repeatedly producing increased amounts of SMR, postsynaptic cells may become more sensitive and consequently the probability of future activation of these cells may be increased. By increasing thresholds for excitation, neurofeedback may have beneficial effects on severity and frequency of seizures in clients with epilepsy. In ADHD, similarly increased thresholds for excitation are believed to be responsible for reductions in cortical and thalamocortical hyper-excitability and accompanying reductions in impulsive tendencies.

Less is known about the neuronal underpinnings of neurofeedback in individuals with autism. Although the autistic brain is an increasing topic of interest in scientific research (e.g. Brambilla, Hardan, Ucelli di Nemic, Perez, Soares, & Barale, 2008), little research has been conducted on the actual consequences of neurofeedback in autism. Studies investigating the EEGs of individuals with autism have revealed abnormal patterns of EEG activity as compared to healthy controls. For example, individuals with autism showed diminished frontal and occipital/parietal alpha power (e.g. Chan, Sze, & Cheung, 2007; Murias et al., 2007) and increased phase consistency between posterior-frontal and anterior-temporal brain areas as compared to healthy controls (e.g., Coben & Padolsky, 2007; Murias et al., 2007). Furthermore, elevated delta and theta power over frontal or fronto-central areas have been found in individuals with autism (e.g. Chan, Sze, & Cheung, 2007; Kouijzer et al., 2009b; Kouijzer et al., 2010; Kouijzer et al., under review; Murias, Webb, Greenson, & Dawson, 2007). Kouijzer and colleagues (2009b; 2010) found reductions in autistic symptoms and improvements in executive functions in accordance with reductions in frontomedial theta power following neurofeedback training. Theta is typically located to the medial prefrontal cortex (MPFC) including the anterior cingulate cortex (ACC; Tsujimoto, Shimazu, & Isomura, 2006) and is inversely related to BOLD (blood-oxygen-level dependence) activation in these structures (Meltzer, Negishi, Mayes, & Constable, 2007). As such, neurofeedback mediated reductions in frontomedial theta power may be directly responsible for improvement in executive functioning and social cognitive abilities, functions that are typically associated with activation of the MPFC (Bush, Luu, & Posner, 2000; Di Martino et al., 2009; Henderson et al., 2006; Mundy, 2003; Ohnishi et al., 2000).

## 5. Efficacy of neurofeedback in autism

Currently, about 10 scientific publications have reported on the efficacy of neurofeedback in autism. Table 1 provides an overview of the studies that investigated the effects of neurofeedback in autism. Some studies described the effects of neurofeedback in one or more participants (Scolnick, 2005; Sichel, Fehmi, & Goldstein, 1995; Thompson, Thompson, & Reid, 2010), whereas other studies compared a group of participants that had neurofeedback with a group of participants that had no neurofeedback or another treatment (Coben & Padolsky, 2007; Jarusiewicz, 2002; Kouijzer et al., 2009b; Kouijzer et al., 2010; Kouijzer et al., under review). Furthermore, in all studies to date, the participants were either children or adolescents. No studies of neurofeedback in adults with autism have been published at this time. About 88% of the participants in all studies that have been published were male. In terms of the autistic spectrum, most studies included participants with a diagnosis autism, Asperger syndrome or PDD-NOS. One study focused on participants with PDD-NOS only (Kouijzer et al., 2009b), whereas two other studies mainly included individuals with Asperger syndrome (Scolnick, 2005; Thompson, Thompson, & Reid, 2010). This paragraph will provide a detailed description of the outcomes of studies investigating the effects of neurofeedback with a consecutive focus on (1) behavioral symptoms as reported by parents and teachers, (2) cognitive functions, and (3) the EEG. The paragraph ends with discussing the long-term maintenance of effects of neurofeedback.

Neurofeedback was found to positively affect autistic symptoms, such as social interaction problems and communication deficits (Coben & Padolsky, 2007; Kouijzer et al., 2009b; Kouijzer et al., 2010; Sichel, Fehmi, & Goldstein, 1995). In addition, improvement in self-esteem, empathy, and flexibility were seen, as well as reductions of anxiety, temper tantrums, and mood changes (Scolnick, 2005). These positive effects of neurofeedback were all reported by parents who filled out questionnaires inquiring about their children's behavior (Coben & Padolsky, 2007; Jarusiewicz, 2002; Kouijzer et al., 2009b; Kouijzer et al., 2010; Thompson, Thompson, & Reid, 2010) or reflected the outcomes of parent interviews (Jarusiewicz, 2002; Scolnick, 2005; Sichel, Fehmi, & Goldstein, 1995). In one study, neurofeedback did not result in a reduction of autistic symptoms (Kouijzer et al., under review). The reason why some studies did find positive effects of neurofeedback on symptom reduction in autism while other studies did not is unclear at this time. Kouijzer and colleagues (under review) suggested that differences in neurofeedback protocols and in sample characteristics between studies may have been responsible for such varying study outcomes. Another possibility may be that variations in study design and thus in the degree of control for nonspecific effects (e.g. the attention that is received by trainees in addition to their training) are responsible. More information about the effects of nonspecific factors and related design issues is provided in the subsequent paragraph entitled 'Quality of neurofeedback research'.

In contrast to the reports of parents, teachers did not report as much improvement in social interactions and communication skills. At the same time, the observations of teachers were included in only three studies (Kouijzer et al., 2010; Kouijzer et al., under review; Scolnick, 2005). In one of these three studies, teachers reported improvement in behavior of adolescents with autism following neurofeedback (Scolnick, 2005). That is, in four out of five cases that were described in this paper, teachers noticed the same behavioral improvement as parents, such as improvement in self-esteem, flexibility, and empathy and reductions in anxiety and temper tantrums. In one case described in this paper, no changes in behavior were reported by the teacher, whereas the parents of that participant did report improvement. In two other studies that investigated teacher reports, teachers did not report any improvement in the behavior of children and adolescents following neurofeedback (Kouijzer et al., 2010; Kouijzer et al., under review).

| Authors and year of publication | n | Study design | Age range (years) | Treatment | Number of sessions |
|---|---|---|---|---|---|
| Sichel, Fehmi, & Goldstein, 1995 | 1 | Case study | 8 | Decrease 4-8 Hz; increase 12-15 Hz; P3, Pz, and P4 | 31 |
| Jarusiewicz, 2002 | 24 | Pretest posttest control group | 4-13 | Decrease 2-7 Hz and 22-30 Hz; increase 10-13 Hz; C4 | 20-69 |
| Scolnick, 2005 | 5 | Case study | 12-16 | Decrease 2-10 Hz and 22-30 Hz; increase 8-11 Hz, 12-15 Hz or 15-18 Hz; Fz, Cz, Pz, C4 or T6 | 24-31 |
| Coben & Padolsky, 2007 | 49 | Pretest posttest control group | 3-14 | Decrease hyperconnectivity | 20 |
| Kouijzer, de Moor, Gerrits, Congedo, & van Schie, 2009 | 14 | Pretest posttest control group | 8-12 | Decrease 4-7 Hz; increase 12-15 Hz; C4 | 40 |
| Kouijzer, van Schie, de Moor, Gerrits, & Buitelaar, 2010 | 20 | Randomized pretest posttest control group | 8-12 | Decrease 3-7 Hz and slight variations; Fz, Cz or F4 | 40 |
| Thompson, Thompson, & Reid, 2010 | 159 | Case study | 5-58 | Decrease 3-7 Hz; increase 12-15 Hz; Cz or CFz | 40-60 |
| Kouijzer, van Schie, Gerrits, Buitelaar, & de Moor, under review | 38 | Randomized pretest posttest control group with blinded active comparator | 12-18 | Decrease 2-7 Hz and slight variations; Cz or CFz | 23-40 |

Table 1. Overview of the studies that investigated the effects of neurofeedback in children and adolescents with autism.

Neurofeedback was demonstrated to have positive effects on cognitive functions of children and adolescents with autism (Coben & Padolsky, 2007; Kouijzer et al., 2009b; Kouijzer et al., 2010; Kouijzer et al., under review). These effects were measured by a series of neuropsychological tasks, which allow a more objective evaluation of the treatment effects than asking parents or teachers what they observed in the behavior of their child or student. A specific cognitive function that was found to be improved after neurofeedback treatment is cognitive flexibility. In three studies, improvement in cognitive flexibility was found in participants who received neurofeedback, whereas participants in the control groups showed no improvement in cognitive flexibility (Kouijzer et al., 2009b; Kouijzer et al., 2010; Kouijzer et al., under review). Cognitive flexibility is defined as the ability to shift to a different thought or action according to situational changes (Hill, 2004). Poor flexibility is one of the core characteristics of everyday behavior of individuals with autism and is often illustrated by a need for sameness. For example, many people with autism have difficulties in switching from one situation to the other or panic if an unexpected event occurs. The positive effects of neurofeedback on cognitive flexibility were found in studies that used the trail making task, which requires the participant to connect letters of the alphabet and numbers in an alternating manner (1-A-2-B-3-C, etc.) on paper. Whether neurofeedback also results in improvement in cognitive flexibility in real life is unknown at this time. Future studies may investigate if the effects of neurofeedback extend to real life conditions. For example by measuring the response of participants with autism in real life scenarios that require cognitive flexibility skills, e.g. a last minute change in schedule. In addition to changes in cognitive flexibility, studies have reported improvements in other cognitive domains. Kouijzer and colleagues (2009b) noted additional improvements in attention, inhibition, and planning, suggesting a more general improvement in executive functions. This finding is supported by Coben and Padolsky (2007) who found a general improvement in executive functions accompanied by improvement in visual perceptual functioning and language skills following neurofeedback treatment.

Another relatively objective way to evaluate the effects of neurofeedback training is QEEG. Since neurofeedback focuses on the change of electrical brain activity, QEEG measures may be used to examine whether the treatment actually influenced the EEG in a structural manner or not. Most studies that examined the effects of neurofeedback in children and adolescents with autism compared pre- and post-treatment QEEGs and found that EEG activity changed after neurofeedback. The specific effects in EEG depended on the neurofeedback protocol that was used. After inhibiting theta power and rewarding beta power, the theta to beta ratios of participants decreased, i.e. changed in the direction of normality on a post treatment measurement (Sichel, Fehmi, & Goldstein, 1995; Scolnick, 2005; Thompson, Thompson, & Reid, 2010). Similarly, neurofeedback that focused on the inhibition of theta power resulted in decreased theta power (Kouijzer et al., 2010) and neurofeedback that aimed to decrease delta and theta power resulted in decreased delta power in subsequent QEEG measurements (Kouijzer et al., under review). A study by Coben and Padolsky (2007) was successful in reducing hyperconnectivity in most participants through the application of neurofeedback. Only one study failed to show effects in the EEGs of children and adolescents with autism who received neurofeedback (Kouijzer et al., 2009b).

The positive effects on autistic symptoms, cognitive flexibility, and EEG activity that were found after neurofeedback are only clinically significant if they are maintained after treatment has ended. That is, if participants would return to pre-treatment levels after the last neurofeedback session, they should continue neurofeedback training for the rest of their lives in order to benefit from its effects. This would be comparable with the structural use of medication for reducing behavioral problems that are co-occurring with autism. Aggressive behavior, for example, can be reduced by the use of atypical antipsychotics (McCracken et al., 2002) and overactivity or disruptive behavior has been decreased with stimulants (Research Units on Pediatric Psychopharmacology, 2005). When the intake of such medication is interrupted, the beneficial effects typically disappear and symptoms return to earlier levels. On the basis of current evidence, however, it appears that neurofeedback in individuals with autism has long term effects on autistic symptoms and leads to long term improvement in cognitive functions. Kouijzer and colleagues used follow-up measures of autistic symptoms and cognitive functions either six months (Kouijzer et al., 2010; Kouijzer et al., under review) or twelve months (Kouijzer et al., 2009a) after the last neurofeedback session was completed. In one study, the effects in EEG theta activity were found to be maintained six months after neurofeedback treatment had ended (Kouijzer et al., 2010), whereas another study found that the initial changes in EEG delta activity that were found directly after the treatment had returned to baseline after six months (Kouijzer et al., under review). The reason why EEG changes were long lasting in one study but not in the other study might be related to the different samples that were used in these studies. The former study included participants of 8 to 12 years old and a broad range of behavioral problems, whereas the latter study included participants of 12 to 18 years old with mainly internalizing problems. Perhaps EEG changes in younger participants or in participants with both externalizing and internalizing behavior problems are more likely to remain over time as compared to EEG changes in older participants or in participants with internalizing behavior problems. Although the changes in EEG activity were not maintained after six months in the study of Kouijzer and colleagues (under review), the positive effects on cognitive flexibility skills that co-occurred after neurofeedback were found to be maintained six months later. This suggests that long term changes in EEG are no requirement for structural improvements in cognitive flexibility. Perhaps a reduction of slow wave power is required for the initiation of cognitive flexibility improvement, whereas continuation of the ability for task switching relies on other mechanisms.

## 6. Quality of neurofeedback research

The efficacy of any treatment program in any specific population can be investigated by experimental research. Such experimental research should meet a number of criteria in order to prevent the study outcomes from being influenced by other factors than the treatment itself. Campbell and Stanley (1963) recommended the use of a pretest-posttest control group design to control for factors that might produce effects confounded with the effects of the experimental treatment such as maturation. In such a randomized pretest-posttest control group design, participants are randomly allocated in two research groups: a treatment group that receives the treatment of interest and a control group that does not receive the treatment. Participants of both groups are assessed at comparable times before and after treatment. The results of the two groups at both times are compared in order to find effects of the treatment. Of the studies that investigated the effects of neurofeedback in individuals with autism, only two studies used random allocation of participants in treatment and control groups (Kouijzer et al., 2010; Kouijzer et al., under review), compared to six studies that did not.

Several authors have suggested that the outcomes of previous studies that investigated the effects of neurofeedback were not a result of neurofeedback per se, but rather reflected nonspecific effects of neurofeedback. Nonspecific treatment effects are positive effects that are caused by other factors than the treatment of interest. In the case of neurofeedback, implicit attention training and intensive one-to-one contact with the therapist might positively affect the results of the treatment. Neurofeedback is a treatment that includes many sessions that are provided twice or thrice a week. In each of these sessions, the client is instructed to focus his or her attention on the computer screen in front of him or her. Several authors have suggested that participants might be positively affected by being involved in such an intensive treatment that requires paying sustained attention to a computer screen (Gevensleben et al., 2009; Heinrich, Gevensleben, & Strehl, 2007; Kouijzer et al., 2010). Furthermore, the long-duration of neurofeedback typically implies intensive one-to-one contact between client and therapist. Therapists pay individual attention to the client and provide warmth, empathy, and acceptance. Furthermore, the contact between client and therapist in neurofeedback sessions has a highly structured character because it often follows a fixed program of alternating training and rest intervals. These factors might be especially important in individuals with autism, who often have difficulties in building a relationship with unfamiliar others. Because neurofeedback offers so many opportunities for the development of the relationship between client and therapist in a structured and predictable environment, there is a good chance for the client with autism to successfully participate in a reciprocal relationship with the therapist. This experience might cause improvement in the social behavior of participants that is unrelated to improvement as a result of neurofeedback training (Gevensleben et al., 2009; Heinrich, Gevensleben, & Strehl, 2007; Kouijzer et al., 2010). In order to control for such nonspecific effects of neurofeedback, a control condition in which participants receive similar amounts of attention training and one-to-one contact with the therapist should be included in the research design.

Another factor that might have played a role in studies that investigated the effects of neurofeedback is treatment expectancy of participants and their parents. The notion of receiving therapy is known to generate expectancy for improvement in participants and their parents (Borkovec & Nau, 1972). Especially if parents have invested time and money in the treatment of their child, these parents may have been inclined towards a positivity bias that matches their investments. Several authors have suggested that the outcomes of previous studies that measured behavioral improvement with parent questionnaires could have been affected by expectancy biases of parents (Gevensleben et al., 2009; Heinrich, Gevensleben, & Strehl, 2007; Kouijzer et al., 2010). In order to control for the effects of expectancy, the expectancy of parents and participants should be measured in each study that evaluates the effects of neurofeedback.

Only one study fully controlled for the nonspecific effects of implicit attention training, one-to-one contact between client and therapist, and treatment expectancy (Kouijzer et al., under review). In this study, an alternative treatment group was created next to the neurofeedback group and the waiting list control group. This alternative treatment was almost identical to neurofeedback training, except for the signal that was fed back to the participants. In the neurofeedback group, the EEG signal was fed back to the client, whereas in the alternative treatment group another bodily signal, i.e. the skin conductance (SC) signal, was fed back. Participants and their parents were blinded and thus not informed about the signal that was used during their training. The participants of the SC group were expected to improve in relaxation and calmness as an effect of the SC training, but not to show reductions in symptoms of autism and to improve in cognitive functions and EEG as much as the participants in the neurofeedback group.

Another option to control for the nonspecific effects of neurofeedback is to use a double-blind placebo controlled study design. Such a study includes one group that receives the treatment of interest and one group that receives a placebo treatment. In the case of neurofeedback, the placebo treatment could include fake feedback that is unrelated to the participants' brain activity. Neither participants nor therapists are aware of the type of feedback that is provided to the participants. For neurofeedback, however, such a design is hard to realize for three reasons. First of all, both the therapist and the participants in the placebo group are likely to discover that the fake feedback is unrelated to the participants' EEG activity. Secondly, high drop-out rates have been found in placebo groups where participants were unable to gain any control over the EEG signal (Orlandi & Greco, 2005). Finally, patients often do not want to take the risk of receiving placebo training for so many sessions and therefore it is hard to include large numbers of participants in double-blind controlled studies. An alternative for placebo feedback is mock-feedback. This training method takes care of extreme situations in which the participant produces extreme muscle activity or in which the electrode detaches from the scalp. The use of mock-feedback dramatically increases the reliability of the feedback and is thus more appropriate to apply in studies evaluating the effects of neurofeedback.

Because most studies that investigated the effects of neurofeedback in children and adolescents with autism did not fully control for the nonspecific effects of neurofeedback, there is a high need for further research that does control for such effects. Therefore, conclusions on the efficacy of neurofeedback for individuals with autism can only be drawn after several such studies have been conducted. Until then, the conclusions of the studies that investigated the effects of neurofeedback should be taken cautiously.

Another aspect that needs attention in future research concerns the treatment protocols that are used in neurofeedback. So far, most neurofeedback studies focused on the reduction of theta power with or without the reward of low beta power (Jarusiewicz, 2002; Kouijzer et al., 2009b; Kouijzer et al., 2010; Kouijzer et al., under review; Scolnick, 2005; Sichel, Fehmi, & Goldstein, 1995; Thompson, Thompson, & Reid, 2010). Furthermore, Coben and Padolsky (2007) used an original approach to use a neurofeedback protocol directed at the normalization of coherence between two or more brain areas. The different treatment outcomes of these and other neurofeedback protocols have not been investigated systematically. It might turn out that some treatment protocols work best for a specific group of individuals with autism, whereas other treatment protocols are most effective for a group of individuals with other characteristics.

A final challenge for future research concerns the identification of responders to neurofeedback. As mentioned earlier in this chapter, some individuals with autism respond well to neurofeedback and are able to change EEG activity during neurofeedback sessions, whereas other individuals do not respond and elicit no EEG changes. Importantly, a recent study (Kouijzer et al., under review) demonstrated that the benefits of neurofeedback only take place in individuals with autism who respond to neurofeedback. It is therefore of crucial importance to identify responders to neurofeedback in an early stage or even better, before treatment starts. Future research should identify demographic, psychological or physiological characteristics of individuals who respond to neurofeedback.

## 7. Future developments in neurofeedback

Neurofeedback as a treatment for clients with various disorders has rapidly expanded in the past years, due to increasing technological developments which made the registration of EEG activity more accurate and available for therapists. Next to the traditional neurofeedback as described previously in this chapter, several other modalities of neurofeedback have been developed. In the next section three of these recent developments are discussed, i.e. LORETA-neurofeedback, ICA-neurofeedback, and fMRI-neurofeedback.

LORETA refers to low resolution tomography and is an inverse technique for reconstructing the source of EEG activity in the three-dimensional brain by electrophysiological models. In LORETA-neurofeedback, feedback reflects EEG activity that is generated by a specific source, which deviates from traditional neurofeedback approaches where feedback reflects spatially nonspecific EEG activity at the sensor level (Congedo, 2003). LORETA-neurofeedback can not be applied in real time, because of time and capacity consuming calculations of the computer. Therefore, LORETA-neurofeedback is applied by using a spatial filter after the EEG activity is recorded. LORETA-neurofeedback can be used to alter EEG activity generated in deep brain structures that can not be recorded accurately by traditional neurofeedback. In a study by Congedo, Lubar, and Joffe (2004) the application of LORETA-neurofeedback was investigated in six healthy students. These participants were trained to decrease beta power and to concurrently increase alpha power generated in the ACC. The results of this study show an increased beta/alpha ratio in the regions of the ACC that were involved in the LORETA-neurofeedback (Congedo, Lubar, & Joffe, 2004). These findings suggest that EEG activity in specific brain areas may be altered by LORETA-neurofeedback.

Related to LORETA-neurofeedback is ICA-neurofeedback. ICA refers to independent component analysis and is a mathematical approach that separates a multivariate signal in independent components. In the case of ICA-neurofeedback, ICA separates the raw EEG signal in separate sources of the signal. This technique can be applied in cases where neurofeedback focuses on specific EEG components that can not be detected easily from the raw EEG signal by traditional neurofeedback devices. ICA- and LORETA-neurofeedback can be used interchangeably, but are not similar. ICA-neurofeedback uses mathematical models to calculate the solutions of the EEG signal, whereas LORETA-neurofeedback is based on electrophysiological models.

A third modality of neurofeedback is fMRI-neurofeedback. FMRI-neurofeedback is an advanced method that uses the BOLD response of regions in the brain. FMRI is a technique that allows measurements of brain activity with a high spatial resolution, but low temporal resolution, as compared to EEG which has a high temporal resolution, but is limited in the spatial domain. At this time, fMRI-neurofeedback is mainly used in research settings and is hardly applied in the treatment of clinical populations. The main reason for this is that fMRI is an expensive technique and that any treatment application will suffer from a long time delay, which lies in the order of several seconds, resulting from the sluggishness of the BOLD response. This delay in feedback makes it especially hard for individuals to relate the feedback to the actual brain activity. Nevertheless, DeCharms and colleagues (2004) successfully applied fMRI-neurofeedback in six healthy participants. They were instructed to imagine hand movements while trying to optimize their strategy to increase activation in a brain area involved in this cognitive process, i.e. the sensorimotor cortex. The participants received continuous information about the strength of activation they were producing in their sensorimotor cortex. After three sessions, participants succeeded in controlling task-specific activation in the sensorimotor cortex.

LORETA-neurofeedback, ICA-neurofeedback, and fMRI-neurofeedback are examples of recent developments in the field of neurofeedback that are expected to gain further scientific interest over the coming years. These techniques hold the potential for changing activation in specific neural regions using neurofeedback. As such, it is more than likely that the clinical application of EEG neurofeedback in the coming years will develop in the direction of EEG source modeling techniques (such as LORETA- and ICA-neurofeedback) to allow the activation or deactivation of specific neural structures that are implicated in neurological conditions such as autism. FMRI-neurofeedback on the other hand may prove a valuable experimental technique for assisting cognitive neuroscience in its aim to uncover the functional organization of the brain.

## 8. Conclusion

Neurofeedback is a technique that is used to alter activity of the brain that deviates from normality in a variety of clinical disorders, such as autism. Recent findings suggest that neurofeedback may provide a beneficial treatment for individuals in the autism spectrum. Indeed several studies have shown that individuals with autism are able to alter their brain activity in specific frequency bands through the use of neurofeedback and that neurofeedback training may be accompanied by prolonged changes in autism symptoms, cognitive functioning and long-term changes in EEG. Although the prospects for the application of neurofeedback in autism spectrum disorders certainly look promising, the scientific evidence for its effectiveness to date is still rather thin. Future studies will have to be conducted using larger samples and appropriate control conditions to allow reliable measures of the efficacy of neurofeedback treatment in autism both in the lab and in clinical practice.

## 9. References

American Psychiatric Association. (2000). *Diagnostic and statistical manual of mental disorders, text revision* (4th ed.). Washington, DC: American Psychiatric Association.

Arns, M., de Ridder, S., Strehl, U., Breteler, M., & Coenen, A. (2009). Efficacy of neurofeedback treatment in ADHD: the effects on inattention, hyperactivity, and impulsivity: a meta-analysis. *Clinical EEG and Neuroscience, 40* (3), 179- 189.

Bair, J.H. (1901). Development of voluntary control. *Psychological review, 8*, 474-510.

Beauregard, M & Lévesque, J. (2006). Functional Magnetic Resonance Imaging Investigation of the Effects of Neurofeedback Training on the Neural Bases of Selective Attention and Response Inhibition in Children with Attention-Deficit/Hyperactivity Disorder. *Applied Psychophysiology and Biofeedback, 31*,(1), 3-20.

Birbaumer, N., Ghanayim, N., Hinterberger, T., Iversen, I., Kotchoubey, B., Kübler, A., Perelmouter, J., Taub, E., & Flor, H. (1999). A spelling device for the paralysed. *Nature, 398*, 297-298.

Borkovec, T.D. & Nau, S.D. (1972). Credibility of analogue therapy rationales. *Journal of Behavior Therapy & Experimental Psychiatry, 3*, 257-260.

Brambilla, P., Hardan, A., Ucelli di Nemic, S., Perez, J., Soares, J.C., & Barale, F. (2008). Brain anatomy and development in autism: review of structural MRI studies. *Brain research bulletin, 61*, 557-569.

Bush, G., Luu, P., & Posner, M. I. (2000). Cognitive and emotional influences in anterior cingulate cortex. *Trends in Cognitive Science, 4*, 215–222.

Campbell, D.T. & Stanley, J.C. (1963). *Experimental and quasi-experimental designs for research.* Chicago, llinois: Rand McNally.

Chan, A.S., Sze, S.L., & Cheung, M. (2007). Quantitative Electroencephalographic Profiles for Children With Autistic Spectrum Disorder. *Neuropsychology, 21* (1), 74-81.

Cherkassky, V. L., Kana, R. K., Keller, T. A., & Just, M. A. (2006). Functional connectivity in a baseline resting-state network in autism. *Neuroreport, 17*, 1687–1690.

Coben, R. & Padolsky, I. (2007). Assessment-guided neurofeedback for autistic spectrum disorders. *Journal of Neurotherapy, 11*, 5-23.

Congedo, M. (2003). *Tomographic neurofeedback; a new technique for the self-regulation of brain electrical activity*. Thesis, Knoxville, TN: The university of Tennessee, Knoxville.

Congedo, M. Lubar, J.F., & Joffe, D. (2004). Low-resolution electromagnetic tomography neurofeedback. *Neural systems and rehabilitation engineering, 12* (4), 387-397.

DeCharms, R.C., Christoff, K., Glover, G.H., Pauly, J.M., Whitfield, S., & Gabrieli, J.D.E. (2004). Learned regulation of spatially localized brain activity using real-time fmri. *Neuroimage, 21*(1), 436-443.

Di Martino, A., Ross, K., Uddin, L. Q., Sklar, A. B., Castellanos, F. X., & Milham, M. P. (2009). Functional brain correlates of social and nonsocial processes in autism spectrum disorders: An activation likelihood estimation meta-analysis. *Biological Psychiatry, 65*, 63–74.

Gazzaniga, M.S. & Heatherton, T.F. (2003). *Psychological Science*. New York: W.W. Norton & Company.

Gevensleben, H., Holl, B., Albrecht, B., Vogel, C., Schlamp, D., Kratz, O., Studer, P., Rothenberger, A., Moll, G.H., & Heinrich, H.. (2009). Is neurofeedback an efficacious treatment for ADHD? A randomised controlled clinical trial. *Journal of Child Psychology and Psychiatry, 50* (7), 780-789.

Greenwald, A.G. (1970). A choice reaction time test of ideomotor theory. *Journal of Experimental Psychology, 86*, 20-25.

Heinrich, H., Gevensleben, H., & Strehl, U. (2007). Annotation: Neurofeedback—train your brain to train behavior. *Journal of Child Psychology and Psychiatry, 48*(1), 3–16.

Henderson, H., Schwartz, C., Mundy, P., Burnette, C., Sutton, S., Zahka, N., et al. (2006). Response monitoring, the error-related negativity, and differences in social behavior in autism. *Brain and Cognition, 61*, 96–109.

Hill, E.L. (2004). Executive dysfunctions in autism. *Trends in cognitive sciences, 8* (1), 26-32.

Jarusiewicz, B. (2002). Efficacy of neurofeedback for children in the autistic spectrum: A pilot study. *Journal of Neurotherapy, 6*, 39–49.

Kamiya, J. (1968). Conscious control of brain waves. *Psychology Today, 1*, 57-60.

Kennedy, D. P., & Courchesne, E. (2008). The intrinsic functional organization of the brain is altered in autism. *NeuroImage, 39*, 1877–1885.

Kouijzer, M.E.J., de Moor, J.M.H., Gerrits, B.J.L., Buitelaar, J.K., & van Schie, H.T. (2009b). Long-term effects of neurofeedback treatment in autism. *Research in Autism Spectrum Disorders, 3*, 496-501.

Kouijzer, M.E.J., de Moor, J.M.H., Gerrits, B.J.L., Congedo, M., & van Schie, H.T. (2009a). Neurofeedback improves executive functioning in children with autism spectrum disorders. *Research in Autism Spectrum Disorders, 3*, 145- 162.

Kouijzer, M.E.J., van Schie, H.T., de Moor, J.M.H., Gerrits, B.J.L., & Buitelaar, J.K. (2010). Neurofeedback treatment in autism. Preliminary findings in behavioral, cognitive, and neurophysiological functioning. *Research in Autism Spectrum Disorders, 4*, 386-399.

Kouijzer, M.E.J., van Schie, H.T., Gerrits, B.J.L, Buitelaar, J.K., & de Moor, J.M.H. (under review). Is EEG-biofeedback an Effective Treatment For Autism? A Randomized Controlled Trial.

Kropotov, J.D., Grin-Yatsenko, V.A., Ponomarev, V.A., Chutko, L.S., Yakovenko, E.A., & Nikishena, I.S. (2005). ERPs correlates of EEG relative beta training in ADHD children. *International journal of psychophysiology, 55*, 23-34.

Lubar, J. F., & Shouse, M. N. (1976). EEG and behavioral changes in a hyperkinetic child concurrent with training of the sensorimotor rhythm (SMR): A preliminary report. *Biofeedback and Self Regulation, 3*, 293-306.

McCracken, J.T., McGough, J., Shah, B. Cronin, P., Hong, D., Aman, M.G., et al. (2002). Risperdone in children with autism and serious behavioral problems. *New England journal of medicine, 5*, 314-321.

Meltzer, J. A., Negishi, M., Mayes, L. C., & Constable, R. T. (2007). Individual differences in EEG theta and alpha dynamics during working memory correlate with fMRI responses across subjects. *Clinical Neurophysiology, 118*, 2419–2436.

Monastra, V.J., Lynn, S., Linden, M., Lubar, J.F., Gruzelier, J., & LaVaque, T.J. (2005). Electroencephalographic Biofeedback in the Treatment of Attention-

Deficit/Hyperactivity Disorder. *Applied Psychophysiology and Biofeedback, 30* (2), 95-114.

Mundy, P. (2003). Annotation: The neural basis of social impairments in autism: The role of the dorsal medial-frontal cortex and anterior cingulate system. *Journal of Child Psychology and Psychiatry, 44*, 793–809.

Murias, M., Webb, S. J., Greenson, J., & Dawson, G. (2007). Resting state cortical connectivity reflected in EEG coherence in individuals with autism. *Biological Psychiatry, 62*, 270–273.

Ohnishi, T., Matsuda, H., Hashimoto, T., Kunihiro, T., Nishikawa, M., Uema, T., et al. (2000). Abnormal regional cerebral blood flow in childhood autism. *Brain, 123*, 1838–1844.

Orlandi, M.A. & Greco, D. (2005). *A randomized, double-blind clinical trial of EEG neurofeedback treatment for attention deficit/hyperactivity disorder (ADHD)*. In ISNR conference.

Raichle, M. E., MacLeod, A. M., Snyder, A. Z., Powers, W. J., Gusnard, D. A., & Shulman, G. L. (2001). A default mode of brain function. *Proceedings of the National Academy of Sciences, 98*, 676–682.

Research Units on Pediatric Psychopharmacology (2005). Randomized, controlled, crossover trial of methylphenidate in pervasive developmental disorders with hyperactivity. *Archives of general psychiatry, 62*, 1266-1274.

Scolnick, B. (2005). Effects of electroencephalogram biofeedback with Asperger's syndrome. *International Journal of Rehabilitation Research, 28*, 159–163.

Sichel, A. G., Fehmi, L. G., & Goldstein, D. M. (1995). Positive outcome with neurofeedback treatment in a case of mild autism. *Journal of Neurotherapy*, 1 (1), 60-64.

Sterman, M. B. (1996). Physiological origins and functional correlates of EEG rhythmic activities: Implications for self- regulation. *Biofeedback and Self Regulation, 21*, 3–33.

Sterman, M.B. & Egner, T. (2006). Foundations and practice of neurofeedback for the treatment of epilepsy. Applied *Psychophysiology and Biofeedback, 31* (1), 21-35.

Sterman, M. B., Macdonald, L. R. and Stone, R. K. (1974). Biofeedback Training of the Sensorimotor Electroencephalogram Rhythm in Man: Effects on Epilepsy. *Epilepsia, 15*, 395–416.

Tan, G., Thornby, J., Hammond, D.C., Strehl, U., Canady, B., Arnemann, K., & Kaiser, D.A. (2009). Meta-analysis of EEG-biofeedback in treating epilepsy. *Clinical EEG and Neuroscience, 40* (3), 1-7.

Thompson, L., Thompson, M., & Reid, A. (2010). Neurofeedback Outcomes in Clients with Asperger's Syndrome. *Applied Psychophysiology and Biofeedback, 35*, 63-81.

Thorndike, E.L. (1933). A proof of the law of effect. *Science, 77*, 173.

Tsujimoto, T., Shimazu, H., & Isomura, Y. (2006). Direct recording of theta oscillations in primate prefrontal and anterior cingulate cortices. *Journal of Neurophysiology, 95*, 2987–3000.

Wyricka, W. & Sterman, M.B. (1968). Instrumental conditioning of sensorimotor cortex EEG spindles in the waking cat. *Physiology and Behavior, 3*, 703-707.

Yucha, C. & Montgomery, D. (2008).*Evidence-Based Practice in Biofeedback and Neurofeedback*. Wheat Ridge, CO: Association for Applied Psychophysiology and Biofeedback.

# 6

# Dietary Interventions in Autism

Yasmin Neggers
*The University of Alabama, Tuscaloosa,
Alabama,
United States of America*

## 1. Introduction

The objective of this chapter is to evaluate the research pertinent to the use of dietary interventions to treat autism. A brief description, rationale, any evidence of efficacy and validity of methodology employed for most frequently used inventions in autism follows.

The number of children diagnosed with autism spectrum disorder (ASD) has increased significantly over the last decades in the U.S. and in other countries. Yet to date, there is no clear etiology or cure for autism. In most cases, specific underlying causes cannot be identified (Cubala-Kucharska, 2010). A number of risk factors being investigated include genetic, infectious, metabolic, nutritional and environmental, but less than 10 to 12% of cases have specific causes known (Srinivasan, 2009). Simultaneously the use of alternative treatment approaches in children with autism has increased, but due to significant methodological flaws, the currently available data are inadequate to guide treatment recommendations (Christison and Ivany , 2006).

It has been suggested that nutritional factors play a major role. Significantly lower levels of various nutrients in blood have been observed in autistic children including low levels of zinc, selenium, vitamin D and omega-3 fatty acids (Elder, 2008). In practice, treatment of ASD usually consists of a comprehensive program of educational intervention, speech therapy, behavioral treatment and developmental therapies. Anecdotal reports and parent surveys and a few research studies have indicated some evidence of diminishing the symptoms of autism by use of diets based on food elimination and rotation, as well as through supplementation and alternative treatments based on intestinal healing (Cubala-Kucharska,2010; Srinivasan, 2009 ). The popularity of these diets indicates a need for more in-depth and rigorous research into their efficacy.

Currently a variety of nutritional interventions are in use, including gluten and casein- free diet (GFCF), ketogenic diet, yeast free diet, restriction of food allergens, probiotics, and dietary supplementation with vitamins A, C, $B_6$, folic acid , $B_{12}$, minerals like magnesium and omega-3 fatty acids (Seung et. al, 2007). In most cases, the dietary interventions discussed below were developed for conditions related to autism, e.g., multiple food sensitivity, inflammatory bowel disease, Candida and viral infections. Wide use of complementary and alternative therapies (CAM) by parents and caregivers has been reported (Elder, 2008). The literature currently available suggests that diets removing both gluten and casein show some efficacy and should be studied further.

## 2. Gluten –Free Casein- Free Diet (GFCF)

One of the most frequently used interventions for ASD is the GFCF diet. Initially focusing on schizophrenia, investigators conducted studies to test the hypothesis that schizophrenia as well as autism was in some way associated with the absorption of "exophrins" contained in gluten and casein (Elder et al., 2006). This diet calls for complete elimination of both gluten and casein, which is found in wheat, rye, barley, and oats, as well as casein, the protein in milk and all milk products.
Rationale: It is hypothesized that some symptoms of autism (e.g., stereotypical and ritualistic behaviors, preservation, excessive activity, speech and language delays) may result from opioid peptides formed from incomplete breakdown of foods containing gluten and casein. It is proposed that increased intestinal permeability, also referred to as "leaky gut syndrome" allows these peptides to cross the intestinal membrane, and cross the blood-brain barrier through entry into the blood stream, thereby affecting the endogenous opiate system and neurotransmission in the nervous system (Cubala-Kucharska , 2010; Milward et al., 2009). This theory is cited to explain why many children with autism have G.I. symptoms, including abdominal pain, diarrhea and gastrointestinal reflex.
Research studies: There have been only a few published studies examining the efficacy of GFCF diets. Most of these studies report some degree of efficacy, yet each has some methodological weakness.

### 2.1 Uncontrolled trials

A literature search using Pubmed and other search engines was conducted to find studies evaluating the efficacy of the GFCF diet as an intervention to improve behavior, cognitive and social functioning in children with autism. Here some of the methodologically superior studies will be discussed briefly and critiqued.

**Reichelt et. al , 1990:**

Authors reported the results of an uncontrolled trial with 15 children, ages 3 to 17 years diagnosed with autism. In 8 children, gluten was eliminated and milk reduced; in three children milk was eliminated and gluten reduced; and in four children, both gluten and milk was eliminated. The children were followed for one year. Behavioral assessment was done by a clinical questionnaire at the beginning and the end of the treatment year. This was compared with the pretreatment year retrospectively. Results showed that at least half of the children improved during the treatment year. This study suffers from several methodological flaws. The subject pool was small and diagnostically heterogeneous. No information was provided about dietary compliance. Also no control group was used.

**Lucarelli et al., 1995**

In an uncontrolled study, 36 children, 8 to 13 years, with a diagnosis of autism were placed on individualized elimination diets for 8 weeks. Cow proteins were eliminated from all diets. In addition, each child received allergen testing, and any food allergen that tested positive was also removed from the diet. At base line and after 8 weeks children were evaluated with the Behavior Summarized Evaluation (BSE). A statistically significant reduction in group scores on 5 of the 7 BSE subscales after 8 weeks on the diet was reported. A lack of controls and relatively short intervention affect the validity of results of this study.

**Cade et al., 2000**

Seventy children with a diagnosis of autism on the GFCF elimination diet for one year were studied. There was no control group of children. Ten children with autism were matched for age, cognitive level and symptom severity. A statistically greater improvement was observed in the diet group on multiple domains of autism symptoms. Problems with the study include uncontrolled design and the outcomes measurement by an invalidated instrument.

### 2.2 Controlled clinical trials

**Knivensberg et al., 2002:**

A single blind study evaluated the effect of the GFCF diet on a group of 20 children with a diagnosis of autism and urinary peptide abnormalities. The authors were testing the hypothesis that products from incomplete digestion of proteins could cause synthesis of caseomorphines and glutomorphines. These compounds could have opioid-like effects when absorbed through a permeable intestine. Evaluation tests conducted before and after a treatment of one year in the areas of communications, language, and motor skills showed significant improvement in the group of children following a GFCF diet (Table 1). Improvements were also noted in social connections, willingness to learn and other areas. The children following the diet had fewer autistic traits after this one year intervention. However, the benefit of using matched controls was diminished by not blinding parents, teachers and subjects to treatment conditions.

**Elder et al. 2006**

A trial of the GFCF diet in 13 children with autism was carried out by Elders et al., 2006. Individual child preferences were taken into account and the participants were provided all meals and snacks from the metabolic kitchen. They evaluated the effect of the GFCF diet on autistic symptoms as measured by the (a) Childhood Autism Rating Scale (b) Urinary peptide levels on gluten free diet. Analysis indicated no significant differences in the behavior of autistic children as measured by emotional expression, body use, peculiarities in object use, resistance to change, activity level and intellectual ability. Also, there was no change in the urinary peptide levels in children on GFCF diet (Table 1).

**Milward et al., 2009 (Cochrane Review,)**

In this comprehensive review an extensive search was carried out to identify any randomized controlled trials (RCT) of gluten and/or casein free diets as intervention to improve behavior, cognitive and social functioning in individuals with autism . Only three papers reporting on three randomized trials were identified which met the rigorous criteria set by the investigators (Table 2). These trials were not mentioned above and are briefly discussed here.

1. Whitely et al., 2010: (The ScanBrit Randomized Single Blind Trial ): This NIH funded study conducted a two stage, 24 month randomized controlled trial in 72 Danish children assigned to diet (A) or non-diet (B) to evaluate core autism behaviors. Results suggested that GFCF had a significant beneficial group effect at 8, 12 and 24 months of intervention on core autistic and related behaviors of children diagnosed with ASD. Due to the absence of a placebo group, this study was unable to eliminate potential effects derived from interventions outside of dietary changes. (Table 2).

2. Diet and Behavior in Young Children with Autism ( Clinical trial No NCT00090428 Ongoing): This ongoing double blind randomized clinical trial is following children on a gluten free and casein free diet for 18 weeks. This long term rigorous trial with adequate sample size may clarify the issues involved with determining the efficacy of GFCF diets (Table 2).
3. Study to Assess the Role of a Gluten Free-dairy Free (GFCF) Diet in the Dietary Management of Autism Associated Gastrointestinal Disorders (ClinicalTrial .gov.Identifier: NCT0116388) (Ongoing, expected completion date April 2011) This ongoing randomized, double blind trial will asses the effect of a GFCG diet on GI symptoms associated with ASD in thirty activities- including physicals, blood samples and allergy testing. Also, an amino acid based supplement drink will be provided at no cost at the MGHFC in Boston, or at the Newton Wellesley Hospital in Newton, or at LADDERS in Lexington MA.

The results of the first trial indicated that a combined gluten and casein free diet reduced the autistic symptoms. The second trial showed no significant difference in outcome measures between the treatment and the control group. The results of the third trial have not yet been published. None of these trials reported an adverse outcome . It is hoped that as these rigorously conducted randomized clinical trials are completed, their results will further clarify the efficacy of GFCF diets in treatment of autism. However, on the basis of limited data available, the current knowledge about the efficacy of GFCF at this time does not merit a recommendation of their use as a standard treatment for autism..

| Investigators | Type of Intervention and Participants | Intervention and duration of study | Outcomes Measured |
|---|---|---|---|
| Elder, 2006 | Randomized, double blind crossover trial. 15 children with autism spectrum disorders (ASDs), ages 2-16. | Gluten and casein free diet adapted to the individual child's food preference vs. matched diet but with gluten and casein 12 weeks | -Childhood Autism Rating Scale (CARS) -Urinary Peptide Levels (UPL) -Ecological Communication Orientation (ECO) - In-home observation of child's behavior |
| Knivsberg, 2002 | Single-blind, randomized trial. 20 children with ASDs and abnormal urinary peptide pattern Ages 62-120 months | Gluten free vs. normal diet 12 months | Autistic traits Cognitive skills (Leiter International performance Scale), Linguistic ability, Motor ability (Movement Assessment Battery for Children) |

Table 1. Characteristics of Studies Which Met the Cochrane Review Criteria

| Investigators | Type of Study and Participants | Intervention and duration of study | Primary Outcomes |
|---|---|---|---|
| | | | |
| ScanBrit<br>Dietary Intervention in Autism<br>(under the remit of a Scandinavian- British collaborative research group)<br>NCT00614198 | Single-blind, randomized-controlled, matched pair adaptive trial.<br><br>72 Danish children ages 4-11 years formally diagnosed for PDD.<br>Exclusion criteria: co-morbid diagnosis for epilepsy, tuberous sclerosis or developmental age < 24 months. | Gluten-and casein - free diet.<br>April 2006-October 2008. | Outcomes: Autism Diagnostic Observation Schedule (ADOS), Gilliam Autism rating scale (GARS), Vineland Adaptive Behavior Scale (VABS)<br>Changes in appearance of multiple compounds in urine |
| Diet and Behavior in Young Children with Autism. National Institutes of Health, Clinical trial No. NCT00090428 | Randomized, Double Blind Placebo Control.<br>30 children, at the University of Rochester Medical Center, Rochester, New York, ages 30-54 months | Gluten-and casein-free diet Vs. Placebo.<br><br>They will also receive uniform educational and behavioral services through their provider.<br>Controlled diet<br>Phase I<br>August 2004-<br>Estimated completion Feb 2009 | Safety and efficacy of the gluten free casein free diet, measured at weeks 18 and 30. |
| A Study to Assess the Role of a Gluten Free-dairy Free (GFCF) Diet in the Dietary Management of Autism Associated Gastrointestinal Disorders.<br>Massachusetts General Hospital.<br>ClinicalTrials .govIdentifier: NCT0116388 | Randomized , double blind Trial<br>Crossover Assignment.<br>Estimated enrollment: 30,<br>ages 2-17 years | Gluten free-Casein-free diet.<br>Study started April 2010.<br>Estimated completion date: April 2011. | To assess if improvements in GI symptoms result in improvements in autistic behavior when using a GFCF diet and dietary management of GI symptoms associated with ASD.<br>To determine the nutritional management of a GFCF restrictive diet.<br>To assess the role of food allergies in the maintenance of GI symptoms. |

Table 2. Characteristics of Recently Completed and Ongoing Randomized Controlled Trials which Met the Cochrane Review Criteria.

## 3. Ketogenic diets

The ketogenic diet was first introduced as a therapeutic method to reduce the number and intensity of epileptic seizures. But it has been reported that in addition, the ketogenic diet is beneficial for mental behavior and hyperactivity. In the classic ketogenic diet, also known as the long-chain triglyceride diet, fat provides the majority of energy, protein is based on minimum daily requirements, and carbohydrates are severely restricted (Kossoff and Zupec-Kana, 2009; Evangeliou et al., 2003).

**Rationale**

It is hypothesized that autistic behavior is associated with a disturbance in glucose metabolism, particularly, mitochondrial energy production, leading to an excess of reduced nicotinamide adenine dinucleotide (NADH) or a lack of nicotinamide dinucleotide (NAD). It is thought that application of a ketogenic diet would produce an improved mitochondrial function by sparing NAD, which will be consumed in the oxidation of glycolytic substrates (Evangeliou et al., 2003; Carroll and Koenigsberger, 1998).

In the past decade, there have been four major meta-analyses of the efficacy of the ketogenic diet. All of these reviews concluded that there is some evidence of seizure reduction and other benefits in children with epilepsy despite the lack of blinded, controlled trials at the time of publications (Keen, 2006; Yeou-Mei et. al, 2003). However, the ketogenic diet has not been shown to be efficacious specifically when used to treat children diagnosed with autism. Also, to our knowledge no randomized clinical trials have been conducted to evaluate the effect of the ketogenic diet for treatment of symptoms of autism.

Research Studies: There is a paucity of data in evaluating the efficacy of the ketogenic diet as a dietary intervention in autism. In a pilot study, Evangeliou et al, 2003 examined the efficacy of the ketogenic diet in autism. Thirty children were put on a ketogenic diet for 6 months .Of the 60% of the patients who adhered to the diet improvement was recorded in several parameters in accordance with the Childhood Autism Rating Scale. These data are very preliminary and better designed clinical trials are needed to test the efficacy of ketogenic diets in the treatment of autism.

## 4. Feingold diet

This diet is based on the benefit of a food-restriction diet for attention deficit and hyperactivity disorder. Scientifically undocumented behavioral improvements after elimination of food colors and flavors have been reported. According to Dr. Feingold's hypothesis elimination of food additives resulted in some cases in dramatic decline in hyperactive symptoms (Feingold, 1985). At this time no rigorous randomized trials have been conducted to evaluate the efficacy of the Feingold diet for easing the symptoms of ASD.

## 5. Antioxidant diets

Antioxidant diets have gained the attention of some investigators who are concerned about oxidative stress in autism and related conditions. Commonly recommended foods are fresh fruits and vegetables, cooked legumes, and whole grains (Jeep et al., 2008). The super foods recommended on this type of diet are broccoli, Brussels sprouts, berries like blueberries and Goji berries. Moderate servings of animal products such as lean meat are allowed. This dietary pattern is part of a healthy diet recommended for the general population but it has not been tested for reducing symptoms of ASD.

## 6. Conclusions

Among the dietary interventions currently in use for treatment of ASD, the gluten-free-casein free diet shows the most promise of efficacy. However, this diet is not without cost in terms of inconvenience and limitation on foods of choice for the affected individual. Due to the potential for nutritional deficiency as a result of long-term dietary exclusion, appropriate clinical and dietetic support should be considered during any attempt to make such dietary changes. The American Dietetic Associations position at this time is that more research is needed to determine the efficacy of dietary therapy approaches (Marcason, 2009).The lack of long term data, preferably life-span data on health risk associated with nutrient limiting diets such as GFCF require further safety study. At present, two double blind, placebo controlled trials are being conducted and results of these trials are likely to provide valid information pertaining to the efficacy of GFCF diet in treatment of autism.

## 7. References

A Study to Assess the Role of a Gluten Free-Dairy Free (GFCF) Diet in the Dietary Management of Autism Associated Gastrointestinal Disorders.Massachusetts General Hospital. ClinicalTrials.govIdentifier: NCT0116388.

Cade R, Privette M, Fregly M. Autism and schizophrenia: intestinal disorders. Nutr. Neurosci. 2000; 3:57-72.

Carroll J, Koenigsberger D. The ketogenic diet: A practical guide for caregivers. J Am Diet Assoc. 1998; 98 (3): 316-321.

Christison GW, Ivany K. Elimination Diets in Autism Spectrum Disorders: Any wheat amidst the chaff? Dev Behav Padiar. 2006; 27 (2): S162-S169

Cubala-Kucharska M. The review of most frequently occurring medical disorders related to aetiology of autism and the methods of treatment. Acta Neurobiol Exp. 2010; 70:141-146.

Diet and Behavior in Young Children with Autism. National Institutes of Health, Clinical trial No. NCT00090428. Clinical trial registry. Diet and behavior in young children with autism. ClinicalTrial.gov.

Elder JH, Shanker M, Shuster J, Douglas T, Burns S, Sherill L. The gluten-free, casein-free diet in autism: results of a preliminary double blind clinical trial. J Autism Dev Disorders. 2006;36(3): 413-420.

Elder JH. The gluten –free,casein-free diet in autism: An overview with clinical implications. Nutr. Clin Pract. 2008; 23 (6):583-588

Evangeliou A, Valchonikolis I, Mihailidou H. et al. Application of a ketogenic diet in children with autistic behavior: Pilot study. J Child Neurol. 2003; 18: 113-118.

Feingold B. Why your child is hyperactive. New York, NY. Random House; 1985.

Jeep R, Couey R, Pittman ES. The super antioxidant diet and nutrition guide. Charlottesville, VA. Hampton Roads Publishing Company; 2008.

Keen DL. A systematic review of the use of ketogenic diet in childhood epilepsy. Pediatr Neurol.2006; 35:1-5.

Knivsberg A, Reichelt KL, Hoten I. A randomized controlled study of dietary intervention in autistic syndrome. Nutr Neurosci. 2002; 5: 251-261

Kossoff EH , Zupec-Kana BA. Ketogenic diets; an update for child neurologists. J Child Neurol. 2009; 24 (8):979-88.

Lucarelli S, Fredianai T, Zingoni AM. Food allergy and infantile autism. Pan Minerva Med. 1995; 37:137-141.

Marcason W. What is the current status of research concerning use of a gluten-free, casein-free diet for children diagnosed with autism? J Am Diet Assoc. 2009; 109.

Milward C, Ferrier M, Calver SJ, Connell-J GG.. Gluten-and casein-free diets for autistic spectrum disorder. Cochrane database of Systematic reviews. 2009 (2): 1-27.CD003498.

Reichelt KL, Ekrem J, Scott H. Gluten, milk protein, and autism: dietary intervention effects on behavior and peptide secretion. J Appl Nutr. 1990; 42:1-11.

Seung HK, Rogalski Y, Shankar M, Elder J. The gluten-and casein- free diet and autism: Communication outcomes from a preliminary double blind clinical trial. J Med Speech-Language Path. 2007; 15(4): 337-345.

Srinivasan P. A review of dietary interventions in autism. Ann Clin Psychiatry. 2009; 21 (4): 237-47

Whitely P, Haracopos D, Knivsberg AM Reichelt KR, Parlar S, Jacobsen J, Seim A, Pedersen L, Schondel M, Shattock M.. The Scan Brit randomized controlled, single blind study of a gluten and casein free dietary intervention for children with autism spectrum disorders. Nutr Neuroscience. 2010; 13 (2): 87-100.

Yeou-Mei CL, Williams S, Basualdo-Hammond C, et al. . A prospective study: Growth and nutrition status of children treated with the ketogenic diet. J Am Diet Assoc. 2003; 103: 707-712.

# Part 2

## Psychosocial Aspects

7

# Intervention Models in Children with Autism Spectrum Disorders

Gonzalo Ros Cervera[1,2], María Gracia Millá Romero[3], Luis Abad Mas[4] and Fernando Mulas Delgado[1,5]
[1]*Invanep, Valencia*
[2]*Elda General Hospital, Alicante*
[3]*Apadis Villena, Alicante*
[4]*Red Cenit, Valencia*
[5]*University Children's Hospital La Fe, Valencia*
*Spain*

## 1. Introduction

Autism spectrum disorders (ASD) are a group of developmental disorders of unknown origin that affect children in many important areas, namely language, communication and social interaction. The burden of the disorder, with an incidence of about one new case in every 100 newborns, makes its early recognition a vital task for all professionals caring for children. Although autism is a chronic condition with no specific cure nowadays, advances in the research in the last 40 years predict new hope and a better prognosis for children and adults with this group of disorders.

ASD affect children's ability to understand and interact with their environment. Our mission as therapists is to recognize their difficulties and try to enter their world in order to increase their communication and relationship skills. Therefore, it is essential to carefully observe the child, taking notes and measuring his or her abilities through the use of ASD-specific and general evaluation scales, such as the Childhood Autism Rating Scale (CARS) for parents or the McCarthy or Battelle scales for children. This initial assessment of the child's situation is critical in order to follow and measure his or her improvements, and focus the therapy based on the results.

The diagnosis of ASD is a difficult issue, not only for the child but also for the parents. Parents of newly diagnosed children need time to understand what is happening. Information is crucial, and it takes time to explain the global aspects of the disease and the planned intervention. Parents are a key element in therapy, not only because they spend the most time with the child and can generalize the new skills taught, but also because a well-informed and supportive environment warrants a better prognosis than a chaotic one.

The Early Intervention setting, with its multidisciplinary richness, is the ideal setting in which to contain and educate the family and establish a positive relationship with the aim of improving the child's abilities. Early intervention programs should pursue these goals:

- An interdisciplinary early diagnosis.
- The design and implementation of specific intervention programs.

- The use of effective resources and methods.
- Communication and interrelation with all health, educational and social services involving the child and his or her family.

Early Intervention Programs can make a difference and produce positive and permanent changes in the child. These specific programs have demonstrated their effectiveness in the containment and extinction of the core symptoms of autism, and in improving the social, communicative, attentional, and cognitive and social skills of the child. They require highly-qualified interdisciplinary professionals with definite skills and enough empathy to be in tune with the child and his or her family's needs. The end goal is not only the improvement of the child's abilities; it is also a question of his or her quality of life and well being and that of his or her family.

From a categorical point of view, there are three kinds of approaches to the intervention in ASD: biomedical, psychodynamic and psychoeducational interventions. The first two are clearly outdated, since they are not based on scientific principles. Only psychoeducational interventions, with special emphasis on behavioral techniques, are the leading approaches nowadays.

In this chapter we will review some aspects of psychological intervention in children with ASD:

- Role of Early Intervention in the management of children with ASD and their families.
- General considerations about intervention models in children with ASD.
- Classification of the intervention models.
- Description of some center-based programs.

## 2. Definition of autism spectrum disorders

ASD are a group of biologically-based neurodevelopmental disorders characterized by impairments in three major domains: socialization, communication, and behavior. Under ASD we refer to the autistic disorder, the pervasive developmental disorder-not otherwise specified (PDD-NOS), and Asperger's disorder. We do not include the other two disorders in the "pervasive developmental disorders" section of the Diagnostic and Statistical Manual of Mental Disorders, Fourth Edition, Text Revision (DSM-IV-TR), i.e., Rett's disorder and childhood disintegrative disorder, because of the poor prognosis and differential approach in the intervention programs (see Table 1). Indeed, we will mostly speak about autism disorder and PDD-NOS, because children with Asperger's syndrome are generally diagnosed at a later age, and they do not require such an intensive behavioral treatment.

The pervasive developmental disorder-not otherwise specified (PDD-NOS) is a diagnosis used to describe patients who show some but not all of the characteristics included in one of the other autistic disorders [APA, 2000]. These children may have milder symptoms or be diagnosed at a later age. This disorder is also known as atypical autism. These children share the core deficits in communication, social behavior, emotion regulation, cognition, and interests that children with other ASD show, but their severity does not fit the restricted criteria for the other diagnoses (Autistic disorder, Asperger's disorder, Rett's disorder or CDD).

## 3. Early diagnosis in ASD

### 3.1 Etiology vs. behavioral phenotype

Discovering the etiologic factors in autism is still a priority for scientists involved in this field of study. Autism spectrum disorder can be due to different causes or a combination of

| |
|---|
| • Mental Retardation |
| • Learning Disorders |
| • Motor Skills Disorder |
| • Communication Disorders |
| • Pervasive Developmental Disorders<br>• Autistic Disorder<br>• Rett's Disorder<br>• Childhood Disintegrative Disorder<br>• Asperger's Disorder<br>• Pervasive Developmental Disorder Not Otherwise Specified |
| • Attention-Deficit and Disruptive Behavior Disorders |
| • Feeding and Eating Disorders of Infancy or Early Childhood |
| • Tic Disorders |
| • Elimination Disorders |

Table 1. Disorders Usually First Diagnosed in Infancy, Childhood, or Adolescence. Reproduced from: American Psychiatric Association. Diagnostic and Statistic Manual of Mental Disorders, 4th ed. American Psychiatric Association. Washington, DC. 1996.

them, like the conjunction of genetics and environment. In the last few years there has been an increase in knowledge about the neurobiological conditions present in this disorder [Mulas et al., 2005]. However, the innate disturbance of affective contact and relationships exhibited in autism still presents a cryptogenic origin in most cases, which greatly hinders early identification and prevention designed to contain its incidence.

In recent years the empirical findings point to establishing the main cause of autism in genetically-based disorders [Díez-Cuervo, 2005]. A group of scientists has found the first clear evidence that a common genetic variation influences the development of autism. The research focuses on single nucleotide polymorphisms, which are a very common variation in the DNA sequence that affects a single base, adenine, thymine, cytosine and guanine in a sequence of the genome. It is estimated that the variants discovered could be behind up to 15% of the cases of ASD in a population [Wang et al., 2009]. Furthermore, neurobiological research on this disorder focuses on increasingly early ages. Based on the results of a study recently published in the BMC Medicine journal [Bols et al., 2011], there appears to be an endophenotype of familiar autism that is particularly evident in the electrical activity of the brain at 9 months.

These scientific advances are opening up new possibilities for early detection and for providing increasingly more accurate and appropriate tools and diagnostic criteria. But while progress is being made in understanding the true etiology of autism, there is a greater need to delve into the diagnosis of early signs and symptoms, identifying prototypical behaviors and indicators that manifest at an early age, the functional diagnosis of all the skills and strengths of children with ASD, and the entire set of consequences associated with the cognitive, linguistic, emotional and social areas.

### 3.2 Early symptoms in autism

Early detection of autism is the first step towards addressing the problems involved in this disorder, in order to influence the child and, if possible, improve his or her development, and enable the family to handle the difficulties arising from this situation with greater knowledge and better strategies. Despite progress in identifying characteristics of autistic traits in the first year of life, ignorance about the presence of autistic signs on the part of the family and health and education staff limits detection and early diagnosis. The first autistic manifestations can be seen, in some cases, after six months, although they usually arise between the age of 18 months and two years [Martos, 2001].

| | | |
|---|---|---|
| | Early signs of autism appearance ⟵⟶ | |
| Primary intersubjectivity<br>Conversational play<br>Play with objects | Secondary intersubjectivity<br>Protolanguage<br>Task cooperation with mother | Symbolic play<br>Language and protodialogue |
| 0 2 8 | 12 | 18 months |

Fig. 1. Normal development and appearance of autism signs [Martos, 2001]

The first symptoms are related to social behavior areas, intersubjectivity and interpersonal relationships. We can find alterations in the response to stimuli that have a strong social component, such as eye contact, looking at the face, maintaining joint attention, pointing behavior, showing objects, or responding in some way when we say the child's name. We can also observe the presence of abnormal sensory and perceptual integration. It must be kept in mind that during the child's first year of life we can identify warning signs that correlate with this disorder (see table 1).

All of these early symptoms can occur with variable intensity and timing of their appearance. They usually anticipate the presence of qualitative impairments in social interaction and the difficulties that these children have in adjusting their behavior to others and sharing the emotional world. Likewise, they can anticipate qualitative changes in the communication skills and difficulties in the development of functional speech. Early on, there is a presence of restricted patterns of behavior and an interest in spontaneous play that tends to be unimaginative and repetitive, as well as showing little or no playing interaction with others. Anxiety expressed about changes in the environment and routines, stereotyped body movements and consolation difficulties are other features that may present at an early age.

### 3.3 Diagnostic process in the child with ASD

First, information about the developmental history of the child will be gathered by interviewing parents and educators. In this first phase of the diagnosis, data will be collected about the child's neurobiological development, status in the achievement of milestones in communication, social competence, receptive response, motor skills, and the onset of the first autistic symptoms. The style of relations, patterns of behavior, interactions with peers and adults, level of participation in structured dynamic groups, and adaptation to nursery or childhood education will also be investigated. To address this part of the analysis, the following tools are very useful:

| Early markers | Clinical characteristics | Associated problems |
|---|---|---|
| -Little or no interest in eye contact.<br>-No orientation response when the child is mentioned.<br>-Lack of protodeclarative pointing.<br>-Absence of protodeclarative showing. | - Indifference toward the parents.<br>- The child is not involved in social interaction games.<br>- No answer or anticipation of beginnings of oral communication.<br>- Absence of babbling and jargon.<br>- Does not imitate sounds, gestures or expressions.<br>- Not interested in toys offered.<br>- Shows fascination with his own hands and feet.<br>- Smells or sucks objects more than expected.<br>- Has fragmented sleep. | - Sleep disturbances.<br>- Problems with food.<br>- Low interest in playing.<br>- Low consolation ability. |

Table 2. Early markers of autism, clinical characteristics and associated problems.

- Autism Diagnostic Interview-Revised (ADI-R) [Lord et al., 1994]: This is a semi-structured interview for parents that makes it possible to obtain meaningful information in three key areas: reciprocal social playing interaction, communication and adaptive behaviors.
- Diagnostic Interview for Social Communication Disorder (DISC) [Wing et al., 2002]: Semi-structured interview that makes it possible to collect developmental information from different sources.
- Diagnosis Checklist for Behavior-Disturbed Children, E-2 [Howlin, 1998]: This is a questionnaire for parents that provides information about the causes and type of behavior disorder of the child.

Subsequently, the clinical examination will be carried out through observation and direct interaction with the child and the application of specific tests. This part of the diagnostic evaluation should objectively determine the child's strengths in several areas of development. The diagnosis of autism should include the use of specific diagnostic instruments of strong sensitivity and reliability. It is necessary to use tools that specifically assess the presence of autistic symptoms [10]. The diagnosis and evaluation of the ASD must be an interdisciplinary task by a specialized and experienced team, using appropriate diagnostic criteria and various procedures, and concluding with a reliable clinical judgment. It is necessary to analyze the developmental history of the child and the autistic symptoms, adaptive behavior, intellectual functioning, communication skills, social competence, interests and activities of the child. The early indicators to be assessed are the following [11]:

1. Child's social relation ability:

- Eye contact,
- Joint attention and action,

- The initiative for interactions,
- Emotional states,
- Reactions to physical contact,
- Response to activities with others,
- Adaptation to social patterns of behavior,
- Intersubjectivity.

2. Communication and language:
- Gestural communication,
- Comprehension and verbal expression,
- Communicative functions,
- Unique language characteristics of the child,
- Presence of echolalia,
- Ability to track orders,
- The ability to differentiate between literal and metaphorical meaning,
- Adequacy of the vocabulary and syntactic constructions.

3. The game:
- Ability to manipulate and functional or stereotyped interaction with objects,
- Imagination and spontaneity,
- Symbolic play.

4. Behavior and mental flexibility:
- Adaptation or opposition to changes in the environment,
- Presence of stereotypes,
- Rituals,
- Presence of limited interests,
- Obsessive behaviors.

### 3.4 Tests for ASD diagnosis in the early years

Currently, there is a series of tests specifically designed for the diagnosis of children with ASD that facilitate the early assessment of the child. Next, we refer to those that are more common and have a higher scientific recognition.

- Checklist for Autism in Toddlers (CHAT) [Baron-Cohen et al., 1992]. Allows early detection of the disorder by observation of deficits in three areas, for children between 18 and 36 months:

a. Social skills: lack of joint reference gaze and significant limitation in the interest in and emotional involvement with others.
b. Communication: absence of protodeclarative function.
c. Imaginative ability: lack of or deficit in social play and symbolic activity.

- Autism Diagnostic Observation Schedule (ADOS-G) [Lord et al., 2000]. This is a tool for the standardized observation of social behavior of children involved with different types of materials and tasks.
- Childhood Autism Rating Scale (CARS) [Schopler et al., 1990]. Evaluates 15 aspects of behavior.
- Gilliam Autism Rating Scale (GARS) [Gillian, 1995]. This is organized into four categories: stereotypes, communication, social interaction and developmental disturbances.

- Behavior Observation Scale for Autism (BOS) [Freeman & Ritvo, 1978]. This is a scale based on the analysis of recorded video sessions.
- ACACIA [Tamarit, 1994]. This is an instrument designed for the assessment and analysis of communicative behavior and social/interpersonal skills in children with serious developmental disorders.
- List of indicators of autism typical of the 18-36 month stage by Rivière [Rivière, 2000], which describes 22 behaviors and traits that can be detected in cases where one can see the presence of this disorder.

| List of indicators of autism typical of 18-36 month stage |
|---|
| 1. Apparent paradoxical deafness. Failure to respond to calls and instructions.<br>2. Not sharing attention hotspots with the gaze.<br>3. Tends not to make eye contact.<br>4. Does not look to adults to understand relational situations that interest or surprise.<br>5. Does not see what people do.<br>6. Does not usually look at people.<br>7. Repetitive or ritualistic play or sort rituals.<br>8. Resists changes in clothes, food, itineraries and situations.<br>9. Greatly alters, especially in unforeseen or unexpected circumstances.<br>10. Novelties upset him or her.<br>11. Watches the same films obsessively, again and again.<br>12. Has tantrums in situations of change.<br>13. No language or, if so, in an echolalic or dysfunctional way.<br>14. It is difficult to "share actions" with him or her.<br>15. Does not point his or her finger to share experiences.<br>16. Does not point his or her finger to ask.<br>17. Frequently "passes through" people as if they were not there.<br>18. Does not seem to understand or "selectively understands" only what interests him or her.<br>19. Asks for things, situations or actions, leading by the hand.<br>20. Does not usually initiate interactions with adults.<br>21. To contact him, you have to "jump over a wall": i.e., requires facing each other, and producing clear and directive gestures.<br>22. Tends to ignore. |

Table 3. Early indicators of autism disorder [Riviere, 2000]

To complement all these tests and obtain further information, where possible, we will use scales of development like the Battelle Developmental Inventory [Newborg et al., 1998], which gives us information on the personal/social, adaptive, motor, communicative and cognitive areas up to eight years of age, and the Bayley Scales of Infant Development (BSID) [Bayley, 1977], with which we can evaluate children up to three years of age in the mental, motor and behavioral domains.

Regarding the assessment of cognitive potential in young children with ASD, tests to be used are:

- Uzgiris / Hunt 's Scales of Infant Development [Dunst, 1980]. Assesses the cognitive development of children less than two years old.

- Merrill-Palmer Scale of Mental Tests [Stutsman, 1931]. From 18 months.
- Leiter International Scale [Leiter, 1948]. Most suitable to evaluate the intellectual profile of people with autism from age two, it is a nonverbal test, including batteries for the assessment of thinking skills, visualization, attention and memory.
- Psychoeducational Profile Revised (PEP-R) [Schopler et al., 1990] Mesibov, Schopler and Caison (1989). An observational instrument used for nonverbal children from a mental age of 2 years.
- McCarthy Scales of Children Abilities [McCarthy, 2006]. They are composed of six scales for children from 2.5 years.
- K-ABC Kaufman & Kaufman [Kaufman & Kaufman, 1997]. This is a battery for the diagnosis of intelligence also from 2.5 years.

### 3.5 Assessment of the familial and social environment

For the child with autism, the environmental aspects have a special meaning, so that it is necessary to perform a systematic analysis of the child's life context. It is, therefore, necessary to understand the reality in which the child lives and his or her requirements by analyzing:

- The functional relationships between the behaviors of the child with autism and the contingencies of the environment in which they occur (e.g., in what situations the temper tantrums occur and the consequences they have.)
- The real opportunities for interaction and learning in the family.
- The perceptions that other people who are related to the child have of him, his level of anxiety, frustration, helplessness or assimilation.
- The degree of structure, directionality and predictability of the contexts in which the child develops.

Knowing about the situation in which the child grows is essential in order to help him develop his knowledge and ability to communicate, so that he connects well with others, and to adapt the settings to suit his needs. An analysis of the fostering environment should serve to improve the adaptation to the physical and relational environment, and to help the family to improve their skills and resources. The family should be aware of the resources available to the child and family and the social, health and education resources at their disposal.

## 4. Role of early intervention in the diagnosis and treatment of ASD

### 4.1 Programs of early intervention in ASD

Early Intervention programs can promote development and produce significant and lasting improvements [McEachin et al., 1993], positively modify the course of development of children with ASD [Dawson, 2003], and improve their individual understanding of the social reality in which they live, their communication and teaching. The effectiveness of these programs and the improvements experienced by children with ASD in terms of their IQ, language and visuospatial abilities have been shown [Smith et al, 2000]. In many cases there is a contention or elimination of the autistic symptoms, as well as significant improvement in perceptual responses and attentional, cognitive, communicative and social skills.

Intervention in the ASD has to target the child, family and environment, and it must be properly coordinated among all the actors involved in this task: Early Intervention Centers

(EICs), family environment, kindergarten, social and health resources and community environment. It aims to promote the adaptation of children with ASD to their living environment and community, respecting their autonomy and individuality. In addition, it must provide the family with the attention they require, so that they can improve their knowledge and strategies to promote a good family atmosphere.

Intervention should begin as soon as possible and must be based on careful individual assessment of the capabilities and difficulties of the child. Implementing an intervention program early on is highly desirable, even before definitively clarifying the diagnosis, in order to promptly manage the autistic symptoms. Interdisciplinary Early Intervention professional teams must develop comprehensive intervention programs working collaboratively with parents. They must also keep in mind that the child with ASD may experience an evolution over time. Therefore, they must respond to changes as they occur in the child due to his or her maturity and changes in capabilities and needs. Based on this, it is necessary to keep in mind the following principles of intervention:

1. Early Intervention programs should be flexible and tailored to each child's individuality and the uniqueness of his family.
2. Each child shall be given a cognitive-behavioral and environmental intervention process.
3. The intervention has to address the child with ASD, the family and all the environments in which the child develops.
4. The intervention has to promote the welfare and quality of life of children with ASD throughout their developmental process.

The working plan has to fit the particular cognitive characteristics and relationships of each child, procuring well-structured environments in which to facilitate the keys to understanding the tasks and anticipating what will be done at each point in time. It is necessary for the program activities to be playful, meaningful and functional, adapted to the child's cognitive potential, with reference to his or her natural surroundings. Empathy and positive reinforcement are of particular significance in the Early Intervention program for children with ASD. We must use those aids, visual, physical or verbal, that can facilitate the child's internalization of the reality and enable improvements in his or her understanding and adaptation.

We believe, as indicated by Juan Martos [Martos, 2005], that any program which provides early intervention with a sufficient and regular external organizational scaffolding that encourages the application of the child's cognitive and self-regulatory capacities in a wide variety of social interaction tasks can be of great benefit to children with autism throughout the preschool years. As long as this intervention is not aversive, the child may benefit from social stimuli, which can mitigate the secondary neurodevelopmental disturbances; such disturbances may be related to the difficulties of the diminished social interaction in the early years of life. Therefore, providing a service of quality which responds fully and satisfactorily to the issues presented by the children, arising from disabilities such as ASD or the risk of suffering them, to their families, and to the environment in which life develops, is a very large and complex task. It requires a set of material resources and highly-qualified human teams [Millá, 2005], in addition to specific skills and the necessary empathy to be in tune with child and family. The intervention must also be conducted in an interdisciplinary way in order to address all aspects of eventual dysfunctions, either in social behavior, in the management of communication and language or in the behavior. The intervention aims to improve the situation and skills of children with ASD, while providing welfare and quality of life.

Professionals working with children with ASD should remember that the intervention will consist mainly of promoting and improving their adaptation to their physical, cultural and social environment and helping their families to participate in this task and improve their skills and resources for dealing with having a child with ASD. Achieving improvements in the conditions of child development requires the involvement of people around the child and the support of social, health and education providers, who foster major changes in the management of this disorder in the child's daily life and in his or her social and family status.

### 4.2 Intervention with the child

The planned intervention from the field of Early Intervention should consider the whole child with ASD, caring for all areas of development. In the intervention program, priorities for action should be established to improve social competences, communication and language skills, play and adaptive and behavior skills.

One of the biggest challenges associated with ASD children is their lack of social approach and the absence of response to the initiatives of others towards them. The intervention means that professionals must make a deliberate intrusion into the child's solitary activities, so that he will be involved with other people in doing his or her favorite activities. This effort should be undertaken in such a way that social interaction is pleasant for the child, structuring interactions to be reciprocal and social rather than isolated and lonely. The active structuration of the early social experiences can lead to significant improvements in social interactions of children with ASD. For more and better social responses of children with this disorder, Early Intervention professionals have to adapt themselves to the idiosyncrasies of the child and family, and direct and be persistent in their interactions and play with the child.

The contents of the intervention program must be established on the basis of the results of the diagnostic evaluation of the child with ASD. It should be based on the skills and competences that the child has, and then continue with the behaviors that begin to emerge and those that, from a developmental standpoint, he should acquire. In the work program for children with ASD, every dimension of child development must be considered and improved globally in all areas: Personal / social, Cognition, Communication, Motor, and Adaptive. However, specifically, we believe that the Early Intervention program for these children has to mainly contemplate perceptual enrichment, and it should put an emphasis on communication and social skills training and intersubjectivity.

Perception and joint attention play a fundamental role in capturing and internalizing the surrounding reality, so that the work on these skills in children with ASD has to be performed from the start of the intervention. The improvement in cognitive abilities by imitating actions, through observational and modeling learning methods, the internalization of concepts or cultural elements, is central to early intervention. We must improve the knowledge the child has of the reality in which he lives through meaningful experiences that will lead him to the reality he should know. Enabling the communication and language of children with ASD is a substantial issue that will improve their skills in symbolic representation and interaction with others. If oral skills cannot be developed, augmentative and alternative systems of communication can help mitigate this limitation. By means of the Early Intervention program, it should be ensured that the child with ASD can improve his or her ability to understand and assimilate interactions with others and improve intersubjective relations, co-regulation and social behavior. To enhance all these skills, the Early Intervention program should [Millá & Mulas, 2009]:

- Create a work environment that offers security to the child in establishing emotional links and enhance empathy.
- Propose an individualized program which starts with the domains and skills the child with ASD has to move forward systematically in his or her area of potential development.
- Carry out the activities in a fun and functional way using as a working model of meaningful learning and incorporating elements of the everyday life context in the child's language.
- Respect the work rate of the children, introducing in the sessions a variety of tasks that meet their learning style, their motivations and interests.
- Use technical aids, visual signs, or augmentative communication systems that allow alternative language to enable the child's language, with the Early Intervention technicians offering a transparent verbal model about the meaning that is simplified in lexical selection and verbal structures.
- Enhance assimilation and adaptation to social situations, encouraging personal interactions with members of the family system, with EIC professionals, and the integration with other children in their environment and kindergarten or school mates.
- Provide children with necessary aid to do the activities of early intervention programs, so that those that will be performed at home or in the school context can be understandable and predictable for him.
- Promote the reduction and elimination of rituals, stereotypes or routines through extinction strategies and behavior modification techniques.
- Following criteria for generalization and individualization and providing structured and predictable environments for children help to obtain better responses from the child, improving his or her skills and quality of life.
- Provide the family with the knowledge and strategies needed to participate in the Early Intervention program and to assist in achieving the objectives.

Systematic and structured Early Intervention Programs demonstrate that they are the most effective intervention from early childhood to improve the prognosis of children with ASD, as most of these children respond favorably, changing the autistic symptoms and improving their attentional, cognitive, communicative and social skills, which contributes significantly to improving their adaptability and their behavior [Grupo de Estudios de Trastornos del Espectro Autista, 2006].

### 4.3 Intervention with the family

The diagnosis of ASD means the beginning of a process of assimilation of a new and complex reality by the family. Having a child with this disorder causes a breakdown of the expectations that were created around having a child. The initial emotional shock of the parents is a sense of personal failure and feelings of confusion. They find it very difficult to understand the new situation, and they need clear and concise information to start adapting to it, accepting it and learning to live with the problems generated by having a child with ASD.

We must consider the family as a partner in developing the intervention program with the child, but at the same time, it also has to be the subject of intervention. The interdisciplinary teams should first seek familiar cohesion and provide the necessary support and the accompaniment in light of the new family circumstances. The main goal of family intervention is to help parents overcome the various phases of the process of assuming the new reality and meet their demands and needs. The information provided about ASD in general, and the situation of the child in particular, should gradually be offered by the Early Intervention professionals, so that the family can properly assimilate and integrate it. It is very important to achieve the adjustment of parental expectations to the real possibilities of the child. Parents need to understand the characteristics of ASD so they can realistically accept symptomatic manifestations of their autistic child. To the extent that parents have a better understanding of the reality of their child and can adapt their environment to the physical, emotional, mental and social needs of the child, the better the child's development will be [Millá, 2005]].

The training we can provide parents reassures them in their parenting role and improves their ability to participate actively in their child's development. Family intervention has to provide guidelines for a structured environment for the child in order to encourage communication and empower his autonomy, to improve family interactions, and to perform daily activities and games to enhance the desired routines, behavior and emotional responses of the child. The family environment is the primary socializing agent of the child with ASD, and in this environment behavioral patterns have to be offered that help in his developmental process and improve the developmental course. Benchmarks to adjust the family situation include the following:

1. Organize the environment to make it more predictable for the child.
2. Use clear gestures and simple language to facilitate understanding.
3. Parents must provide the child with experiences in a fun and safe environment, fostering his or her emotional development.
4. Avoid complex environments that are noisy, very stimulating or unstructured.
5. Be patient and have strategies for setting limits on behavioral disturbances and stereotyped behaviors or rituals.

EICs should also ensure the families the support they need to improve the functioning of the family system, providing them with available community resources, financial assistance, respite services, etc.

The presence in the family of a child with ASD can be an awkward situation for siblings. They suffer from broken expectations, expecting a sibling with whom to play and share, but having to deal with a very different reality. The Early Intervention program should also offer support for siblings of children with ASD, creating a space in which to express their concerns and anxieties, where they can feel supported and acquire knowledge, skills and strategies to interact more effectively with their sibling. In this sense, it is necessary to explain and educate them about the difficulties of the child with ASD, request their participation in simple tasks of the intervention program, make them feel they are very important people and responsible for acting with their brother or sister, and set aside time to stay and play with him or her and express their affection.

### 4.4 Intervention with the environment

Children with ASD, like the rest of the child population, are involved in idiosyncratic social contexts where they have to incorporate cultural references, language or behavior particularities, and where they will grow in the company of their families. As some of the major characteristics of ASD are the social deficits and the difficulty in interacting with the environment, it must be ensured that these children have access to community resources in a manner that fits their style of relationships and their adaptive possibilities. It is very important that from a young age they become familiar with the physical and social environment where they live, the home, neighborhood, park, kindergarten, etc., as a way to join the social life that corresponds to them by age. From the Early Intervention teams, it is necessary to influence the participation of the elements and agents of the child's world and the suitability of the environment to the individual characteristics of the child.

As for health services in general and pediatric neurology services in particular, there has to be a close collaboration and coordination among professionals and the EIC, in order to address the diagnostic and intervention planning. It is necessary to maintain this coordination while carrying out the specific program of Early Intervention, which will unify criteria for action and offer common information to the family, avoiding confusion and contradictions.

Toddlers with ASD are usually enrolled in kindergartens or nursery schools; for that reason, professionals in these centers and Early Intervention professionals together must agree on the objectives and methodology to be followed, the most suitable adaptation of the environment, the selection of teaching contents, and the support in the school setting. The relationship between infant school and EIC must be based on collaborative attitudes, and it has to provide resources and advice to facilitate the integration process and the maximum development of the child. It tries to procure a context as normalized as possible and adopt measures that encourage the incorporation of the child into normal dynamic activities.

In certain cases, it may be necessary to use the social services to provide support for the child or the family in certain circumstances of socioeconomic disadvantage or difficulties. It can also be necessary to use, in the presence of specific problems, mental health services for children and adolescents. In sum, the specific program of Early Intervention also has to address all the factors from the environment that can contribute to improving the living conditions and opportunities for the development of the child with ASD.

## 5. Common features of an effective intervention program

There are dozens of intervention programs suggested in the literature. All of them claim benefits from their use. The problem lies most of all in the generalization of the benefits, because children with ASD do learn new skills, but they often fail to use them in settings other than the educational or center-based ones.

In general, there is a consensus that education and community help are key elements to promote communication and social skills in children with ASD [Fuentes-Biggi et al., 2006]. Core features that a successful autism educational program should include have been suggested [Dawson & Osterling, 1997; Myers & Jonson, 2007; NRC, 2001]:

- A high staff-to-student ratio (1:1 or 1:2).
- Individualized programming for each child.
- Teachers with special expertise in working with children with autism.
- Ongoing program evaluation and adjustment.
- A curriculum emphasizing attention, imitation, communication, play, and social interaction.
- A highly supportive teaching environment.
- Predictability and structure.
- Functional analysis of behavior problems.
- Transition planning.
- Family involvement.
- Close monitoring and modification as the child's needs change.

## 6. Classification of the intervention models

Intervention in children with ASD has changed a lot since the early beginnings in the 1950s, when the psychodynamic theories were predominant. Until the 1980s, most ASD children didn't go to school; they were simply rejected or institutionalized, as if they were fools or insane. A bad relationship between children and parents was assumed as an explanation for the disorder. Since then, the Special Needs Education Program has offered a curriculum for all these children, which nowadays is called the Individualized Education Program (IEP).

The IEP is a paradigm that exists in the United States, following the Individuals with Disabilities Education Act (IDEA), which is a law from 2004 intended to protect children with disabilities and ensure them a correct education plan [IDEA, 2004]. It is a multidisciplinary, team-developed plan required for every child receiving special education services, and should include: the present level of the child's development, the annual goals and how they will be measured, the school personnel needs and how long the child will participate with children without special needs. With variations, the idea of a curriculum for people with ASD is developed in all countries managing these children.

In general, there is a secular trend toward improvement in the ASD symptomatology with the intervention programs. Howlin categorizes the outcome of the ASD programs as good, fair and poor (see Table 3), depending on the independence achieved by the children after the intervention (Howlin, 2005). There has been a change from the initial interventions before the 1980s to the later ones [Volkmar, 2011]. Of course, the outcome is related to the initial severity of the core symptoms, and a higher IQ and better language capabilities of the child at the time of diagnosis have been correlated with a better prognosis in communication and social competence [Sigman & McGovern; Szatmari et al., 2003].

| |
|---|
| Good: moderate to high levels of independence living/job, some friends/ acquaintances |
| Fair: need support at work/home but some autonomy |
| Poor: living in situation with close supervision in most activities |

Table 4. Classification of outcomes in the ASD intervention studies

There is a general lack of good scientific validation of the effectiveness of the various intervention methods [Seida et al., 2009]. The scientific approach, with random assignment to the groups and even separation into treatment and no treatment groups, makes it difficult and sometimes illegal to keep autism children from receiving treatment.

In order to classify the intervention programs, there are different criteria to use. For example:

- According to the setting where it is instructed:
  - Center-based programs.
  - Home-based programs.
  - School-based programs.
- According to the target age of the children:
  - Early Intervention programs (until 3-4 years, depending on the country).
  - School age programs.
  - Adult age programs.

In this review, we will summarize the intervention models based on the type of intervention, i.e., according to its nature. Each model focuses on some or all of the aspects involved in the definition of ASD, in trying to:

- Increase social skills.
- Increase communication skills.
- Decrease maladaptive behaviors.

We will not discuss whether school-based, home-based or center-based interventions are best because there are many issues that make it difficult to interpret and generalize the results about the efficacy of the different intervention programs [Matson, 2007; NRC, 2001; Ospina et al., 2008]:

- ASD represents a complex diagnosis, involving a wide repertory of symptoms. Therefore, each intervention program can focus on improving some symptoms but not others. Thus, it is important to be aware of this while evaluating the study population and the outcomes of each paper reported.
- Interventions in children with ASD, by their nature, are complex and varied. There are many components suitable to be implemented in different ways and by different personnel (sometimes not professional) and in different settings, making it difficult to generalize the outcomes.
- Group comparison can be delicate because there are many studies that compare an active group receiving treatment with a no treatment or waiting list group, thus overestimating the intervention effect, due to the negative perspective of the no intervention group.
- Outcome variations can be accounted for by a different follow-up period. The time to follow-up must be in accordance with the nature of the intervention, and it must be studied whether the effects remain in the long term.
- Results should be rated according to the methodological quality and its bias potential (over or underestimation of the treatment effect). Furthermore, the publication bias tends to publish fewer studies with no or a negative effect.

A main classification of the intervention models follows [Roberts, 2004], which we will use to discuss the main intervention models (see Table 4 for details):

- Biologically Based Interventions
- Psychodynamic Interventions
- Educational Interventions

### 6.1 Biologically based interventions

Although educational interventions seem to be the most effective approach in the rehabilitation of children with ASD, there has been a continuous sprouting of new controversial treatment approaches that claim to "cure" the autism [Weiss et al, 2008]. Of course, there is a role for medication in treating challenging behaviors (i.e., typical and atypical antipsychotics) and attention-deficit (stimulants and non-stimulants), and for the treatment of epilepsy-associated problems. We will briefly discuss some medications or medical interventions that are supposed to be aimed at treating the core deficits in ASD [Weissman et al., 2010]:

- Melatonin: we are not referring to its use in sleep regulation in children with ASD after trying behavioral interventions, where it can be of benefit [Garstang & Wallis, 2006; Paavonen at al., 2003]. Although some studies suggest an abnormal production of melatonin in children with ASD [Johnson et al., 2009], there is no evidence that its use improves the core deficits in ASD.

- Biologically Based Interventions
    - Medication
    - Complementary and alternative medicine
- Psychodynamic Interventions
- Educational Interventions
    - Behavioral Interventions
        - Early intensive behavioral intervention (EIBI)
        - Contemporary Applied Behavior Analysis
            - Pivotal Response Training (PRT)
            - Natural Language Paradigm (NLP)
            - Incidental Teaching
    - Developmental Interventions
        - Floor Time (DIR)
        - Responsive Teaching (RT)
        - Relationship Development Intervention (RDI)
    - Therapy Based Interventions
        - Communication Focused Interventions
            - Visual Strategies and Visually Cued Instruction
            - Manual Signing
            - The Picture Exchange Communication System (PECS)
            - Social Stories
            - Speech Generating Devices
            - Facilitated Communication (FC)
            - Functional Communication Training (FCT)
        - Sensory-Motor Interventions
            - Auditory Integration Training (AIT)
            - Sensory Integration
    - Combined Interventions
        - The SCERTS Model
        - Treatment and Education of Autistic and related Communication Handicapped Children (TEACCH)
        - Learning Experiences-An Alternative Program for Preschoolers and Parents (LEAP)
    - Family Based Interventions
        - Family-Centered Positive Behavior Support (PBS) Programs
        - The Hanen Program (More than Words)

Table 5. Classification of the intervention models in ASD.

- Naltrexone: is an opiate antagonist that has been hypothesized to be helpful in reducing the symptoms of autism by blocking endogenous opioids that may be released during self-injurious repetitive behaviors, but it has not been effective in improving the core deficits in autism, although it can ameliorate the challenging behaviors [Posey et al., 2008].
- Secretin: is a gastrointestinal hormone that inhibits intestinal mobility and release of gastric acid and stimulates secretion of pancreatic fluid and bicarbonate. It has been studied because of the frequent complaints of abdominal pain in children with ASD, but it has shown no evidence in multiple studies [Williams, KW et al., 2005].
- Antifungal agents: based on a supposed urinary candida overgrowth in children with ASD, there have been several antifungal agents used (e.g., nystatin or fluconazole). There are no systematic reviews of the efficacy of this treatment, and most clinical guidelines do not recommend its use.
- Intravenous immunoglobulin: based on the fact that fetal brain development is related to a prenatal immune response, its use has potential adverse effects, and it has not shown any improvement in the core deficits in ASD [DelGiudice-Asch et al, 1999; Pliopys, 1998]. It is not recommended as a treatment for autism [Feasby et al, 2007].
- Chelation: is the process of administering substances (like ethylene diamine tetra-acetic acid [EDTA] for example), to remove heavy metals from the body. Linked to the thimerosal and vaccines theory, there is no evidence to suggest that these treatments are effective [Demicheli et al., 2005; Madsen et al., 2003].
- Hyperbaric oxygen: based upon the hypothesis that increasing atmospheric pressure enhances oxygen delivery to the brain, there was an initial interest in its use for treating the core deficits in ASD [Rossignol, 2007], but a recent study [Jepson, 2011] failed to replicate the benefits.
- Dietary Interventions: there have been multiple proposals of avoiding or supplementing diets in order to benefit ASD symptoms. From omega-3 fatty acids [Bent et al., 2009], B6-magnesium supplementation [Nye & Brice, 2005], dimethylglycine [Kern et al., 2001], probiotics [Parr, 2008], folinic acid [Main et al., 2010], methycobalamin, vitamin C, zinc, digestive enzymes [Levy & Hyman, 2008], to gluten-free or casein-free diets, none of them has achieved significant and clinical relevance in ameliorating the core ASD deficits [Millward et al., 2009].

### 6.2 Psychodynamic interventions

Psychodynamic therapies are based on the assumption that autism is the result of the exposure of a developing child to a "cold" ambient, i.e., the cause of the symptoms would be found in the way parents had raised their child. This explanation was raised in the psychoanalytic years, where Kanner [Kanner, 1943] described his first patients, and it reached its height with Bettelheim [Bettelheim, 1967], who sometimes treated them with a "parentectomy", putting them in residential institutions.

Psychodynamic therapies are seldom used today, as there is strong evidence to support the perspective that autism is a developmental and cognitive disorder, rather than an emotional disorder, and there is little empirical evidence demonstrating the effectiveness of psychodynamic interventions. Today there are still some authors who support these theories [Hobson, 1990], and intervention models like "Holding Therapy" [Tinbergen & Tinbergen, 1983] or "Pheraplay" [Des Lauriers, 1978] were developed, although there is no evidence of their utility.

### 6.3 Educational interventions

The importance of early intensive and educational interventions in improving the core deficits in ASD is well-documented [Howlin et al., 2009; Ospina et al., 2008; Seida et al., 2009; Spreckley & Boyd, 2009]. The goals of treatment are to maximize independent functioning and improve quality of life. Nowadays, there is no doubt that certain behavioral and educational treatment strategies improve the core deficits in ASD (behavior, language and peer interaction) and intelligence scores, so the questions are how soon to begin a particular intervention program and how to choose the appropriate method for each child [ Reichow & Wolery, 2009; SIGN, 2007].

The educational interventions can be described as behavioral, developmental, therapy-based or combined.

#### 6.3.1 Behavioral interventions

Behavioral interventions are now considered an "established" treatment for ASD children, although they should not be expected to lead to normal functioning [National Autism Center, 2009; Spreckley & Boyd, 2009]. They may improve the core symptoms of ASD, mainly in the first 12 months of treatment. Behavioral interventions are those in which instrumental learning techniques constitute the predominant feature of the intervention approach, based on the principles of behavior modification.

Ivar Lovaas and colleagues pioneered one of these intensive behavioral interventions, Applied Behavioral Analysis (ABA) in the 1960s [Lovaas & Simmons, 1969]. It seeks to reinforce desirable behaviors and decrease undesirable behaviors, teaching new skills and generalizing them through repeated reward-based trials. It requires a low student-to-therapist ratio and very intensive intervention (at least 25 hours a week). At this time, this is the only evidence-based approach to intensive early intervention for children with autism [Frea & McNerney., 2008].

Discrete trial training (DTT), originally developed by Ivar Lovaas, is the most structured form of intensive therapy. It consists of breaking down skills into more discrete components to be taught in a stepwise fashion: the therapist presents an instruction (stimulus), prompts a response, waits for the child's response, and provides an appropriate consequence depending on the response [Francis, 2005]. The original behavioral interventions, based almost exclusively on DTT techniques, were developed at the University of California, Los Angeles under the Young Autism Project [Lovass, 1987; Lovaas, 2003], and although they have demonstrated benefits in attention, imitation, obedience and discrimination, they have been criticized because of the lack of generalization and because the structured setting does not represent more naturalistic interactions between adults and children [Myers, 2007].

For this reason, contemporary ABA programs have been developed, which are taught in more naturalistic settings, with methods like Pivotal Response Training (PRT), the Natural Language Teaching Paradigm [Koegel et al., 1998] or Incidental Teaching [Hart & Risley, 1975], where the child initiates the interaction, improving the generalization of the skills [Schreibmann & Ingersoll, 2005]. In the current literature, the term Early Intensive Behavioral Interventions (EIBI) has arisen to summarize all these approaches, and it is accepted that they promote changes in the intelligence quotient and positive changes in adaptive skills and expressive and receptive language skills. New trends in the Contemporary ABA techniques include Positive Behavioral Support [Horner et al., 1993], Functional Assessment [O'Neill et al., 1997] and Functional Communication Training [Durrand, 1993], with its "errorless" teaching.

### 6.3.2 Developmental interventions

Also known as normalized interventions, they focus on the ability of the child to form positive relationships with other people. They focus on teaching essential skills (social communication, emotional relationships, cognitive abilities) that were not learned at the expected age, and include the Denver model, the Developmental Individual Difference Relationship-based approach (DIR or Floor Time) [Greenspan, 1998] and Responsive Teaching [Myers & Johnson, 2007].

### 6.3.3 Therapy based interventions

The Communication Interventions are strategies that promote communication skills in order to improve overall functioning. They include the use of behavioral strategies like Functional Communication Training, or the use of augmentative communication strategies.

The Sensory-Motor interventions are based on the hypothesis that various sensory experiences (e.g., visual, tactile, auditory) will help to guide development. The studies have not clearly demonstrated significant benefits [Parr, 2008].

### 6.3.4 Combined interventions

They include more than one interventional model, but mainly based on a specific approach. For example, the Social Communication, Emotional Regulation, Transactional Support (SCERTS) program is a developmentally-based model [Wetherby & Prizant, 2000]. The Early Start Denver Model (ESDM) uses a mixture of a clear behavioral approach with a relationship-based model, and it uses the parents as therapists [Dawson et al., 2010]. Another approach is the Learning Experiences-An Alternative Program for Preschoolers and Parents (LEAP), with a developmental basis and behavioral instruction for parents [Strain & Hoyson, 2000].

The Treatment and Education of autistic and related Communication-handicapped CHildren (TEACCH) method is a "whole life" approach, and focuses on structuring the environment in order to facilitate skill development and independence. It is currently an "established" model in interventions with children with ASD [Panerai et al., 2002]. The principles of the TEACCH model are (www.teacch.com/whatis.html):

- Understanding the culture of autism
- Using an individualized person- and family-centered plan
- Organizing the physical environment
- A predictable sequence of activities
- Visual schedules
- Routines with flexibility
- Structured work/activity systems
- Visually structured activities

## 7. Conclusion

The intervention in the child with ASD will be mainly based on promoting a better adaptation to his physical, cultural and social environment, and helping his family to participate of this labor and improve the skills and resources with which to confront having a child with this disorder.

Early intervention programs for children with ASD should be aimed at improving the overall situation of the child, his abilities and skills, but they must also try to improve his

quality of life and that of his family. These programs produce significant and lasting improvements, but this intervention must be carried out with a holistic and interdisciplinary approach, addressing all issues that pose dysfunctions.
There are multiple intervention models, most of them claiming clear benefits. There is a lack of good, controlled, unbiased studies with a large enough population to establish good scientific evidence that would recommend one intervention or another. Of all the models, the behavioral one has shown some benefits, although the developmental and communication-focused approaches can also improve the social and relation skills of the child with ASD. Nowadays, the trend is to combine the best of various models in a structured fashion and with testing to measure the benefits achieved. The prognosis of children with ASD has improved in the last 50 years, when some children were institutionalized as the only treatment.

## 8. References

American Psychiatric Association (2000). Pervasive Developmental Disorders. In: *Diagnostic and Statistical Manual of Mental Disorders, Fourth Edition, Text Revision (DSM-IV-TR®).* American Psychiatric Association, Washington, DC. p.70.

Autism and Developmental Disabilities Monitoring Network (2009), United States, 2006. *MMWR Surveill Summ*; 58:1.

Baron-Cohen S, Allen J y Gillberg C (1992). Can autism be detected at 18 months? The needle, the haystack, and the CHAT. *Br J Psychiatry*; 161: 839-843.

Bayley N (1997). Escalas Bayley de Desarrollo. *Ed. TEA.*

Bent et al (2009). Omega-3 fatty acids for autistic spectrum disorder: a systematic review. *J Autism Dev Disord*; 39:1145.

Bettelheim, B. (1967). The empty fortress: Infantile autism and the birth of the self. *New York Free Press.*

Bols W et al (2011). EEG complexity as a biomarker for autism spectrum disorder risk. *BMC Medicine.* http://www.biomedcentral.com/1741-7015/9/18.

Dawson, G, Osterling, J (1997). Early intervention in autism: effectiveness and common elements of current approaches. In: *The effectiveness of early intervention: Second Generation Research*, Guralnick, MJ (Ed), Paul Brookes, Baltimore. p.307.

Dawson G (2003). *Autism Summit Conference Session 3: early intervention research.* Washington DC.

Dawson et al (2010). Randomized, controlled trial of an intervention for toddlers with autism: the Early Start Denver Model. *Pediatrics*; 125:e17.

DelGiudice-Asch et al (1999). Brief report: a pilot open clinical trial of intravenous immunoglobulin in childhood autism. *J Autism Dev Disord*; 29:157.

Demicheli et al. (2005). Vaccines for measles, mumps and rubella in children. *Cochrane database of systematic reviews* (Online: Update Software), CD004407.

Des Lauriers. (1978). Play, symbols, and the development of language In M. Rutter & E. Schopler (Eds.), *Autism: A reappraisal of concepts and treatment* (pp. 313-326). New York: Plenum.

Díez-Cuervo A (2005). Estado actual de la investigación genética en los trastornos de espectro autista. En Martos J., González P., Llorente M. y Nieto C. eds. *Nuevos desarrollos en autismo: el futuro es hoy.* Madrid: APNA-IMSERSO. P. 373-411.

Dunst CJ (1980). Clinical and Educational Manual for use with the Uzgiris-Hunt Scale. *Univ Park Pr.*

Durand VM (1993). Functional communication training for challenging behaviors. *Clin Commun Disord.*;3(2):59-70

Feasby et al. (2007). Guidelines on the use of intravenous immune globulin for neurologic conditions. *Transfus Med Rev.* Apr;21(2 Suppl 1):S57-107.

Fombonne, E. (2009). Epidemiology of pervasive developmental disorders. *Pediatr Res*; 65:591.

Francis, K. (2005). Autism interventions: A critical update. *Developmental Medicine and Child Neurology* 47(7), 493-499.

Frea & McNerney (2008). Early intensive applied behavioral analysis intervention for autism, In: *Effective practices for children with autism*, J.K. Luiselly et al. (Ed.), 83-110, Oxford University Press, ISBN 978-0-19-531704-6, New York, United States.

Freeman BR y Ritvo ER. (1978). Behaviour Observation Scale for Autism. *Psychological Association Meeting New York, NY.*

Fuentes-Biggi, J., et al. (2006). [Good practice guidelines for the treatment of autistic spectrum disorders]. *Rev Neurol.* 43(7): p. 425-38.

Garstang & Wallis (2006). Randomized controlled trial of melatonin for children with autistic spectrum disorders and sleep problems. *Child Care Health Dev*;32(5):585-9.

Gilliam JE. (1995). Gilliam Autism Rating Scale. *Pro-Ed* Austin TX.

Greenspan, S. I. (1998). A developmental approach to problems in relating and communicating in autistic spectrum disorders and related syndromes. *SPOTLIGHT on Topics in Developmental Disabilities*, 1(4), 1-6.

Grupo de Estudios de Trastorno del Espectro Autista (2006). Guía de buena práctica para el tratamiento de los trastornos del espectro autista. *Rev Neurol*; 43 (7): 425-438.

Hart, B., & Risley, T. (1975). Incidental teaching of language in the preschool. *Journal of Applied Behavior Analysis*, 8, 411-420.

Hobson, R. P. (1990). On psychoanalytic approaches to autism. *American Journal of Orthopsychiatry*, 60, 324-336.

Horner, R., O'Neill, R., & Flannery, K. (1993). Building effective behavior support plans from functional assessment information. In M. Snell (Ed.), *Instruction of persons with severe handicaps* (4th ed., pp. 184-214). Columbus: OH: Merrill.

Howlin, P. (1998) Psychological and educational treatments for autism. *Journal of Child Psychology and Psychiatry and allied disciplines.* 39, 307-32.

Howlin P. (2005) The effectiveness of interventions for children with autism. *J Neural Transm Suppl.*;(69):101-19.

Howlin, P, Magiati, I & Charman, T. (2009) Systematic review of early intensive behavioral interventions for children with autism. *Am J Intellect Dev Disabil*; 114:23.

Individuals with Disabilities Education Act. (2004). Building the legacy: *IDEA*. Retrieved April 29, 2008 from http://idea.ed.gov/.

Jepson et al. (2011) Controlled evaluation of the effects of hyperbaric oxygen therapy on the behavior of 16 children with autism spectrum disorders. *J Autism Dev Disord.*;41(5):575-88.

Johnson, KP, Giannotti, F, & Cortesi, F. (2009) Sleep patterns in autism spectrum disorders. *Child Adolesc Psychiatr Clin N Am*; 18:917.

Kanner, L. (1943). Autistic disturbances of affective contact. *Nervous Child*, 2, 217-250.

Kaufman AS, Kaufman NL. (1997) K-ABC Batería de Evaluación de Kaufman para niños. Madrid: *TEA*.

Kern, JK et al. (2001) Effectiveness of N,N-dimethylglycine in autism and pervasive developmental disorder. *J Child Neurol*; 16:169.

Koegel, L. K., Koegel, R. L., & Carter, C. M. (1998). Pivotal responses and the natural teaching paradigm. *Seminars in Speech and Language*, 19(4), 355-372.

Leiter RG. (1948) Leiter international performance scale. Chicago: *Stoelting Company*.

Levy, SE, Hyman, SL. (2008) Complementary and alternative medicine treatments for children with autism spectrum disorders. *Child Adolesc Psychiatr Clin N Am*; 17:803.

Lord C, Rutter M, Le Couteur A. (1994) Autism Diagnostic Interview-Revised: A revised version of a diagnostic interview for caregivers of individuals with possible pervasive developmental disorders. *J Autism Dev Disord.*; 24(5): 659-685.

Lord C et al. (2000) The Autism Diagnostic Observation Schedule-Generic: A standard measure of social and communication deficits associated with the spectrum of autism. *J Autism Dev Disord.*; 30(3):205-223.

Lovaas, O. I., & Simmons, J. Q. (1969). Manipulation of self-destruction in three retarded children. *Journal of Applied Behaviour Analysis*, 2, 143–157.

Lovaas, O.I. (1987) Behavioral treatment and normal educational and intellectual functioning in young autistic children. *J Consult Clin Psychol*. 55(1): p. 3-9.

Lovaas, O.I. (2003) Teaching individuals with developmental delays: basic intervention techniques. 2003, Austin, TX: *Pro-Ed*.

Madsen, K. M., Lauritsen, M. B., & Pederson, C. B. (2003). Thimerosal and the occurrence of autism: Negative ecological evidence from Danish populationbased data. *Pediatrics*, 112, 604-606.

Main, PA et al. (2010) Folate and methionine metabolism in autism: a systematic review. *Am J Clin Nutr*; 91:1598.

Martos J. (2001) Autismo. Definición, instrumentos de evaluación y diagnóstico. En *Autismo: enfoques actuales para padres y profesionales de la salud y la educación*. Daniel Valdez (coord). Buenos Aires: Fundec. Serie Autismo.

Martos J. (2005) La intervención educativa desde las posiciones educativas neuropsicológicas en el autismo. En Mulas F. (ed). *Autismo infantil*. Barcelona: Viguera Editores. p. 276.

Matson, J.L. (2007) Determining treatment outcome in early intervention programs for autism spectrum disorders: a critical analysis of measurement issues in learning based interventions. *Res Dev Disabil*. 28(2): p. 207-18.

McCarthy D. (2006) Escalas McCarthy de Aptitudes y Psicomotricidad. Madrid: *TEA Ediciones* (1972) adaptation 2006.

McEachin J, Smith T, et al. (2003) Longterm outcome for children with autism who received early intensive behavioral treatment. Am J Ment Retard 1993; 97: 35972; discussion, 37391. En C.A. Gadia, R.F. Tuchman. *Manejo de los niños con trastornos del espectro autista* Rev neurol; (36) 2.

Millá MG. (2005) Centros de Desarrollo Infantil y Atención Temprana. En MG Millá y F Mulas. *Atención Temprana. Desarrollo infantil, diagnóstico, trastornos e intervención*. Valencia: Promolibro. p.311.

Millá MG. (2005) Centros de Desarrollo Infantil y Atención Temprana. En MG Millá y F Mulas. *Atención Temprana. Desarrollo infantil, diagnóstico, trastornos e intervención*. Valencia: Promolibro. p.321.

Millá MG y Mulas F. (2009) Atención temprana y programas de intervención específica en el trastorno del espectro autista. *Rev Neurol;* 48 (Supl 2): S47-S5

Millward C et al. (2008) Gluten- and casein-free diets for autistic spectrum disorder. *Cochrane Database Syst Rev.* 16;(2):CD003498.

Mulas F. et al. (2005) Bases clínicas neuropediátricas y patogénicas del trastorno del espectro autista. En F. Mulas ed. *Autismo infantil.* Barcelona: Viguera Editores. p. 57.

Myers, SM, Johnson, CP. (2007) Management of children with autism spectrum disorders. *Pediatrics;* 120:1162.

National Autism Center's National Standards Report. (2009) *National Autism Center,* Randolph, MA. Available at: www.nationalautismcenter.org/pdf/NAC%20Standards%20Report.pdf. (Accessed on April 23, 2011).

National Research Council (2001). *Educating Children with Autism.* Washington D.C.: National Academy Press.

Newborg J, Stock JR y Wnek L. (1998) Inventario de Desarrollo Battelle. Madrid: *TEA Ediciones.*

Nye, C, Brice, A. (2005) Combined vitamin B6-magnesium treatment in autism spectrum disorder. *Cochrane Database Syst Rev;* :CD003497.

O'Neill, R. et al. (1997). *Functional assessment and program development for problem behavior: A practical handbook.* Pacific Grove: CA: Brooks/Cole.

Ospina, M.B., et al. (2008) Behavioural and developmental interventions for autism spectrum disorder: a clinical systematic review. *PLoS ONE.* 3(11): p. e3755.

Paavonen et al. (2003). Effectiveness of melatonin in the treatment of sleep disturbances in children with Asperger disorder. *J Child Adolesc Psychopharmacol;*13(1):83-95.

Panerai, S, Ferrante, L, Zingale, M. (2002) Benefits of the Treatment and Education of Autistic and Communication Handicapped Children (TEACCH) programme as compared with a non-specific approach. *J Intellect Disabil Res;* 46:318.

Parr, J. (2008) *Autism. Clinical Evidence Handbook.* BMJ Publishing Group London. p.69.

Plioplys, AV. (1998) Intravenous immunoglobulin treatment of children with autism. *J Child Neurol;* 13:79.

Posey et al. (2008). Developing drugs for core social and communication impairment in autism. *Child Adolesc Psychiatr Clin N Am.* Oct;17(4):787-801, viii-ix.

Reichow, B, Wolery, M. (2009) Comprehensive Synthesis of Early Intensive Behavioral Interventions for Young Children with Autism Based on the UCLA Young Autism Project Model. *J Autism Dev Disord;* 39:23.

Rivière A. (2000) ¿Cómo aparece el autismo?. Diagnóstico temprano e indicadores precoces del trastorno autista. En Rivière A y Martos J comp. *El niño pequeño con autismo.* APNA Madrid.

Roberts JM. (2004) A review of the research to identify the most effective models of best practice in the management of children with autism spectrum disorders. Sydney: *Centre for Developmental Disability Studies.* Sydney University. Department of Ageing, Disability and Home Care.

Rossignol, DA. (2007) Hyperbaric oxygen therapy might improve certain pathophysiological findings in autism. *Med Hypotheses;* 68:1208.

Schopler E, et al. (1990) Individualized assessment of autistic and developmentally disabled children: Psychoeducational Profile Revised (PEP-R). Austin, TX : *PRO-ED.* Vol 1.

Schreibman, L. and B. Ingersoll (2005) Behavioral interventions to promote learning in individuals with autism, in *Handbook of autism and pervasive developmental disorders*, F. Volkmar, et al., Editors, John Wiley & Sons: Hoboken, NJ. p. 882-896.

Seida, JK, et al. (2009) Systematic reviews of psychosocial interventions for autism: an umbrella review. *Dev Med Child Neurol*; 51:95.

SIGN (2007), Scottish Intercollegiate Guidelines Network. Assessment, diagnosis and clinical interventions for children and young people with autism spectrum disorders. A national clinical guideline. *Scottish Intercollegiate Guidelines Network*, Edinburgh. Available at www.sign.ac.uk. (Accessed on April 22, 2011).

Sigman M, McGovern CW. (2005) Improvement in cognitive and language skills from preschool to adolescence in autism. *J Autism Dev Disord*;35(1):15-23.

Smith T, Groen AD, Wynn JW. (2000) Randomized trial of intensive early intervention for children with pervasive developmental disorder. *Am J Ment Retard*; 105: 269-85.

Spreckley, M, Boyd, R. (2009) Efficacy of applied behavioral intervention in preschool children with autism for improving cognitive, language, and adaptive behavior: a systematic review and meta-analysis. *J Pediatr*; 154:338.

Strain, P. S., & Hoyson, M. (2000). The need for longitudinal intensive social skill intervention, leap follow-up outcomes for children with autism. *Topics In Early Childhood Special Education*, 20(2), 116-122.

Stutsman R. (1931) Guide for administering the Merril-Palmer scale of mental tests. In L.M. Terman (Ed.), *Mental measurement of preschool children*. New York: Harcourt, Brace & World: 139-262

Szatmari P et al. (2003) Predictors of outcome among high functioning children with autism and Asperger syndrome. *J Child Psychol Psychiatry*;44(4):520-8.

Tamarit J. (1994) Prueba ACACIA. Madrid: *Alcei-6*.

Tinbergen, N., & Tinbergen, E. A. (1983). *Autistic children: A New Hope for a Cure*. London: Allen and Unwin.

Volkmar, F. (2011). Treatment for autism: Overview of model programs, In: *Understanding Autism*, Retrieved March 21, 2011, Available from: http://autism.yale.edu/initial-topics/2

Wang K, Zhang H et al. (2009). Common genetic variants on 5p14.1 associate with autism spectrum disorders. *Nature Rev*. april. doi:10.10.1038/nature07999.

Weiss et al. (2008). Evidence-Based Practice for Autism Spectrum Disorders. *Clinical Assessment and Intervention for Autism Spectrum Disorders*, Pages 33-63.

Weissman et al. (2010). Autism spectrum diroders in children and adolescents: Complementary and alternative therapies. *UpToDate*, 2010. (Accessed on April 23, 2011).

Wetherby, A. W., & Prizant, B. M. (2000). *Autism Spectrum Disorders: A Transactional Developmental Perspective* (1st ed. Vol. 9). Baltimore: Paul H Brookes.

Williams, JG et al. (2006) Systematic review of prevalence studies of autism spectrum disorders. *Arch Dis Child*; 91:8.

Williams, KW. et al. (2005). Intravenous secretin for autism spectrum disorder. *Cochrane Database Syst Rev*; CD003495.

Wing L et al. (2002). The Diagnostic Interview for Social and Communication Disorders: background, inter-rater reliability and clinical use. *J Child Psychol Psychiatry*; 43 (3): 307-327.

8

# Philosophy of Caring in the Psychotherapy with Children and Adolescents Diagnosed with ASD

Anna Bieniarz
*Medical University of Lublin*
*Poland*

## 1. Introduction

This chapter attempts to build a bridge merging theoretical foundations and practical issues with a view to finding a better understanding of helping patients with autistic spectrum. The disorder is not only seen as a severe medical problem, but also as a socially neglected issue. A family with a disabled child or adolescent must cope with different problems depending on physical, psychological or economic conditions to name only a few of them. There must be a complex treatment for the disorder. It consists of many specialist methods, e.g. "holding therapy" techniques based on the TEACCH model, educational and behavioral programs pointed at social skills training or a psychotherapy directed at the psychological problems of a child or his/her parents if necessary.

The psychotherapeutic method employed for autistic children and adolescents may become effective if there is a high level of functioning acquired. Nevertheless, there are some difficulties inherent when including individuals diagnosed with mental retardation into psychotherapy (Berry, 2003). The disorders of autistic spectrum are mostly chronic conditions and therefore require long-term therapeutic treatment. It seems natural that psychodynamic psychotherapy as additional help offered to an autistic person would be considered.

The present content is to recognize potential connections between psychotherapy (mainly focusing on a psychodynamic approach) with individuals of ASD and the basis of the caring concept, primarily attributed to a nursing theory.

On describing and adopting the thesis and philosophy of caring into psychotherapeutic practice on a psychodynamic work with children and adolescents of autistic spectrum the perspective of the relationship available within therapy is expected to be widened.

## 2. Place of care in treatment

Caring is an important factor and should always take place in a curing process. It produces a recovery, leads to well-being or creates the circumstances to exist a sense of safety and then emotional change may be possible.

There are many concepts of it available among various disciplines. Each of them tries to explain why people care for others. Biologists classify caring into instinctive behaviour, sociologists stress social expectations and suggest that caring is simply a consequence of the social process. Anthropologists connect caring with ritual behavior, religion, commitment or power (Wiseman, 1997).

Morse et al. proposed considering caring through five perspectives: caring as a human trait; as a moral imperative; as an effect; as an interpersonal relationship and as a therapeutic intervention (Morse et al., 1990 cited in: McCance et al., 1997). The latter is understood in the terms of a patient's outcomes, but it is hard to use a specific measure to know the care concept better (Sourial, 1997).

### 2.1 Roots of caring

"Care theory" has existed in social scientific discourse with the work of Carol Gilligan, named "In a Different Voice" and published in 1982. Two years later another book was published, "Caring" by Nel Noddings. Both of them were focused on the ethical thinking about giving care to others and put in the feminist context of understanding the phenomenon (Levy, 2006).

Gilligan and Noddings perceived caring as female attribute. Caring is equal to women's work and thus devalued in the patriarchal society. Traditionally, care-giving has been ordered to the ability of building close relationships, usually belonging to a woman's nature. Gillian pointed out that masculinity is valued through separation, while femininity through attachment, which leads to the conclusion that women judge themselves according to the ability to care (Gilligan, 1982 cited in: Poole & Isaacs, 1997). Noddings has stressed the interpersonal character of care and its role in the ethical response in people. Her ideas were carried over mainly to nursing theory and clinical practice (Dyson, 1997).

#### 2.1.1 Philosophy

The philosopher who centralised his theory on the term "care" was Heidegger in a book 'Being and Time' (Heidegger, 1962). He thought of 'care' (Sorge), 'concern' (Besorgen) and 'solitude' (Fursorge), but he did not actually referred the words to ethics (Paley, 2000). The meaning of care based on his philosophy is close to worry about something, which corresponds with the situation of chronic distress, as in families with an autistic child.

There is an important differentiation between caring 'for' others and caring 'about' others. The first implies some action, it is associated with tending to someone's needs. The second is connected with having particular feelings for another person (Graham, 1983; Ungerson, 1983; Blustein, 1991, all cited in: Wiseman, 1997).

Gaut (cited in: McCance et al., 1997) proposed three general meanings of care, which are: attention to or concern for; responsible for or providing for; regard, fondness, or attachment, we can see all of them in the clinical practice on the medical field.

The philosophy of caring is a part of professional ethics, which is the basis for standards for fulfilling its function towards the people requiring the assistance of experts. The requirements of caring are formalized in professional legal regulations, describing the rules of proper fulfillment of its function. Every country has its own regulations in that matter, which should be used in practice and should be treated as a decisive factor in case of dilemmas and doubts.

#### 2.1.2 Medicine

There are many models of care in the medical background. Most of them can be found in nursing theory. The first one, which will be mentioned in this chapter, is the theory of trans-cultural caring proposed by Madeleine Leininger: *Caring refers to actions to assist, support, or facilitate another individual or group with evident or anticipated needs to ameliorate or improve human condition or life ways* (Leninger, 1985 cited in: Tuck et. al., 1998, p. 92). To specify her concept of care, Leininger has given 11 assumptions of caring, that are:

1. Human caring is a universal phenomenon, but the expressions, processes and patterns vary among cultures;
2. Every nursing care situation has transcultural caring behaviours, needs and implications;
3. Caring acts and processes are essential for human development, growth and survival;
4. Caring should be considered the essence and unifying intellectual and practice dimension of professional nursing;
5. Caring has biophysical, psychological, cultural, social and environmental dimensions which can be studied and practiced to provide holistic care to people;
6. Transcultural caring behaviours, forms and processes have yet to be verified from diverse cultures, when this body of knowledge is procured, it has the potential to revolutionize present-day nursing practices;
7. To provide therapeutic nursing care, the nurse should have knowledge of caring values, beliefs and practices of the client(s);
8. Caring behaviours and functions vary with the social structure features of any designed culture;
9. The identification of universal and non-universal folk and professional caring behaviours, beliefs and practices will be important to advance the body of nursing knowledge;
10. Differences exist between the essence and essential features of caring and curing behaviours and processes;
11. There can be no curing without caring but there may be caring without curing (Leininger, 1988 cited in: Cohen, 1991, p.901).

The care may be perceived differently according to the culture, where it appears. It may also take different forms, depending on the cultural background.

A second model of caring has been proposed by Jean Watson. She describes human caring and puts it into intersubjective perspective. Caring is presented as sharing one's personal, spiritual, moral and social self (Watson, 1985 cited in: Tuck et. al., 1998, p. 93). Watson (Watson 1978, 1988 cited in: Cohen et. al., 1991, p. 906) mentions 10 'carative factors' which are:

1. The formation of humanistic-altruistic value system;
2. The instillation of faith and hope;
3. The cultivation of sensitivity to self and others;
4. The development of help – trust relations;
5. The expression of positive and negative feelings;
6. The creation of a problem-solving caring process;
7. The promotion of transpersonal teaching/learning;
8. Supportive, protective, and/or corrective mental, physical, societal, and spiritual environments;
9. Assistance with human needs;
10. The allowance for existential- phenomenological- spiritual forces.

In Watson's view of caring, it requires two people (nurse and patient) and leads to the spiritual growth of each of them. The model draws the attention to the problem of perception and adequate response to one's needs.

A third model of caring was proposed by Simone Roach (McCance et. al., 1999 cited in: Ślusarska et. al., 2008), who describes in her "5 C" theory, five qualities of caring:

1. compassion,
2. competence,
3. confidence,
4. conscience and
5. commitment.

Caring is treated as part of being in the world, a basic element of the human condition. In Roach's opinion, compassion is the answer to a special need of the care-receiver. The competence arises from knowledge, common sense, practical abilities, professional experience and the motivation element. Confidence is understood as a basis for caring, it is always present, thus the relationship composed by respect is possible to achieve. The forth quality of caring, which is conscience, connects with a moral judgement and controls human behaviour. The last one, commitment, is regulated by emotional tension between personal desires and duties and the choices between them (Tschudin, 1992 cited in: Dobrowolska, 2006).

### 2.1.3 Psychology

There is an abundance of models associated with "care" in the field of social as well as on developmental and clinical psychology. From the point of view of social psychology, care appears during interpersonal interactions between people and can be analyzed as a social exchange of goods (understood as positive emotions). It involves people who are mutually part of a particular relationship and direct friendly feelings towards the other side of the contact.

Developmental perspective focuses on care as one of the most powerful factors that influence developmental changes, especially of infancy and early childhood.

Erich Fromm treats care as one of the components of love. The other elements constituting love are: respect, responsibility and knowledge (Fromm, 1947).

John Bowlby describes maternal care and its functions in building an attachment (Bowlby, 1969 cited in: Bell & Richard, 2000). He uses the term attachment to emotional bond that child creates with an adult person, his carer, which is mother in mostly cases. The situation implies presence of a dependent and caregiver.

## 2.2 Practical aspects

Care is the basic element in the maternal relationship with a newborn child. Winnicott has stressed that the way a mother holds her child is in essence a transmission of her feelings and it produces a strong bond between them. In the opinion of Winnicott, the three main functions of the mother in relation to her child are: holding, caring and showing objects. These tasks can help to integrate an ego of the child, at first weak and vulnerable to any traumas (Winnicott, 1994).

The dyadic relationship connecting the mother and the newborn child is seen to be a prototype of the caring. The character of the first caring activities responds to the capacity of giving care to others and receiving it from them later in life. It is questionable, whether one can learn and teach others the capacity and whether it is possible to achieve the competence of caring during a psychotherapy process. It seems to correspond with the receptivity of the therapist and the ability to regress on the part of the patient. There is an additional feature of the psychotherapist needed, in the case of the treatment of an autistic person. Patience is the most important and exacting component within this kind of therapy.

### 2.2.1 Care in psychodynamic psychotherapy

The presented description of psychotherapy is mainly based on the psychodynamic approach. Psychotherapy with children and adolescents diagnosed with ASD is generally a difficult task and should be preceded by long-term training, which includes many observations of the normal mother-infant interactions in their natural environment, and theoretical knowledge about human development and its psychopathology. The clinical illustration of early interactions of autistic children must be also present. The supervision and experience of a working team consisting of a variety of specialists would be an imperative element when preparing to work with ASD conditions. The psychotherapist must be trained to listen to and try to understand the meaning of the patient's communication. Beyond the formal demands, he ought to find and practise, within himself, a natural ability to take care of his patients.

An autistic spectrum disorder is seen as a defense mechanism used by individuals, who are too sensitive to defend themselves against the deficit or excess of traumatizing stimuli (Bettelheim, 1972). Another therapist, Tinbergen, noticed that autism may be a reaction of the individual, who experiences strong anxiety in opposition to surrounding external world (Tinbergen, 1986).

Direct observation of autistic children may result in a conclusion that they do not wish for an excessive intrusion into their lives from other people, and a best carer for them would be a carer who does not care. This, however, does not seem true, when we take into account their behavior while playing with dolls, when they copy their mothers' gestures and behaviour. It can be specifically observed during a first consultation with a specialist. Moreover, the need for proper care can be indicated by the frequent repetition of words used by the carer, especially the words of the mother.

The signs of caring should be included in every phase of the psychotherapy, especially with children and adolescents with autism, because of the high level of loneliness which these young people meet in their lives (Bauminger et al., 2004). The care is to be recognized in its verbal and nonverbal forms. A verbal character of caring is identical with the encouragement to social communication, producing the supporting comments, naming the successes and the positive emotions that the patient shows to the therapist, but also verbalizing difficult or negative attitudes toward psychotherapy and psychotherapist in order to help the child or adolescent to face it and cope with it.

Nonverbal signs of caring are needed in the therapist's behaviour and the emotional and physical environment where the therapy takes place. The attentiveness to stable conditions in the therapy room (an arrangement of the chairs, a configuration of papers on the desk or keeping the toys in the same position in the cardboard box, which belongs to a particularly young patient) should be present. The setting is an extremely important factor in the contact with children with autism.

Children with autism do experience emotions, but they have difficulties in identifying them (Ruberman, 2002). The therapist should clarify the child's and adolescent's emotions and behaviours, by using appropriate interpretations according to the developmental level of the patient. The clarifications refer to emotional states and behaviours by the patient and others to ease the disability of reading the minds of others.

The therapy is supposed to help integrate the child's and adolescent's fragmented experiences with himself and the others. Tustin treated autistic spectrum disorder as a part of a child psychosis, which is responsible for a confusion symptom observed in some autistic cases (Tustin, 1990 cited in: Morra, 2002). The non-autistic part of the personality on which psychotherapy process would be based must be found (Alvarez & Reid, 1999). Referring to healthy parts of the personality creates the possibility of change in the functioning of a child Ruberman argues that psychotherapeutic treatment of children with pervasive developmental disorders ought to be directed to a younger, rather than older age group (Ruberman, 2002). He states that psychodynamic psychotherapy ought to be modified if it is to reach the developmental needs of the young patient.

The care of the therapist is seen in the attempts made to interest the child and to involve him in a mutually meaningful relationship. Sometimes a therapist has to develop a special language to communicate with his patients. It is most noticeable during the role play, in which the adult is invited to take a part.

There should also be some kind of balance of caring and frustration in the therapeutic encounter. The dominance of care interventions familiarises the child with the therapy and prolongs the autonomy process. On the other hand, too much frustration can only be a destroying force and increase the anxiety of the child. As Greenspan states, one of the main goal of the psychodynamic psychotherapy is to develop a connection between an affect, a language and a cognition of the child or the adolescent (Greenspan, 1997 cited in: Ruberman, 2002).

Wolff has proposed four basic psychotherapeutic tasks in psychotherapeutic work with children:

1. To create a non-critical and secure relationship with the child;
2. To enable the child to express freely his inner thoughts and feelings;
3. To understand and underlying meaning of the child's communications;
4. To reflect this back to him (Wolff, 1992, s. 236).

The creation of secure relationships functions as a basis for the therapy and it is connected with increased caution on providing caring interventions, especially at the beginning of the psychotherapeutic process.

Care may be reflected as a cognition of a particular patient. To be aware of any signal of one's emotions, the therapist should be able to recall his knowledge and experiences as well as being open-minded to a new understanding of therapy dynamics.

The psychotherapy with adolescents can activate strong feelings both, on a patient's and psychotherapist's side. The youngsters experience a general conflict between aggression and closeness (Erikson, 1968). They search for caring and avoid it, as well. The therapist is to confront with the difficult and contradictory needs of an adolescent. An important task for psychotherapy is the providing of help to integrate the spheres where the young patient has problems, as within family relations or peer contact. One of the developmental tasks mentioned by Havighurst indicates a tendency to achieving emotional independence of parents and other adults (Havighurst, 1972 cited in: Gander & Gardiner, 1981). Although the adolescent with autism may not reach this developmental stage in the same time as his peers do, he would be also faced with some kind of a separation-individuation process, in his life. Throughout the process, a care is transferred from the family to the outside word. It is helpful to catch the traits of it and support the youngster to handle different feelings associated with the attempts of reaching an autonomy. The psychotherapeutic work must be always connected with supervision, that helps to obtain a better understanding of symptoms, their role in an actual therapeutic relation and to notice the care signals within a curative process. It serves as to capture the possible lack of energy to care for the patients and prevent a burn-out syndrome.

The role of the care concept according to psychotherapy with children and adolescents with ASD is centered on acting to meet patient's needs. There are two ideas of psychodynamic psychotherapy strongly linked to the care theory. The first one belongs to Winnicott's concept of holding and the second to Bion, the author of the container-contained phenomenon. The holding concept takes place in unspecific and constant relationship between patient and therapist. It is based on the rituals like coming to the therapy room of precise hour, one or several times a week. The repetitiveness is intended to smooth the different kinds of traumas. It also enables the experience of the omnipotence of the child or an adolescent. The therapist acting like a mother (an object) who satisfies patient's primary needs or serves as the safe environment, but he is the representative of the reality too, which is sometimes resisted of patient's unconscious desires. Bion's concept of container is seen as understanding and modifying the patient's communications by the therapist. The mother-child relation is likewise a foundation of these actions. The therapist (like a mother in the first months of infant's life) changes the primitive elements of infant's thinking and participates in creation of the infant's self-image process. The original verbal material is to be transformed in the therapist's mind and then turned back to the patient's in a changed form (Bion, 1994).

The caring is incorporated with every step of the two above mentioned therapeutic experiences. There must be an estimation of the patient's ability to accept and acquire the content of the psychotherapeutic intervention.

### 2.2.2 Care in cognitive-behavioral treatment

Cognitive-behavioral therapy is reserved for patients with anxiety and depressive problems. It was modified to be suited for children and adolescents diagnosed with ASD and an anxiety or depressive symptoms.

The approach is time-limited and it focuses on the present. The treatment is time-limited, usually lasting from 12 to 16 sessions. There is a rational element strongly stressed in the treatment. The goal of the therapy centres on the behavioral change and reduction of a dysfunctional thinking.

Due to the CBT (Cognitive Behavioral Therapy) approach, the autistic disorder is connected with a triad of impairments: social, behavioral and the failures in communication (Rhode, 2010). The cognitive deficits caused by brain defect play an important role in the method selection. The CBT shows a therapist as an active person, involved in the process of changes in the patient's cognitive and behavioral sphere. The way he acts, supports the child or adolescent with autism is essential to the psychotherapeutic effects.

As a model for the disabled child or adolescent, the directive therapist needs to teach the patient the social meaning of care behaviour. He should be able to show care-giving and care-receiving as a part of social interaction. There ought to be a stress put on the patient's thoughts and attitudes including an ability of self-care. Care towards others would be considered as one of the home tasks.

### 2.2.3 Care in humanistic approach

Within the humanistic field of psychotherapy Virginia Axline proposed eight principles for non-directive therapists:

1. the rapid creation of a warm and friendly relationship with the child;
2. total acceptance of the child exactly as he is;

3. establishing permissiveness so that the child is free to express his feelings openly in the relationship with the therapist;
4. alertness to the feelings the child expresses and reflecting these back to him so that he gains insight into his behaviour;
5. a deep respect for the child's capacity to solve his own problems if given the opportunity, and leaving him with the responsibility for choices and the initiation of changes;
6. no attempt to direct child's behavior or conversation: where the child leads the therapist follows;
7. no attempt to hurry the treatment along;
8. the setting of limits only to the extent of anchoring the treatment in reality and making the child aware of his responsibility in the relationship (Wolff, 1992, s. 228).

The humanistic point of view treats care in terms of subjective category. Similarly to humanistic understanding, there is an existential meaning of care. In the heideggerian standpoint, care is considered as "being with", "being beside" , assist in one's experience of loneliness (Heidegger, 1962).

The humanistic components are present in every therapeutic encounter, but that approach does not exist as a separated method for treating ASD conditions.

### 2.2.4 Care in family therapy

The treatment of an autistic child or adolescent should be complex and it ought to take care of his family, too. In the family session, there is a need for a neutral posture by the therapist. There is a general rule, not to use the word "patient" about the particular person. Instead it is the norm to treat the disabled child or adolescent as "indicated patient" and to reserve the term "patient" for the whole of the family. That is why, the care is directed to the family viewed as an integral system, which has its own basic rules, its own borders protecting it from an external world, its specific structure and its communication within.

The therapist has the opportunity to see and analyze the dynamics of the care-giving and care-receiving processes between the family members. There is a chance to observe and discuss the conflicts and methods of solving them. Autistic spectrum disorder is an important component of the family system and it influences the whole of the relationship inside and outside the system.

Similarly to the situation of the family with a chronic disability affecting their child, the family with an autistic child meets the same problems. The sense of guilt occurring on the parental side, may be recognized as an irritation towards the medical staff. Also there is a sense of loss of a "normal" child development and the plans for his or her future. These feelings can block the transferring to the next development level of the family's life cycle.

There may be an overdose of the maternal caring of the disabled child, that makes it impossible to take the next step and it results in the isolation of the child and also the family, which cannot find enough support from the social environment. The disorder of the child may divert attention from the marital problems of parents. If one parent takes care of the autistic child, the rest of the family may distance themselves from the situation and suffer from a lack of attention to their problems. They might also be accused by the disabled member's carer, of a deficit of caring ability and a lack of involvement in looking after the child. The siblings might feel rejected and can demonstrate unaccepted forms of behaviour. Sometimes the siblings are the main cause of the application of a particular family to the therapy or consultation (Furgał, 2010).

The autistic spectrum disorder may activate unresolved problems of the family. That is why the therapist must work on problems connected with the actual situation and past problems influencing the present.

There can be two main phases of therapy with a family raising an autistic child (Furgał, 2010). Crisis is the first one. It starts before the final diagnosis is given. The family tries to cope with a difficult situation, future plans are changed, a new daily schedule is organized. At that phase the family is concerned with establishing a sense and value in living with the disabled member. The main feeling is sadness, but the family tries to cope with the problem and creates a flexible readiness for future challenges. The second step seen in therapy, is the chronic phase, that takes place after the final diagnosis. The whole family strives to adapt to the present situation. Acceptance of the changes in family life is achieved. There are new roles of caring negotiated, but it does not mean that the members do not miss the former state, and preview the identity of the family. As new information about autism is delivered, the members of the family balance their needs in accordance with that of caring for the autistic child. The family strives to live in a normal way in spite of the presence of the autistic spectrum(Furgał, 2010).

An important factor influencing the quality of therapeutic work is the attitude of the family to the specialists. If there is an unsatisfactory experience due to the contact with the medical staff, the family might not cooperate with the therapist well. Sometimes the situation arises, where the therapist is seen as a great caregiver and the family members feel free from the duty of offering additional care to the disabled child.

Burn-out syndrome is the most seen problem of a family with an autistic child. The parent (usually the mother) is exhausted by the caring of her disabled child and she needs some rest. The cooperation between the therapist and other specialists who can help (for instance by providing the addresses of useful institutions) is a very important issue. The main problem present in almost every family with an ASD member is connected with different losses (the loss of freedom, the loss of preview activity, sometimes the loss of the money, the loss of the health etc). The therapist should carefully confront the family with these losses and the feelings associated with them.

There can be unaccepted emotions associated with an autistic child, which produces feelings of shame and the tendency to omit the subject during a therapy discussion. Parents may experience conflicts about their situation, the treatment and methods of education of the autistic child. They may have trouble with expressing their thoughts, the problems connected with revealing their feelings.

The treatment is centered on the stimulation of the development of the family. There should be a therapeutic work on increasing the family's sense of control of the treatment. The empowerment of the family serves as additional care. One of the therapeutic tasks belongs to the concentration of the family activity outside the autistic spectrum theme (Furgał, 2010). The family life should extend to the sphere where the autistic spectrum does not appears. It does not mean that the family is introduced to the resignation of care-giving, but there ought to be a sphere where members can develop their own interests, hobbies or activities, to look after the autistic child with renewed energy. Attention to the strong features of the family during the therapy process is necessary. The family may feel confused or surprised, in the beginning. They are not used to listening or analyzing these types of trials, but it can be a chance to see their situation from another perspective.

## 3. Conclusion

This chapter has presented the concept of caring according to psychotherapy with children and adolescents diagnosed with ASD. Psychotherapy is an additional form of treatment and will never be used as the only way of providing help to the children. It can be implemented especially with children with autism who suffer from co-existing psychological problems, anxiety disorders or depression.

The inspiration for the work was the practical problem of emotional fatigue in professionals because of the ineffectiveness of treatment of the subjects with ASD condition and the need for improvement. As one of the participants in the study of the caregivers living with the autistic child had stated: "Professionals in the medical field lack the patience and understanding of dealing with persons with autism" (Phelps et al., 2009, p. 31). Intellectual consideration of the subject of caring and caring behaviours, including both the children or adolescents with autism and their parents or caregivers, results in paying more attention to the various manifestations of care in the specialists' own actions or conduct. It also allows for distancing oneself from the negative emotions of parents of autistic children referred to specialists and helps to overcome the negative feelings of the specialist, caused by the difficult emotions of the caregivers.

This has been a review of the literature connected with "caring" and an attempt to suit the results to psychotherapeutic background due to the treatment of pervasive developmental disorders. Special attention was dedicated to the psychodynamic approach and its involvement in the understanding of ASD during the therapy process. Children and adolescents treat the therapist like their parent, and have similar expectations concerning the care or the lack of care. The therapist should assess the level of expectations and modify it aiming at strengthening the autonomy of the young patient.

The care is firstly considered to be a part of natural human development seen in the mother-child relationship.

The concept of care was introduced to the scientific field by the nursing practitioners and described from the feminist perspective. The application of the concept to psychotherapy practice is worth considering. As Botticelli states, there is a female-dominated profession of psychotherapy. She notes that the treatment was defined to be a provision of care (Botticelli, 2006). Although the psychodynamic approach was much criticized for its inappropriate etiology of the autism (Bettelheim, 1972), one might find a useful understanding of the disorder and its mechanisms.

There were proposals for a linkage between the psychodynamic and humanistic approaches on the basis of concept of care (Bondi, 2008). This content tries to present the characterization of the role of caring in the treatment of children and adolescent suffering from autistic spectrum disorder.

There were described the philosophical frames and practical aspects of the care dynamics. Different views on the care concept may help to broaden the subtle meaning of the social interactions. Care seems to be an important theme in psychotherapeutic work with autistic subjects and it deserves to be part of future research. It is an important task in therapy to make or improve the ability for self-care in the children and adolescents diagnosed with autism, because of their deficits in social development. The ability can be helpful in surviving in today's world.

The research focusing on the concept of care would enrich the understanding of the needs of the individuals with ASD conditions.

## 4. References


Alvarez A., Reid S. (1999). *Autism and personality. Findings from the Tavistock Autism Workshop*. Routledge.Taylor and Francis Group. ISBN 978-0-415-14602-9, London and New York.

Bauminger N., Shulman C., Agam G. (2004). The link between perceptions of self and of social relations in high-functioning children. *Journal of Developmental and Physical Disabilities*. Vol.16, No. 2, pp.193-214, ISSN 1573-3580.

Bell D.C. & Richard A.J. (2000). Caregiving: The Forgotten Element in Attachment. *Psychological Inquiry*, Vol. 11, No. 2, pp. 69- 83, ISSN 1532-7965.

Berry P. (2003). Psychodynamic therapy and intellectual disabilities: dealing with challenging behavior. *International Journal of Disability, Development and Education*, Vol. 50, No. 1, pp. 39-51, ISSN 1465-346X.

Bettelheim B. (1972). *The empty fortress. Infantile autism and the birth of the self.* The Free Press. ISBN 0-02-903140-0, New York, USA.

Bion W. R.(1994) Clinical seminars & other works. Karnac Books.ISBN 1855750619, London.

Bondi L.(2008). On the relational dynamics of caring: a psychotherapeutic approach to emotional and power dimensions of women's care work. *Gender, Place and Culture.* Vol. 15, No. 3, pp. 249-265, ISSN 1360-0524.

Botticelli S. (2006). Globalization, psychoanalysis and the provision of care. *Studies in Gender and Sexuality*. Vol. 7, No. 1, pp. 71-80, ISSN 1940-9206.

Cohen J.A. (1991). Two portraits of caring: a comparison of the artists, Leininger and Watson. *Journal of Advanced Nursing*, Vol. 16, No. 8, pp. 899- 909, ISSN 0309-2402.

Dobrowolska B. (2006). Troska jako kategoria etyki medycznej [Care as a category of medical ethics]. *Pielęgniarstwo XXI wieku*, Vol. 17, No.4, pp. 15- 20, ISSN 1730- 1912.

Dyson L.(1997). An ethic of caring: conceptual and practical issues. *Nursing Inquiry*. Vol. 4, No. 3, pp. 196-201, ISSN 1440-1800.

Erikson E. (1968). *Identity, youth and crisis*. W.W. Norton & Company, ISBN 0-393-31144-9, New York & London.

Fromm E. (1947). *Man for Himself: An Inquiry into the Psychology of Ethics*. Rinehart, ISBN 0415-21020-8, New York

Furgał M. (2010).Terapia rodziny z dzieckiem autystycznym [The family therapy with the autistic child]. In: *Autyzm – epidemiologia, diagnoza i terapia* [Autism - epidemiology, diagnosis and therapy]. Pietras T., Witusik A., Gałecki P. (eds), pp. 219-225, Wydawnictwo Continuo, ISBN 978-83-89629-99-9, Wrocław, Poland.

Gander M.J., Gardiner H.W. (1981). *Child and adolescent development*. Little Brown and Company, ISBN 0-316-303224, Boston, USA.

Heidegger M. (1962). *Being and Time.* Macquarrie J.& Robinson E. (trans.), Blackwell Publishing, ISBN 0-631-19770-2, Oxford & Cambridge.

Levy T. (2006). The Relational Self and the Right to Give Care. *New Political Science*, Vol. 28, No. 4, December 2006, ISSN 1469-9931.

McCance T.V., McKenna H.P., Boore J.R.P. (1997). Caring: dealing with a difficult concept. *International Journal of Nursing Studies*. Vol. 34, No. 4, pp. 241-248, ISSN 0020-7489.

Morra M. (2002). Some considerations about personality structure in child psychosis. *Journal of Child Psychotherapy*. Vol. 28, No. 3, pp. 283-303, ISSN 1469-9370.

Paley J. (2000). Heidegger and ethics of care. *Nursing Philosophy*, Vol. 1., No. 1, pp. 64-75, ISSN 1466-769X.

Phelps K.W., Hodgson J.L., McCammon S.L., Lamson A.L. (2009). Caring for an individual with autism disorder: A qualitative analysis. *Journal of Intellectual & Developmental Disability,* Vol. 34, No.1, pp. 27-35, ISSN 1469-9532.

Poole M., Isaacs D. (1997). Caring: a gendered concept. *Women's Studies International Forum.* Vol. 20, No. 4, pp. 529-536, ISSN 0277-5395.

Rhode M. (2010). Child psychotherapy with children on the autistic spectrum. In: *Child and adolescent psychotherapy. Psychoanalytic approaches.* Lanyado M. & Horne A. (eds)., pp. 287-299. Routledge.Taylor & Francis Group, ISBN 978-0-415-46369-0, London & New York.

Ruberman L. (2002). Psychotherapy of children with pervasive developmental disorders. *American Journal of Psychotherapy*. Vol. 56, No. 2, pp. 262-273, ISSN 0002-9564.

Sourial S. (1997). An analysis of caring. *Journal of Advanced Nursing*. Vol. 26, No. 6., pp. 1189-1192, ISSN 0309-2402.

Ślusarska B., Dobrowolska B. & Zarzycka D. (2008). Teoretyczne podstawy kategorii „opieka" w pielęgniarstwie [Theoretical basis of the category of „care" in nursing]. *Problemy Pielęgniarstwa,* Vol. 16, No. 4, pp. 384- 389, ISSN 1233-9989.

Tinbergen E.A.., Tinbergen N. (1986) *Autistic children. New hope for cure.* Routledge. ISBN 0041570111, London.

Tuck I., Harris L., Renfro T. & Lexvolds L. (1998). Care: A Value Expressed in Philosophies of Nursing Services. *Journal of Professional Nursing,* Vol. 14, No. 2, pp. 92- 96, ISSN 8755-7223.

Winnicott D.W. (1994). *Dzieci i ich matki* [Babies and their mothers].Wydawnictwo WAB, ISBN 83-85554-30-0, Warszawa, Poland.

Wiseman V. (1997). Caring: the neglected health outcome? or input? *Health Policy.* Vol. 39,No. 1, pp. 43- 53, ISSN 0168-8510.

Wolff S. (1992). Child psychotherapy. In: *An Introduction to the Psychotherapies.* Bloch S.(ed.), pp. 222-251, Oxford University Press , ISBN 0-19-261469-X,Oxford, New York, Tokyo.

World Health Organization (1992). *Manual of the International Statistical Classification of the Diseases and Related Health Problems: Diagnostic criteria for research* (10th edition). ISBN 92-4-154649-2, Geneva, Switzerland: Author.

# 9

# TEACCH Intervention for Autism

Rubina Lal and Anagha Shahane
*Department of Special Education, SNDT Women's University, Mumbai, India*

## 1. Introduction

Education is one of the fundamental factors for development. It enriches people's understanding of themselves and the world. It improves quality of life and leads to broad social benefits to the people and society. Education raises people's productivity, creativity and promotes entrepreneurship and technological advances. No country can achieve sustainable economic development without investing in education. The ultimate goal of education is to help a person become responsible, independent, and contributing member of the community to which he or she belongs. For children with special educational needs, education aims to maximize their potential and help them become well adjusted individuals.

Autism is a developmental disorder that affects a child's perception of the world and how the child learns from his or her experiences. Even among the most complex disabilities, autism remains an enigma. Autism is the most frequently occurring form of a group of disorders known as Autism Spectrum Disorders (ASD). The Autism Society of America (2006) defines autism as a complex developmental disability that typically appears during the first three years of life and is the result of a neurological disorder that affects the normal functioning of the brain, impacting development in the areas of social interaction and communication skills. Both children and adults typically show difficulties in verbal and nonverbal communication, social interactions, and leisure or play activities. One should keep in mind however; that autism is a spectrum disorder and it affects each individual differently and at varying degrees. Autism affects essential human behaviors such as social interaction, ability to communicate ideas and feelings, imagination, and establishment of relationships with others (National Research Council, 2002). Children with autism may also show abnormal responses to sensory stimuli, such as touch, sounds and sights.

There are several goals for the education of children with autism. These goals emerge from the universal belief in education for all children and what can be taught to children with autism. Education provides opportunities for acquiring knowledge and abilities that enhance personal independence and socially responsible behaviour. In comparison with neurotypical children, a child with ASD may need to be taught different behaviours in order to manifest independence and responsible participation in the community.

Neurotypical children learn many behaviours without direct teaching, but this is not so with children who have autism. A young autistic child may have rote learned to count but may not be able to name things that he uses daily. As he grows older, he may be able to operate electronic equipment but not be able to dress appropriately. Hence, educational goals for these students, as part of addressing independence and social responsibility, needs to address language, social, and adaptive goals that are not part of standard curricula. Education must foster acquisition of not only academic but also social adaptive skills, language and communication and reduction in problem behaviour in such children (Lal, 2005).

Studies show that children with autism respond well to structured educational program tailored to their specific needs. The severe challenges that some of them face is best addressed by an educational program that follows the behavioural approach, and is implemented in one to one or small group sessions (Vismara & Rogers, 2007; Lal & Lobo, 2007). Children with autism have difficulty with abstract, language-based, conceptual tasks that require sequencing and organization. Typical methods of teaching such as verbal explanation, demonstration and modelling may not be successful due to social, communication and limited imitative behaviours in the children. Conversely, tasks that are visual in nature and rely more on eye-hand integration, spatial, or motor capacities are better comprehended and enjoyable for them. It is possible to capitalize on these strengths while remediating the weaknesses. Thus, if tasks, even those that are verbal and conceptual in nature, are structured for the child so that both what is expected and how to achieve it is apparent from visual characteristics, teaching and learning the tasks is easier (Schopler et al, 1998). Structure in teaching and teaching environment addresses the unique features of autism. It enables to children to understand what is expected of them, encourages self control and enhances skills to cope with the ever changing and dynamic social situations. Structured teaching approaches provide familiar, predictable and structured environments that reduce anxiety, promote independence, increase flexibility and tolerance for change (Quill, 2000, as cited in Simpson & Smith Myles, 2008).

TEACCH (Treatment and Education of Autistic and related Communication handicapped CHildren) is a program designed to provide the structure and predictability that children with autism require to function successfully. This chapter presents the findings of a research study conducted in Mumbai, India, to determine the effect of TEACCH based intervention on development of independent work skills in children with autism.

## 2. TEACCH

TEACCH is an evidence-based service, training, and research program for individuals of all ages and skill levels with autism spectrum disorders. Established in the early 1970s by Eric Schopler and colleagues, the TEACCH program has worked with thousands of individuals with autism spectrum disorders and their families. The TEACCH approach includes a focus on the person with autism and the development of a program around the person's skills, interest, and needs. The TEACCH priorities centre on understanding autism, making necessary adaptations, and selecting strategies for intervention that utilize the person's existing skills and interests. The TEACCH program emphasizes individual assessment for understanding the person. It also believes in the 'culture of autism', suggesting that people with autism are part of a distinctive group with common characteristics that are different, but not necessarily inferior to others (Mesibov et al, 2004). Understanding the culture of autism requires understanding persons with autism as they are and to develop program to suit each person's functioning level.

By accepting the culture of autism TEACCH program works toward changing the structural norms to facilitate inclusion of persons with autism, rather than moulding them into an

existing normal model. Because some of the neurological issues that contribute to autism characteristics are irreversible, TEACCH intervention does not aim to 'normalize' a child with autism. In stead, the long term objective is to help the child develop into an adult who can function well in the environment.
Structured teaching is an important component of the TEACCH program. This is because structure suits the 'culture of autism' more than any other technique.

### 2.1 TEACCH principles

Given the cognitive and behavioural features of autism, the TEACCH program has developed ways to help children with autism function in the culture that surrounds them. The educational program recommended by TEACCH is founded on principles discussed below.

- Strengths and interests:
  All children have strengths and interests that can be used for teaching them. In case of autism, the child's attachment to certain colour, for example, may be made functional by marking the key aspects of his/her work in that colour. Preferred activities/objects can be used as rewards when the child completes or learns a task that is new or complex in nature. Similarly, a child's compulsion to complete tasks in a set sequence may be tapped for teaching him or how to use checklists for a range of activities such as, personal care, household chores and classroom routines etc.
- Ongoing assessment:
  All children have the potential to develop and learn. From the severely intellectually impaired nonverbal autistic child with issues in personal care and aggression, to the high functioning child with autism who can read, write and function satisfactorily in school, all of them have gaps in skills and have potential for progress. The TEACCH educational program is designed by observing children's approach to a variety of materials, directions, and activities, presented in different modalities and different amounts of structure. Special attention is paid to communication, self care, vocational and recreation skills (TEACCH Autism Program, 2011).
- Assistance in Understanding:
  Children with autism have difficulty in understanding the meaning of their experiences. This often is central to the problems faced by them. Teachers and caregivers cannot assume that the children would automatically understand why they have been asked to do certain things, or how the behaviours taught to them are related to what is being expected from them. Even the high functioning children are uncertain about expectations and customs in a particular social situation. The educational program supports and enables the children to deal with confusing and hard to interpret situations. This also reduces challenging or noncompliant behaviours that may emerge due to lack of understanding about expectations.
- Parent collaboration:
  Parents and family are important to the educational planning. The program is sensitive to the home environment. Hence, it includes the wishes and life styles of the child's family as significant elements. Parents are consulted with regard to specific ways to dressing, eating, or spending leisure time, and these are incorporated in the program as teaching goals for the child. This helps the children in functioning effectively in environments other than the classroom.

- Individualization:
  Providing for individual differences is a key element of TEACCH educational program. Children with autism often do not learn well in a group due to the differences in skills, difficulty in learning by imitation, and idiosyncrasies. Also, strength on one area may not correlate with performance in other areas. For example, good visual perception may not correspond with their ability to read facial expression. Similarly, expressive ability can mask significant receptive language deficits. Many children who are able to do grade level academic work may not know how to other functional tasks such as personal care and hygiene. On the other hand, some children with significant intellectual disability may have abilities (e.g. solving puzzles, painting, and singing etc.) that do not match with their cognitive functioning. A teacher using the program should know the children well and be prepared to teach them at different levels in different areas.

### 2.2 Structured teaching

Structured teaching is an approach in instructing children with autism. Structure, according to dictionary, is the action of building or constructing--arranging things in a definite pattern of organization. Structured teaching allows for implementation of a variety of instructional methods (e.g., visual support strategies, Picture Exchange Communication System - PECS, sensory integration strategies, discrete trials etc.). Structured teaching is based upon an understanding of the unique features and characteristics associated with the nature of autism. It describes the conditions under which a person should be taught rather than 'where' or 'what'. It is a system for organizing environments, developing appropriate activities, and helping people with autism comprehend what is expected of them. Structured teaching utilizes visual cues which help children with autism focus on the relevant information which can, at times, be difficult for the person with autism to distinguish from the non-relevant information.

Structured teaching addresses behavioral deficits in a proactive manner by creating appropriate and meaningful environments that reduce the stress, anxiety and frustration which may be experienced by children with autism. Deficits in behavior may occur, due to the following characteristics of autism:

- Language and communication difficulties:
  Autistic children have great difficulty in understanding spoken words. They have trouble understanding that words relate to objects and activities. Abstract words are extremely challenging because they are not linked to something tangible that can be inspected and pointed to. Without concrete visual connections to objects or activities, words are nearly impossible for them to understand. Processing language involves taking in speech sounds that one hears and converting them into patterns of understanding. Children with receptive language difficulties and language processing problems may not be attentive when someone is teaching and/or may not be able to follow long strands of directions. When given a task to complete, they may forget what they were asked to do or be able to complete only a few steps
  Several researchers have identified *joint attention* and *symbol use* as the core deficits in the area of language and communication (Sigman & Ruskin, 1999; Wetherby, et al., 1998; Jordan, 2003) for children with autism. Joint attention reflects the difficulty in coordinating attention between people and objects and is evident by deficits in

orienting and attending to a social partner; shifting gaze between people and objects; sharing feelings with another person etc. Symbol use reflects difficulty in learning conventional and shared meanings for symbols and is evident in deficits in using conventional gestures; learning conventional meanings for words; and using objects functionally and in symbolic play.

- Social relations difficulties:
  As they grow, babies learn how to be social and interactive by watching how others talk, play and relate to each other. They enjoy the give-and-take of social engagement and will initiate, maintain and respond to interactions with others. In fact, they seek out these interactions. Children with autism, however, often do not show the expected development of early social interaction skills. They seem not to have the same "drive" to interact socially as their peers do. These social impairments affect children's interactions with adults as well as with other children. They affect children's ability to initiate interactions with others as well as to respond to interactions that are initiated by others. Many children also show profound *empathy* deficits. They develop a limited appreciation or no appreciation at all, of other people's feelings and ideas. To the severely autistic children, their own feelings and ideas are the only feelings and ideas that appear to exist. Autistic children may have no reaction to another person's crying, for example. They may have no idea that their words and actions affect other people. Many autistic children are completely unaware of their surroundings and other people in their surroundings. It is impossible for some autistic children to take another person's perspective without deliberate training. For individuals with autism, it does not come naturally to consider other people's perspective. This makes it difficult for them to understand how others think and feel (Richard 2000). Clinicians and researchers call this inability to consider others' perspective as deficit in *theory of mind*. Theory of mind, the ability to attribute mental states to self and others in order to understand and predict behaviour, is an area of weakness among individuals on the autism spectrum. *Play* is considered a key social behavior. As children with autism have trouble in symbol use, joint attention and understanding others' perspective, participating in pretend play and using imitative skills are difficult for many of them.
- Sensory processing difficulties:
  Sensory processing is the way our central nervous system receives and understands the meaning of sensations (Miller, 2000). Children with autism tend to have extreme reactions to sensory stimulation. Their senses may become hypersensitive (over-sensitive) or hyposensitive (under-sensitive). *Hypersensitive* children find themselves overloaded with even moderate levels of sensation, and work to block out sensory inputs such as light, sound and touch. *Hyposensitive* children, on the other hand, are not stimulated enough by normal sensory inputs and typically seek out extra stimulation. Children who are hypersensitive to touch sensations may tantrum when they are touched, while hyposensitive children may crave and seek out strong hugs that provide deep pressure. Children with high pain tolerances may injure themselves quite significantly but carry on as though nothing has happened, while oversensitive children may find simple touches or textures to be intolerable.
- Resistance to change:
  Children with autism have a propensity to establish and enforce routines. A lack of completion of the activity in a routine can lead to distress and anxiety. Researches indicate that insistence on completing an activity in a particular way may be the child's

attempt to find patterns and look for rules and organization within environment (Baron-Cohen, 2002). Once a pattern has emerged it must be maintained. Thus, establishment of a routine ensures that there is no opportunity for change. Clinical evidence suggests that the routine becomes more dominant and elaborate when the person has recently experienced changes in the key people in their life, accommodation, daily routine and expectations or when they display signs of anxiety. The anxiety may be due to apprehension that they are unsure how to socialize and may make a mistake, and not knowing if there will be a change in routine or expectation. The students may resist the change by complaining or resist with their behaviour by becoming aggressive or defiant. They may tantrum or become agitated. Too many unexpected changes in the day may cause them to be overwhelmed and experience a 'melt-down.'As a person matures, the insistence on routine tends to diminish, but change is never easily tolerated.

- Organizational difficulties:
  Organization requires integration of several elements and arranging them so as to achieve a preset objective. Since children with autism experience problems in integration of information into a cohesive whole, they have poor organizational skills. It is difficult for them to focus on the immediate task and the desired outcome (Mesibov & Shea, 2003). Sequencing requires similar skills. Hence, it is not unusual for such children to perform a series of tasks in illogical order, and to be unaware of it. This shows that while they have learned the steps of a complex process, they do not understand the relationship among the steps or the importance of each step with regard to the final outcome.
- Distractibility:
  It is common for children with autism to experience problems in attending to specified stimuli such as, colours or shapes etc. Paying and sustaining attention to a task is difficult. Similarly, knowing what to attend to and shift attention from one stimulus to another when required is a challenge too. This is especially problematic when fast and multifaceted social exchanges take place (Simpson, et al., 2008). Distractibility is also caused by the inability to integrate sensory information. A child may pay attention to a teacher's hand rather than what he/she is showing him; or pay attention away from the task to a sound that is so soft that the teacher does not even hear. At times, need for repetitive behaviours also cause distractibility in such children. Whatever the source of distraction, the children have difficulty in prioritizing the importance of external stimulation or internal needs in the process of doing a task.
- Concrete thinking:
  Regardless of their cognitive level, children with autism experience problems with symbolic or abstract language concepts. Straightforward facts and descriptions are grasped better. They often do not understand that word meanings may change according to the situation in which they are used. Hence, it is difficult for them to follow the humour in jokes, criticism in sarcastic remarks, and the message in idioms and adages. A high functioning student with autism may explain the meaning of "a bird in hand is better than two in bush" as "it is easier to hold one bird in the hand. A bush is big, so it is not easy to hold birds while they are in the bush. Our hands are not so big"
- Difficulty with generalizations:
  Children with autism are often unable to apply to learned skill to different situation. For instance, a child who has learnt to put on socks may refuse to put them on if the

socks given are of different colour than the ones used during training. Similarly, the children may learn to wash plates, but do not understand that dirty trays can be washed in the same manner. They also often learn the literal wording of a rule, but not understand its underlying purpose, and so have problems applying the rule in different settings. A child who did not understand physical space, used to stand very close to people when talking to them. He was told to stop four feet away from them before speaking to them. He understood this, but became concerned with measuring how far he was from people than speaking with them. Also, he insisted on keeping this distance even while talking to his parents. He had obviously not understood the concept of physical space behind this rule, and that the rule did not apply to all situations in a similar manner.

### 2.2.1 Elements of structured teaching

The use of structured teaching has been central to TEACCH program since its inception more than four decades ago. The elements of structured teaching include physical organization, schedules, work systems, and task organization. A brief description of each is provided below.

- Physical Structure:
  Physical structure refers to the actual layout or surroundings of a person's environment, such as classroom, play room, home etc. Children with autism have difficulty differentiating between dissimilar events and seeing how distinct activities relate to one another. The physical boundaries are clearly defined with activity labels like music, work, play, snacks. The use of consistent, visually clear areas and boundaries for specific activities enables children with autism to better understand their environments and relationships between events. The teacher should consider classroom goals for the child and then allocate specific areas for major activities. Planning physical structure depends on curricular goals and child's individual needs. Since children with autism have difficulty differentiating between dissimilar events and seeing how distinct activities relate to one another, a clearly organized classroom helps in learning important concepts. It also teaches independence and alleviates anxiety caused by ambiguity and transition. Physical structure is essential for a number of reasons: Physical structure provides environmental organization for children with autism; clear physical and visual boundaries help the person to understand where each area begins and ends; and the physical structure minimizes visual and auditory distractions. The amount of physical structure needed is dependent on the level of self-control demonstrated by the child, not his cognitive functioning level. As children learn to function more independently, the physical structure can be gradually lessened.
- Schedules:
  Schedules are important aspect of structured teaching. They are visual cues that tell the children what to expect through the day. They explain the sequence of activities that would occur during the day. Like the physical structure schedules help the children in comprehending the difference between events and how each event relates with another. Visual schedules are beneficial for children with autism in improving the sequential memory, receptive language, and attention problems. Schedules help children in predicting daily or weekly events. They aid in transitions which are often very difficult for autistic children. Schedules can motivate children to complete a task that they do not want to do because they can see a favorite activity follows soon after the less

preferred tasks. Visual schedules can be presented in written (for more capable children) and pictorial (for non readers) forms. Those children who need a high degree of concrete structure may use object schedules.

- Work Systems:
  Physical structure and schedules enable children with autism to understand where to go and what to expect during the day, work systems tell them what they should do in their assigned physical areas. Work systems are essential for teaching independent work behavior. Through work systems children know the behavior expected of them in work activities. Systems help in organization and completion of tasks. Work systems provide four types of information: work that is to be done; how much work to be done; indication of when the work is completed, and what happens after a given is done. Work systems can be made to suit the needs of children on individual basis. Like schedules, work systems can be presented in written as well as pictorial forms. This is helpful as the visually clear task components with predetermined number of material and defined end points enable children to understand how to start and complete the tasks. This organization facilitates independent work behavior.
- Visual Structure:
  Children with autism are visual learners (Lal & Bali, 2008). They do their work better when instructions are presented visually. Visual structure refers to visual organization, clarification and instruction pertaining to tasks. When a task is presented in clear visual form it is easier for the children to identify its features. Since visual information is concrete and less dynamic, children learn the task easily. Similarly, visual organization also facilitates information processing. Task elements can be so organized that sensory overload is avoided. Visual instructions are graphic representation of task steps. Visual instructions are also helpful in explaining the daily routine to the children.

### 2.3 TEACCH teaching method

The TEACCH instructional method is broadly based on the principles of applied behavioural analysis. It recommends breaking the learning task into small steps that must be taught with prompts and the learning behaviour to be shaped with use of reinforcers

- *Instructions*: They consist of directions given to a child regarding the task that has to be done. Instructions may be verbal or nonverbal. The mode is instruction is selected to suit the functional level of the child. If instructions are verbal, the teacher should avoid using too many words or long and complex sentences. Use of phrases and telegraphic language help the child focus on key element of the instruction. For example, in stead of saying 'I want you to go to the wash room and clean your hands well before sitting down for lunch' the teacher may instruct a child to 'wash hands, and then eat'. This telegraphic statement will be understood better by the child than the earlier long sentence. When instructions are given nonverbally they are accompanied by contextual and visual cues. Providing only the materials that the child needs to use for a specific task and presenting them sequentially enable the child to understand not only their relevance for each step of the task, but also learn to work independently. For example, if paper, paint brushes and colours are kept on the work table, it is easy for the child to understand that the teacher expects him/her to paint.
- *Prompts*: A teacher uses prompts to shape a child's behaviour to the desired level. Prompts help a child to complete a new task. Different types of prompts may be used.

Physical prompts are used to give manual assistance in task completion; verbal prompts are reminders for a task; gestural prompts are signs or actions that point to or demonstrate the task; and visual prompts may use pictures/symbols/colour cards to cue the child to the task. Prompts should be used systematically. They must be offered before the child responds incorrectly. Decision regarding the prompt level depends on the child's functioning. It is important for the teacher to ensure that unintentional prompts are not given (e.g. slight movement of head, eyes or hand may amount to gestural prompt when such a prompt is not planned). It is as important to withdraw the prompts when the child learns to do the task in order to prevent prompt dependence in the children.

- *Reinforcement*: Behaviours that are reinforced positively are likely to be repeated. Typically growing children are motivated to work because of the praise they may receive from others, intrinsic satisfaction of working and a sense of achievement when the task is completed well. Children with autism may not be motivated by any of these. However, there are items and activities that do motivate these children. The teacher needs to determine what interests and motivates a child. Some children may like a particular toy, a book, an object, or a food item where as others may find activities more interesting. An important aspect of reinforcement is that it should be given immediately after the child emits a correct response. Praise and social rewards should accompany tangible reinforcers. This pairing increases the desirability of personal contact for the children with autism and makes people greater sources of reinforcement in the future.

## 3. Research support for TEACCH

As an intervention approach for autism, TEACCH program has been well researched. Several empirical studies, conducted across countries have established the program's efficacy for children with autism and other severe developmental disabilities. In a longitudinal study, Tsang and colleagues (2007) evaluated the usefulness of TEACCH program on 34 children from a pre-school in Hong Kong. This experimental research provided TEACCH intervention to 18 children while 16 control children continued with the regular training. The study lasted for 12 months. Children's cognitive, social adaptive functioning and developmental abilities were measured prior to intervention, during intervention and post intervention. The intervention group children showed better outcomes at post test. They also showed progress in developmental domains during intervention. Hume, et al (2009) examined the effects of work system on independent work and play skills of students with autism. A Single subject 'withdrawal of treatment' design, with replications across three participants, was used to assess the effect of intervention over on task behaviour and work completion skills of the students in classroom and employment settings. Observational data indicated that all students showed increases in on task behaviour and in the number of task completed or play material used, and reduction in teacher prompts. Siaperas & Beadle-Brown (2006) report the outcomes of a study conducted by the Greek Society for the Protection of Autistic People in which 12 autistic residents in an institution were taught using the structured teaching approach. After the 6 month intervention period the subjects showed significant improvement in personal independence, social abilities, and functional communication abilities. Kusmeirski & Henckel (2002) determined the effectiveness of TEACCH program on reduction of maladaptive behaviour and enhancement of independence in functional activities. Four children with autism, of 8 to

13 years, residing in a residential institute were studied. Baseline data were collected for 30 days followed by 30 days of intervention to two children. Results indicated that use of TEACCH schedule decreased maladaptive behaviour in one child, while the other child improved on the ability to independently complete functional tasks.
Some studies have assessed the benefits of TEACCH program in family environment. Hungelmann (2001) evaluated a home program in which parents of children with autism were taught how to implement structured teaching in the home. The study included baseline sessions, treatment sessions, home visits and follow up sessions. Results indicated that children demonstrated significant gains in task mastery as they progressed through the TEACCH program. Parents who participated perceived the program as an effective means to remediate their child's deficits. Similarly, Malhotra, et al. (2002) published the results of a study conducted with parents of children with autism. The treatment methods were drawn from TEACCH protocol. The parents were taught how to use behavioural strategies for enhancing eye contact, reduction of maladaptive behaviour, structuring time, activities, and physical environment. Parents were trained in using the techniques, educated about the nature of their children's disorder, and counselled to deal with the emotional fall out of the diagnosis. Subsequently, 5 children were given TEACCH based intervention for 3 to 6 sessions of 45 to 60 minutes each. Results showed that the parents found the intervention helpful for the children and themselves.

## 4. Method

The study employed a one group - pre test - post test experimental design, and was conducted on children with autism enrolled in schools in Mumbai.

### 4.1 Subjects

Children enrolled in four schools were considered for the study. As per the school records a total 27 children manifested autistic features. Administration of DSM –IV and Childhood Autism Rating Scale identified 21 of the 27 children as having autism. A random selection of 12 children was made from this group. The selected children were within the age range of 8 to 12 years.

### 4.2 Instruments

The Scale of Independent Work Skills (SIWS) and TEACCH based intervention program were the main instruments used in the study. They were developed for the purpose of the research. A brief description of both is given below.

- *Scale of Independent Work Skills*: SIWS was used as a measure at pre and post tests. The instrument measured behaviour under four main domains, namely conceptual skills, daily living skills, pre-vocational skills and self engagement activities. Each domain consisted of items stated in behavioural terms. The authors used the following steps in the development of SIWS: (a) *generation of item pool* was effected by reviewing instructional goals and objectives of educational programs followed in inclusive schools in Mumbai. In addition, observation of classroom work and social behaviours, and discussion with teachers contributed to the process of item generation; (b) *review of items* was done by experienced teachers and domain experts. This was done for determining the content validity of the instrument. Items that were accepted by all reviewers were retained; (c) The draft was subsequently *pilot tested* on children with autism. This resulted in addition, deletion or modification of some items. Two items were changed within the daily living domain; a few more were added to the pre-vocational domain. The SIWS consisted of several items based on educational goals pre set for the children. Hence, the ability to sort and arrange objects according to shapes, colours, sizes and patterns were assessed under conceptual skills; daily living skills were measured by manifestation of such behaviours as self care, cleaning and washing of items of daily use; pre-vocational skills included the ability to fold, cut, insert, string and staple etc., and finally solving puzzles and completing given task on worksheet comprised the activities of self engagement. The SIWS used a 5-point scale to measure children's response on the basis of the level of prompts required by them. The rating was given as per independent response, symbol prompt, picture prompt, gesture prompt, and physical prompt, with independent response earning 5 points and physical prompt 1 point respectively. The SIWS had a total of 34 items, with a maximum attainable score of 170. The scale had a test - retest reliability coefficient of 0.82.

- *TEACCH based intervention program*: The program was premised on the principles of structured teaching. Though structured teaching has several components such as physical organization, schedules, work systems and visual structure and information, the study used only two components, namely work systems and visual structure. Since the children were selected from different educational settings and were available only for intervention sessions, it was not possible to accommodate changes in either physical organization or daily schedules of the respective settings. The intervention consisted of teaching of independent work behaviours. For each child at least 5 activities were selected with at least an activity each from what could be included under conceptual, daily living, pre-vocational and self engagement skills. A child's functioning level also determined the selection of activities for him/her. For example, making of sets (as per a given number) was not chosen as an activity for a child who had not learned counting. Each child was given 15 sessions of structured teaching. A session was of 30 minute's duration. The first two sessions were used for demonstration of skills to be learned. Task material was presented in boxes/trays (refer to figures 1,2,3,4,&5) that provided definite boundaries. Boxes/trays had visual cues, and the material within were so arranged that activity moved from left to right. Generally, a task had a 'finished' symbol placed at the extreme right to indicate completion of the task. Reinforcement was chosen as per individual preferences of the children

### 4.3 Procedure

The intervention began after the children were pre tested on SIWS. A typical intervention session proceeded in the following manner:

- Work table was prepared in advance with only task material set on the table
- Teacher sat next to the child and gave telegraphic instructions, e.g. 'sort beads'
- Each task had a visual symbol that denoted the activity, e.g. sorting task had coloured symbols, matching with that of the beads, near the bowls where sorted beads would be kept
- The child was prompted (pictorial, gestural or physical) to comply with the instruction.
- Rewards were presented after the child had reached 'finished' symbol

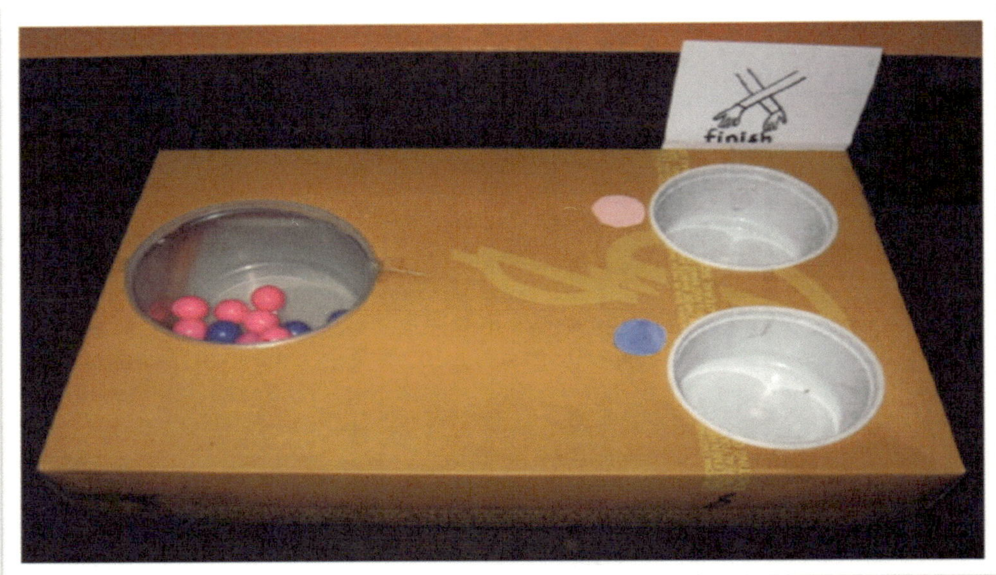


Fig. 1. Colour Sorting Task

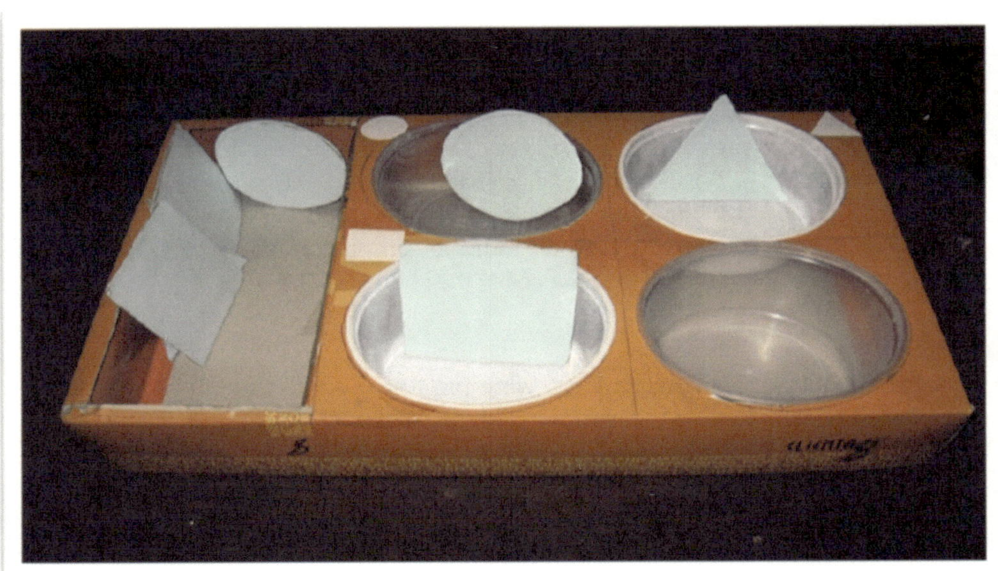

Fig. 2. Shape Sorting Task

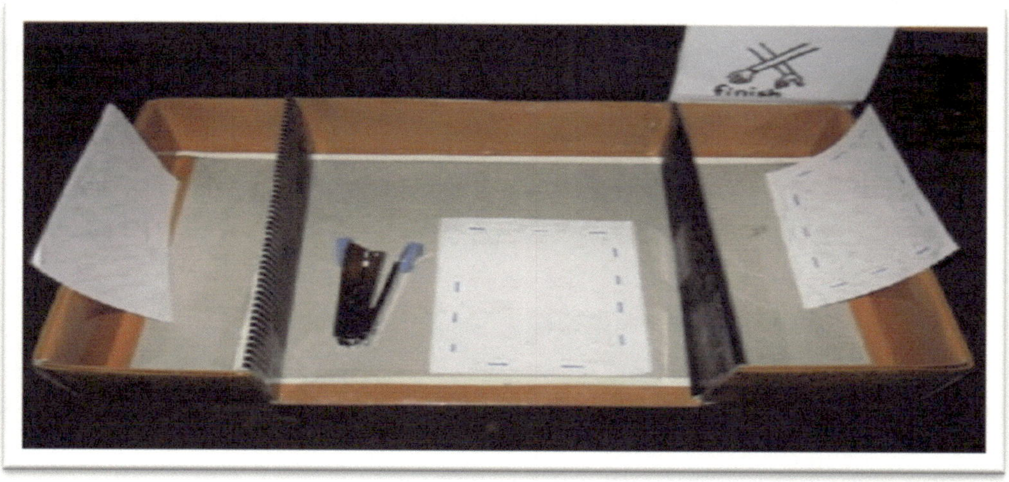

Fig. 3. Paper Stapling Task

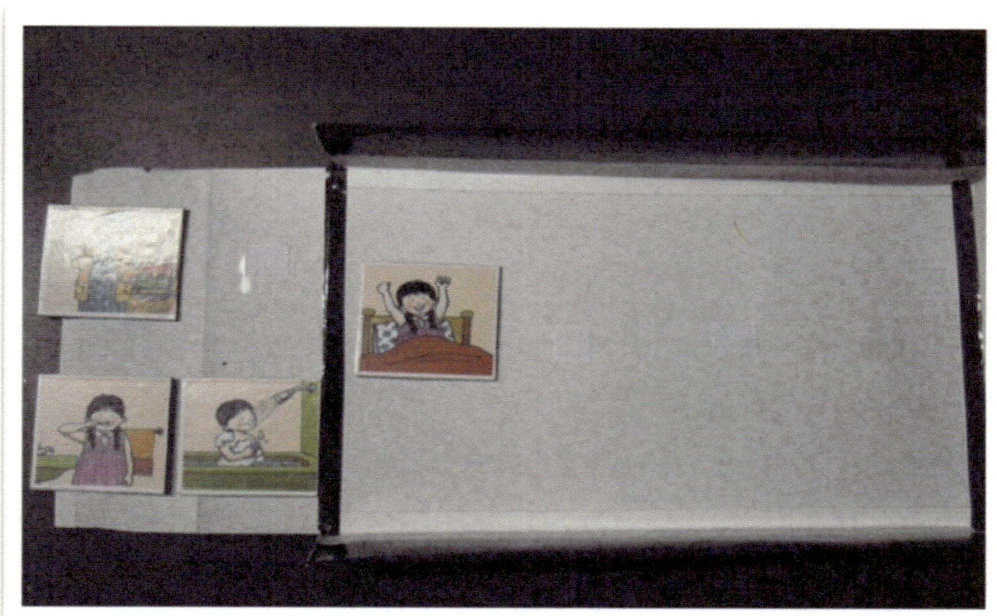

Fig. 4. Daily Living Task

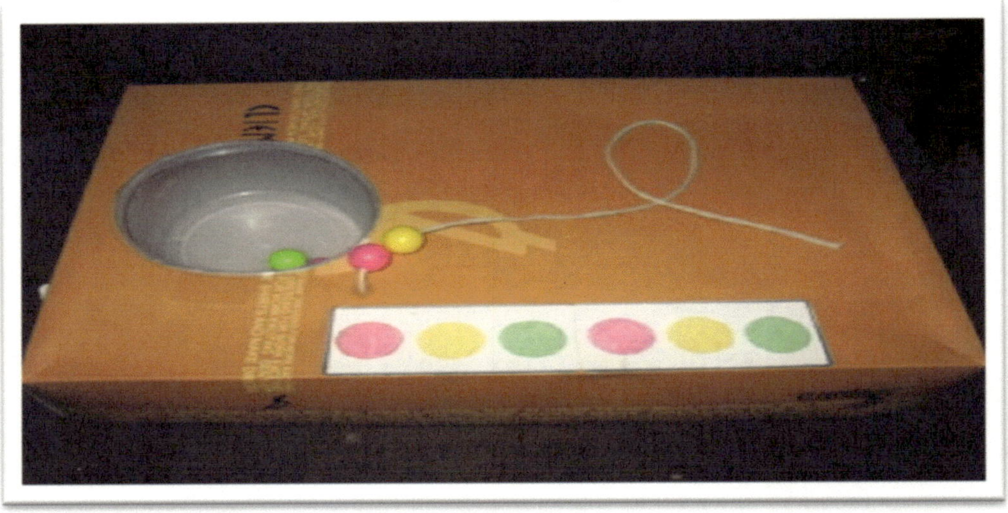

Fig. 5. Bead Stringing Task

Each activity was done twice during a session. The intervention focussed on teaching the skills measured by SIWS. However, the activities selected for intervention were different from those in SIWS. As the children learned the activities, they were asked to do the activity once with the task tray and then without the task tray during a session. A record of behaviour was maintained for each child. At the completion of 15 sessions, SIWS was administered again.

## 5. Results

The study aimed to determine the effect of TEACCH intervention on independent work behaviour of 12 children with autism selected as subject. At the end of intervention period the authors could see the change in the children's ability to understand and perform selected tasks independently. This general observation was supported by the data from SIWS re administration. The use of t-test was justified as the children were selected randomly. The SIWS measured behaviour on four subareas consisting of conceptual skills, daily living skills, pre-vocational skills and self engagement activities. An analysis of the composite mean score on SIWS at pre and post tests along with the scores on each subarea is presented below.

| MEAN | N | df | t-value | Significance |
|---|---|---|---|---|
| 113.17 | 12 | 11 | 8.4 | P<0.001 |
| 129.67 | 12 | | | |

Table 1. Comparison of Composite Mean Scores on SIWS at Pre and Post Tests

The composite mean score on SIWS at pre test was compared with that at post test (refer Table 1.). The post test mean (129.67) was significantly higher than mean (113.17) at pre test as shown by the resultant t-value (8.4, df=11, $p<0.001$). In Figure 6, a detail comparison of each child's performance shows the positive effect of TEACCH intervention.

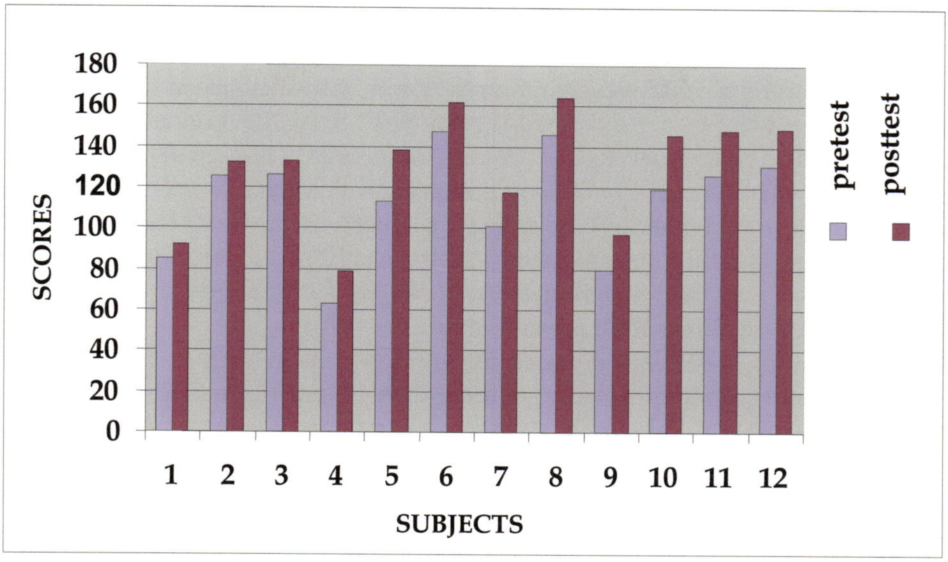


Fig. 6. Children's Composite Scores on SIWS at Pre and Post Tests

As seen in Figure 6, TEACCH intervention enhanced the independent work skills of all children. Each of the 12 children improved their performance, though some gained more than the others. This variance in gain could be due to the initial differences in their functioning levels.

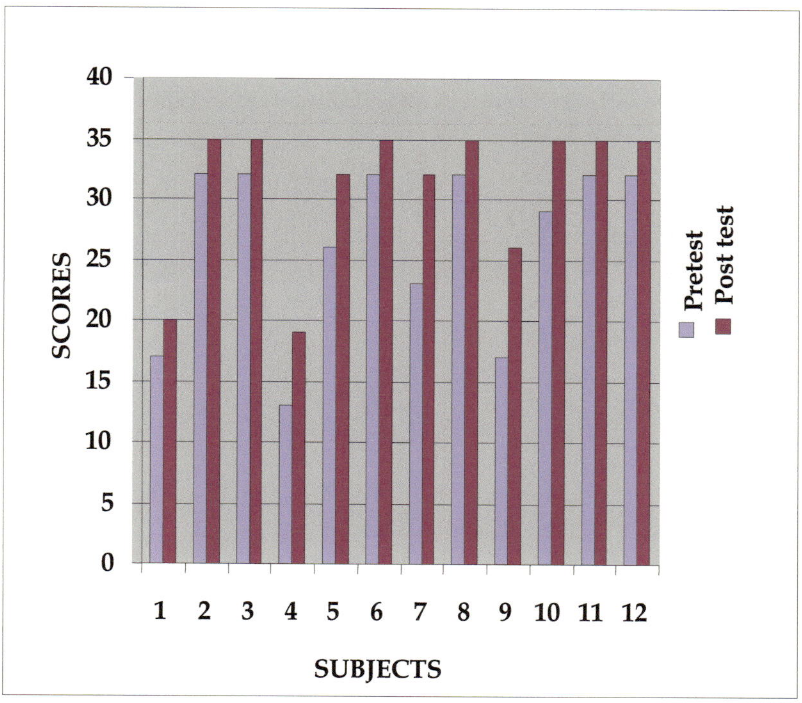


Fig. 7. Children's Scores on Conceptual Skills at Pre and Post Tests

The children's scores on selected component skills of independent work behaviour were analysed to assess the effect of intervention across all components. On conceptual skills, the pre test mean score of 26.42 was significantly lower than their mean score of 31.17 post intervention as evident from the derived t- value (6.92, $p<0.001$). A description of how each child performed on conceptual skills at pre and post tests may be seen in Figure 7.
A positive change in conceptual ability was seen in all children. For some children the gain conceptual skills were higher in ratio to their composite scores (ref. Fig 6). Subject 1 and subject 9 showed a marked improvement (increments of 3 and 9 points respectively) in this area in comparison to their overall gain on SIWS. Similarly, subject 4 and subject 7 also showed considerable change from pre to post test.
Further analysis of SIWS data revealed an improvement in daily living skills too. The children showed a gain in mean score of more than 4 points from 36.25 (pre test) to 40.33 (post test). This gain was found to be statistically significant (t value= 2.56; $p<.05$). Analysis of individual raw scores at pre and post tests brought out a gain pattern different from that for conceptual skills. Figure 8 represents this gain graphically.

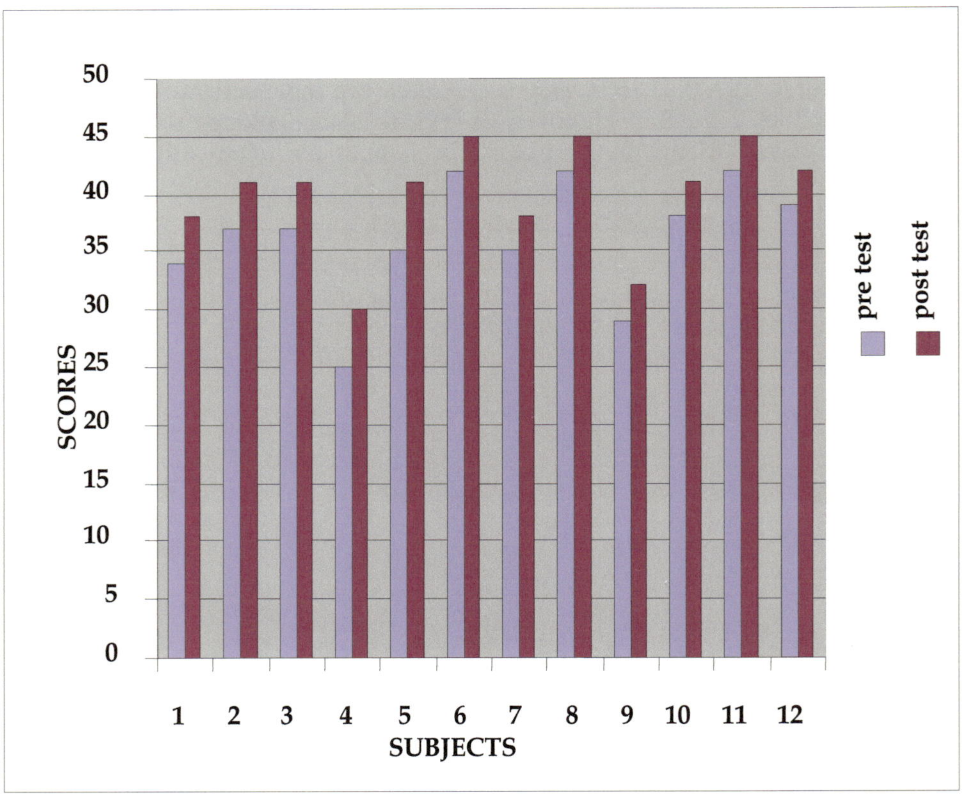


Fig. 8. Children's Score on Daily Living Skills at Pre and Post Tests

As can be seen from Fig.8 the gain in daily living skills was almost uniform. Though all children improved their score post intervention, the difference between the pre and post test score was not as much as seen in other areas.

With reference to pre vocational and self engagement activities too, the children showed an overall gain. Individual performance of each child on pre vocational activities is presented in Figure 9.

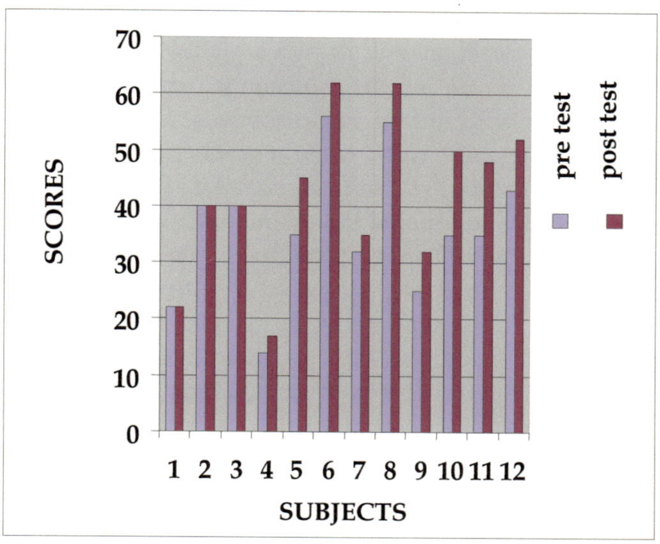


Fig. 9. Children's Score on Pre Vocational Activities at Pre and Post Tests

The pre test mean score (36.00) on pre vocational activities was lower than the mean (42.08) post intervention. Though some children did not show any change in their performance post treatment, the overall gain was statistically significant (t value=4.16; $p<.002$). On self engagement activities too improvement in behaviour was evident. However, this was not found statistically significant. Individual performance is presented in Figure 10.

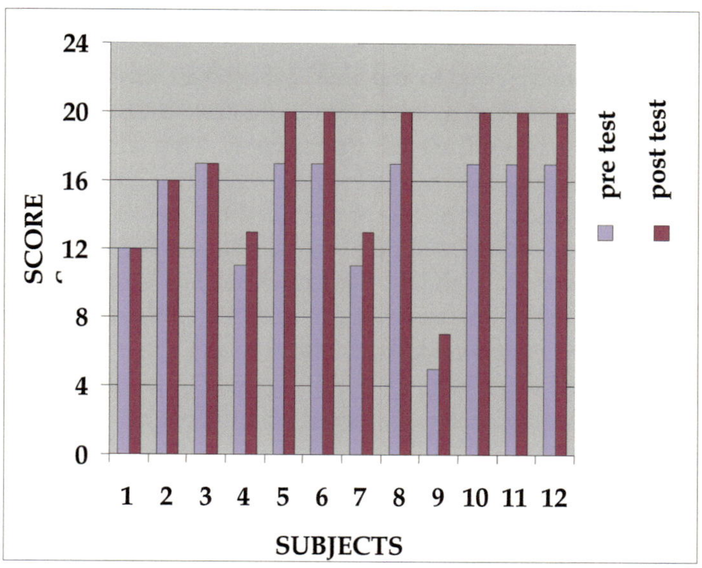


Fig. 10. Children's Score on Self Engagement Activities at Pre and Post Tests

## 6. Discussion

There are behaviours that neurotypical children learn on their own, but children with autism require to be taught. Increased independence and the ability to manage one's own behaviour and task performance continue to be areas of concern for children with developmental disabilities. Development of work skills, positive work attitude and acceptable work behaviour is one of the educational aims for students with special educational needs. Students with autism have difficulty independently initiating work; continue working and seeking new work when a given task is completed. Independent work behaviour does not persist without supervision. Hence, early development of independent functioning skill is considered important for children with autism.

An effective classroom for such children provides a physical structure that facilitates learning, and teaching methods that help language acquisition, social and academic skills and behaviour management. Educational strategies that provide structure and predictability to the learning process, allowing children to anticipate task requirements and set expectations, and teach a variety of skills across content areas in the natural environment are useful for children with autism (Earles-Vollrath, et al. 2008).

Children with autism are visual learners. Environmental supports that include use of labels, boundary settings, visual schedules, behaviour based communication tools and activity completion signals enable them to respond more appropriately in day to day activities by increasing independence and conceptual understanding. The specific learning characteristics of children with autism, namely, distractibility, difficulty in organization, sequencing and generalization, require that intervention be designed around specific strengths (e.g. visual-spatial organization) and needs (e.g. structure and predictability) of such children (Mesibov, et al. 2003). Work systems and visual structure, the two elements of TEACCH approach used by the authors in this study, are premised on these strengths. Effective work systems visually present information so that the child understands what is expected to be done. The authors used pictures, symbols, colours and objects to indicate the task at hand. For a shape sorting task, each shape would be placed in a separate bowl. This would make the task visually clear to the child who when given a collection of shapes, would know what was expected of him/her. Similarly, tasks were visually clear, organized and wherever required included visual instructions. This visual structure enhanced independent work behaviour. Sorting tasks had visually clear shapes or beads that improved visual discrimination easier. Use of trays and bowls (refer fig1 and 2) for keeping the materials rather than spreading materials out on table, helped visual organization. Task instructions were often given through jigs. Jigs are visual representation of how a task is to be carried out. They are helpful because they provide instructions in the way that is easiest for children with autism to understand. As can be seen in Figure 3, the bead stringing task visual instructions included a partial model of the activity to be done and a picture cue for the pattern to be followed. Visually presented stimuli enable the children to process information more efficiently (Lal, 2010). The significant difference between the children's pre and post test scores on SIWS may be attributed to these factors. According to some researches, children with autism experience central coherence deficits (Frith, 1996, Jarrold et al., 2000). The inability to hold information in mind in order to use it later in other tasks is what causes the autistic children to lack central coherence. They cannot hold one piece of information in mind while manipulating the next step in a sequence (Grandin, 1995). This affects their ability to form concepts. Visually organized and systematic presentation of simple tasks aids development of conceptual skills as the children are able to process information better. Evidence of significant gain in conceptual skills indicated the positive effect of work systems and visual structure used in this research. Oral instructions augmented by visual cues strengthen cooperation and understanding of daily living activities. Pre teaching of such tasks is useful. Pre teaching consists of providing clear reminders to the learner before the skill is to be used (Wheeler, 2007). The authors used picture cards and symbols to denote steps of selected daily living activities. These were pre taught and later used as recall aids when children were asked to do the activities. This visual support enhanced memory and improved independence in task performance. Similarly, work systems, visual clarity, visual organization and visual instructions contributed to the positive change in children's score from pre to post test in pre vocational and self engagement activities. Independent functioning in the four sub variables was evident as children maintained the performance level even when the prompts were gradually faded.

## 7. Conclusion

Cultivating strengths and interests, rather than emphasizing on deficits is an important aspect of person centred teaching. In case of autism, it is central to intervention. TEACCH based teaching subscribes to this. It respects the "culture of autism" and recognizes that the difference between children with autism and others may work in favour of the former. Their basic strengths in visual skills, recognition of details, and memory, among other areas, can serve as a foundation for independent functioning in adulthood. Drawing on children's interests, however peculiar they may appear to most people, helps increase their understanding and motivation for tasks (Mesibov & Shea, 2003). The results of this study support the above findings. TEACCH based intervention was effective in enhancing independent work behaviour in children with autism. The results of this research may be useful for parents and teachers who are in need of evidence based and suitable intervention for children with autism.

## 8. Acknowledgment

The authors wish to thank the children who participated in this study, and are grateful to the children's parents, teachers and school administrators for their support.

## 9. References

Autism Society of America (2006). *Defining Autism.* Retrieved Oct. 8, 2008. Available from http://www.autismsociety.org

Baron-Cohen, S. (2002). The extreme male brain theory of autism. *Trends in Cognitive Science.* 6, 248-254 Retrieved Mar 2011. Available from http://www.cell.com/trends/cognitive-sciences/abstract/S1364-6613(02)01904-6

Earles-Vollrath, T.L., Cook, K. T., Robbins, L., and Ben-Arieh, J. (2008). Instructional strategies to facilitate successful

Learning outcomes for students with autism spectrum disorders. In *Educating children and youth with autism: strategies for effective practice*. (2nd edition) Simpson, R. L, Smith Myles, B. (Eds.) pp 93-178 Pro Ed. ISBN -13: 978-1-4164-0210-7. Texas (2008)

Frith, U. (1996). Cognitive explanations of autism. Acta Pediatrica Supplement 416, 63-68

Grandin, T. (1995). *Thinking in Pictures and Other Reports from My Life with Autism* Vintage Books, ISBN 0-679-77289-8, New York

Hungelmann, A. M. (2001). An Analysis of TEACCH based home programming for young children with autism. Retrived Jan. 2011. Available from http://sitemaker.umich.edu/365.bernstein/teacch

Jarrold, C., D.W. Butler, E.M. Cottington, & F. Jimenez (2000). Linking theory of mind and central coherence bias in autism and in the general population. *Developmental Psychology* 36(1) , 126-138 Retrieved Mar, 2011 Available from http://www.sciencedirect.com/science?_ob=Publication

Jordan, R. (2003). Understanding autism spectrum disorders *Proceedings of International Conference on Autism: Alternative Strategies* New Delhi, Sept., 2003

Hume, K., Loftin, R., and Lantz, J. (2009) Increasing independence in autism spectrum disorders: A review of three focussed interventions. *Journal of autism and Developmental Disorders* 39 (9), 1329-38. ISSN: 0162-3257

Kusmeirski, S.and Henckel, K. (2002). Effects of TEACCH program on maladaptive and functional behaviours of children with autism. Retrieved Apr. 2008. Available from
http://researchautism.net

Lal, R (2005). Effect of inclusive education on language and social development of children with autism. *Asia Pacific Disability Rehabilitation Journal*. 16, 1:77-88 ISSN: 2211-5242

Lal, R and Lobo, S. (2007). Discrete trial training and development of pre learning skills in intellectually impaired children with autism. *Journal of Rehabilitation Council of India*. 3, 1&2: 15-23 ISSN 0973-2497

Lal R, Bali M (2008). Effect of visual strategies on development of communication skills in children with autism. In *Exploring Autism* Pillai, M.V.(Ed.) pp 155-166 Icfai University Press ISBN 978-81-314-1588-7, Hyderabad.

Lal, R. (2010). Effect of alternative and augmentative communication on language and social behavior of children with autism. *Educational Research and Reviews* 5(3)119-125 ISSN 1990-3839

Malhotra, S., Chakrabarti, S. and Nehra, A. (2002). Psychological interventions with parents of autistic children. *Indian Journal of Psychiatry* 44 (2) 108-117

Mesibov, G.B., Shea, V., and Schople, E. (2004) *The TEACCH Approach to Autism Spectrum Disorders*. Springer, ISBN 978-0-306-48646-3, New York

Mesibov, G.B., Schopler, E., and Hearsay, K. A. (2003) Structured Teaching *Proceedings of International Conference on Autism: Alternative Strategies* New Delhi, Sept., 2003

Miller, L. L. S. (2000). Toward a consensus in terminology in sensory integration theory and practice: part 1: taxonomy of neurophysiological processes. *Sensory integration Special Interest Section Quarterly,* 23 (1), 1-4 Retrieved April, 2011. Available from http://www.spdfoundation.net/pdf/TowardaConcensus-Part1.pdf

National Resource Council, (2002). *Educating Children with Autism.* National Academic Press, ISBN 0-309-07269-7 Washington

Richard, G.J. (2000). The source for treatment methodologies in autism. East Moline, IL,: Lingui Systems Inc. Retrieved Jan.2009. Available from http://www.eiu.edu/~commdis/

Schopler, E, Mesobov, G.B., & Kunce, L. J. (Eds.). (1998). *Asperger's Syndrome or High Functioning Autism?* Plenum Press, ISBN 0-306-45746-6 New York

Siaperas, P., Beadle-Brown J. (2006). A case study of a structured teaching approach in adults with autism in residential home in Greece. Retrieved Apr. 2011. Available from http://www.researchautism.net/autism_research_journal_articles_publications_study.ikml?ra=1782&s=1

Sigman M, Ruskin E (1999). Continuity and change in the social competence of children with autism, Down syndrome, and developmental delays. *Monographs of the Society for Research in Child Development* 64 (1): v-114 ISSN: 1540-5834

Simpson, R. L, Smith Myles, B. (Eds.) (2008) *Educating children and youth with autism: strategies for effective practice.* (2nd edition) Pro Ed. ISBN -13: 978-1-4164-0210-7. Texas

Simpson, R. L., Smith Myles, B., and LaCava, P.G. (2008). Understanding and responding to the needs of children and youth with autism spectrum disorders. In *Educating children and youth with autism: strategies for effective practice.* (2nd edition) Simpson, R. L, Smith Myles, B. (Eds.) pp 1-60 Pro Ed. ISBN -13: 978-1-4164-0210-7. Texas (2008)

TEACCH Autism Program (2011) Retrieved April, 2011. Available from http://teacch.com/educational-approaches

Tsang, S.M., Shek, D.T.L., Lam, L.L., Florence, L.Y.T., and Cheung, P.M.P. (2007). Brief report: Application of the TEACCH program on Chinese pre school children with autism - does culture make a difference? *Journal of autism and Developmental Disorders* 37 (2), 390-396. ISSN: 0162-3257

Vismara, L. and Rogers, S. (2007). Early intervention: Teaching approaches with demonstrated success. Retrieved Mar.2011. Available from http://support.autism-society.org/site/News2?page=NewsArticle&id=9829

Wetherby, A., B. Prizant, and T. Hutchinson (1998). Communicative, social-affective, and symbolic profiles of young children with autism and pervasive developmental disorders. *American Journal of Speech-Language Pathology,* 7, 79-91 ISSN: 1058-0360

Wheeler, M. (2007). *Toilet Training for Individuals with Autism or other Developmental Issues* ($2^{nd}$ edition) Future Horizons ISBN 1-932565-49-3, Texas

# 10

# Applied Behavior Analysis: Teaching Procedures and Staff Training for Children with Autism

Carolyn S. Ryan
*Institute for Children with Autism and Related Disorders and Queens College of the City University of New York, CUNY, United States of America*

## 1. Introduction

The current chapter will present an overview of current effective teaching methods for children with autism. Applied behavior analysis has been referred to as the treatment of choice for those with autism (United States Surgeon General, 1999; New York State Department of Health, 1999a, 1999b, 1999c). At its core, applied behavior analysis is the data- and research-based application of behavioral principles to socially relevant behavior (Baer, et al., 1968; Cooper, et al., 2007; Wolf, 1978). Additional key components of applied behavior analysis are generalizability, conceptually systematic, technologically sound, practical, and effective (Baer, et al., 1968). These key components will be described below.

Due to the pervasive nature of autism that results in dramatic impairments in communication and social behavior, along with restricted and repetitive behavior – the primary goals of treatment are to improve the child's communication and social behavior as well as reduce the occurrence of restricted and repetitive behavior (American Psychiatric Association, 2000). Applied behavior analysis has been demonstrated to be the treatment of choice for students with autism based on over 40 years of supportive evidence in improving social behavior and communication and reducing levels of problem behavior (Lovaas, 1987). The methods used in applied behavior analysis focus on targeting specific behavior, defining the behavior, designing an intervention to meet the goal of behavior change, implementing the intervention, analyzing the effectiveness of the intervention, and continuing the intervention or designing a procedure to maintain the behavior change (Cooper et al. 2007).

Research approaches for teaching students with autism have been effective across social, communication, and problem behavior areas (Smith, 2001). Teaching methods will be reviewed in the current chapter along with staff training methods for building effectiveness and competency with those who teach students with autism (Reid & Green, 1980; Ryan & Hemmes, 2005, Ryan, et al., 2008).

## 2. Applied Behavior Analysis - key components

This section of the chapter presents key terms as a review in applied behavior analysis (ABA). The brief review describes terms that are important for understanding the remainder of the chapter. ABA is a scientific method of teaching that is based on the principles of

learning and behavior in which each target behavior is operationally defined and modified. Key components of ABA will be described below.
ABA is the systematic, controlled, and empirical investigation of socially important behavior using empirically validated research-based and socially acceptable practices (Baer, et al., 1968; Cooper, et al., 2007, Newman et al., 2003). When we consider how socially important behavior change is, some considerations for a given individual, include: chronological age, behavioral repertoire, community, developmental age, family background, religious values, ethnicity, and other factors important to the individual. In addition, we consider approaches to behavior changes that are socially valid (Wolf, 1978).
A second key component is that ABA is behavioral (Baer, et al, 1968; Newman et al., 2003). Practitioners of ABA studies observable, measurable responses. Data are collected in an ongoing manner. In teaching situations, repeated measurement and graphing of performance in a systematic way assists in monitoring progress over time. This allows continuous assessment of the effectiveness of teaching methods to guide trainers and teachers to modify programs and curricula to increase learning. In addition, monitoring and modifying staff behavior is crucial to a successful program. Furthermore, because objectivity is essential to science, reliability measures of all those involved are systematically obtained through inter-observer agreement data collection.
ABA is analytic, meaning, empirical demonstration of functional relations between antecedent events, behavior, and consequent events (Baer, et al, 1968). All teaching methodology stems from research empirically demonstrating the effectiveness of stimuli presented by teachers before and after student performance. Furthermore, functional analysis of problem behavior is performed before implementation and continuation of behavior reduction programs.
ABA is technological (Baer, et al, 1968). All behavior that needs to be changed is precisely defined, and all procedures and methods used are explicitly described in a step-by-step fashion. ABA is also conceptually systematic, since all of its technology is directly related to the field of the experimental analysis of behavior.
ABA is committed to teaching skills that are practical, effective, and can generalize to other responses, people, or settings (Baer, et al, 1968). Every educational program is selected according to whether it is appropriate, meaningful, and functional for the individual student. Research in applied behavior analysis strives to answer questions, such as:

- Is the skill likely to be maintained in the everyday, natural environment?
- Are the responses going to help improve the quality of the person's life?
- Can programming be conducted for generalization of skills to be used outside the teaching situation or learning environment?
- Can skills be taught so that generalization is shown spontaneously?

Continuous research is directed toward answering the above questions and to measure and to increase the effectiveness and generality of applied behavior analytic methodology.
In terms of how ABA may benefit students with autism, there are several considerations (New York State Department of Health, 1999a, 1999b, 1999c). Each student is systematically observed for current behavioral functioning. Based on the student's behavior repertoire, behavior excesses and deficits are identified and long-term and short-term goals are devised. Each student is taught using an individualized curriculum using positive reinforcement to encourage accurate responding. Programs and treatment plans are research- and data-based. Programs include an individualized teaching strategy. The effectiveness of teaching and treatment implementation is evaluated in an ongoing manner

using specific data-collection procedures, including visual displays, such as, graphs or charts. Data collection is used to evaluate the progress of the student and the teaching professionals.

In summary, ABA is critical in the education and intervention for students with autism. Some important factors in the realm of ABA as related to students with autism are as follows. There is a strong emphasis on defining problems in terms of behavior that can be operationally defined and measured. Increases or decreases in the target behavior indicate the extent to which behavior changed or improved. Teaching and treatment procedures are designed to assist each person to function more fully in society. Methods and rationales are described and defined. Socially important changes are demonstrated using scientific demonstrations that are explicated using single-subject research designs. In addition, there is a very high value placed on all those involved in the education of students with autism.

## 3. Applied Behavior Analysis - forms of behavior

Two forms of behavior are respondent and operant behavior (Cooper et al., 2007). Respondent behavior refers to reflexive responses that are elicited by certain stimuli and over which individuals have little or no control (e.g., sneezing, blinking, or emotional responses). New reflexive behavior can be learned by pairing the stimulus or unconditioned stimulus (US) that controls the reflexive response or unconditioned response (UR) with a new stimulus that is initially the neutral stimulus (NS). Based on pairing the NS with the US, the NS then becomes the conditioned stimulus (CS) that will elicit the conditioned response (CR). The CR will be similar, in most cases, to the UR; however, there may be differences in the magnitude, latency, topography, and/or other response measures. Associations between stimuli can be learned; reflexive behavior can occur in response to new stimulus associations. Reinforcer inventories and assessments involve respondent behavior, in that, individuals act pleasantly, unpleasantly, or neutral when presented something preferred, nonpreferred, or neutral, respectively. Emotions are often described in terms of respondent behavior. Unconditioned and conditioned emotional responses are terms used in the same manner as described above.

Operant behavior refers to behavior that is emitted as a result of its history of consequences. Operant behavior is different from respondent behavior because operant behavior is selectively targeted and maintained by the consequences that it has produced. New operant behavior can be learned and maintained using consequences. Providing a preferred activity immediately after a response occurring will most likely increase the response occurrence in the future. For example, if a student says, "Can I listen to music?" and earns listening privileges, most likely the requesting behavior will occur again in the future. On the other hand, providing a non-preferred activity to a student immediately after a response occurring will most likely not increase the response occurrence in the future; in fact, the response may not occur again in the future. For example, if a student attempts to gain someone's attention by throwing puzzle pieces on the floor that is then followed by the teacher's request to have the student clean up (if she does not enjoy cleaning up), most likely the throwing behavior will not occur again in the future.

These features imply that students may be taught appropriate, functional responses that may be new responses or replacements for problem responses. In addition, the deficits or lack of appropriate skills shown by students with autism may be related to physiological, covert events, as well as a lack of appropriate educational practice.

Operant behavior is modified by antecedent and consequent events. Antecedent events are those that precede responses. Discriminative stimuli are events that set the occasion for a response to occur. Consequent events are those that follow behavior; these may be reinforcing, punishing, or neutral. Preferred events that follow a response can be viewed as reinforcers if they increase the probability of the future occurrence of the response. Nonpreferred events that follow a response can be viewed as punishers if they decrease the probability of the future occurrence of the response. Neutral events that follow a response do not affect the probability of the future occurrence of the response. In effective educational procedures, consequences are contingent on behavior; the responses should produce the consequences contingently. As a result of the modification of antecedent and consequent events in order to influence the occurrence of responding, the diagnostic label for an individual is not useful.

Direct behavioral observation can allow one to describe the target behavior or response by specifying, in written form:

- what the behavior is,
- how much, how well, or how often the behavior is done, and
- the circumstances (when and where) under which the behavior is done.

After the target behavior or response is described, measurement of the target behavior on an ongoing basis can be conducted. Decisions about educational procedures are made according to the data collected. Continuation, modification, or discontinuation of educational procedures is conducted according to behavioral progress.

## 4. Applied Behavior Analysis - five step model

The following five step model may be used as a guide in understanding ABA (Cooper et al., 2007):

1. Select behavior to be analyzed:
    - Assess behavior of interest
    - Operationally define the target behavior
    - Establish priorities, goals, and objectives
    - Analyze the system, obtain involvement and support from intervening agents
2. Measure the behavior:
    - Select measurement procedures
    - Collect data, including baseline data
    - Continue data collection on an ongoing basis
3. Select treatment procedures:
    - Identify current contingencies
    - Select materials, equipment, and setting
    - Negotiate treatment plans as needed
4. Implement procedures:
    - Monitor effects based on data collection
    - Modify procedures as needed
5. Evaluate effects of treatment:
    - Data collect
    - Modify or fade treatment

## 5. Applied Behavior Analysis - reinforcement and punishment

Figure 1 displays antecedent and consequent events as related to reinforcement and punishment procedures. Positive reinforcement is a procedure by which a stimulus or positive reinforcer is delivered, given, shown, or otherwise presented, immediately following a target response that serves to increase the future occurrence of that response. There is a positive contingency between a target response and an appetitive stimulus (See Figure 1).

Negative Reinforcement is a procedure by which a stimulus is removed, taken away, turned off, or otherwise withdrawn immediately following a target response that serves to increase the future occurrence of that response. There is a negative contingency between a response and an aversive stimulus (See Figure 1).

There are two types of negative reinforcement trials: escape and avoidance. In escape trials the target response terminates the aversive stimulus, e.g., a student may request a break during a difficult reading task to delay the aversive stimulus of the task. A short-term escape consequence may be taking a 5-min coffee break, whereas, a long-term escape consequence may be leaving an aversive job position and never returning. In avoidance trials the target response prevents the delivery of the aversive stimulus, e.g., before beginning a teaching program, a student may request to use the bathroom and avoid the aversive stimulus of the teaching program. For example, a short-term avoidance consequence may be calling in sick to work, whereas, a long-term avoidance consequence may be never returning to work.

*Important Factors for Reinforcement:*

- Age-appropriate events
- Choice of reinforcers
- Duration of reinforcing event
- Functionality
- Immediacy
- Motivating operations (establishing and abolishing operations, e.g., deprivation/satiation)
- Varied events

There are several types of reinforcers (Cooper et al., 2007; Newman, et al., 2003). These terms and descriptions follow below.

a. Primary reinforcers are items that are naturally reinforcing, e.g., edible reinforcers, such as food or drink; temperature.
b. Secondary or conditioned reinforcers are items that acquire reinforcing properties through learning and pairing the new items with an already established reinforcer, e.g., activities, candy, games, snacks, toys, or time with a favorite person; sensory reinforcers, such as, auditory, olfactory, tactile, visual, or vibratory.
c. Generalized reinforcers are items that acquire reinforcing properties through consecutive pairing with established reinforcers and can be generally effective in producing behavior change, e.g., grades, money, praise, or stars; social reinforcers, such as, smiling, praise, attention, or otherwise friendly remarks.
d. Positive reinforcers refer to the stimuli involved in positive reinforcement procedures in which an item or stimulus is presented immediately following the target response in order to increase the future probability of that target response e.g., adult attention, hug, or smiles.

e. Negative Reinforcers refer to the stimuli involved in negative reinforcement procedures in which an item or stimulus that is aversive or unpleasant is removed from the situation immediately following the target response in order to increase the future probability of that target response, e.g., complete a task, finish a difficult chore, or turn off loud music.

There are two motivating operations (MOs) that can be used to describe a level of effectiveness of a reinforcer, i.e., establishing operation (EO) or deprivation and abolishing operation (AO) or satiation (Cooper et al., 2007). Deprivation refers to the establishing operation for which reinforcers have been withheld to the point that the specific reinforcer is effective in increasing or maintaining behavior. Satiation refers to the establishing operation for which reinforcers have been presented to the point that the specific reinforcer is no longer effective in increasing or maintaining behavior.

There are a variety of methods of obtaining reinforcers for a student. Reinforcers are individually-based, meaning that a reinforcer may be a preferred item that a particular student likes or will work towards obtaining.

**Diagram of consequences**

The following diagrams are presented to further the understanding of the use of reinforcement. In the case of reinforcement, this procedure involves the presentation (positive reinforcer) or removal (negative reinforcer) of a stimulus immediately following the target response in order to increase the future likelihood of the target response occurring.

| | | STIMULUS | |
|---|---|---|---|
| | | PRESENTED | WITHDRAWN |
| PROBABILITY | INCREASE | POSITIVE REINFORCEMENT ($S^{R+}$) | NEGATIVE REINFORCEMENT ($S^{R-}$) |
| OF BEHAVIOR | DECREASE | POSITIVE PUNISHMENT ($S^{P+}$) | NEGATIVE PUNISHMENT ($S^{P-}$) |

The diagram above Fig. 1. shows the relation between types of stimuli and the two reinforcement procedures. In positive reinforcement, an appetitive stimulus or event is presented (positive reinforcer) immediately following the target response to increase the future likelihood of the target response occurring. In negative reinforcement, an aversive stimulus or event is removed immediately following the target response to increase the future likelihood of the target response occurring.

Reinforcers for some students may be playing with bubbles, dolls, games, and toys; hearing praise, seeing someone smile, obtaining tickles, and eating crackers; some other students may prefer playing with racecars, making objects from clay, playing a chase game, obtaining high-fives, and eating apples.

The following methods may be used for obtaining reinforcers:

a. Identify Reinforcers: reinforcers can be assessed based on the general effects that particular items have on the behavior of people similar to the target person, e.g., attention, money, praise, privileges, snacks, toys. Age-appropriateness of the reinforcers should be determined. Preferred items may be obtained by:

| | | | |
|---|---|---|---|
| | Reinforcement | | |
| Positive, + | Appetitive **Stimulus (↑)** | **Aversive Stimulus (↓)** | **Negative, -** |
| | **Aversive** Stimulus (↑) | Appetitive **Stimulus (↓)** | |
| | Punishment | | |

Fig. 2. Diagram of consequences in applied behavior analysis. The upper diagram displays the manner in which a stimulus may be presented or withdrawn immediately following a given target behavior in order to affect the future probability of behavior. The lower diagram displays the qualitative description (appetitive or aversive) of stimulus that may be presented (↑) or removed (↓) immediately following a target behavior along with its associated procedure, namely reinforcement or punishment.

- Asking the person.
- Observing the person.
- Observe similar people.
- Use the Premack Principle*
- Use reinforcer sampling

b. *Premack Principle: A response frequently performed by a student can be used to reinforce a response that the student performs infrequently. A more likely or preferred activity can serve to reinforce a less likely activity, e.g., riding a bike can reinforce homework completion.

c. Reinforcer or Preference Assessment: Indirect and direct methods of assessing preferences are conducted in order establish items that are most favorable for the student. Ultimately, reinforcers may be assessed within a teaching situation based on the student's later frequency of showing the target behavior. If the target response is shown, then the action, item, or other stimulus presented immediately following the target response served as a reinforcer for that target response.

*Some Important Factors in the Effective Use of Reinforcers:*

- Anticipate generalization by (a) shift from frequent to occasional reinforcement and (b) shift from artificial to natural reinforcement.
- Avoid satiation through (a) the use of a variety of reinforcers and (b) use small amounts.
- Do not allow the reinforcer apart from the teaching situation, or when the target response occurs.
- Establish conditioned reinforcers.
- Make reinforcers contingent on the performance of the target response.
- Present the reinforcer immediately following the target response.
- Reinforcers should be easily administered and rapidly consumed.
- Use conditioned reinforcers to bridge the gap between other reinforcers delivered or the next trial.
- Vary the pace of reinforcement: allow a short interval (2- to 3-second intervals) for reinforcement and change it next time to a longer interval (6- to 10-second intervals).
- Vary the tone of voice used: for the most part, use an enthusiastic voice for reinforcers; however, other tones, may include whisper, deep tones, and loud voice.

- Vary words and gestures: use different words and expressions, as well as actions and activities to make the session fun and exciting.

Punishment is another behavior analytic procedure that affects the future probability of behavior (see Figure 1). Positive Punishment or Type 1 Punishment is a procedure by which a stimulus or positive punisher is delivered, given, shown, or otherwise presented, immediately following a target response that serves to decrease the future occurrence of that response (Cooper et al, 2007). A stimulus is delivered, given, shown, or otherwise presented immediately following a target response that serves to decrease the future occurrence of that response. There is a positive contingency between a target response and an aversive stimulus.

For example, saying, "No," to a student after he throws a toy on the floor can be assessed as a punisher by measuring the effects on behavior. If "No" decreases the probability of throwing the toy on the floor in the future, then it serves as a positive punisher.

Negative punishment or Type II Punishment is a procedure by which a stimulus is removed, taken away, turned off, or otherwise withdrawn immediately following a target response that serves to decrease the future occurrence of that response (Cooper, 2007). A stimulus is removed, taken away, turned off, or otherwise withdrawn immediately following a target response that serves to decrease the future occurrence of that response.

For example, taking away a preferred toy contingent upon a student screaming can be assessed as a punisher by measuring the effects on behavior. If the toy taken away decreases the probability of screaming in the future, then it serves as a negative punisher.

For purposes of this chapter, reinforcement is explained in detail because the teaching procedures described below relay on reinforcement procedures and simple correction procedure. The description of punishment procedure is limited.

## 6. Applied Behavior Analytic teaching procedures

Teaching procedures based on applied behavior analysis are most effective for students with autism and other related disorders (Cooper et al., 2007; Lovaas, 1987; Sundberg & Partington, 1998). The purpose of ABA teaching procedures is to understand, improve, and solve behavior issues. Teaching methods are based on research findings. As a science, applied behavior analysis is constantly changing its teaching methods according to scientific evidence. Effective methods of teaching have incorporated the principles of applied behavior analysis. Two methods include discrete-trial teaching and incidental teaching. Both teaching methods are conducted by systematically breaking down the target behavior into smaller components and addressing each response. Each one of these teaching approaches is data-based and research-based procedures. Research has documented that each one of these procedures are effective for teaching specific behavior goals.

### 6.1 Discrete-trial teaching

One effective instructional method for teaching students with autism is discrete-trial teaching (Sarakoff & Sturmey, 2004; Smith, 2001; Sundberg & Partington, 1998; Touchette & Howard, 1984). In discrete-trial teaching, programming is arranged by dividing a large behavior goal into small, component target responses. Those small, component target responses are then taught in a clear, distinct manner. The manner by which the small component responses are taught takes advantage of the three-term contingency in ABA. The three-term or ABC contingency properly distinguishes among key elements of teaching (see

Figure 3). The three-term contingency represents the interdependency of three components (Cooper et al., 2007).

| Three-Term or ABC Contingency | | | | |
|---|---|---|---|---|
| **$S^D$** | → | **R** | → | **$S^{r+/-}$** |
| (Discriminative Stimulus) | | (Response) | | (Reinforcer) |
| **A** | → | **B** | → | **C** |
| (Antecedent Stimulus) | | (Behavior) | | (Consequence) |

Fig. 3. Three-term contingency

The upper portion of Figure 3, depict the terms in the ABC contingency. The terms used in the ABC contingency are as follows: antecedent stimulus (A), followed by a given behavior (B), immediately followed by a consequence (C). The ABC contingency is generally interchangeable with the three-term contingency. The terms used in the bottom portion of Figure 3 represent the three-term contingency. The three-term contingency is comprised of the presentation of a discriminative stimulus ($S^D$), followed by a given target response (R), immediately followed by a positive or negative reinforcer ($S^{r+/-}$). For purposes of the current chapter, the three-term contingency will be used to describe the components of discrete-trial teaching.

Discrete trial teaching is the teaching methodology that incorporates the principles of ABA by breaking down tasks into smaller parts and presenting them in a simplified, repeated manner to best facilitate learning (Newman, et al., 2003; Sarokoff & Sturmey, 2004; Sundberg & Partington, 1998). Data are collected on each trial to measure and evaluate progress over several trials and teaching sessions. A discrete trial consists of the events depicted in Figure 3, before making use of the Three Term or ABC Contingency.

Important factors for discrete-trial teaching are considered in its accurate implementation. Discrete-trial teaching makes assessment of progress efficient. In addition, the teaching conditions and requirements are consistent across trials and teaching sessions. There are clear expectations about the requirements of the student. Additionally, discrete-trial teaching makes data collection and observation of the student and the teacher's responses clear and easy to measure.

Discrete-trial teaching is therefore used to: (a) allow data collection and assessment of student and instructor behavior, (b) clarify what is expected of the student and instructor, and (c) maintain consistent teaching conditions and requirements. Green (1996) and Smith (2001) noted that discrete-trial teaching is an effective strategy for teaching new skills with students with autism.

The following describe the required discrete-trial teaching target responses from Ryan & Hemmes (2005).

"*Distraction-free*: make the teaching area distraction-free by removing extraneous stimuli, such as sounds, toys, people; reinforcers are within the reach of the instructor and out of the reach or direct view of the child.

*Materials*: have teaching materials used for the program within reach of the instructor and as needed, the child; containers or boxes should be open or ready for use; items such as edible or tangible reinforcers are within reach of the instructor.

*Attending*: establish appropriate attending responses by having the child sit or stand with hands and feet still in a position facing the instructor or task materials while making eye contact with the instructor or looking at the task materials in anticipation of the delivery of a direction.

*Verbal Direction*: present a clear, brief, and appropriate instruction appropriate to the program; one particular direction should be presented, with or without a prompt, that was brief in word length; the words should be clearly spoken, concisely presented, and not repeated.

*Voice tones*: differential voice tones used, i.e., a neutral, directive tone of voice for instructions; an enthusiastic tone of voice for reinforcer words and sounds; a firm voice for corrective feedback.

*Wait*: allow appropriate amount of time for the child to respond to instruction, approximately 5 s, after an instruction was presented by the instructor, as appropriate to the program.

*Praise statement*: immediately following a correct response, the instructor will deliver a behavior-specific praise statement specific to the correct target response made by the child, within 2 s - 4 s, e.g., "Great (specified behavior)."

*Contingent reinforcers*: present primary or secondary reinforcer(s), e.g., tangible, social, or edible, for a brief duration during praise statement, contingent on correct responses.

*Prompting and correction procedure*: provide an appropriate prompting procedure within 5 s after the child's failure to respond or an appropriate correction procedure as a predetermined gestural, verbal, and/or physical prompt, immediately following an incorrect response, as appropriate to the program and target response.

*Pause for inter-trial interval*: allow a brief pause in instruction, up to 5 s, following delivery of the consequential stimuli after a target response and during the inter-trial interval, prior to presenting the next trial.

*Incidental or additional teaching*: present additional or incidental teaching responses, during the interval following the consequential stimuli presentation, the instructor may make a response related to the reinforcing stimulus or event.

*Data recorded*: record data for correct or incorrect responses following each of the child's responses, after each trial on the data sheet. " (Ryan & Hemmes, 2005)

It is critical that the above discrete-trial teaching responses be conducted in the manner described so that teaching is effective and efficient. Staff training on required discrete-trial teaching responses will be described below.

### 6.2 Incidental teaching

Incidental teaching is an applied behavior analytic teaching technique that is used to increase the spontaneous use of language. Incidental teaching occurs within the context of the interactions between two people. An incidental teaching episode begins with an initiation by the first person (the student) who specifies an individual reinforcer; the second person presents a prompt for a language response from the first person and differentially reinforces that language response by the delivery of the reinforcer previously specified by the first person (Hart & Risley, 1974, 1975, 1980, 2000). Incidental teaching is also one component of naturalistic language training (Hart & Risley, 1980). Incidental teaching has been used in a variety of ways to promote generalization of language skills (Hart & Risley, 1974, 1975, 1980, 2000; McGee, et al., 1992). Incidental teaching can be used in a variety of situations and contexts. The important feature is that incidental teaching assists in maintaining language responses. It has been effective for individuals in teaching and maintaining language of students with autism.

The following required incidental teaching target responses are as follows. A *student initiation* is

"defined as an unprompted nonverbal or verbal response that indicated a preferred item or activity. Correct performance of incidental teaching, given a student initiation, is demonstrated by five target responses:
(a) *watch,*
(b) *remove,*
(c) *ask,*
(d) *pause,* and
(e) reward.
Incidental teaching is required to begin within 5 s of a student initiation. *Watch* for an initiation was defined as: the instructor is sitting or standing within 1- to 1.5-m of the learner. *Remove* the desired item was defined as the instructor's making eye contact with the learner for at least 1 s after a learner initiation, and keeping the requested item or activity away from the learner. *Ask* for a correct response was defined as the instructor's using an expectant look and one statement or one question to ask the learner to say more about the initiation made. *Wait* for a correct response was defined as the instructor's allowing up to 10 s for the learner to respond independently, or providing a prompt after 10 s. *Reward* was defined as the instructor's presenting behavior-specific praise about the learner's initiation, using an enthusiastic tone of voice, along with access to the object or activity that the learner requested" (Ryan, et al., 2008).

## 7. Staff training procedures

In addition to the research documenting the effectiveness of discrete-trial teaching and incidental teaching procedures, research has supported the effectiveness of staff training procedures to teach the methodology of each of these procedures (Ryan & Hemmes, 2005; Ryan et al., 2008).

Staff training procedures that are well-established and accepted in the research literature, include: verbal, written, and video instructions; modeling; role-playing; in-vivo practice; and performance feedback (Cullen, 1988; Delamater, et al., 1984; Demchak et al., 1992; Fielding, et al., 1971; Fleming, et al., 1996; Gardner, 1972; Gladstone & Spencer, 1979; Greene, et al., 1978; Harchik, et al., 1989; Harris, et al., 1975; Johnson & Fawcett, 1994; Krumhus & Malott, 1980; Matson, 1990; Neef, et al., 1986; Page, et al., 1982; Parsons & Reid, 1995; Parsons, et al., 1996; Parsons, et al., 1987; Reid & Green, 1990; Richman, et al., 1988; Sepler & Meyers, 1978; Touchette & Howard, 1984). These established training methods can be used alone or in conjunction with more than one method to promote skill development. In addition, behavior skills training takes advantage of several aspects of the methods mentioned above to train in a concise manner (Sarakoff & Sturmey, 2004).

### 7.1 Staff training on discrete-trial teaching

Ryan & Hemmes (2005) examined instructor performance of discrete-trial teaching responses after a performance-based training procedure with a stringent criterion in which instructor were required to show criterion-level performance on written and oral quizzes and on performance demonstrations. Training topics used in the Ryan & Hemmes procedure are noted below.

a. Autism
b. Applied Behavior Analysis
c. Reinforcement
d. Discrete-Trial Teaching
e. Schedules of Reinforcement
f. Teaching Techniques
g. Generalization and Maintenance
h. General Programming Procedures
i. Professionalism
j. Observational Learning
k. Incidental Teaching
l. Peer Interaction
m. Activity Schedules
n. Group Direction Following
o. Functional Analysis of Behavior
p. Punishment
q. Behavior Reductive Approaches
r. Collecting and Graphing Data
s. Troubleshooting and Problem Solving
t. Initial Curricular Areas and Skills

The following training procedures were used: (a) verbal instructions in a lecture format, (b) videotaped instruction, (c) role-playing, and (d) in-vivo training (Arco, 1991; Demchak, et al., 1992; Gardner, 1972; Harris, et al., 1975; Johnson, & Fawcett, 1994; Matson, 1990; Quilitch, 1975; Sepler, & Myers, 1978). Discrete-trial teaching responses were labeled and operationally defined as noted above: (a) distraction-free, (b) materials, (c) attending, (d) verbal direction, (e) voice tones, (f) wait, (g) praise statement, (h) contingent reinforcer(s), (i) prompting and correction procedure, (j) pause for inter-trial interval, (k) incidental or additional teaching responses, and (l) data recorded. Systematic measurement of the discrete-trial target responses were obtained during home-based early intervention teaching sessions with young students with autism. The author provided specific performance feedback to instructors after each session.

Instructors were trained on the above training topics. In addition, instructors were specifically trained to emit discrete-trial teaching responses. Following training, accuracy of discrete-trial teaching behavior was assessed during home-based teaching sessions for young students with autism. Feedback for teaching performance was presented following each teaching session during the Post-training phase.

The author scored videotapes of all sessions conducted by each instructor using the datasheet shown in Figure 4. The author then provided feedback to the instructor on accuracy in emitting the 12 responses required for discrete-trial teaching. Video was used in order to decrease the likelihood of reactivity (Hay, et al., 1977). Each session was defined as the presentation of one educational program using 10 discrete trials. One of three categories of educational programs was used: (a) receptive language, (b) expressive language, and (c) nonverbal imitation. Educational programs were devised in accord with each child's educational needs and behavioral repertoire. Educational programs targeted a specific behavior goal. The instructions, prompting procedures, and consequences for an educational program were identical across goals. The consequences for correct responses were behavior-specific praise and an additional reinforcer.

For a receptive language program, the target response was a nonverbal response specified in the instruction. The instruction for receptive language was, "Point to (item)," with the target item(s) located near the student. The prompting procedure delivered when the student did not respond, was brief physical guidance to have the student use a pointing finger to point. The error correction procedure for an incorrect response was, "This is 'point to (item)'," along with modeling and physical guidance of the response.

For the expressive language program, the target response was a verbal utterance specified in the instruction. The procedure for the expressive language program included a question, e.g., "What do you want?" The appropriate response was "(*item*)." The prompting procedure was the initial sound of the target response, such as, "ja" for "juice," for the student to repeat the utterance required. The error correction procedure was, "Try again, '(*item*)'," emphasizing the sound(s) of the word(s) for the student to repeat.

For the nonverbal imitation program, the target response was a nonverbal response that matched the action shown by the instructor. The procedure for the nonverbal imitation program included, "Do this," while modeling the action. The prompting procedure involved physical guidance of the appropriate body part(s) to move as modeled. The error correction procedure was, "This is 'do this'," with physical guidance to have the student perform the target response.

All of the target discrete-trial teaching responses were scored on each trial. Feedback was presented by the author following each videotaped session observation. Praise was provided for accurate target responses. Inaccurate responses were described along with a rationale for change. In addition, a description of correct responding was presented. Acknowledgment from the staff member was requested along with practice of the correct responses. Additional practice using role-play or in-vivo techniques were used in order to demonstrate accurate responses. The author requested instructors to ask questions for clarification. The feedback ended with an appreciation statement.

The results of the discrete-trial teaching staff training procedure showed that each instructor performed at criterion level for all of the quizzes and performance demonstrations. Figure 5 displays the percentage of accuracy for each of the discrete-trial teaching responses recorded for the three Instructors involved in training. Across all three instructors, the mean percentage of accurate responding pooled across 10 sessions was above 89%. Without this level of training, instructors observed as a normative sample showed as low as 48% accuracy.

Ryan & Hemmes (2005) assessed the effects of an intensive training package designed to produce high levels of accurate discrete-trial teaching responses through the use of performance criteria. The instructors who participated in the study performed at high mean levels. The importance of requiring performance criteria was explicated from the normative data collected from four instructors of students with autism in a special education setting. Data from the normative sample were considerably lower than those of the instructors from the Ryan & Hemmes study.

The Ryan & Hemmes findings concur with those of the literature on the effectiveness of training procedures using verbal and video instruction, modeling, role-playing, in-vivo practice and instruction, and performance feedback in producing accurate teaching performance (Arco, 1991; Cullen, 1988; Fleming, et al., 1996; Harchik, et al., 1989; Krumhus & Malott, 1980; Parsons, et al., 1996). Reid & Green, 1980; Sepler, & Myers, 1978). The Ryan & Hemmes results are consistent with the findings that individual feedback with praise is crucial in the maintenance of teaching responses (Adkins, 1996; Harchik, et al., Reid & Parsons, 1995).

**Discrete-Trial Teaching Data Sheet**

**Observer #/Name:**______________________________ **Session#:**_____
**Teacher name:**______________________ **Educational Program:**_____
**Session start time and end time (duration):** ________________________

1. Teaching area **distraction-free**?
2. Teaching **materials** available?
3. **Attending** responses established?
4. One **verbal direction** only?
5. **Voice tones** differential, appropriate, and contingent?
6. **Wait** $^{D}$?
7. **Praise statement** after correct response?
8. **Contingent reinforcers**?
9. **Correction procedure**?
10. **Pause** prior to the next trial?
11. **Incidental or additional teaching** during pause?
12. **Data recorded**?

**Trial Number**

| **Responses** | **1** | **2** | **3** | **4** | **5** | **6** | **7** | **8** | **9** | **10** | |
|---|---|---|---|---|---|---|---|---|---|---|---|
| Distraction Free | | | | | | | | | | | |
| Materials | | | | | | | | | | | |
| Attending | | | | | | | | | | | |
| Verbal Direction | | | | | | | | | | | |
| Voice Tones | | | | | | | | | | | |
| Wait | | | | | | | | | | | |
| Praise Statement | | | | | | | | | | | |
| Reinforcers | | | | | | | | | | | |
| Correction/ Procedure | | | | | | | | | | | |
| Pause | | | | | | | | | | | |
| Incidental/ Additional | | | | | | | | | | | |
| Record Data | | | | | | | | | | | |
| Mean % | | | | | | | | | | | |

Fig. 4. Discrete-trial teaching datasheet use din conducting the Ryan & Hemmes (2005) study.

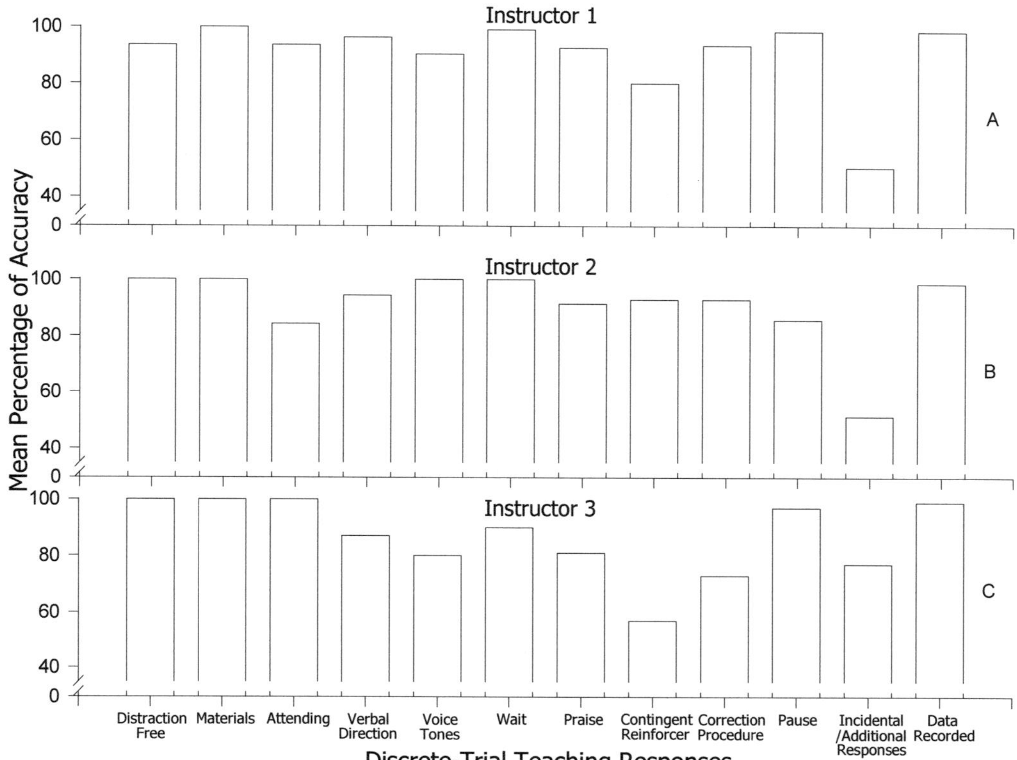


Fig. 5. Figure reprinted with permission from Ryan & Hemmes (2005). Percentage of accurate responding across the 12 discrete-trial responses for Instructors 1, 2, and 3 as displayed in Panels A, B, and C, respectively.

Mean accuracy of performance for the staff was 92% or above across 10 sessions. These data were contrasted with the substantially lower levels of accuracy from normative data of instructors conducting sessions in a comparable setting. These data suggest the importance of requiring criterion-level performance during training.

Instructors in Ryan & Hemmes study showed low accuracy levels of *incidental or additional teaching responses.* Incidental teaching has been found to be important for arranging opportunities for spontaneous variety and generality in speech in a various settings (Hart & Risley, 1974, 1975, 1980, 2000; McGee, et al., 1983; McGee, et al., 1985). Instructors were trained to show incidental or additional teaching responses; however, further instruction, as noted below in the following section, may be required to improve performance.

### 7.2 Staff training on incidental teaching

The Ryan & Hemmes (2005) study highlighted the need for staff training on incidental teaching responses. Due to the nature of incidental teaching, the requirements for stimulus and response generalization in implementing incidental teaching accurately are high (Hart & Risley, 1974, 1975, 1980, 1982, 1985). At the time of the Ryan et al. (2008) study, there was no research on training staff to implement incidental teaching. Ryan et al. (2008) assessed the effects of a brief group staff training procedure on instructors' use of incidental teaching responses and on student initiations. In Experiment 1, instructors of students with autism were provided with an instruction session during which a training package on incidental teaching was presented. The training package included a videotape example of incidental teaching, written text including the definitions and descriptions of incidental teaching, and written incidental teaching scenarios. Posters and wallet-sized cards indicating the required incidental teaching responses were displayed and provided to the instructors (see Figure 6). The data sheet presented in Figure 7 was used during training.

During each session, incidental teaching performance was scored upon the occurrence of each student initiation (see Figure 8 for datasheet). Ryan et al. (2008) labeled and described the terms and definitions of incidental teaching responses as mentioned in the above section. After an initial assessment phase and training session, the author requested that the instructors, "Do this in your classroom." Prior to each session, the author requested that the assistant instructors, "Do your best to get as much language from the students as possible."

Instructors from Ryan et al.'s (2008) Experiment 1 showed an increase in the proportion of incidental teaching responses. In addition, improvement in incidental teaching was accompanied by an increase in student initiations. Their data provide evidence for an effective and efficient training method for instructors in setting the occasion for incidental teaching episodes.

A large-scale systematic replication of Experiment 1 was conducted in Experiment 2 in order to evaluate the generality of the findings observed. In addition to the training components of Experiment 1, Experiment 2 included role-playing with feedback during training. Pre-training sessions were conducted prior to training; post-training sessions were conducted within one week after Training. After training, the author asked each participant to demonstrate incidental teaching in the classroom. The author provided feedback to instructors using a four-part feedback-delivery model.

> "The components were: (a) praise for correct responses; (b) description of the incorrect responses; (c) description and role-playing of alternative correct responses; and (d) empathetic statement for practice." (Ryan et al., 2008).

Immediately following training and prior to recording Post-training data, one incidental teaching training poster was placed in each classroom. There was an increase in dependent responses in Experiment 2. The findings suggest that brief staff training is an important initial step in improving incidental teaching and student initiations.

The Ryan et al.'s (2008) Experiments 1 and 2 provided evidence for the effectiveness of a brief staff training procedure for incidental teaching which was demonstrated on a small-scale and then a large-scale basis.

## 8. Conclusion

In summary, applied behavior analysis (ABA) is the treatment of choice for students with autism. ABA is the scientific approach to teaching that specifies the importance of individualized programming and data-based decisions that is critical in the education for students with autism. Two effective ABA teaching procedures were discussed in the current chapter. Discrete-trial teaching and incidental teaching have been found to improve the rate of learning by students with autism. Both teaching procedures are designed to target specific goals for the student. Each procedure systematically improves upon learned responses by the student. Staff training research has been conducted in order to teach others how to use discrete-trial and incidental teaching procedures. Effective training procedures were reviewed in the current chapter. The Ryan & Hemmes (2005) method described for training discrete-trial teaching responses was successful in training a high level of accuracy. The two experiments described from Ryan, et al. (2008) provide evidence for the effectiveness of brief staff training procedures implements on a small-scale and on a large-scale in a school for students with autism. The author suggests that training on teaching procedures described within the chapter is feasible, practical, and efficient in educational programs for students with autism.

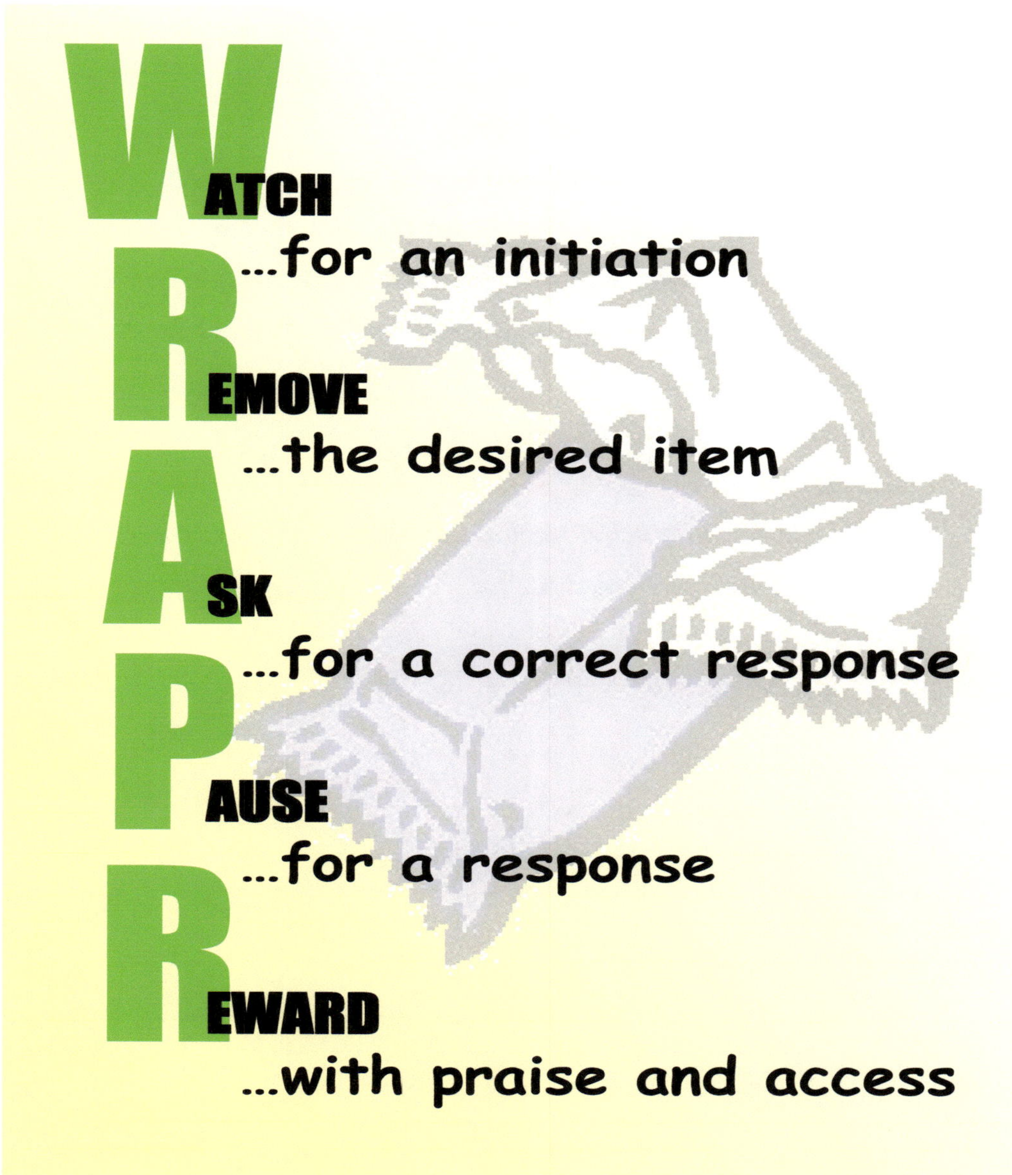


Fig. 6. Diagram of poster and wallet-sized handouts for staff training on incidental teaching responses using in the Ryan, et al. (2008) study.

**Data Sheet for Scoring Incidental Teaching Responses**

Observer name:__________________ Session # Reviewed:__________________

Teacher name:__________________ Educational Program: __________________

Session start time and end time (duration): __________________

1. Watch for an initiation: the instructor is available an looking down or away from the student while working.
2. Remove the desired item: after the student makes a verbal or nonverbal initiation for an object, activity, or other event, the instructor removes the item(s) and makes eye contact with the student.
3. Ask for a correct response: the instructor uses an appropriate statement or question to ask the student to say more about the initiation made.
4. Pause for a correct response: the student responds independently or is prompted to respond within 10 s of the instructor s request.
5. Reward: the instructor presents behavior specific praise about the student s initiation along with access to the object or activity that the student requested.

| Responses | 1 | 2 | 3 | 4 | 5 | 6 | 7 | 8 | 9 | 10 | Total | % |
|---|---|---|---|---|---|---|---|---|---|---|---|---|
| Watch | | | | | | | | | | | | |
| Remove | | | | | | | | | | | | |
| Ask | | | | | | | | | | | | |
| Pause | | | | | | | | | | | | |
| Reward | | | | | | | | | | | | |
| Total | | | | | | | | | | | | |
| % | | | | | | | | | | | | |

Fig. 7. Incidental teaching data sheet used in Ryan et al. (2008) during training. Reprinted with permission of the author.

**Data Sheet for Scoring Incidental Teaching Responses: Instructor & Learner**

Date:____________________ Session#/Tape#/Duration:____________________ Program:____________________

Instructor (Teacher TA) Name/Code: ____________________ Student Name/Code:____________________

Observer Name/Code:____________________

***W**atch for an initiation*: the instructor is available and waits for the student s initiation; the instructor is looking down or away from the student while working.

***R**emove the desired item*: after the student makes a verbal or nonverbal initiation for an object, activity, or other event, the instructor removes the item(s) and makes eye contact with the student.

***A**sk for a correct response*: the instructor uses an appropriate statement or question to ask the student to say more about the initiation made.

***P**ause for a correct response*: the student responds independantly or is prompted to respond within 10 s of the instructor s request.

***R**eward:* the instructor presents behavior specific praise about the student s initation along with access to the object or activity that the student requested

*L.In*: Learner Initiation; *LR*: Learner Response; *Pr:* Prompted response; *Er*: Error response; S: Successful episode; U: Unsuccessful episode

| | 1 | 2 | 3 | 4 | 5 | 6 | 7 | 8 | 9 | 10 | 11 | 12 | 13 | 14 | 15 | Total + | Total - |
|---|---|---|---|---|---|---|---|---|---|---|---|---|---|---|---|---|---|
| ***W*** | + - | + - | + - | + - | + - | + - | + - | + - | + - | + - | + - | + - | + - | + - | + - | | |
| ***#L.In*** | | | | | | | | | | | | | | | | | |
| **R** | + - | + - | + - | + - | + - | + - | + - | + - | + - | + - | + - | + - | + - | + - | + - | | |
| **A** | + - | + - | + - | + - | + - | + - | + - | + - | + - | + - | + - | + - | + - | + - | + - | | |
| **P** | + - | + - | + - | + - | + - | + - | + - | + - | + - | + - | + - | + - | + - | + - | + - | | |
| ***LR*** | + - | + - | + - | + - | + - | + - | + - | + - | + - | + - | + - | + - | + - | + - | + - | | |
| ***Pr*** | + - NA | + - NA | + - NA | + - NA | + - NA | + - NA | + - NA | + - NA | + - NA | + - NA | + - NA | + - NA | + - NA | + - NA | + - NA | | |
| ***# Pr*** | | | | | | | | | | | | | | | | | |
| ***Er*** | + - NA | + - NA | + - NA | + - NA | + - NA | + - NA | + - NA | + - NA | + - NA | + - NA | + - NA | + - NA | + - NA | + - NA | + - NA | | |
| ***# Er*** | | | | | | | | | | | | | | | | | |
| ***R*** | + - | + - | + - | + - | + - | + - | + - | + - | + - | + - | + - | + - | + - | + - | + - | | |
| ***Episode*** | S U | S U | S U | S U | S U | S U | S U | S U | S U | S U | S U | S U | S U | S U | S U | | |
| **Total S** | | | | | | | | | | | | **Total Correct Responses:** | | | | | |
| **Total U** | | | | | | | | | | | | **Total Incorrect Responses:** | | | | | |
| **Type of Info Asked** | Request ______ Comments______ Object Id.______ | | | | Yes/No ______ Number Id. ______ Taste Questions______ | | | | Conversation______ Color Id.______ Body Part Id. ______ | | | | Other______ Praise______ | | | | |

Fig. 8. Incidental teaching datasheet used after training. Reprinted with permission of the author.

## 9. Acknowledgment

The author wishes to acknowledge her former and current colleagues and students from whom she has learned so much. She also expresses her gratitude for her professors from Queens College and the Graduate School and University Center of the City University of New York, CUNY for their inspiration and guidance.

## 10. References

Arco, L. (1991). Effects of outcome performance feedback on maintenance of client and staff behavior in a residential setting. *Behavioral Residential Treatment, 6,* 231-247.

Baer, D. M., Wolf, M. M., & Risley, T. R. (1968). Some current dimensions of applied behavior analysis. *Journal of Applied Behavior Analysis, 1,* 91-97.

Cooper, J. O., Heron, T. E., & Heward, W. L. (2007). *Applied behavior analysis.* Upper Saddle River, NJ: Pearson Education, Inc.

Cullen, C. (1988). A review of staff training: The emperor's old clothes. *Irish Journal of Psychology, 9,* 309-323.

Delamater, A. M., Conners, C. K., & Wells, K. C. (1984). A comparison of staff training procedures: Behavioral applications in the child psychiatric inpatient setting. *Behavioral Modification, 8,* 39-58.

Demchak, M., Kontos, S., & Neisworth, J. T. (1992). Using a pyramid model to teach behavior management procedures to childcare providers. *Topics in Early Childhood Special Education, 12,* 458-477.

Fielding, L. T., Errickson, E., & Bettin, B. (1971). Modification of staff behavior: A brief note. *Behavior Therapy, 2,* 550-553.

Fleming, R. K., Oliver, J. R., & Bolton, D. M. (1996). Training supervisors to train staff: A case study in a human service organization. *Journal of Organizational Behavior management, 16,* 3-25.

Gardner, J. M. (1972). Teaching behavior modification to nonprofessionals. *Journal of Applied Behavior Analysis, 5,* 517-521.

Gladstone, B. W., & Spencer, C. J. (1977). The effects of modeling on the contingent praise of mental retardation counselors. *Journal of Applied Behavior Analysis, 10,* 75-84.

Greene, B. F., Willis, B. S., Levy, R., & Bailey, J. S. (1978). Measuring client gains from staff-implemented programs. *Journal of Applied Behavior Analysis, 11,* 395-412.

Harchik, A. E., Sherman, J. A., Hopkins, B. L., & Strouse, M. C. (1989). Use of behavioral techniques by paraprofessional staff: A review and proposal. *Behavioral Residential Treatment, 4, 331-357.*

Harris, V. W., Bushell, D., Jr., Sherman, J. A., & Kane, J. F. (1975). Instructions, feedback, praise, bonus payments, and teacher behavior. *Journal of Applied Behavior Analysis, 8,* 462.

Hart, B. (1985). *Naturalistic language training techniques.* In S. Warren, & A. Rogers-Warren (Eds.), *Teaching functional language* (pp. 63-88). Baltimore: University Park Press.

Hart, B., & Risley, T. R. (1974). Using preschool materials to modify the language of disadvantaged children. *Journal of Applied Behavior Analysis, 7,* 243-256.

Hart, B., & Risley, T. R. (1975). Incidental teaching of language in the preschool. *Journal of Applied Behavior Analysis, 8,* 411-420.

Hart, B., & Risley, T. R. (1980). In vivo language intervention: Unanticipated general effects. *Journal of Applied Behavior Analysis, 13,* 407-432.

Hart, B., & Risley, T. R. (1982). *How to use incidental teaching for elaborating language.* Lawrence, KS: H & H Enterprises.

Hart, B., & Risley, T. R. (2000). *Meaningful differences in the everyday experience of young American children*. Baltimore, MD: Paul H. Brookes.

Hay, L. R., Nelson, R. O., & Hay, W. M. (1977). The use of teachers as behavior observers. *Journal of Applied Behavior Analysis, 10,* 345-348.

Johnson, M. D., & Fawcett, S. B. (1994). Courteous service: Its assessment and modification in a human service organization. *Journal of Applied Behavior Analysis, 27,* 145-152.

Krumhus, K. M., & Malott, R. W. (1980). The effects of modeling and immediate and delayed feedback in staff training. *Journal of Organizational Behavior Management, 2,* 279-293.

Lovaas, O. I. (1987). Behavioral treatment and normal educational and intellectual functioning in young autistic children. *Journal of Consulting and Clinical Psychology, 55,* 3-9.

McGee, G. G., Krantz, P. J., & McClannahan, L. E. (1985). The facilitative effects of incidental teaching on preposition use by autistic children. *Journal of Applied Behavior Analysis, 18,* 17-31.

McGee, G. G., Krantz, P. J., Mason, D., & McClannahan, L. E. (1983). A modified incidental-teaching procedure for autistic youth: Acquisition and generalization of receptive object labels. *Journal of Applied Behavior Analysis, 16,* 329-338.

Matson, J. L. (1990). *Handbook of behavior modification with the mentally retarded.* New York: Plenum Press.

Neef, N. A., Parrish, J. M., Egel, A. L., & Sloan, M. E. (1986). Training respite care providers for families with handicapped children: Experimental analysis and validation of an instructional package. *Journal of Applied Behavior Analysis, 19,* 105-124.

New York State Department of Health (1999a). *Clinical practice guideline on autism/pervasive developmental disorders assessment and intervention for young children: Review of recommendations.* New York: Author.

New York State Department of Health (1999b). *Clinical practice guideline on autism/pervasive developmental disorders assessment and intervention for young children: Quick reference guide.* New York: Author.

New York State Department of Health (1999c). *Clinical practice guideline on autism/pervasive developmental disorders assessment and intervention for young children: The guideline technical report.* New York: Author.

Newman, B., Reeve, K. F., Reeve, S. A., & Ryan, C. S. (2003). *Behaviorspeak.* New York: Free Press.

Page, T.J., Iwata, B.A., & Reid, D.H. (1982). Pyramidal training: A large-scale application with institutional staff. *Journal of Applied Behavior Analysis, 15,* 335-351.

Parsons, M. B., & Reid, D. H. (1995). Training residential supervisors to provide feedback for maintaining staff teaching skills with people who have severe disabilities. *Journal of Applied Behavior Analysis, 28,* 317-322.

Parsons, M. B., Reid, D. H., & Green, C. W. (1996). Training basic teaching skills to community and institutional support staff for people with severe disabilities: A one-day program. *Research in Developmental Disabilities, 17,* 467-485.

Parsons, M. B., Schepis, M. M., Reid, D. H., McCarn, J. E., & Green, C. W. (1987). Expanding the impact of behavioral staff management: A large-scale, long-term application in schools serving severely handicapped students. *Journal of Applied Behavior Analysis, 20,* 139-150.

Quilitch, H. R. (1975). A comparison of three staff-management procedures. *Journal of Applied Behavior Analysis, 8,* 59-66.

Reid, D. H., & Green, C. W. (1980). *Staff training.* In J. L. Matson (Ed.), *Handbook of Behavior Modification with the Mentally Retarded (pp. 71-90).* New York: Plenum Press.

Richman, G. S., Riordan, M. R., Reiss, M. L., Pyles, D. A. M., & Bailey, J. S. (1988). The effects of self-monitoring and supervisor feedback on staff performance in a residential setting. *Journal of Applied Behavior Analysis, 21,* 401-409.

Ryan, C. S., & Hemmes, N. S. (2005). Post-training discrete-trial teaching performance by instructors of young children with autism in early intensive behavioral intervention. *The Behavior Analyst Today, 6,* 1-12.

Ryan, C. S., Hemmes, N. S., Sturmey, P., Jacobs, J. D., & Grommet E. K. (2008). Effects of a brief staff training procedure on instructors' use of incidental teaching and learners' frequency of initiation toward instructors. *Research in Autism Spectrum Disorders, 2,* 28-45.

Sarakoff, R. A., & Sturmey, P. (2004). The effects of behavioral skills training on staff implementation of discrete-trial teaching. *Journal of Applied Behavior Analysis, 37,* 535-538.

Sepler, H. J., & Myers, S. L. (1978). The effectiveness of verbal instruction on teaching behavior-modification skills to nonprofessionals. *Journal of Applied Behavior Analysis, 11,* 198.

Smith, T. (2001). Discrete trial training in the treatment of autism. *Focus on Autism & Other Developmental Disabilities, 16, 86-92.*

Sundberg, M. L., & Partington, J. W. (1998). *Teaching language to children with autism or other developmental disabilities.* Pleasant Hill, CA: Behavior Analysts, Inc.

Touchette, P. E., & Howard, J. S. (1984). Errorless learning: Reinforcement contingencies and stimulus control transfer in delayed prompting. *Journal of Applied Behavior Analysis, 17,* 175-188.

U.S. Department of Health and Human Services. *Mental Health: A Report of the Surgeon General – Executive Summary.* (1999).

Rockville, MD: U.S. Department of Health and Human Services, Substance Abuse and Mental Health Services Administration, Center for Mental Health Services, National Institutes of Health, National Institute of Mental Health.

Wolf, M. M. (1978). Social validity: The case for subjective measurement, or how applied behavior analysis is finding its heart. *Journal of Applied Behavior Analysis, 11,* 203-214.

# 11

# Creating Inclusive Environments for Children with Autism

Dagmara Woronko and Isabel Killoran
*York University*
*Canada*

## 1. Introduction

Although the prevalence rate of Autism Spectrum Disorders (ASD) varies, recent figures suggest that close to 1% of children (Autism Society Canada, 2009; CDC, 2006) are identified with ASD. With inclusive philosophies paving the way for education in mainstream classrooms, attention must be given to equitable opportunities and practices for this growing population in our school systems (Killoran & Adams, 2006; Sapon-Shevin, 2003; United Nations, 2006). The research on inclusion and children with ASD is fairly limited; however, it has shown that in some regions at least, these students are excluded from school at a "significantly higher rate than students with other [special education needs]" (Humphrey & Lewis, 2008, p. 132). Children with ASD are "considered more difficult to include effectively than those with other SEN" (Humphrey & Lewis, 2008, p. 133). While there is much diversity with respect to strengths, abilities, functional levels and challenges among children with ASD, a core set of universal concerns exist. Some of these include sensory responsiveness, communication, and socialization. This chapter will focus on creating a sensory responsive environment, developing effective verbal and/or non-verbal communication, and fostering genuine relationships.

Using the three main principles of Universal Design for Learning (UDL) as an overarching assumption, this chapter will explore how educators can provide effective opportunities for multiple means of representation, expression, and engagement to address common areas of need (CAST, 2011; Hehir, 2009). By following these principles, an educator is able to create a community that welcomes all while addressing students' specific needs. Many educators have been overwhelmed with the past practice of individualization in isolation, a task that left many students alone and disconnected from their peers. The current practices of differentiation and universal design for learning enable educators to plan for their students in such a way that all are integral, contributing, valued members of the learning community.

This chapter provides a synthesis of current research on evidence-based classroom interventions and accommodations for learners with ASD in inclusive settings, at all age levels, with respect to sensory environments, assisted communication, and facilitation of social relationships. Emphasis is placed on accommodations that meet UDL requirements. A comprehensive search of the Education Resources Information Center (ERIC) database was conducted using keywords for, and related to, autism, universal design for learning and sensory, communication, and social skills interventions. Empirical research was reviewed, as well as qualitative studies and narratives. Manual searches of the reference lists were conducted to identify additional sources.

## 2. Creating a sensory responsive environment

Children with ASD often display atypical sensory processing. "Sensory processing" refers to the relationship between neurological thresholds and self-regulatory strategies for adaptive behaviour (Hocchauser & Engel-Yeger, 2010). From a clinical perspective, sensory under-responsiveness and/or over-responsiveness can lead to behaviours, which either generate or avoid sensory stimulation in an effort to help the child with ASD cope with environmental stimuli (Iarocci & McDonald, 2006). In order for inclusive education practices to be effective for children with ASD, a deeper awareness of sensory processing needs must be acquired by educators, and classroom environmental accommodations implemented.

Sensory integration dysfunction, or "sensory perceptual issue", is defined as a disruption in the process of organizing sensational information gathered from the seven senses: smell, taste, touch, sight, sound, vestibular (movement), and proprioceptive (muscle and joint receptors) senses (Ayres, 1979; Bogdashina, 2003; Howe, Brittain, & McCathren, 2004; Myles, Cook, Miller, Rinner, & Robbins, 2000; Yack, Aquilla, & Sutton, 2002). Sensory integration difficulties have been reported in 42 to 88% of children with ASD (Baranek, 2002, p. 398). These difficulties can influence a child's gross and fine motor development, balance, coordination, visual perception and self-help skills, thus having a potential impact on the ability to engage in social activities and develop feelings of success and mastery in the classroom (Baranek, Boyd, Poe, David & Watson, 2007; Howe, et al., 2004). The Ziggurat model, an intervention program for learners with ASD, stipulates that a student's sensory needs must be met before effective and engaged learning can take place (Murray, Hudson Baker, Murray-Slutsky, & Paris, 2009; Myles, Grossman, Aspy, Henry & Bixler Coffin, 2007).

No two children are alike, and this is especially true for children with ASD. Because there is much variation with respect to sensory responsiveness, educators need to acquaint themselves with their students' *specific* sensory needs before the school year commences, thus giving them time to make any necessary accommodations to the classroom environment (Killoran, 2005). Often children with ASD will require a sensory diet delivered during the school day (Baranak 2002; Yack, et al., 2002). Below is a synthesis of evidence-based environmental accommodations for a variety of sensory integration responses and behaviours. Each student with ASD will present with his or her own unique set of responses, behaviours and needs.

Hochhauser and Engel-Yeger (2010) have found an association between smell over-responsiveness and a reduced amount of participation in certain classroom activities in children with ASD. Common classroom activities such as crafts, colouring, drawing and snack/lunch periods can be particularly distressing for children with odour over-responsiveness (Hochhauser & Engel-Yeger, 2010). Making classrooms scent-free environments and purchasing odourless craft supplies can help not only those with ASD, but also any children with odour sensitivities in the classroom (Case-Smith & Arbesman, 2008). Encouraging children to bring in snacks and lunches that are not response-inducing will eliminate the need for removal of students with ASD from the classroom during these particularly socially engaging periods in the school day.

Children with ASD who have an over-responsive tactile sense may exhibit negative emotional reactions to specific consistencies of solids and fluids, and/or to intentional or accidental touch. Tactile over-responders will engage in sensory avoiding behaviours, aimed at people, situations, tasks and activities that are anxiety inducing (Killoran, 2004; Myles et al., 2000; Murray, et al, 2009). These learners may need preferential seating within the classroom to give them distance from others who may contribute to touch that may be distressing (Murray, et al., 2009). When lining up for recess or other activities, educators should assign these students to the back or front of the line, thereby minimizing opportunities for unwelcome touch (Howe, et al., 2004; Killoran, 2004). The UDL guidelines call for multiple tools for expression, communication, composition and construction in the inclusive classroom (CAST, 2011). For learners with tactile over-responsiveness, educators should consider the use of tools rather than hands for craft and other messy classroom activities (Howe, et al., 2004). These tools can be used by all students in the inclusive classroom, not only those with ASD.

Children with ASD who are tactile under-responders must have their needs accommodated within the inclusive classroom environment as well. These children require consistent tactile stimulation throughout their school day. They respond well to the use of weighted or vibrating pencils and the use of sandpaper placed under written work (Myles et al, 2000; Murray, et al, 2009; Yack et al, 2002). Providing an under-responsive tactile learner with a fidget toy to hold can reduce potentially disruptive sensory seeking behaviour, such as touching peers at inappropriate times (Friedlander, 2008; Howe, et al, 2004). Placing a rice-filled or inflated cushion on their chair can provide needed tactile stimulation as well (Friedlander, 2008). These classroom accommodations respond to the UDL's requirement for the provision of tools for self-regulation and optimize access to tools and assistive technologies for students with ASD in inclusive classroom settings (CAST, 2011).

Learners with ASD who are sight and sound over-responders may be distracted by classroom stimuli such as fluorescent lights that buzz or flash, an overabundance of colours in the classroom, noise from fans or air conditioners, the clinking of dishes in the cafeteria down the hall, or a line tapping against a metal flagpole outside (Friedlander, 2008; Howlin, 2005). Environmental accommodations in the classroom are needed to calm their nervous systems by eliminating extraneous noise and visual distraction (Case-Smith & Arbesman, 2008; Murray, et al., 2009).

Hochhauser and Engel-Yeger (2010) found that children with ASD who have high visual and auditory sensitivity work best one-to-one rather than in groups, as the opportunity for visual and auditory distraction is minimized. The UDL guidelines highlight the need for educators to provide options for self-regulation that facilitate personal coping skills and strategies (CAST, 2011). One such strategy is the use of Auditory Integration Training (AIT). AIT is based on the concept that electronically filtered music provided through earphones may be helpful in remediating auditory hypersensitivities (Baranek, 2002; Case-Smith & Arbesman, 2008; Dawson & Watling, 2000). Auditory Integration Therapy was developed in 1993 by Berard and Tomasis. It involves listening to electronically modified music which has had the peak frequencies to which an individual with ASD is hypersensitive, dampened (Baranek, 2002; Dawson & Watling, 2000). Children typically listen to 2 half-hour daily sessions for a total of 10 hours (Dawson & Watling, 2002). Recorded music is individualized according to specific needs, and can be kept in the classroom for use when sensory over-responsive behaviours are peaking.

Additional sound dampening accommodations such as tennis balls on chair legs, floor carpeting and vent covers may be helpful in decreasing background noises in the classroom as well (Myles et al., 2000; Murray et al., 2009; Yack et al., 2002). Visual schedules can help over-responders to focus their attention to the task at hand (Case-Smith & Arbesman, 2008; Humphrey, 2008). These environmental accommodations can be useful in minimizing sound and visual distractions for all learners in the inclusive classroom, not just those with ASD.

The vestibular system is located in the inner ear. Accurate processing of vestibular information allows individuals to successfully regulate posture, balance, and eye movement (Howe et al., 2004; Yack et al., 2002). Children with ASD who are over-responders to vestibular input are fearful, cautious or avoidant of movement; those who are under-responders seek excessive vestibular input (Howe, et al, 2004; Myles et al., 2000; Yack et al., 2002). Hocchauser and Engel-Yeger (2010) found that children who are over-responsive to vestibular input tend to be clumsy, have motor difficulties, low muscle tone and low levels of energy. Consequently, they may be reluctant or unable to participate in physical education classes (Hocchauser & Engel-Yeger, 2010). Howe, et al.,(2004) caution against forcing these children into participating in physical activities. Instead, they suggest offering the student opportunities for self-directed movement. Additionally, it is important to provide over-responsive vestibular learners with secure seating in the classroom, given their difficulties with balance. In place of traditional seating, educators should consider providing these students with alternative forms of seating such as bean bag chairs that mould to the student's body (Howe, et al., 2004).

Children with ASD who are under-responsive to vestibular input require regular opportunities for physical exercise and stimulation (Baranek, 2002; Yack et al., 2002). Daily routines and classroom accommodations may include sensory-motor breaks or movement breaks to improve attention spans, social skills and work performance (Howlin, 2005; Murray, et al., 2009). These can be built in to the daily physical activity that all children should be getting. The use of therapy balls in the classroom on which students can bounce to stimulate the vestibular system is another strategy that other children in the inclusive classroom may benefit from (Howlin, 2005; Wong Bonggat & Hall, 2010).

Finally, attention must be paid to the proprioceptive system of children with ASD. The proprioceptive system is located in the muscles and joints, and notifies the brain with respect to body position (Howe, et al.,2004; Killoran, 2004; Yack et al., 2002). The brain uses this information to move in a coordinated manner and to plan movements for a new task (Howe, et al., 2004). Children with proprioceptive difficulties can appear clumsy when completing tasks; they may bump into their surroundings in an effort to collect needed input for the body with respect to position (Howe, et al., 2004; Yack et al., 2002). Murray, et al., (2009) point out the need for strong sensory input that provides meaningful sensory feedback. Songs with gestures, high-energy rhythmic activities, jumping on a trampoline, stretching activities, or other activities to wake up the sensory systems should be integrated into the learners' day (Murray, et al., 2009). These activities will not only benefit the students with ASD in the classroom, but all children learning in the inclusive classroom.

All of the accommodations discussed above satisfy CAST's (2011) guidelines for UDL. The accommodations mentioned above support inclusive learning environments, as they do not necessitate the removal of children with ASD from general education classrooms. These accommodations can benefit many learners in the classroom, as they are designed for universal use and multifaceted situations. They provide the sensory responsive environment necessary for children with ASD to learn in an engaging and inclusive classroom. Coupled with effective communication programs, strategies and accommodations, the foundation for fostering genuine relationships is laid.

## 3. Developing effective communication

Children with ASD can live relatively secluded lives with little social interaction outside of school hours (Hochhauser & Engel-Yeger, 2010). Social isolation stems in part from qualitative impairments in reciprocal social interaction and communication, and a tendency for restricted, repetitive, and stereotyped patterns of behavior, interest, or activity (Walker & Berthelsen, 2008). Communication challenges are most pronounced in children with ASD who are non-verbal; however echolalia, expressive language delay, receptive language difficulties and literal interpretations of idioms and colloquial language contribute to communication difficulties even among high-functioning, verbal children with ASD. The ability to communicate effectively, be it through the medium of spoken language, sign language, PECS, or computer assisted communication, is the foundation upon which meaningful social relationships are built. This section will examine the communicative challenges of children with ASD, and the role of the classroom teacher in creating an inclusive classroom environment in which various forms of communication are valued and explored. Effective communication programs, strategies and accommodations will be discussed, with an emphasis on their contribution to opportunity for social and academic success in the general education classroom.

The ability to communicate effectively contributes to meaningful, reciprocal and satisfying social relationships. Children with ASD who are nonverbal require effective communication programs, strategies and accommodations within the inclusive classroom in order to have an equitable opportunity for social engagement with peers and educators (Freeman, Perry, & Bebko, 2002). Through the use of gestures, vocalizations and/or augmentative and adaptive communication systems, children with ASD are able to interact meaningfully and reciprocally with their peers and their classroom environment (Mastrangelo & Killoran, 2007). A universally designed classroom is one in which multiple modes of communication and expression are explored, encouraged and given value (CAST, 2011).

Children with ASD who are nonverbal can use a number of strategies and assistive technologies in order to communicate more effectively with the world around them. One such assistive strategy is the use of the Picture Exchange Communication System (PECS). PECS teaches spontaneous communicative skills within a social context through the use of pictures or symbols (Howlin, 2004; Magiati & Howlin, 2003). In a universally designed inclusive classroom, these pictures or symbols can be used throughout the room as an assistive technology for use with all learners, not only specifically those with ASD. Teaching all children in the classroom how to communicate using the PECS binders of peers with

ASD can help to facilitate reciprocal communication (Simpson, 2005). Educators who have incorporated the use of PECS in their inclusive classrooms report positive outcomes not only for children with ASD, but for the entire classroom population. They cite increased independence and confidence, improvement in the use of words for learners with ASD, reduced tantrums and frustrations over the inability to communicate, and improved teaching practices (Case-Smith & Arbesman, 2008; Magiati & Howlin, 2003). Mirenda (2003) notes increased reciprocal communication exchanges and social interactions with peers as additional benefits to symbolically augmented communication.

Training in Sign Language (SL) can result in quicker and more complete learning of vocabulary among children with ASD than does speech training (Goldstein, 2002; Mirenda, 2003; Yoder & Layton, 1988). The presentation of speech training programs is particularly ineffective among those children with ASD who have poor verbal imitation skills (Yoder & Layton, 1988). Incorporating SL gestures into the inclusive classroom setting serves to benefit all learners (Bonvillian, Nelson & Rhyne, 1981; Tincani, 2004). Teaching typically developing children SL has become commonplace in mainstream society, as a means to pair spoken language with gestures. Typically developing school-aged children often learn second languages through the pairing of speech and SL gestures (Iverson & Goldin-Meadow, 2005; McCafferty, 2002). This use of SL can thus be expanded within the inclusive classroom setting to teach both learners with ASD and those without how to reciprocally communicate with one another. This satisfies CAST's (2011) UDL guidelines for provision of multiple options for perception and comprehension, use of multiple types of media for communication, and fostering a sense of collaboration and community.

The use of speech generating devices (SGD) with children with ASD is an emerging field. SGDs are an assistive technology that can help children with ASD who are non-verbal or language emergent, communicate with peers and educators in the classroom. Despite the small number of studies conducted with respect to SGD's success as an accommodation in the inclusive classroom, researchers are finding that the use of SGDs with some children with ASD can lead to verbal imitation of SGD output and a desire to use more communicative tools/devices in general (Blischak, Lombardino & Dyson, 2003; Franco et at., 2009; Thunberg, Ahlsen, & Dahlgren Sandberg, 2007). Implementation of SGD use in the inclusive classroom provides children with ASD an option with respect to expression and communication, and optimizes access to assistive tools and technologies, all of which are part of the UDL guidelines (CAST, 2011).

Assisted communication for non-verbal children with ASD is a necessary component of the inclusive classroom. Inclusive classrooms promote social interactions between children with ASD and their typically developing peers, leading to improved educational outcomes and greater learning and social competencies (Mastrangelo & Killoran, 2007). Opportunities for increased and successful social interactions are strongly correlated with the achievement of communicative competence (Prizant, Wetherby, Rubin, & Laurant, 2003). Research indicates that limited communication skills are strongly associated with peer rejection for children with ASD in inclusive classroom settings (Fujiki & Brinton, 1996; Humphrey, 2008; Walker & Berthelsen, 2008). A universally designed classroom is one which provides options for language, optimizes access to assistive technologies and fosters collaboration and community (CAST 2011). A universally designed classroom is the setting necessary for the creation of meaningful and genuine friendships for children with ASD.

## 4. Fostering genuine relationships

Children with ASD often face challenges socializing in general education classroom settings and have trouble interacting with others (Embregts & van Nieuwenhuijzen, 2009; Fujiki & Brinton, 1996; Humphrey, 2008). Inclusive school settings should set the development of social competence as one of their primary goals (Walker & Berthelsen, 2008). The World Health Organization defines participation in meaningful social activities and relationships as a vital part of human development and life experience, through which children acquire skills and competencies, and find purpose and meaning in life (Hochhauser & Engel-Yeger, 2010). Research indicates that increasingly, children with developmental disabilities are being socially isolated, bullied and excluded in general education classroom settings (Humphrey, 2008; Wang & Parrila, 2008).

Children with ASD require individual and appropriate support to engage in positive play experiences and social interactions with their peers (Mastrangelo & Killoran, 2007; Walker & Berthelsen, 2008). The degree to which they are supported in acquiring peer-related social skills is a consequence of their classroom teacher, who has a significant role in creating a learning community within which all children are valued (Mastrangelo & Killoran, 2007; Walker & Berthelsen, 2008). UDL guidelines specifically outline the need for creating classroom environments which foster community and collaboration (CAST, 2011). These inclusive classroom settings make the development of genuine friendships a possibility for children with ASD.

Too often, peer helpers are mistaken as "friends" for children with ASD in inclusive classroom settings. Group seating plans and group work activities often perpetuate the idea that typically developing peers who help students with disabilities, or merely sit next to them, are akin to "friends." Peer-mediated strategies have long been used by educators to increase the rate of social interaction by reinforcing and prompting a typically developing peer to initiate interactions or shape the social responding of a student with disabilities (Haring & Breen, 1992; DiSalvo & Oswald, 2002; McConnell, 2002). However, genuine friendships are those that translate into the after-school settings of home and community activities; peer-mediated strategies do not always see this translation materialize. As such, children with ASD remain socially isolated despite having a network of peer support in the classroom setting. A strategy that is effective at building up more intimate relationships at all age levels is Circle of Friends, or Circle of Support (Falvey, Forest, Pearpoint, & Rosenberg, 2000; Forest, Pearpoint, & O'Brien, 2000).

One opportunity often available to educators who have children with disabilities in their classes is the chance to work with an educational assistant (teacher aide, paraprofessional, support worker). Research has shown, however, that this resource is often misused and the results on socialization, particularly, are detrimental to the students (Giangreco, Edelman, Luiselli, & MacFarland, 1997; Malmgren, & Causton-Theoharis, 2006). With very little in-service, an educational assistant is able to make a significant difference to peer interactions and socialization (Causton-Theoharis & Malmgren, 2005). Among the strategies/accommodations that an educational assistant can provide for a student with ASD in the classroom are:

- Increasing physical proximity to peers
- Fading assistance to allow for more natural peer interaction opportunities

- Partnering student with ASD with peers during academic tasks
- Verbally highlighting similarities between student with ASD and peers
- Creating communication cards focused on social exchanges
- Teaching peers how to communicate with target student using sign language gestures
- Utilizing interactive technology
- Giving student with ASD classroom responsibilities that encourage interaction with peers (Causton-Theoharis, J., & Malmgren, 2005, p. 436)

Social skills training programs are another possible response to the need for individualized training in reciprocal play and conversational skills for children with ASD. While social skills training programs have been shown to have a positive effect on problem-solving skills in children with ASD (Embregts & van Nieuwenhuijzen, 2009; McConnell, 2002; Wolfberg & Schuler, 1993), these programs can lack social validity in terms of generalization of skills outside of the training sessions (Haring & Breen 1992; Ozonoff & Miller, 1995). Haring and Breen (1992) found that social skills training packages, while useful in terms of determining existing levels of social competence, may not translate into friendship relationships outside of the training context. Thus, attention should be turned toward the acquisition and development of social skills within the inclusive classroom environment, rather than in clinical training settings.

Research indicates that children with ASD who have at least one reciprocal, genuine friendship are more involved in their classroom social networks and more accepted by peers overall (Rotheram-Fuller, Kasari, Chamberlain & Locke, 2010). In the younger and middle elementary school years, inclusion alone appears to be sufficient in integrating some children with ASD into the social structure of classrooms; however, changing cognitive and physical skills, coupled with emerging and evolving competitive games, leave children with ASD needing assistance in facilitating true social involvement in the older grades (Howlin, 2005; McConnell, 2002; Rotheram-Fuller, Kasari, Chamberlain & Locke, 2010).

Children with ASD often lack the conversational skills necessary to develop effective reciprocal social speech. A possible response to this problem is through the use of pre-determined scripts. Pre-determined scripts teach children with ASD role-specific dialogue in socio-dramatic play situations (Causton-Theoharis, J., & Malmgren, 2005; Charlop-Christy & Kelso, 2003; Thiemann & Goldstein, 2001). Activities can be incorporated into the inclusive classroom in which the whole student population participates in dramatic role-playing activities. Educators model role-appropriate behaviour and speech, and provide opportunities for verbal and social exchanges between children with ASD and those without (Charlop-Christy & Kelso, 2003; Thiemann & Goldstein, 2001). Research indicates that following pre-determined script teaching sessions, role-appropriate speech and play in play settings increases among children with ASD (Charlop-Christy & Kelso, 2003; Ganz, Kaylor, Bourgeois, & Hadden, 2008; Thiemann & Goldstein, 2001). Pre-determined script teaching provides children with ASD with options for fostering collaboration and building fluencies, with graduated support for practice and performance, guidelines recommended by the UDL (CAST, 2011).

Other evidence-based teaching strategies/accommodations that may be useful in the creation of genuine friendships for children with ASD, especially younger children, include:

- Pre-linguistic Milieu Teaching (PMT) (McCathren & Watson, 2001)
- Using AAC systems with peers (Garfinkle & Schwartz, 2001)
- Peer interaction play centres (PALS) (Chandler, 1998)
- Can-do Thinking (Hull, Venn, Lee, & Buren, 2000).

(adapted from Mastrangelo & Killoran, 2007, pp. 81-82).

Ultimately, educators are the ones responsible for creating universally designed classrooms that circumvent barriers, provide opportunities for positive and reciprocal social interactions, and foster the development of specific skills (Mastrangelo & Killoran, 2007; Walker & Berthelsen, 2008). Children with ASD have the right to learn in equitable, sensory responsive classrooms that value multiple means of communication and expression. When these vital conditions are met, children with ASD will have the foundation necessary to create meaningful, lasting and genuine friendships. Through using the suggestions discussed within this chapter, educators have the opportunity to create a mutually beneficial learning community, one in which all students are included and valued. It is our responsibility to do so and it is our students' right to expect it of us.

## 5. References


Autism Society Canada. (2009). *Prevalence in Canada*. Retrieved November 15, 2010, from http://www.autismsocietycanada.ca/asd_research/research_prevalence/index_e.html

Ayres, A.J. (1979). *Sensory integration and the child*. Los Angeles, CA: Western Psychological Services.

Baranek, G. T. (2002). Efficacy of sensory and motor interventions for children with autism. *Journal of Autism and Developmental Disorders,* 32 (5), 397-422.

Baranek, G. T., Boyd, B. A., Poe, M. D., David, F. J., & Watson, L. R. (2007). Hyperresponsive sensory patterns in young children with autism, developmental delay, and typical development. *American Journal on Mental Retardation*, 112 (4), 233-245.

Blischak, D., Lombardino, L., & Dyson, A. (2003). Use of speech-generating devices: in support of natural speech. *Augmentative and Alternative Communication*, 19 (1), 29-35. doi:10.1080/0743461032000056478

Bogdashina, O. (2003). *Sensory perceptual issues in Autism and Asperger Syndrome: Different sensory experiences, Different perceptual worlds.* London, UK: Jessica Kingsley Publishers.

Bonvillian, J. D., Nelson, K. E., & Rhyne, J. E. (1981). Sign Language and Autism. *Journal of Autism and Developmental Disorders*, 11 (1), 125-137.

CAST. (2011). *UDL Guidelines: Educator Checklist Version 2*. Retrieved March 15, 2011 from http://www.udlcenter.org/aboutudl/udlguidelines/downloads.

Case-Smith, J. & Arbesman, M. (2008). Evidence-based review of interventions used for autism used in or of relevance to occupational therapy. *American Journal of Occupational Therapy*, 62 (4), 416-429. doi: 10.5014/ajot.62.4.416

Causton-Theoharis, J., & Malmgren, W. (2005). Increasing peer interactions for students with severe disabilities via paraprofessional training. *Exceptional Children, 71*(4), pp. 431-444.

Centre for Disease Control. (2006). *Prevalence of Autism Spectrum Disorders --- Autism and Developmental Disabilities Monitoring Network,* United States. Retrieved November 16, 2010 from http://www.cdc.gov/mmwr/preview/mmwrhtml/ss5810a1.htm.

Chandler, L. (1998). Promoting positive interaction between preschool age children during free play: The PALS Center. *Young Exceptional Children, 1*(3), 14-19.

Charlop-Christy, M. H., & Kelso, S. E. (2003). Teaching children with autism conversational speech using a cue card/written script program. *Education and Treatment of Children,* 26 (2), 108-127.

Dawson, G. & Watling, R. (2000). Interventions to facilitate auditory, visual and motor integration in autism: a review of the evidence. *Journal of Autism and Development Disorders,* 30 (5), 415-421.

DiSalvo, C.A., & Oswald, D. P. (2002). Social interaction of children with autism: consideration of peer expectancies. *Focus on Autism and Other Developmental Disabilities,* 17 (4), 198-207. doi: 10.1177/10883576020170040201

Embregts, P. & van Nieuwenhuijzen, M. (2009). Social information processing in boys with autistic spectrum disorder and mild to borderline intellectual disabilities. *Journal of Intellectual Disability Research,* 53, 922-931. doi: 10.1111/j.1365-2788.2009.01204.x

Falvey, M. A., Forest, M., Pearpoint, J., & Rosenberg, R. L. (2000). *All my life's a circle: Using the tools: Circles, MAPS & PATHS.* Toronto: Inclusion Press.

Forest, M., Pearpoint, J., & O'Brien, J. (2000, July). Circle of friends: Not a program. *Inclusion News 2000.* Toronto: Inclusion Press.

Franco, J. H., Lang, R. L., O'Reilly, M. F., Chan, J. M., Sigafoos, J., & Rispoli, M. (2009). Functional analysis and treatment of inappropriate vocalizations using a speech-generating device for a child with autism. *Focus on Autism and Other Developmental Disabilities,* 24 (3), 146-155. doi: 10.1177/1088357609338380

Freeman, N. L., Perry, A., & Bebko, J. M. (2002). Behaviour is communication: Nonverbal communicative behaviour in students with autism and instructors' responsivity. *Journal on Developmental Disabilities, 9*(2), 145-155.

Friedlander, D. (2008). Sam comes to school: Including students with autism in your classroom. *The Clearing House,* 82 (3), 141-144.

Fujiki, M., & Brinton, B. (1996). Social skills of children with specific language impairment. *Language, Speech, and Hearing Services in Schools,* 27, 195-202.

Ganz, J. B., Kaylor, M., Bourgeois, B., & Hadden, K. (2008). The impact of social scripts and visual cues on verbal communication in three children with autism spectrum disorders. *Focus on Autism and Other Developmental Disabilities,* 23 (2), 79-94. doi: 10.1177/ 1088357607311447

Garfinkle, A., & Schwartz, I.S. (2001). "Hey! I'm talking to you": a naturalistic procedure to teach preschool children to use their AAC systems with their peers. In M. Ostrosky & S. Sandall (Eds.), *Teaching strategies: What to do to support young children's development. Young Exceptional Children, Monograph Series, No. 3* (pp. 47-57). Longmont, CO: Sopris West.

Giangreco, M., Edelman, S., Luiselli, T., & MacFarland, S. (1997). Helping or hovering? Effects of instructional assistant proximity on students with disabilities. *Exceptional Children, 64*(1), 7-18.

Goldstein, H. (2002). Communication intervention for children with autism: a review of treatment efficacy. *Journal of Autism and Developmental Disorders,* 32 (5), 373-396.

Haring, T. G., & Breen, C. G. (1992). A peer-mediated social network intervention to enhance the social integration of persons with moderate and severe disabilities. *Journal of Applied Behaviour Analysis,* 25 (2), 319-333.

Hehir, T. (2009). *Policy foundations of universal design for learning.* Wakefield, MA: National Centre on Universal Design for Learning. Retrieved March 21, 2011 from http://www.udlcenter.org/sites/udlcenter.org/files/Hehir_Policy_Foundations_of_Universal%20Design_for_Learning_0.pdf.
Originally published as Hehir, T. (2009). Policy foundations of universal design for learning. In D. T. Gordon, J. W. Gravel & L. A. Schifter (Eds.), A policy reader in universal design for learning (pp. 35-45). Cambridge, MA: Harvard Education Press.

Hochhauser, M., & Engel-Yeger, B. (2010). Sensory processing abilities and their relation to participation in leisure activities among children with high-functioning autism spectrum disorder (HFASD). *Research in Autism Spectrum Disorders,* 4, 746-754. doi:10.1016/j.rasd.2010.01.015

Howe, M. B., Brittain, L. A., & McCathren, R. B. (2004). Meeting the sensory needs of young children in classrooms. *Young Exceptional Children,* 8 (1), 11-19.

Howlin, P. (2005). The effectiveness of interventions for children with autism. *Neurodevelopmental Disorders,* 101-119. doi: 10.1007/3-211-31222-6_6

Hull, K., Venn, M., Lee, J., & Van Buren, M. (200). Passports for learning in inclusive settings. In S. Sandall & M. Ostrosky, (Eds.), *Natural environments and inclusion. Young Exceptional Children Monograph Series No. 2* (p. 69-77). Longmont, CO: Sopris West.

Humphrey, N. (2008). Including pupils with autistic spectrum disorders in mainstream schools. *British Journal of Learning Support,* 23 (1), 41-47. doi: 10.1111/j.1467-9604.2007.00367.x

Humphrey, N., & Lewis, S. (2008). What does 'inclusion' mean for pupils on the autistic spectrum in mainstream secondary schools? *Journal of Research in Special Educational Needs,* (8), 3, 132.140.

Iarocci, G., & McDonald, J. (2006). Sensory integration and the perceptual experience of persons with autism. *Journal of Autism and Developmental Disorders,* 36 (1), 77-90. doi: 10.1007/s10803-005-0044-3

Iverson, J. M., & Goldin-Meadow, S. (2005). Gesture paves the way for language development. *Psychological Science,* 16 (5), 367-371. doi: 10.1111/j.0956-7976.2005.01542.x

Killoran, I., & Adams, N. (2006). Why inclusion? In I. Killoran & M. Brown. *There's room for everyone: Accommodations, supports and transitions infancy to postsecondary*. Wheaton, MD: ACEI.

Killoran, I. (2005). Transition planning: The key to successful inclusion. *Focus on Inclusive Education Quarterly, 2*(4), 5-8.

Killoran, I. (2004). Understanding the child with sensory integration dysfunction. *Focus on Inclusive Education Quarterly, 2*(1), 3-7.

Magiati, I., & Howlin, P. (2003). A pilot evaluation study of the picture exchange communication system (PECS) for children with autistic spectrum disorders. *Autism*, 7 (3), 297-320.

Malmgren, K., & Causton-Theoharis, J. (2006). Boy in the bubble: Effects of paraprofessional proximity and other pedagogical decisions on the interactions of a student with behavioral disorders. *Journal of Research in Childhood Education, 20*(4), 301-312.

Mastrangelo, S., & Killoran, I. (2007). Play and the child with disabilities. In C. Jeandheur Ferguson & E. Dettore (Eds.), *To play or not to play: is it really a question?* (pp. 73-86). Olney, MD: Association for Childhood Education International.

MCathren, R. B., & Watson, A. L., (2001). Facilitating the development of intentional communication. In M. Ostrosky & S. Sandall (Eds.), *Teaching strategies: What to do to support young children's development. Young Exceptional Children, Monograph Series, No. 3* (pp. 25-35). Longmont, CO: Sopris West.

McCafferty, S. G. (2002). Gesture and creating zones of proximal development for second language learning. *The Modern Language Journal*, 86 (2), 192-203. doi: 10.1111/1540-4781.00144

McConnell, S. R. (2002). Interventions to facilitate social interaction for young children with autism: review of available research and recommendations for educational intervention and future research. *Journal of Autism and Developmental Disorders*, 32 (5), 351-372.

Mirenda, P. (2003). Toward functional augmentative and alternative communication forstudents with autism: manual signs, graphic symbols, and voice output communication aids. *Language, Speech and Hearing Services in Schools*, 34, 203-216.

Myles, B., Tapscott Cook, K., Miller, N., Rinner, L., & Robbins, L. (2000). *Asperger Syndrome and sensory issues: Practical solutions for making sense of the world. Kansas: AAPC.*

Murray, M., Hudson Baker, P., Murray-Slutsky, C., & Paris, B. (2009). Strategies for supporting the sensory-based learner. *Preventing School Failure*, 53 (4), 245-251.

Myles, B. S., Grossman, B. G., Aspy, R., Henry, S. A., & Bixler Coffin, A. (2007). Planning a comprehensive program for students with autism spectrum disorders using evidence-based practices. Education and Training in Developmental Disabilities, 42 (4), 398-409.

Ozonoff, S., & Miller, J. N. (1995). Teaching theory of mind: a new approach to social skills training for individuals with autism. Journal of Autism and Developmental Disorders, 25 (4), 415-433.

Prizant, B. M., Wetherby, A. M., Rubin, E., & Laurant, A. (2003). The SCERTS model: a transactional, family-centered approach to enhancing communication and socioemotional abilities of children with autism spectrum disorder. *Infants and Young Children*, 16 (4), 296-316.

Rotheram-Fuller, E., Kasari, C., Chamberlain, B., & Locke, J. (2010). Social involvement of children with autism spectrum disorders in elementary school classrooms. *The Journal of Child Psychology and Psychiatry*, 51 (11), 1227-1234. doi:10.1111/j.1469-7610.2010.02289.x

Sapon-Shevin, M. (2003). Inclusion: A matter of social justice. *Educational Leadership, 61*(2), 25-28. Retrieved on March 11, 2011 from http://pdonline.ascd.org/pd_online/inclusiveclassroom/el200310_saponshevin.html

Simpson, R. L. (2005). Evidence-based practices and students with autism spectrum disorders. *Focus on Autism and Other Developmental Disabilities*, 20 (3), 140-149. doi: 10.1177/10883576050200030201

Thiemann, K. L., & Goldstein, H. (2001). Social stories, written text cues, and video feedback: effects on social communication of children with autism. *Journal of Applied Behavioural Analysis*, 34 (4), 425-446. doi: 10.1901/jaba.2001.34-425.

Thungren, G., Ahlsen, E., & Dahlgren Sandberg, A. (2007). Children with autistic spectrum disorders and speech generating devices: communication in different activities at home. *Clinical Linguistics and Phonetics*, 21 (6), 457-479. doi: 10.1080/02699200701314963

Tincani, M. (2004). Comparing the picture exchange communication system and sign language training for children with autism. *Focus on Autism and Other Developmental Disabilities*, 19 (3), 152-163. doi: 10.1177/ 10883576040190030301

United Nations, (2006). The Convention on the Rights of Persons with Disabilities. Retrieved on March 20, 2011 from http://www.un.org/disabilities/convention/conventionfull.shtml

Walker, S., & Berthelsen, D. (2008). Children with autistic spectrum disorder in early childhood education programs: A social constructivist perspective on inclusion. *International Journal of Early Childhood*, 40 (1), 33-51.

Wang, S., & Parrila, R. (2008). Quality indicators for single-case research on social skill interventions for children with autistic spectrum disorder. *Developmental Disabilities Bulletin*, 36, 81-105.

Wolfberg, P. J., & Schuler A. L. (1993). ntegrated play groups: a model for promoting the social and cognitive dimensions of play in children with autism. *Journal Of Autism and Other Developmental Disorders*, 23 (3), 467-489.

Wong Bonggat, P., & Hall, L. J. (2010). Evaluation of the effects of sensory integration-based intervention by a preschool special education teacher. *Education and Training in Autism and Developmental Disabilities*, 45 (2), 294–302.

Yack, E., Aquilla, P., & Suttton, S. (2002). *Building bridges through sensory integration: Therapy for children with autism and other pervasive developmental disorders.* TX: Future Horizons.

Yoder, P. J., & Layton, T. L. (1988). Speech following sign language training in autistic children with minimal verbal language. *Journal of Autism and Developmental Disorders,* 18 (2), 217-229.

# 12

# Creating a Mediating Literacy Environment for Children with Autism - Ecological Model

Shunit Reiter[1], Iris Manor-Binyamini[1],
Shula Friedrich-Shilon[2], Levi Sharon[2] and Milana Israeli[2]
[1]*University of Haifa,*
[2]*Ofer School for students with Autism,*
*Israel*

## 1. Introduction

Positive long-term outcomes for individuals with autism spectrum disorders are strongly correlated with social communicative competence (National Research Council, 2001). Thus, when developing a comprehensive educational program, intervention should be across everyday social contexts and a range of social partners', not just the initial teaching situation. Although a range of methodologies call for the implementation of supports at specific times of the individuals day, vulnerabilities in social communicative competence are evident across every activity, every social partner and every social contest (Rubin et al, 2009. P-195).
Literacy in this broad sense is a vital tool for students with autism to understand their life-environment and integrate in the community as adults (Alberto et al, 2007). Therefore we extend the meaning of "literacy" in the context of autism beyond the ability to read and write texts, to the more fundamental processes of production and reception of information between the individual and the environment, which fulfill communicational, social, educational and recreational needs. Theoretical literature emphasizes visual perception as a major way of learning for students with autism, and is crucial in the development of literacy.
Interest in the literacy experiences and achievements of children with autism is relatively new. The impetus for this interest has evolved from a variety of sources, including the inclusion of more children with atypical levels of disabilities into the general education schools (Kaderavek and Rabidoux, 2004, p-237). Despite the increased attention directed to promoting literacy for inclusion, we currently have limited theoretical and practical models. The goal of this chapter is to present a working model that illustrates the process of constructing a visual literacy environment in an inclusion program at a school for autistic students over the course of five years. The model development is the product of a systematic thought process and it has important contribution in a few fields:

1. The educational model is the main outcome granted by the school to the Special Education system. The model can be easily replicated as a consequence of the methodological display of its components.
2. A common language: the educational model insures that the communication will be based common use by of the of teaching methods by the school staff.

3. An ecological system vision: the long term systematic development enables the study of the pattern of links and that exist between the different elements in the school.

This five year study was funded by the Department of Experimental Schools, Ministry of Education, Israel

## 2. Methodology

### 2.1 Research method

Case study is a common array in qualitative research. According to Stake (Stake, 1995), when the research goals are the understanding of human experience, case study is the appropriate method. Stake notes that the most interesting cases in education and social studies are of people who operate within interactive organizational settings. In this study, the organizational setting is an entity with boundaries that are set by a given timeframe - the timeframe is five years of learning. The place - the place investigated is the Ofer Special Education School for children with autism. The participants - the participants are all the participating professionals, the families of the students and the community at large. The change presented in this article is a complex change. Vosniadou and his colleagues (Vosniadou et al., 2001) claim that change processes occur gradually. The investigation of a long-range ethnographic case makes it possible to follow the gradual change processes, define the change and gain an insight to those the professionals working within the educational system. The choice to investigate pedagogical change in a special education school is due to a number of reasons: the first one is that it is possible to learn from this school since it is an experimental school. In addition, an investigation of this kind of school makes it possible to present a comprehensive description including a large number of details, thus enabling us to gain new insights. Finally, as Shulman notes (Shulman,1986), case study is appropriate for educational research when the situation is complex and when it is difficult to operate a methodology of controlled variables within the given situation.

Ethnography - This is a scientific field dealing with the study of the customs of a single society. The ethnographic approach is focused on direct personal observation of social behavior within a specific culture in terms that are as close as possible to the way that the members of that particular culture perceive the world (Geerts, 1973: 1983). Ethnography was chosen as the methodology for this study due to various reasons: first, ethnographic research requires a wide, in-depth and comprehensive view, as much as possible, while stressing what is called in research "self-explanatory understanding". Schutz (Schutz, 1971) stresses that the self-explanatory understandings turn into social and cultural understandings manifested in the context of that particular culture only. The current study focuses on the development of a social culture within an educational organization for students with autism. Secondly, the ethnographic methodology makes it possible to focus on interactive systems and on processes related to behavioral patterns in situations involving complex psychological dynamics (Manor-Binyamini, 2010). It can be assumed that the development of the topic investigated follows the definition of complex psychological dynamics. Thirdly, this methodology, requiring a long range daily involvement in the research field, make it possible to use "Thick Description" (Geerts, 1973), i.e. a rich description of reality.

## 2.2 Research process

The study presented in this article followed the work of approximately 70 professionals as well as 90 students and their families at a special education school attended by students with autism at the age of 6-21. The study conducted between 2004-2009 made use of interviews, observations, documentation of interdisciplinary team meetings and videos of lessons. The data collection was made in a number of centers: the students, the school, the parents and the community.

## 2.3 Research tools

Interviews - The type of interview used in this study was a semi-structured interview. The advantage of an interview of this type is that it is guided and focused according to the topics associated with the research goals, and at the same time, it makes it possible for the interviewee to have the freedom of wide range responses. In addition, this type of interview makes it possible to effectively utilize time. This type of interview is methodical in its essence and it makes it possible to compare the responses of different interviewees (Zabar Ben-Yehoshue , 1999). Another major/important point is that an interview of this type is most suitable for the clarification of a research question that does not focus on the actual existence or non-existence of the objective reality but rather on the meaning given to it by the person investigating. The interviews were narrative. The interviewees were educators, aides and parents. Each interview lasted approximately one hour. All interviewees were asked the same questions and all of them expressed their consent to participate in the study. The interview and the observation are the main data collection tool in qualitative studies (Friedman, 2005).
Data collection through observation included approximately 30 observations of lessons that took place in each classroom once a week. The population present at the lessons were the teacher, the aides and the students. The aides were instructed on how to work during these lessons.
At addition to observations of lessons, video recording were made of approximately ten lessons at different classrooms in the school. Video recording make it possible to see the participants' body language, the classroom atmosphere as well as the communicative and behavioral aspects, such as: gestures and the students' initiative beyond the words pronounced during the lesson. Video recording are an additional source of information
The study has also recorded approximately 40 meetings of the interdisciplinary team / the educators on this topic. The meetings were documented throughout the five years of the study. Each meeting lasted for approximately two hours and regularly took place on Tuesdays. Each meeting was attended by the school's entire multi-professional team. The meetings were part of the team's institutional learning courses each year.

## 2.4 Analysis of the data

Analysis of the data was based on the processes of grounded theory. This analysis included three phases:
**The first phase of the analysis - initial analysis.** It started with the ongoing reading and observation of the research materials collected. The reading and observation activities were conducted by the two researchers and an additional professional. They read and observed all the research findings individually. In addition, three meetings took place, during which a joint analysis of the interviews was made. Also, each of the researchers observed on her own the lessons that had been recorded, while focusing on the participants' body language and the

classroom atmosphere. The goal of the ongoing and complete reading and observation was to provide us with a wide and comprehensive orientation without losing the context of the data (Dey, 1993: Charmaz, 2000). At this phase, we divided the data into data segments, each of them serving as a 'meaning unit'. Each 'meaning unit' was a segment of data that dealt with a certain topic. We named each of the meaning units by names that reflected the name of the segment. The names were as close as possible to the language of the population investigated, involving almost no conceptualization, without attempting to find a common denominator with equivalent meaning units. At this phase, we carefully examined the data, verbatim, line after line and sentence after sentence. In each line, we asked what the topic of the line/sentence was - without losing the whole picture of the entire information.

**The second phase of the analysis - mapping analysis.** We examined each meaning unit that we had created in the initial analysis as well as the names accompanying them, and we searched for the connections and/or relationships existing between them. We formulated categories and sub-categories by combining meaning units having the same topic and giving the same name to all the units that had been diagnosed as having the same topic. These meaning units were identified as belonging to sub-categories, and later on, to one category (Pidgeon & Henwood, 1996). We made comparisons while searching for relationships between the meaning segments, and searching for associations between the categories. In addition, we combined categories into themes.

**The third phase of the analysis - focusing analysis.** At this phase of the analysis, we focused the categories and the data segments attributed to them into a coherent explanation for the themes and we analysed them. The product of this phase is the ethnographic model that will be presented later on. Since the study is ethnographic, we analysed the findings of the study. The research team presented the findings to the entire school team throughout the years of research and received feedback from them.

## 3. Findings

It is possible to present the research findings in a summarizing model. We will present the model and explain each of the spheres involved in it, including examples that will demonstrate the practice existing in the school that is being investigated (See figure number 1)

The model is as follows:

The model presented consists of three spheres:

The first sphere, which is the external sphere, is focused on the participants of the educational activity. They include the following: students-classroom, family, school and community. The second sphere, which is more internal, presents three major themes upon which the school work is based. These themes are as follows: literacy, inclusion and mediation (this sphere is the basis for the school work and we will therefore discuss it at length in this article). The last sphere, which is the most experienced internal developmental transition present throughout the years by the students of this school starting from first grade up to the transition into the community. This sphere has five types of Transition Phases.

### 3.1 The first sphere

**Details on the population taking part in the educational activity**

**Student/classroom -** The school population has on the autism spectrum disorders varying degrees of intellectual disability - from mild intellectual disability to intermediate

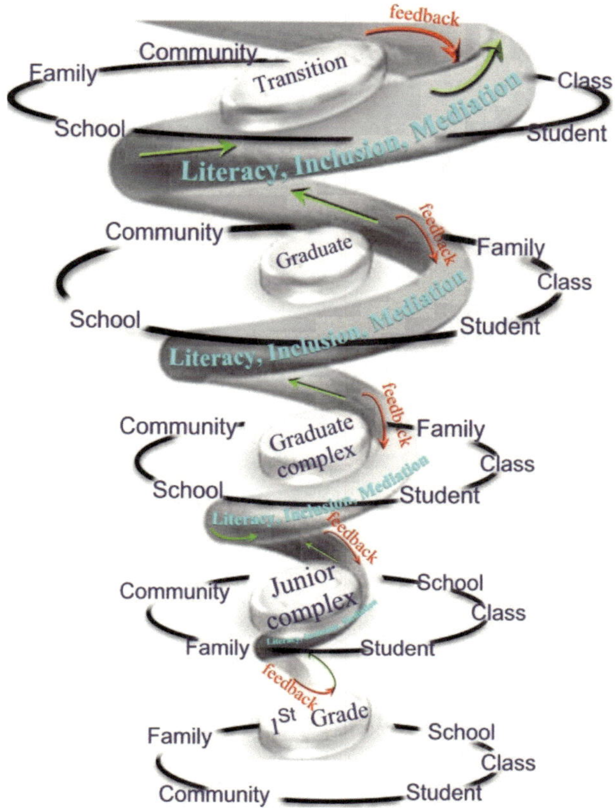


Fig. 1. Mediating Literacy Environment for Children with Autism- Ecological model

intellectual disability. The main diagnosis of the students is autism. Approximately 50% of the students are non-verbal. Approximately 80% of the students are assisted by Augmentative and Alternative Communication (AAC) at varying levels of complexity. Approximately 85% of the students acquire reading skills with the help of PCS symbols. Some of them make progress towards the acquisition of phonetic reading.

**The classroom -** There are approximately 13 classrooms in the school. Each class has approximately 8 students. There is a teacher and an aide in each class. Each class has a homeroom teacher and complementary teacher. The school has a school syllabus from which the team assembles the classroom syllabus at the beginning of each school year. In addition, the classroom team prepares the IEP for each student, which is based on the strength and needs according to the school and class syllabuses. The IEP is written in collaboration with the family, the group home (in case the student that lives outside the family home), additional caregivers within the community, if there are any, taking into account the difficulties and needs of the family. The discussions on the students/class progress are conducted with the multi-professional team which includes the class educational team, the aides, the Para-medical, professional and care-giving team.

**The school -** The school investigated was founded 15 years ago. It was recognized as an experimental school by the Department of Experimental Schools, Ministry of Education, Israel. At the time of the study, there were approximately 90 students learning in eleven homerooms. The team includes 70 persons (including administrative personnel). The school operates for eleven and a half months during the school year, five days a week between 8:00 am and 4:45 pm, and on Fridays between 8:00 am and 12:45 pm. There is an additional activity in school operated by the Alut Club (Alut - The Israeli Autism Society) on days when there is no activity conducted by the Ministry of Education (on holiday eves and holiday breaks). 25% of the students are girls and 75% are boys. 30% of the students live in group homes outside their family homes. The age of students is between 6-21. They are divided into two age divisions: the younger division (age 6-13), the older division (age 13-21). The divisions are distinguished according to the level of the contents being taught as well as the emphasis on daily activities. For example: emphasis within the older division is on the inclusion in work within the community. The school provides ongoing training and guidance of teaching interns as well as student/teachers and para-medical professions. The school is a regional school accepting students from approximately ten districts. In addition, the school accepts students from a variety of cultural backgrounds (secular, religious, Jewish, Christian, Muslim and new immigrants from different countries).

**The family -** According to professionals, the role of the school is to create a sense of parental capability and equip the home with tools that make it possible to cope with the students in their home as well. The school is attentive to the needs of the families. It accompanies the families with the help of the school's educational, care-giving and medical (pediatrician, psychiatrist, neurologist) team. A social worker and psychologist are available in the school for the parents, helping them to cope throughout the years of study in the school.

During the experiment, the team became aware of the great importance of the family's involvement in the students' educational and therapeutic progress. Therefore, several family workshops have been developed. These workshops are intended to provide the enormous needs of the families and to strengthen the dyadic contact between the parents and their children. In addition, the team members became aware of the significance of the relationship between the siblings of children with autism, and the need to provide support to the siblings as well. (See details later on).

**The community -** The community includes all the entities with which the students are in contact with outside the school, such as: inclusion schools, the Children's Library at the University of Haifa, the Art Museum, the IDF (Israel Defense Forces), dentists, residential facilities within the community, workplaces etc.

### 3.2 The second sphere

As can be seen in Illustration No. 1, this sphere is the base of the school activity, and therefore we are going to discuss it in-depth. The experiment involved three major topics throughout the five years of the research duration: literacy, inclusion and mediation. Throughout these years, it was possible to follow the three themes and the way that they were structured into the school work. We are going to present each theme including examples in each of them.

*Literacy*

Literacy is a communicative tool for students with autism. Literacy within the school investigated includes a variety of visual means, including visual reading, the global identification of words and graphic symbols assisting the students decipher the environment in which they live and act in it according to acceptable codes. Table No. 1 presents the literacy centers in school in regard to the transition stages. We stress that for each age group, there are adjustments made according to the students' level and ability.

| Transition stages | Alternative supporting communication | Reading & writing | Listening & speaking | Genres |
|---|---|---|---|---|
| Entering first grade | | Emphasis on different reading methods and adjusting them for the school students. Using accepted symbol system to produce written communication | Responding to initiated communication | Following directions |
| Younger age group | | Attempting to teach phonologic awareness and not only logo-graphic awareness. Writing the alphabet Writing words and expanding the written vocabulary | Responding to initiated communication. Initiative for communicative social interaction | Greetings Songs Short story Fables |
| Older age group | | Emphasis on the use of global words (identification, comprehension of meaning, ability to choose a word and use it in daily living. Writing words and expanding the written vocabulary. Writing sentences, if possible. | Responding to initiated communication. Initiative for communicative social interaction. Initiated participation in learning processes and social processes | Newspaper? Advertisements in all of the media channels. Supermarket list. Invitation. Note. Announcement. |
| Preparing to go into the community | | Guiding the community on the topic of autism, the importance of visual support, and the existing tools intended to improve the students' comprehension and expression. The communities learn about the tools and structure the environment for the students. | | |

Table 1. The Literacy Centers in Each of the Transition Stages

*Inclusion*

The model guiding the experiment in the school investigated is the ecological model. This model assumes that the student is not the source of the problem, and that therefore he/she is not the only change agent. Therefore, in order to create change in the quality of inclusion, the school team should carry out the change - the adjustments required - within the close and faraway environment, assuming that this change would affect the student's functioning. This means that the goal of the school is that the community carrying out the inclusion (the nuclear and extended family) the homeroom class in special education, the inclusion class, the class given at the community center, the Sick Fund physician, the residential place, the workplace etc.) will eventually be able to take up the school's role in guiding the student and in assisting him/her in the best and safest absorption into it while providing support and guidance by the school team. Due to the awareness of the difficulties involved in the field and the desire to make the inclusion process more effective for the school students as well as the teacher and students in the regular schools, a new role has been created in the school - the coordinator of inclusions. The position of the coordinator of inclusions involves the following:

- The preparation of the teacher and students carrying out the inclusion prior to the arrival of the students with autism at the inclusive setting.
- Follow-up of the students' progress and guidance of the teacher carrying out the inclusion throughout the inclusion process.
- The formation of contact between the homeroom teacher carrying out the inclusion and the homeroom teacher of the student being included for the purpose of adjusting the teaching materials, the continuation of work within the classroom and the provision of assistance to the team carrying out the inclusion.
- Ongoing training for the aides carrying out the inclusion on behalf of the school.

According to the analysis of the research findings, the way in which the school team perceives the inclusion within the community is that first of all it is related to the inclusion of the students within their **homes**, and with **the students' family members.** The school's role is to create a sense of parental capability and equip the home with the tools required to cope with the students at home too. The school attends to the needs of the families. There are support groups (parents, siblings) and a variety of dyadic workshops (agriculture, leisure time) intended to serve as support as well as enrich the parents' toolbox.

There are different types of inclusions in the school intended to "adjust" the "appropriate attire" to each student, out of the awareness that inclusion is important and that the students are capable of being in an inclusion setting. The school assumes responsibility and it mediates between the various inclusion spheres since the inclusion activities require collaboration between the classroom teams, between the school teams and the teams outside the school as well as between the parents and the school team. Details of the inclusions existing in the school are given below. Table No. 2 presents the nature and spheres of inclusions existing in the school in the transition phases.

*Mediation*

Mediation in the school is manifested in making the environment accessible to students with autism. During the years when the experiment was conducted, the school professionals perceive the concept of making the environment accessible by including the following elements:

| Transition Phases | Inclusion Forms | Inclusion Spheres |
|---|---|---|
| Entering first grade | Forming a class within a new setting | Inclusion within the classroom's students<br>Dyadic activities in collaboration with parents and under the guidance of a music therapist. |
| Younger age group | Learning inclusions<br>Social inclusions<br>Parties for age groups<br>Going out into community public institutions (university, museums, supermarket etc.) | • Inclusions within the school - the students learn outside their homeroom classes, i.e. they are placed in other classes according to their level, ability and fields of interest. For example: a student who likes English and this subject is not being taught in his/her homeroom class, is placed in another class during English lessons.<br>• Inclusions in regular schools in a variety of subjects (Hebrew, mathematics, English, computers, art, music, gym etc.).<br>• Inclusions within the school - students from regular schools arrive at a lesson/therapy in the school.<br>• Inclusion of a student in another class - outside his/her homeroom class.<br>• A variety of therapies given to pairs of students (art, music, movement, yoga, animals, communication etc.).<br>• Mentoring activities: one student serves as a mentor to another student;<br>• An older age group class serves as mentors to a younger age group class. This mentorship serves as a way to learn to assume responsibility, to be able to provide explanations, accompaniment and assistance to others. (It is important to note that sometimes inclusion starts as full mentorship provided by the older student to the younger one, and as the process continues, |

| | | |
|---|---|---|
| | | it is possible to see how both of them grow, and at he end - there is no difference between the mentor and the trainee). |
| Older age group | Learning and social inclusions<br>Parties for age groups<br>Going out into community public institutions (university, museums, supermarket etc.)<br>Workshops: jewelry, chorus, orchestra<br>Preparation for going out to live in group homes<br>Inclusions within the workplace | • Inclusions in regular schools in a variety of subjects (Hebrew, mathematics, Bible, English, computers, art, music, gym etc.).<br>• Inclusions within the school - students from a regular school arrive to lessons/therapy within the school.<br>• Inclusion of a student in another class - outside his/her homeroom class.<br>• A variety of therapies given to pairs of students (art, music, movement, yoga, animals, communication etc.).<br>• Mentorship activity; one student serves as mentor fro another student; an older age group class serves as mentor for a younger age group class. |
| Preparation to go out into the community | Providing guidance to the community carrying out the inclusion on the topic of the autistic disorder, the importance of visual support and the tools existing for the improvement of the students' comprehension and expression. The community learns how to use the tools and structure the environment for the students. | |

Table 2. The nature and spheres of inclusions existing in the school in the transition phases

1. An environment that is clear and structured for the student, based upon literacy means due to being familiar with the characteristics of the autistic disorder, and the visual channel being the strength of these students.
2. A safe and familiar environment that minimizes anxiety.
3. An environment that enables the students to express themselves and is responsive to them, i.e. it is flexible enough to "follow" the students.
4. An environment requiring that the students utilize their potential, i.e. an environment presenting challenges and new situations to the student and encouraging them to adjust.
5. An environment that provides the students with the tools to adjust and gives them the time required to adjust safely and successfully. The team enables the student to have the

experience, make mistakes, ask and request help prior to helping the child. According to this perception, doing things rather than letting the students do it themselves would only serve the short-term goals for the students but would cause long-term damage. Mediation helps students understand and internalize the material studied.

Based upon this definition, the work carried out in the school as part of this experiment, as observed and documented during the year of the research simultaneously, by each of the participants was as follows:

1. **On the student and class level** - teaching communicative tools, the way to act within the family and community, and coping with transitions, difficulties and frustrations. As part of the initiative, the students are provided with literacy tools required for communication (communication boards, social stories, behavioral codes etc.). Unlike other schools that teach literacy for the purpose of obtaining information and enrichment, the teaching of literacy at the Ofer School is not only the goal but mainly a means of achieving communication - for the purpose of improving the students' comprehension and expression.
2. **On the team level -** professionalism on the topic of autism, the implications of this disorder, the characteristics of learning and the ways to bypass the communication and language difficulties. Learning occurs within workshops and team meetings through the literature review of articles, joint learning, the teaching of colleagues etc.).
3. **On the family level -** Guidance and consultation, participation in professional workshops given to the educational team, empowerment of parental capability, active participation in the school activities. Full participation of the family in the work process, guidance by the educational and therapeutic team, dyadic workshops, workshops for siblings and sending supportive communication cards and teaching materials to the students' homes. Continuous updating through the school website and forum - it is difficult for many parents to go out when their son/daughter is home, and therefore, many parents do not participate in meetings, courses and parent-teacher meetings. The school website and forum serve as an important tool in maintaining contact with the school: the forum provides professional answers to parents' questions. There are many links on the school website to other websites on autistic disorder and there is a database of symbols for home use by the parents.

   There is ongoing contact with **residential settings outside the home** (group homes and workplaces within the community) according to need.
4. **On the community level -** Guidance and consultation (on autism, the implications of this disorder, the characteristics of learning and the ways to overcome the communication and language difficulties), accompaniment of the settings carrying out the inclusion (the principals, teachers and students) - prior to, during and after the completion of the students' studies at the school, being in touch with additional educational settings prior to the students' entrance into school (kindergartens, schools), presenting the school work model: in professional conferences dealing with autism, communication and literacy, participation in a number of experimental schools on behalf of the Department of Experimental Schools, Ministry of Education, Israel, establishing district courses in educational settings for students with autism in order to expose the work method practiced in the school and provide instruction to educational and therapeutic teams, hosting the visits of university students studying in the departments of communication and special education of the universities and colleges in the region, instruction of special education and communication interns studying at the universities and colleges in the region.

| Transition Phases | Literacy means to making the environment accessible | The importance of accessibility for students with autism |
|---|---|---|
| Entering first grade | Structuring the daily agenda with words or alternative supportive communication.<br>Dividing the lesson into defined and measurable units; beginning, middle and end.<br>Providing details of the products expected at the end of the task (for example; two worksheets; gluing 10 labels continuously; inserting cards into 20 envelopes etc.).<br>Preparing ahead of time to anticipated changes (for example: a substitute teacher, going out on a trip, a guest arriving at the classroom) through the use of symbols and social stories. | Concern over the unknown and unexpected make the students with autism feel tense and distract them. A change in their daily routine (even change that is perceived by us as being "a change for the better") can cause emotional turmoil and anxiety. Structuring the daily agenda visually at the beginning of each day, clarifying what is to be expected every hour and every lesson, and preparing the students ahead for time for each change helps calm them down and enable them to focus on the task ahead of them. |
| Younger age group | The "Café Ofer" menu - the students order drinks and food from the waiters by using menus with symbols.<br>Defining the behavioral rules in inclusion while using clear rules or symbols for the purpose of clarifying what is expected from the students who are going through the inclusion process: what is allowed, what is prohibited, recess time, when inclusion begins and ends. | The use of menus makes it possible for students experiencing difficulty in speech to realize their right of choice and reduce their dependence upon the accompanying teacher/aide.<br>Clear behavioral rules reduce anxiety and help the students understand what is to be expected of them at the place that carries out the inclusion process. |
| Older age group | The "Café Ofer" menu - the waiters receive orders from students who experience difficulties with speech through the menu that includes symbols.<br>The use of a menu with symbols at the dining room - each student orders his/her lunch from the menu.<br>The work rules or behavior rules expected at the place of inclusion are presented ahead of time and placed in a location that is accessible to the students.<br>Defining the beginning and end of the work, the daily agenda and the production expected (in school or at | The use of menus - the waiters mediate to their colleagues rather than the teaching team. |

| | | |
|---|---|---|
| | the workplace) – all of this is done through the use of visual cues that the students are able to comprehend. | |
| Preparation to go out into the community | Prior to the inclusion process, the community learns about the purpose of having the environment structured for students with autism and its importance for utilizing the students' potential.<br>This is a WIN-WIN situation: the community gains a person who is less dependent. The community is capable to cope with the difficulty on its own, and the students gain a community that includes them due to being willing rather than by being coerced to do so out of the Special Education Law.<br>As the inclusion process proceeds, the school representative fades out and transfers the responsibility for structuring the environment and mediating the environment to the students and to the representatives of the community carrying out the inclusion. | |

Table 3. Mediation as a means to making the environment accessible

- **A Dictionary of Symbols** has been developed by the school, the goal of which is to enable the multi-professional team to use a uniform language in all of the classes and age groups. The use of a uniform language is essential mainly at the time of transition from one class to another, between age groups, between different teachers and upon going out into the community. The uniformity of symbols makes it possible to have a continuum. It leads to uniformity for both the team and the students.
- Clarification: additional means for the accessibility of the environment are added at each age group – this is done in addition to continuing the use of the means learned in the earlier classes according to need and the extent of detail that each student requires.

**The third sphere** – as can be seen in the illustration, No. 1 forms the inner sphere of the school work and it represents the transitions. The professionals perceive the transitions as a continuum of learning and development in regard to each student starting from the first day in school up to the age of 21. According to this perception, the school team establish a transition plan. We are going to expand the discussion on two major transitions for the family and the students: the transition from kindergarten to the Ofer School, and the transition from the school into the community. The reason for the focus on these two transitions is as follows: the first grade is the entrance into school. The class resembles a kindergarten setting at the beginning of the year. During the year, the students acquire learning habits and a school setting. The students begin to take part in the activity of the entire school. In the second grade, the students move to a phase in which they are part of the school and then, they start going out to inclusion within the community. The different between sixth grade and seventh grade is in the contents of their studies and in the topics emphasized. The focus starts to be on the anticipation towards the training for adult living as well as working and living within the community. This includes functional relatedness to the academic lessons such as reading (for example: reading a recipe, writing a supermarket list), arithmetic (for example: the use of money and , reading the clock and telling the time of day.) and civics (receiving an Israeli Identity Card is one example).

A practical description of the two programs is as follows:

**The program of the transition from kindergarten to school:**

a. Inviting the kindergarten children to activities throughout the school year.
b. Inviting the parents of the kindergarten children to an introduction meeting with the school.
c. Prior to the arrival of students from kindergarten to first grade, the school team receives the child's file from the kindergarten teacher (diagnoses, observations) - and the entire information enters the school at the same time. The relevant information is also transferred to the social worker in the municipality. (According to the Privacy Protection Law, the transfer of information is made only following the parents signed written consent).

**The program of transition from school to the community:**

a. An occupational team has been established in the school. This team includes an occupational therapist, professional teachers and an educational team of the older age group which has prepared a study array for the students towards going out to work within the community.
b. Instruction and accompaniment for the students when they go out to a workplace that is suitable to their ability and fields of interest. There is instruction and accompaniment at the workplace by the educational team on behalf of the school. The instruction of the team includes explanation on the essence of making the environment accessible to the students through the use of literacy means and the provision of tools for the right accessibility.
c. As part of the learning of occupation and work experience, the "Café in School" was established. The students learned about the management and operation of a Coffee Shop in a theoretical and practical manner. The food at the Coffee Shop was prepared and served by the students. The Coffee Shop served the students and the team once a week. The students' parents are invited during events that take place at school to sit at the Coffee Shop and enjoy what their sons/daughters had prepared.

## 4. Discussion and summary

The discussion will focus on the contribution and limitations of the model presented in this chapter. This model has a number of theoretical and practical contributions:

a. This model demonstrates that children with autism as well as children with multiple-problems and complex disorders develop to a great extent according to normal developmental stages. As the environment would make it possible to have a variety of options and would adjust to the student instead of expecting the student to adjust to the environment, so would the students' development be better and their inclusion within society would be of greater quality.

b. The model developed at the school shows that a comprehensive educational environment that applies a variety of therapeutic methods, i.e. an environment that is familiar with a wide variety of treatment methods of autism and that knows how to make an educated decision that is suitable to the needs of each student (rather than work according to a single method) in a flexible manner in the learner's natural environment, advances the learner's development.
c. Some of the activities that have taken place at the school throughout the years of the research are group activities (unlike one-on-one work). In other words: the school setting makes it possible to establish groups of students according to subject, age, the students' fields of interest. This is impossible to do in a one-on-one intervention.
d. In the practical aspect, the model serves as a contribution to the inclusion of students with autism within schools that carry out the inclusion since it can be implemented in schools that are inclusive.
e. The study and the school's entrance into a research-based experimental process lead to the development of a professional team. This kind of team asks questions and is aware of the need for different solutions for both the individual student and for the same student during the different spheres of his/her life.
f. The research work along the work at school leads to the development of a multi-professional team possessing professional humility and collaboration with the parents.

### 4.1 Limitations of the study

The model presented does not provide an answer to multi-cultural conditions, to immigrants from Russia, to Arab children, to differences in culture. This is a topic that needs an answer. There are several students of Ethiopian origin in the school. There are Arab students in the school where the school has no interaction/contact with their communities. There are also Ethiopian children for whom there is no knowledge or tools for cultural issues and challenges that a child with autism would raise in this community, and the same is true for the religious community.

It would be desirable to expand the work and research on this work with the family, starting from the nuclear family and the extended family. Following this study, the need to expand the work model with the nuclear and extended family was raised. This topic was raised during meetings with parents who pointed out the challenge that they are facing from the moment that their child is diagnosed as being on the autistic spectrum.

## 5. References


Alberto, P, A,. Fredrick, L,. Hughes, M,. McIntosh, L,. & Cihak, D. (2007). Components of Visual Literacy: Teaching Logos. *Focus on Autism and other Developmental Disabilities.* 22(4).

Charmaz, . ( 2000). Grounded theory: Objectivist and constructivist methods. In N. K. Denzin & Y. S. Lincoln *Handbook of qualitative research* (Second edition) (pp. 509-535). London: Sage Publications

Dey, I. (1993). Qualitative data analysis. London: Rutledge.

Friedman, Y., (2005). Measuring and evaluating the social and educational programs. Jerusalem: Henrietta zold Institute.

Geertz, C. (1973). *The Interpretation of Culture.* Basic Books. New York.

Geertz, C. (1983). *Local Knowledge*. Basic Books. New York.

Kaderavek, J,. & Rabidoux, R,.(2004). Interactive to independent literacy: a model for designing literacy goals for children with atypical communication. *Reading& Writing Quarterly,* 20. 237-260.

Manor-Binyamini, I. (2011). A Model of Ethnographic Discourse Analysis for an Interdisciplinary Team. *Journal of Pragmatics,* 43. 1997-2011.

National Research Council. (2001). *Educating children with autism.* Committee on Educational Interventions for Children with Autism, Division of Behavioral and Social Sciences and Education. Washington, DC: National Academies Press.

Pidgeon, N. & Henwood, K. (1996). Grounded theory: practical implementation. In John T. R. Richardson (Ed.), *Handbook of qualitative research methods* (pp.86-101). Leicester: The British Psychological Society Books.

Schutz, A,. (1971). The stranger: In : Schutz, A. (Ed.), *School and Society*. Open University Press

Stake, R.E. (1995). *The art of case study research*. Thousand Oaks, CA: Sage.

Shulman, L. (1986). "Those who understand: knowledge growth in teaching". *Educational Researcher* 15/2 pp 4-14.

Rubin, E,. Laurent, A, C,. Prizant, B, M,. & Wetherby, M. (2009). AAC and the SCERTS MODEL. In Mirenda, P. & Lacono, T. *Autism Spectrum Disorders and AAC*. Paulh Brookes Publishing.

Zabar Ben-Yehoshue. N. (1999). *Qualitative research in Teaching and Learning* . Massada Publishing (Hebrew).

Vosniadou, S., Ioannides, C., Dimitrakopoulou, A. & Papademetriou, E. (2001). Designing learnig environment to promote conceptual change in science. *Learning and Instruction,* 36, 381-419.

# 13

# Self-Regulation, Dysregulation, Emotion Regulation and Their Impact on Cognitive and Socio-Emotional Abilities in Children and Adolescents with Autism Spectrum Disorders

Nader-Grosbois Nathalie
*Catholic University of Louvain*
*Belgium*

## 1. Introduction

The literature about typically developing children describes the development of models and the results of empirical studies focusing on self-regulation, emotion regulation and co-regulation during interactions with adults or peers. By contrast, it is only in the last decade that these processes have been examined in atypical children, including children with ASD. Infantile autism is a pervasive developmental disorder characterized by disturbances concerning not only the areas of socialization and communication but also the ability to modify and change behaviour. In recent studies on children with ASD, in order to better understand their deficits in cognitive and social activities, the specificities of their ability or inability to manage and regulate their own behaviour and emotions have been considered. Before the appearance of conceptual models and studies on regulation processes in children with ASD, several models of their deficits or specificities in the mobilization of their executive functions had previously been developed; these models cannot be ignored for the understanding of new conceptions of regulation.

This chapter focuses on the impact of specificities of executive functioning, self-regulation and dysregulation on cognitive and socio-emotional abilities in children and adolescents with autism spectrum disorders (ASD). Firstly, we define self-regulation and emotion regulation and explain briefly how these processes develop during typical childhood, and what factors play a role in this evolution. This may help to identify more accurately the differences that appear in children with ASD. Secondly, we present several conceptual models of executive function and regulation in children with ASD, in order to approach their atypical micro-genetic functioning and macro-genetic development, as well as some empirical studies that have confirmed these models. The impact of deficits of self-regulation and dysregulation on their functional abilities and on their development in different areas is highlighted. In particular, we point to the specificities of children with ASD in the area of emotion regulation. On the basis of this literature, we propose an integrative model of functioning and development of children with ASD. Finally, we suggest some perspectives for future research and we give guidelines for assessment and intervention.

## 2. Self-regulation, emotion regulation and executive functions: definitions

Particularly over the last two decades, self-regulation has often been studied in typically developing people, generating a range of conceptions and methodological approaches in the areas of developmental psychology, learning psychology and cognitive education (Bandura, 1997; Boekaerts, 1999; Boekaerts et al., 2000; Bronson, 2000; Vygotsky, 1978; Zimmerman, 2000). Self-regulation uses executive functions, which are neuropsychological processes that permit the physical, emotional and social self-control necessary to maintain goal oriented-actions; they include inhibition of responses, working memory, shifting attention, cognitive flexibility, planning of actions and fluency (Corbett et al., 2009; Mottron, 2004; Ozonoff et al., 1991; Rajendran & Mitchell, 2007; Russell, 1997).

On the basis of a review of literature generated by various theories of self-regulation in the areas of developmental psychology, learning psychology and cognitive education, an integrated model of self- and other-regulation has been developed (Nader-Grosbois, 2007a; Nader-Grosbois et al., 2008). This model approaches self-regulation as a dynamic process that mobilizes one's personal resources and resources in the material and social environment in order to solve various goal-oriented problems. It distinguishes seven self-regulated strategies in the learner (operationally described in a validated coding grid): identification of objective, planning or exploration of means, self-regulated attention, self-motivation, joint attention, behaviour regulation and self-evaluation; it also distinguishes seven corresponding other-regulation strategies that could be displayed by the partner or the adult. This other-regulation could be favourable or unfavourable to the development of self-regulation in children, depending on its adjustment (Nader-Grosbois et al., 2008).

In addition, emotion regulation corresponds to a set of processes by which an individual assesses, controls and modifies his or her spontaneous emotional responses in order to accomplish his or her goals or to express socially adequate emotional behaviour (Eisenberg et al., 2000, 2006, 2007; Gross & Thompson, 2007; Luminet, 2002; Mikolajczak et al., 2009; Nader-Grosbois, 2009; Thompson, 1994). According to these authors, by his or her manner of mentally conceiving an emotional situation, a person may modify the type of his or her emotional states and the duration of his or her emotional responses or their intensity: the regulation may amplify or inhibit emotional responses, using various strategies[1]. Various levels of regulation come into the picture: emotions may act as regulators themselves, or they may be regulated or it could at any rate be desirable to regulate them in social interactions (Rimé, 2007). Emotion regulation is therefore regarded as an element in emotional intelligence[2], which plays a role in the construction of social intelligence (Salovey et al., 1993). Emotion regulation has implication for social communication, in which emotions have the function of organizing the relationships of individuals to their environment, and are the basis of socialization, and also of social sharing (Eisenberg et al., 2000, 2006; Rimé, 2007; Thompson, 1994). The regulation contributing to individuals'

[1]In this instance, the person may select the situation (according to the probability of desirable or non desirable emotions); modify the situation (according to emotional impact); focus her attention only on particular aspects of the situation; operate a cognitive change about the meaning of this situation in order to appreciate her abilities to cope with it; and finally, regulate her emotional, behavioural, verbal and physiological responses (Eisenberg et al., 2006; Gross, 1998; Luminet, 2002).

[2]Emotional intelligence corresponds to the ability to control and differentiate between our own emotions and those of others, and to use these indications to guide our actions and thoughts.

adjustment to the environment activates internal and external processes responsible for supervising, assessing and modifying emotional reactions in the course of realization of goals (Brun & Mellier, 2004[3]; Thompson, 1994).

## 3. Self-regulation and emotion regulation in typically developing children

### 3.1 How does self-regulation develop in typically developing children?

The ability to identify objectives and to plan sequences of actions emerges when the child becomes capable of mental representation around the age of two years, and develops in later periods of life. In various contexts, even in daily scripts, the child aims at more and more complex goals; his or her planning becomes more systematic and varies depending on the requirements of the task (Bronson, 2000; Chang & Burns, 2005; Friedman & Scholnick, 1997; Gardner & Rogoff, 1990; Gauvain, 1999; Hudson & Fivush, 1991; Hudson et al., 1995; Nader-Grosbois, 2007a; Parrila et al., 1996; Prevost et al., 1995; Sethi et al., 2000; St-Laurent & Moss, 2002). Strengthened by the metacognitive awareness of the child's own cognitive process, self-regulated attention enables attention to the task to be controlled by removing distractions (Chang & Burns, 2005; Friedman & Scholnick, 1997; Zimmerman, 2000) and helps with planning (Parrila et al., 1996; Silverman & Ippolito, 1997). By identifying errors, the learner adjusts his or her actions, inhibits inadequate responses and initiates alternative strategies; he or she self-evaluates (Boekaerts, 1996; Nader-Grosbois, 2007a; Pintrich, 1999; Stipek et al., 1992; Wood & Wood, 1999; Zimmerman, 2000). Self-motivation guides the choice of goals, and implies the maintenance of a plan of action despite obstacles and required effort; the learner self-administers consequences for his or her behaviour, displays positive self-reinforcement, and experiences emotional reactions depending on the feeling of self-efficacy (Boekaerts, 1996; Chang & Burns, 2005; Nader-Grosbois, 2007a; Pintrich, 1999; Wolters, 2003; Zimmerman, 2000).

Moreover, the learner may adapt conditions in the learning environment (Zimmerman, 2000). Depending on his or her difficulty in solving tasks, the learner mobilizes the social environment, through communicated requests. He or she regulates the partner's behaviour by requesting help or a demonstration, or by seeking approval for his or her actions; he or she initiates referential joint attention toward the partner (Bandura, 1997; DeCooke & Brownell, 1999; De la Ossa & Gauvain, 2001; Nader-Grosbois, 2007a; Puustinen, 1998; Stipek et al., 1992; Szepkouski et al., 1994; Wood & Wood, 1999; Zimmerman, 2000).

According to Perry (1998), several conditions help the development of self-regulated learning strategies in children: challenges in complex meaningful tasks, the possible modification of the task and of assessment criteria in order to obtain an optimal challenge, potential support from others, and opportunities for self-evaluation. In empirical studies, the most frequent contexts used for studying self-regulation have been: planning of daily tasks (Hudson & Fivush, 1991; Hudson et al., 1995) or of itinerary (Nader-Grosbois &

---

[3]Brun and Mellier (2004) conceived an evolution of three types of emotion regulation. First, "intra-personal regulation" includes vigilance, regulation of stress and the application of emotional representations. Second, "inter-individual regulation in imaginary situations" refers to the recognition of facial expressions, evocation, identification of mental states and the understanding of emotional terms; it reflects the child's level of emotional knowledge. Third, "interpersonal regulation in interactive situations" concerns emotional language, shared and joint attention, empathy and looking for social references on other people's faces.

Vieillevoye, 2011; St-Laurent & Moss, 2002), Tower of Hanoi (Klahr & Robinson, 1981; Welsh, 1991), labyrinths (Gardner & Rogoff, 1990), problem-solving or learning situations (De la Ossa & Gauvain, 2001; Nader-Grosbois & Thomée, 2007; Nader-Grosbois & Lefèvre, 2011; Puustinen, 1998; Winnykamen, 1993), computer tasks (Chang & Burns, 2005; Nader-Grosbois et al., 2008; Nader-Grosbois & Lefèvre, 2011) or standardized assessment situations of cognitive functioning (Nader-Grosbois, 2007b, 2007c) and various situations of pretend play in dyads of peers (Nader-Grosbois & Vieillevoye, 2011; Vieillevoye & Nader-Grosbois, 2008). Some of these empirical studies have shown inter-situational variability of self-regulation and of mobilization of specific self-regulatory strategies, not only in typically developing children, but also in children or adolescents with intellectual disability (see Nader-Grosbois & Lefèvre, 2011; Nader-Grosbois & Vieillevoye, 2011; Vieillevoye & Nader-Grosbois, 2008).

In addition, a child's self-regulation may help to increase his or her level of mastery of the task (Wolters, 1999). Some self-regulated strategies are more efficient in specific contexts: notably goal-oriented planning, sustained by proper self-attention and by the control of on-going actions and results (Bauer et al., 1999; Cuskelly et al., 1998; Focant et al., 2006; Gauvain & Rogoff, 1989; Gilmore et al., 2003; Parrila et al., 1996; Pintrich, 2000). Moreover, fewer requests for help by a child during a teaching session were predictive of good performance (Wood & Wood, 1999). Higher achievers easily identify when they need help from the adult, and in this way the child-adult dyad may function at the upper bounds of the child's zone of proximal development (as observed by Nader-Grosbois et al., 2008; Puustinen, 1998; Winnykamen, 1993; Wood & Wood, 1999).

### 3.2 How does emotion regulation develop in typically developing children?

#### 3.2.1 Evolution of strategies of emotion regulation

In typically developing babies, the emotions are expressed in early social interactions by means of various cues that induce reactions from the caregivers. They produce more and more differentiated expressions of emotions, such as interest, disgust, joy, sadness, anger and fear, which are recognizable to those around them (Harris et al., 1989; Haynie & Lamb, 1995; Izard & Malatesta, 1987; Lewis & Sullivan, 1996). From early infancy, they respond to emotions in their interactions with others. At the beginning of the second year of life, they become able to express "social emotions" such as empathy (Lewis et al., 1989). During the first three years of life, infants increase their expressiveness of emotions and they begin to verbally express their emotional states (Harris et al., 1989; Malatesta-Magai et al., 1994).

From the age of 3 years, the child starts to modify the intensity of her or his emotional expression depending on the situation, in conformity to social rules (Cole et al., 2009; Nader-Grosbois & Baurain, 2011; Saarni, 1999). From preschool age, children intentionally control their emotional expressions, in order to induce a false belief in their partner (Perron & Gosselin, 2004) or in order to avoid hurting others' sensibility or to protect their own feelings (Saarni, 1999). Although children develop skills to express their emotions, the imperatives of social life imply that they learn to dissimulate, control their own emotional states and regulate their expressive behaviour in particular contexts; children begin to distinguish between real and apparent emotions at 3 to 4 years old, and the dissimulation of emotions develops particularly from 6 to 10 years old (Banerjee, 1997; Gosselin, 2005; Harris et al., 1989; Nader-Grosbois & Baurain, 2011; Perron & Gosselin, 2004; Sissons Joshi & McLean, 1994; Zeman et al., 2006).

By the end of the preschool period, when the child feels negative emotions, he or she is able to use diverse strategies of emotion regulation: to regulate the expression of emotions, to comfort himself or herself, to self-distract by redirecting his or her attention away from whatever is causing him or her stress or engage in some other activity, to manage his or her frustration, to inhibit emotional behaviours which are socially inappropriate, to postpone a waiting, to approach or withdraw from situations, to stay organized when he or she faced with powerful emotional events, or to negotiate with others (Denham et al., 2002; Dennis & Kelemen, 2009; Macklem, 2008; Stansbury & Sigman, 2000).

The development of emotion regulation has a potential role in social interactions between preschoolers and in the evolution of their social competence (Cole et al., 2004; Dennis, 2006; Dennis et al., 2009a-b; Eisenberg et al., 1995, 1997a-b, 2006; Eisenberg & Spinrad, 2004; Fabes et al., 1999; Nader-Grosbois & Baurain, 2011; Rieder et al., 2007; Spinrad et al., 2006). In other words, the children's abilities to regulate and control their emotional and behavioural responses could help them to have good interactions with peers, and could contribute to social adjustment, including in school (Eisenberg et al., 1995, 1997a-b; Fabes et al., 1999). Emotion regulation comprises intra-individual processes related to cognitive and control processes (Dumas & Lebeau, 1998; Harris et al. 1989; Stein et al., 1993) and inter-individual social processes (Campos et al., 1989; Eisenberg & Fabes, 1992; Eisenberg et al., 1997a-b, 2000; Walden & Smith, 1997), both of which play a basic role in the stable development of social competence during preschool and school age (Sallquist et al., 2009).

### 3.2.2 What are the factors in the development of emotion regulation?

First, social interactions with peers offer children opportunities to exercise their emotion regulation; emotional and behavioural responses from peers should provide them with feedback on their own abilities (Bronson, 2000; Dunn, 2003; Nader-Grosbois & Baurain, 2011; Parker & Asher, 1987). The less they regulate their emotions, the more they have difficulties in establishing relationships with peers (Eisenberg & Fabes, 1995a; Eisenberg et al., 1997a), the more they focus on themselves, the less they are empathic toward others' distress (Eisenberg et al., 1998a) and more they display poor social abilities, in the form of intensely externalized or stressed behaviours (Fabes et al., 1999). Depending on the interactive context, emotion regulation in preschoolers could potentially vary, in order for their emotions to be adequately adjusted. For example, during cooperative play between peers, children display exchanges, are emotionally expressive and positive, or are particularly engaged towards their partner and express joy (Gottman, 1986; Herbé et al., 2007).

Second, through social referencing behaviour and socio-cognitive development, the child acquires an understanding of emotions (causes and consequences), ToM emotions, and a knowledge of social rules that allows him or her to determine which emotion should be expressed when, towards whom and in what circumstance. Social abilities in children are linked with their skills at expressing and recognizing emotions and at understanding others' emotions and intentions (Denham & Burton, 2003; Dodge et al., 1986; Fabes et al., 1999; Nader-Grosbois, 2011). Effectively, the understanding of emotions should favour emotion regulation by the child, because the identification of his or her feelings and emotions becomes conscious; this consciousness allows him or her to link his or her emotions with events and helps him or her to regulation his or her emotions appropriately (Denham & Burton, 2003; Gottman et al., 1997; Liew et al., 2004). The understanding of emotions is a mediator in the link between emotion regulation and social adjustment (Izard et al., 1999, 2000; Lindsey & Colwell, 2003). Conversely, the level of regulation in preschoolers predicts their understanding of emotions (Schultz et al., 2001).

Third, among cognitive processes that could support emotion regulation, we would draw attention to executive functions allowing inhibition, planning and persistence. Although theoretically and in the definition of emotion regulation, the link between executive functioning and emotion regulation is present, most empirical studies examine them separately. In the model of Zelazo and Cunningham (2007), emotion corresponds to a motivational aspect of cognition in goal-oriented problem-solving, and emotion regulation may be primary or secondary, but is always at least partially linked with executive functioning. In problem-solving in daily life, emotion regulation is considered as secondary in relation to executive functioning, in sustaining motivation or self-control in order to persevere or to suppress frustration. By contrast, in other situations, the problem that needs to be solved is disturbing for the child, who must remain calm; in this case, emotion regulation is considered as primary if it is linked to executive functioning throughout the goal-oriented behaviour. In this model, reciprocal relations are postulated, since the two processes influence each other in variable ways depending on the type of problem to be solved. Empirical studies need to be conducted in order to improve our knowledge of this subject, in the same vein as some recent studies. Carlson and Wang (2007) observed in 3- to 5-year old children a positive link between the development of inhibition controlling attention and motor responses and emotion regulation (even when age and verbal abilities were controlled for), whatever the expression of positive or negative emotions. By means of a battery of direct tests administered to 7- to 8-years old children and of reported assessments by parents and teachers, Garcia-Andres et al. (2010) found that socially popular children obtained better scores in both emotion regulation and executive functioning than socially rejected children. Lengua (2002) reported that emotionality and self-regulation (sustained by executive functioning) predicted social adjustment in children: negative emotionality predicted problems in adjustment and positive emotionality predicted positive adjustment; moreover, self-regulation both predicted and moderated the effect of multiple risks of vulnerability *versus* resiliency.

Fourth, the child's language also helps him or her to understand his or her emotions, to self-regulate, to learn adequate manners, to manage his or her emotions and to regulate them. However, its role varies depending on the period of infancy and childhood (before three years, from three to six years, and of school age) (Eisenberg et al., 2005). Empirical studies highlighted that preschoolers' language abilities were positively linked with their ability to distract themselves in frustrating situations (Stansbury & Zimmerman, 1999) and a specific impairment in language was associated with difficulties in emotion regulation (Fujiki et al., 2002[4], 2004[5]).

Fifth, pretend play offers opportunities to experience emotional and social situations, to control negative emotions, to solve conflicts and to negotiate rules with partners (Fantuzzo et al., 2004; Howes et al., 1992; Lemche et al., 2003). In their study, Galyer and Evans (2001)

---

[4] Children with specific language impairment (aged from 6 to 9 years and from 10 to 13 years) had significantly lower levels of emotion regulation than typically developing children.

[5] Emotion regulation and level of language skills in children with specific language impairment (aged from 5 to 8 years and from 9 to 12 years) were significant predictors of their reticence as measured by their teachers.

found that the level of involvement in pretend play by preschoolers with their parents was positively linked with their capacity for emotion regulation. Lindsey and Colwell (2003) reported that girls who engaged in a high level of pretend play regulated their emotions better, according to their mothers.

Sixth, family or parental factors could also have an impact on the child's emotion regulation. The parents contribute to the socialization of their child's emotion regulation by means of supportive strategies, displayed through verbal and non-verbal behaviours in response to the child's emotions, including distress. The parents may facilitate emotion regulation in their distressed child by means of supportive strategies, by encouraging him or her to turn his or her attention away from the sources of distress, or by comforting him or her; conversely, the parents may display non-supportive strategies[6] such as punitive attitudes, minimization or expression of anger, that impede emotion regulation in the child and consequently, increase his or her distress (Calkins & Johnson, 1998; Calkins et al., 1998; Daffe & Nader-Grosbois, 2011; Davidov & Grusec, 2006; Mirabile et al., 2009; Scaramella & Leve, 2004; Thompson & Meyer, 2007).

### 3.2.3 How can emotion regulation be assessed in children?

Several studies concerning the process of emotion regulation have used questionnaires[7] completed by parents and/or teachers of typically developing children of preschool or school age (Contreras et al., 2000; Eisenberg et al., 1995b, 1997a-b, 2000a-b, 2001a; Eisenberg et al., 1996b; Guthrie et al., 1997; Rydell et al., 2003). Some other studies have analyzed direct observations[8] of typically developing children of preschool or school age (Cole et al., 2009; Dennis, 2006; Dennis et al., 2009a; Eisenberg et al., 1997a-b, 2000a-b, 2001a; Spinrad et al., 2006).

A review of instruments used (for details, see Baurain & Nader-Grosbois, 2011, in press) has emphasized the variety of components and types of behaviour taken into account by researchers interested in emotion regulation, as well as the lack of instruments enabling nuanced observations of young children in various contexts. The authors have pointed out that there were good reasons to work out a methodological design[9] allowing the observation

---

[6] For example, Spinrad et al. (2004) found that maternal questioning of the child's emotions was related to his or her lack of self-regulation skills during a disappointment task.

[7] Emotion Regulation Checklist (ERC, Shields & Cicchetti, 1997), Emotional Regulation Rating Scale (ERRS, Carlson & Wang, 2007), Emotion Regulation Subscale of the Social Competence Scale (Conduct Problems Prevention Research Group, 1999).

[8] Children on their own confronted with tasks inducing frustration or disappointment, or requiring persistence or the simulation of positive emotions; dyads of children occupied in cooperative or competitive play; or a child playing with an adult (parent or examiner) and being confronted with situations inducing distress. The coding is performed by macro-analysis or by micro-analysis of behaviours involving positive or negative emotional expressions, verbal and non-verbal behaviours reflecting cues of emotion regulation; or strategies of emotion regulation.

[9] To this end, Baurain and Nader-Grosbois (2007, 2011, in press) have designed a coding grid for observations, featuring the distinct categories of behaviour identified in the literature. These categories are as follows: (1) the child's behaviour with respect to social rules; (2) the child's social behaviour while playing (prosocial behaviour, behaviour showing respect for the task); (3) emotional expressions (positive and negative; joy, anger, sadness, fear) by the child while playing, and adaptation of emotion; (4) consciousness of the felt emotion and evocation at the end of game. These categories were also constructed according to the types of situations and interactive contexts in which the children could be

of the variability of emotion regulation in interactive contexts (cooperative, competitive and neutral) in typically developing children and in atypical children, in order to allow future comparative studies to be performed.

## 4. Self-regulation, dysregulation and emotion regulation in children and adolescents with autism spectrum disorders (ASD)

Few studies have examined the variability of self-regulation in people with ASD or other developmental disorders, depending on contextual and environmental factors and on their individual characteristics, although such studies could generate guidelines for improving interventions oriented towards the development of their self-regulated learning. Several theories and hypotheses have been developed about people with ASD to explain deficits in executive functioning, self-regulation, emotion regulation or dysregulation and their impacts on cognition, emotional abilities or social cognition, including theory of mind.

### 4.1 Executive control dysfunction

According to the "executive control dysfunction" hypothesis, a deficit in their executive control system[10] generates a set of problems in people with ASD, including lack of flexibility in behaviour, disorders in inhibition, difficulties to postpone immediate goals, deficits in planning, in strategy selection, in shifting attention (Corbett et al., 2009; Griffith et al., 1999; Hugues et al., 1994; Joseph et al., 2005; Mc Evoy et al., 1993; Mottron, 2004; Ozonoff et al., 1991; Ozonoff, 1997; Russell, 1997; Turner, 1997[11]); they could create obstacles in several areas of development (notably in cognitive domains, such as pretend play[12], or in communicative domains, such as joint attention[13]) and in the construction of social cognition, including the development of theory of mind (ToM)[14].

---

observed during the "Dyadic Game of Socio-Emotional Problem-Solving". This game aims to make children engage in socio-emotional problem-solving (by means of 13 challenges) in different interactive climates in order to observe and analyze their behaviour in a direct way. This game is designed like a Snakes and Ladders game, but presents socio-emotional situations and problems, illustrated by pictures, that are situated along four possible courses drawn on a plate. The purpose of the game is to resolve several problems in order to reach the end of a course (represented by a star), by engaging in an interactive climate which varies according to the context: neutral (the child plays only with an adult), or competitive and cooperative (the child plays with another child-partner). This game was designed in order to assess two aspects: (1) performance in socio-emotional problem-solving; (2) variation of socio-emotional regulation depending on the interactive context, assessed by means of the "coding grid of socio-emotional regulation" (applied by viewing videos of the children's performance in the game).

[10] For a review, see Hill (2004).

[11] Turner (1997) explained that the repetitive behaviours of people with ASD are a consequence of their difficulties with generating alternative actions, managing their attention, and monitoring their own actions, particularly in new situations; their executive dysfunction could make them less flexible, slow in their activity or too impulsive.

[12] In an empirical study, Jarrold (1997) emphasized that during pretend play, children with ASD encountered difficulties in goal selection and in executive control, notably inhibition of dominant response.

[13] For example, there is a link between joint attention and set-shifting (Stahl & Pry, 2002).

[14] For a review of emotional competences in children with ASD, see Begeer et al. (2008). Specifically for a review of emotional cognition, theory of mind and specificities of face recognition in children with ASD, see Nader-Grosbois and Day (2011).

Russell (1997) suggests that early dysfunction in the action-monitoring system and in developmental features of executive functioning, and memory problems, have an impact in children with ASD in terms of their self-awareness, their development of knowledge regarding their own actions, their regulation through inner speech, and their imitation of others' actions, as well as their understanding of others' intentions and minds.

Some researchers argue that executive abilities may be linked with ToM; conversely, others suggest that executive abilities are needed for ToM. There is a debate as to whether ToM tasks can be reduced to executive processes (e.g. Russell, 1997; Russell et al., 1991; Russell & Hill, 2001; Russell et al., 2003; Pellicano, 2007) or whether ToM is required for executive control (e.g. Perner et al., 2002).

A study led by Fischer and Happé (2005) compared three groups of children with ASD: ten who received training in ToM beliefs (using "photos in the head"); ten who were trained in set-shifting using cards; and seven children in a control group who received no intervention. Both types of individual training (25 minutes per day, for five to ten days) led to an improvement in ToM skills based on beliefs.

The link between executive functions and ToM was examined by Pellicano (2007) in thirty children with ASD (5 to 6 years old) and in forty typically developing children, matched for chronological age, in order to examine issues of developmental primacy. These children were assessed by means of a battery of tasks measuring ToM (first- and second-order false belief tasks) and components of executive functioning (planning, set shifting, inhibition). A significant correlation was obtained between ToM and executive function components in the ASD group, independent of age and ability, while ToM and higher-order planning ability remained significantly linked in the typically developing group. Examination of the relational pattern of ToM executive functioning impairments in the ASD group showed dissociations in only one direction: impaired ToM with intact executive functioning. Even if these results support the view that executive functioning may be an important factor in the acquisition of ToM in children with ASD, it is not enough on its own to explain their difficulties with ToM. In their studies, Pellicano and his colleagues (2007; Pellicano et al., 2006) showed that as children with ASD present differentiated executive profiles in taking into account several processes (assessed by means of a set of tasks), it could implicate specific links between their particular executive (dys)functions and their particular (dis)abilities in ToM.

This hypothesis of dysfunction in executive control may help to explain several features in cognitive strategies and behaviour in people with ASD. However there is variability in their executive function profiles, and certain executive problems are not specific to them, but are shared by people presenting other disorders (Rajendran & Mitchell, 2007).

### 4.2 Cognitive complexity and control theory

In the "Cognitive complexity and control theory" (CCC, Frye et al., 1995; Zelazo & Frye, 1997; Zelazo et al., 2001, 2002), executive functioning is related to ToM in typically developing children and atypical people because both ToM and measures of executive functions include higher-order rule use (leading to a correct judgement in belief tasks, for example). Three main arguments are advanced by Zelazo et al. (2001) in favour of the potential utility of the CCC approach in order to understand people with developmental disorders. First, they argue that each developmental disorder may have an impact on consciousness, control of behaviour and rule complexity, and that researchers should not overlook the fact that a large proportion of people with ASD in particular are intellectually impaired. This intellectual deficit may interact with other inabilities to account for various findings observed in studies of both their executive functioning and their ToM development. Second, they suggest that the CCC conception makes it possible to identify, in people presenting distinct disorders (including ASD), what the specificities are in particular components of executive functions and in ToM. Third, the CCC approach enables participants' performance to be observed in various tasks from different domains, in order to assess the specificity in each developmental disorder. Some empirical studies support the CCC conception. In their study of children with ASD and with Down syndrome, Zelazo et al. (2002) reported that individual differences in ToM are correlated with individual differences in performance in two tests of rule use, except in children with ASD who present a severe intellectual deficit (VIQ <40). This study was replicated by Colvert, Custance, and Swettenham (2002) with other samples, in which children with high functioning ASD were compared with two typically developing groups.

### 4.3 "The development of autism: a self-regulatory perspective"

In his model "the development of autism: a self-regulatory perspective", Whitman, (2004) emphasized the essential role of self-regulation in several processes of development and functioning in children with autism, including sensory, motor, cognitive, emotional, communicative and social processes. Whitman (2004, pp.153-164) explains several characteristics of this dynamic model. It corresponds to a multivariate theory that takes into account multiple factors to understand the development of autism in its various manifestations. It is based on the triad of symptoms of the Diagnostic and Statistical Manual of Mental Disorders (DSM-IV) (deficits in social interaction, in communication and language, stereotypical responses) and on symptoms described in several specific theories about their specificities in all areas of development. As shown in Fig. 1, the self-regulatory construct refers to adaptive and maladaptive coping processes of various natures: motor[15], cognitive[16], linguistic[17], and social[18]. Each of these processes may be considered either directly or indirectly as a "cause" that could influence other processes (primarily, secondarily or minimally) and it could constitute a complex system or chain of causal factors in the emergence of symptomatology of autism (see Fig. 1. inspired by the diagram in Whitman, 2004, p.156). The changes in each process over time involve a reorganization of this dynamic system. All these constructs are considered at either a psychobehavioural level

[15] Repetitive stereotypic movements, such as rocking, hand flapping, and head banging; poor motor imitation (Receveur et al., 2005); overall clumsiness (Ghaziuddin & Butler, 1998); and atypical gait (Hallett et al., 1993). Gepner and Mestre (2002) reported dissociation between the motor system and visual input of children with ASD: they are less reactive posturally to visually perceived environmental motion than typically developing children; their hyporeactivity to such visual input is linked with motor impairments.

[16] Notably, deficits in attention (Allen & Courchesne, 2001) and in joint attention (Filipek et al., 2000; Maestro et al., 2002) were described in infants and in children. Their cognitive style is characterized by its extreme concreteness: they solve tasks requiring rote memory well but they have more difficulties in tasks requiring abstraction or higher-order conceptual processes (Filipek et al., 2000).

[17] For example, their deficits in joint attention are linked to their later language deficits and to their difficulties in understanding and inferring others' states of mind (Phillips et al., 1992).

[18] Ruble (2001) observed that they engage less frequently in goal-directed behaviours in social situations, and these behaviours are less self-initiated and simpler (than those of typically-developing children).

or a neurobiological level. Whitman indicated that it is possible to identify individual dynamic trajectories of development by applying this approach.

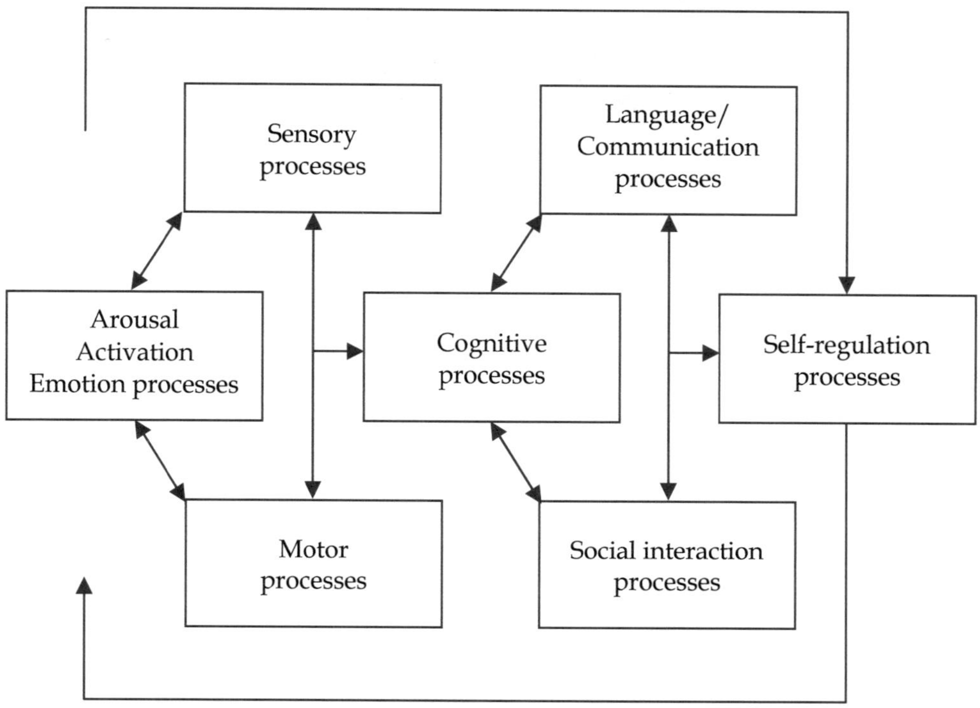


Fig. 1. Whitman's model of self-regulation in the development of autism.

Whitman (2004, p.155) specifies: "although individuals with autism differ in their specific pattern of symptoms, they share in common an inability to self-regulate". Observation of persons with ASD reveals that even if they are sometimes able to use some self-regulatory strategies, they mobilize these strategies with low efficiency or by means of unconventional behaviours.

More specifically, this author suggests that emotions and self-regulation must be taken into account in conjunction, because they can be either risk factors or protective factors in the social adjustment of children with ASD. He specifies that children with ASD may be vulnerable to stress if their arousal[19] and state-regulation dysfunction, if their self-regulatory

[19] Arousal is defined as a physiological state of readiness, an overall state of nervous excitation that could be influenced by the environment and by the individual's perception of the environment. It is situated on a continuum from hypo-arousal (low excitation, associated with inattention, even sleepiness, apathy, indifference) to hyper-arousal (high excitation, associated with high distractibility, intensity of feelings). The middle of the continuum corresponds to moderate arousal with focused attention and alertness. On basis of the numerous findings on arousal-activation problems in individuals with ASD, Huebner and Dunn (2001) postulated that they have an inability to modulate or regulate arousal. According to them, hyper-arousal can be associated with avoidance or immobility. Paris (2000) also hypothesized that regarding abnormalities in their arousal, if over-stimulated, they display disorganized, impulsive or even inhibited responses as a consequence of avoidance or withdrawal. According to Whitman (2004, p.116), they could differ in the way they experience stimuli

system is poorly developed or if environmental stressors are too intense or prolonged. His theory also describes how the emotions in children with ASD indirectly influence the development of self-regulation through their impact on sensory, motor, social, cognitive, and language or communicative processes. Not only do these latter processes directly affect the development of self-regulatory behaviour (through the tools they provide for self-regulation), but self-regulation provides individuals with the capacity to control their emotions.

According to Whitman (2004, p.167), children with ASD could present different self-regulatory styles; in particular he refers to "over-controlling" and "under-controlling" styles. "Over-controlling" children are described as obsessive, self-protective, wary, socially withdrawn, uncomfortable with ambiguities, preferring a structured environment, and reactive to new situations. By contrast, "under-controlling" children do not develop complex form of self-regulation (such as planning or self-monitoring), ask for more social support and are impulsive, distractible and disturbed by unexpected events, and seek immediate gratification.

In order to integrate reciprocal influences between the neurobiological and psychobehavioural characteristics of children with ASD and the social and parental environment, Whitman (2004, p. 168-170) also proposes multiple bi-directional inter-relations between these factors. When parents are confronted with a child who displays peculiar and ambiguous behaviour (for example, behaviour that is hypersensitive, socially avoidant, communicatively and cognitively delayed or ritualistic), they have little insight into why he or she acts in this way and how they could help or support for him or her. This situation induces parental stress that could lead to assistance being sought. This author gives several guidelines for intervention with respect to children with ASD and their parents, in connection with his model, including support with self-regulation development. On basis of the theoretical model of Vygotsky (1978), Whitman suggests that the scaffolding provided by parents and social workers should induce engagement with challenging task; they should do this by adjusting their physical guidance, verbal prompting and modelling and reducing their other-regulation in order to allow the child to assume responsibility and learn to self-regulate. Gradual support and the encouragement of self-instruction in problem-solving help the child to acquire new cognitive and behavioural abilities to self-regulate.

#### 4.4 The dysregulation model

Based on studies of autism in the fields of neurophysiology, neuropsychology and developmental psychopathology, Adrien's model (1996, 2005) designates all deficits in regulation processes in autism using the concepts of "functional dysregulation" and "developmental dysregulation". Adrien distinguishes between the micro-genesis of autistic children's dysregulation that occurs in problem-solving contexts, during activities, and the macro-genesis of dysregulation that has an impact in various developmental domains. This model represents part of a similar approach to that of the model devised by Whitman.

---

and their intensity, in the way they react to stimuli, and in their sensitivity (hyper- or hypo-sensitive) and coping style (such as withdrawal). When variations in routines occur, negative emotional hyper-reactivity can be displayed; basic sensory stimuli (such as noise, smells, or light touch) can be emotional triggers. By contrast, hypo-responsiveness can be displayed in response to other stimuli, in particular social stimuli (such as one's name being called, facial reactions, or praise, O'Neill & Jones, 1997; Volkmar & Pauls, 2003).

### 4.4.1 Functional dysregulation

In ASD, functional dysregulation could be explained by basic neurophysiological disorders such as cerebral modulatory insufficiency (Lelord, 1990), or by disorders with regard to sensory modulation (focusing on a stimulus, filtering its relevant information and processing overall stimulus information, Ornitz, 1985). Several empirical studies have shown that this deficient modulation is observed in the irregular morphology and amplitude of cortical responses to sound stimuli and in the unstable inter-modal "sound-light" association[20] recorded by means of cortical evoked potentials (Bruneau et al., 1999; Martineau et al., 1992a, 1992b). A link has been emphasized between a deficit in maintaining cross-modal associative responses and disturbances in regulatory behaviour: children with ASD who presenting the highest functional dysregulations, take few initiatives to play or to interact and do not finish their activities, have a deficiency in inter-modal cortical associations (Martineau et al., 1998). Difficulties in temporal cortical regions implicated in the regulation of auditory perception and vocal information processing are identified in children with ASD (Gomot et al., 2002; Khalfa et al., 2001; Zilboviscius et al., 2000).

Specifically, in problem-solving situations, five types of dysregulation[21] of activity are distinguished by Adrien et al. (2001a): "breaking off" of action sequences; "perseveration" of some actions; "slowness" in the rhythm of activity; "variability" in levels of behaviour during the activity; and "lack of synchronization" between actions usually coordinated in a sequence of actions. These disorders may appear at three phases of activity: initiation (becoming involved in the activity by producing actions), maintenance (maintaining the initiated activity) and achievement (completion of the action sequence).

In cognitive activity such as object permanence tasks, children with ASD display a pervasive difficulty in maintenance, make more perseverative errors when the abstraction degree of task was higher (tasks at sensory-motor Piagetian stage VI, prevision of actions), and are more variable in their behavioural strategies (Adrien et al., 1995); they produce an incomplete and atypical sequence of actions in searching for an object hidden by a screen (Adrien, 2005). In symbolic play activities, functional dysregulation affects the quality of pretend play in limiting the diversification of actions and of sequences of behaviours (Blanc et al., 2001). Instead, children with ASD may tenaciously perseverate with respect to specific features of a toy, and they often play with it according to a very specific routine. In joint attention episodes, at 10 and 24 months, infants with ASD present visual-motor discordances, perseveration, slowness and a significant variability in their responses to joint attention elicited by others (Gattegno et al., 1999).

### 4.4.2 Developmental dysregulation

In order to explain intra- and inter-domain heterochrony in the development of children with ASD, Adrien (1996, 2005) conceptualized developmental dysregulation. He postulated that the importance of heterochrony in their developmental profiles is linked with the intensity of their dysregulation.

---

[20] The methodological design is as follows: a sound and a flash of light were presented several times to the child; responses in the auditory and visual cortex and also in inter-modal associations were recorded.

[21] In order to measure them, they have devised the Regulation Disorders Evaluation Grid (RDEG, Adrien et al., 2001). The fifteen items are divided according to five types of disorders and three phases of activity.

Adrien's view (1996, 2005) is supported by the results of some empirical studies and also by clinical observations, showing the impact of dysregulation on the cognitive, socio-emotional and interactive development of children with ASD (Adrien et al., 2001a; Blanc et al., 2005; Huebner & Dunn, 2001; Nader-Grosbois, 2007b; Paris, 2000; Rossignol et al., 1998; Seynhaeve, 2006; Seynhaeve & Nader-Grosbois, 2008a, Seynhaeve et al., 2008b[22]). Some studies have highlighted negative relations between dysregulation and several developmental domains such as social interaction, joint attention, behaviour regulation (Blanc et al., 2005), language understanding, emotional expression, affective relationships, schemes, symbolic play (Adrien, 1996; Blanc et al., 2005) and theory of mind (Rossignol et al., 1998) in children with ASD.

In a comparative study of 18 children with ASD, 18 children with intellectual disabilities and 18 typically developing children (matched for developmental age), Adrien et al. (2001a) emphasized the presence in the ASD group of frequent and numerous types of dysregulation disorders, occurring at all times in sensory-motor actions during the performance of object permanence tasks[23]. They also discovered significant links between the intensity of regulation disorders and developmental levels in the initiation of and in response to social interaction: perseveration and lack of achievement were higher in children with ASD presenting the lowest developmental level (level 1 simple, from 4 to 7 months) or the highest developmental level (level 4 symbolic including the use of verbal communication with two words, from 20 to 30 months). These last two subgroups of children with ASD usually displayed previous action schemata in new situations. These authors interpret this observation as a defect of flexibility and a central executive dysfunction (as was suggested by Hugues et al., 1994).

These results are coherent with the classical diagnostic criteria of ASD, which refer to impairment in reciprocal social interactions and in verbal and non-verbal communication as well as a restricted repertoire of activities and interests (DSM-IV, APA, 1994).

### 4.5 Emotion regulation in children with ASD

Because of late reliable diagnoses of ASD, it is usually around the age of 6 to 12 years that children with ASD are studied (Dumont-Mathieu & Fein, 2005). However, in order to study emotional abilities (in expression, response, regulation and understanding of emotions) of young "autistic" infants and children, it is possible to use delayed diagnoses. Studies focusing on emotion regulation in atypical children are rare. However, poor emotion regulation is a characteristic frequently associated with autistic profiles (Southam-Gerow & Kendall, 2002). How do their emotional expression and emotion regulation evolve?

During the first year of life, although infants with ASD show similar expressions of emotions, they are less attentive to faces and their affective behaviour is less oriented towards others than that of control TD or ID infants matched for IQ or mental age (Baranek, 1999; Maestro et al., 2002, 2005; Osterling et al., 2002; Palomo et al., 2006; Werner et al., 2000). Although children with ASD are sensitive to emotional cues emitted by others, such as distress (Nadel et al., 2000; Sigman et al., 1992), they do not easily express their own emotions appropriately (Brun et al., 1998; Loveland et al., 1994; Snow et al., 1987; Yirmiya et al., 1992).

[22] Studies led by Nader-Grosbois and Seynhaeve will be detailed in a later section of this chapter.
[23] Assessed by means of the object permanence scale (Infant Psychological Development Scales, IPDS, Uzgiris & Hunt, 1975).

Preschoolers with ASD, compared with children matched for MA, display similar emotional expressiveness in social interactions or when they are watching video sequences illustrating others' emotional expressions (Capps et al., 1993). By using the "Maximally Discriminative Facial Movement Coding System" (MAX), Yirmiya et al. (1989) observed that although children with ASD show a similar quantity of positive and negative emotions to TD children, their facial movements often incongruously express more than one emotion (for example, joy and sadness). By contrast, Snow et al. (1987) reported that young children with ASD display fewer expressions of positive emotions than TD and ID children. Poorer emotional expressiveness in children with ASD was emphasized, in comparison with TD and Down syndrome children (Kasari & Sigman, 1996; Loveland et al., 1994). At preschool age, during social exchanges, children with ASD barely modify their emotional reactions in response to others (Konstantareas & Stewart, 2006), they show poor emotional coordination and timing of affect (Scambler et al., 2007) and they hardly initiate shared attention with others (Mundy et al., 1990; Travis et al., 2001; Warreyn et al., 2005). According to Saarni (1999), because of their cognitive specificities or deficits in the way they interpret their own emotional experiences and those felt by others, children with ASD are unlikely to convey their emotions conventionally.

At school age, they respond with less concern and comforting or empathic behaviours to others' emotional expressions; they do not easily share their emotional states with a partner (Bacon et al., 1998; Corona et al., 1998; Dawson et al., 2004; Kasari et al., 1990; Sigman et al., 1992). This weak responsiveness to others' emotions remains stable over a 5-year period (Dissanayake et al., 1996). This lack of empathy in children and adolescents with ASD has been widely reported, although it seems possible to specifically train them to make empathic responses in social scenarios (Argott et al., 2008; Charman et al., 1997, 1998; Dyck et al., 2001; Gena et al., 1996; Hudry & Slaughter, 2009; Sigman et al., 1992; Travis et al., 2001; Yirmiya et al., 1992). However, empathic behaviour may vary according to the individuals with ASD (McGovern & Sigman, 2005) and also according to specific emotional context, or familiarity with social agents (as is reported by parents who indicate that their children display empathy towards familiar agent, Hudry & Slaughter, 2009). At school age, in contrast with TD or ID children who spontaneously display their positive emotions in social interactions, children with ASD share their emotional expressions with others in a less spontaneous way (Attwood et al., 1988; Bieberich & Morgan, 2004; Snow et al., 1987), notably in unstructured situations in which the caregiver does not initiate the interaction (Kasari et al., 1993a). The combination of emotional expression on their part, eye contact and expressiveness in response to their caregiver's expressions is also exhibited less by them than by control groups (Dawson et al., 1990b). They therefore appear less expressive because they have neutral, flat or idiosyncratic expressions more frequently than MA controls; this continues into later life (Czapinski & Bryson, 2003; Hobson & Lee, 1998; Kasari et al., 1990; Loveland et al., 1994; Yirmiya et al., 1989). For example, these children displayed less attention and fewer smiles than children with Down syndrome when other children were laughing in play situations (Reddy et al., 2002). Sometimes, children with ASD display happy expressions in solitary or unpleasant situations more often than in social situations (Whitman, 2004). Individuals with ASD do not experience complex emotions such as embarrassment, pride and guilt in the same way as TD people (Grandin, 1995).

According to Begeer et al. (2008), in comparison with TD children, children with ASD present similar elementary emotional expressiveness and experiences, but differ in the inter-

and intra-personal integration of their emotions. These authors also specify that "empirical evidence found for the influence of age, intelligence and context factors on the level of emotional expressiveness in children and adolescents with ASD refines the marked impairments of emotional expressive behaviour that are suggested in the diagnostic manuals" (Begeer et al., 2008, p. 346). Tardif et al. (2007) reported that studies of emotional expressiveness have emphasized a deficit in expression, in modulation and in internal and external regulation of emotions in children with ASD. They are described as easily stressed, anxious and fearful. They have difficulty in self-regulating their emotions when their feelings become excessive.

Several authors postulate that there is a significant impairment of emotion regulation that could explain a set of inabilities in children with ASD in their social interactions (Gulsrud et al., 2009; Konstantareas & Stewart, 2006). Trevarthen (1989) suggests that autism is due to an early basic deficit in the production of emotions and of emotion regulation in reaction to environmental stimulations. He hypothesized a biological origin of this impairment: a dysfunction of central regulator systems. Children with ASD do not feel emotions related to exchanges initiated by others or to experiences they have in connection with objects. Moreover, poor, absent or unexpectedly excessive emotion in children with ASD does not play its role of regulator, as a means of seeking, producing, maintaining, inhibiting, and interrupting behaviours with respect to others or to objects (Tanguay, 1990). According to Adrien (1996), this deficiency of emotionality in children with ASD is more apparent in situations requiring regulation, due to the interruption, maintaining, amplification or reduction of emotional affects. These children prefer to resist change and conserve their initial state in order to avoid new social situations that may be sources of amplification or reduction of felt emotions, requiring regulation.

We consider that the study of specificities in emotion regulation in children with ASD should be included in a dynamic and integrative approach taking account of different levels of cognitive and socio-emotional competences or deficits (as suggested by Yeates et al. 2007, Nader-Grosbois, 2011): perceptual information processing[24], executive and cognitive abilities (attention, inhibition, etc.), social information processing (including ToM, making it possible to understand one's own and others' emotions), social problem-solving abilities, social interactions and social adjustment. To infer what other people think or feel and to regulate one's emotions in social interactions requires the perception of subtle face, voice and body movements, the processing of various sources of information simultaneously and in an integrated way, the selection of the most important and pertinent information in the context and the inhibition of an already given response in a similar situation in order to find another, more appropriate one. Emotion regulation in social situations could therefore depend on such factors, in which children with ASD present deficits.

### 4.6 Dysfunction in co-regulation

Environmental conditions, including parental strategies of social regulation or of socialization of emotions toward their child with ASD could contribute to support his or her emotion regulation or self-regulation, or conversely could help induce dysregulation. As children with ASD display maladaptive behaviours that predict maternal stress (Tomanik et al., 2004), it is plausible that stress may also interfere with the maternal support of emotion

[24] As suggested by Mottron (2004).

regulation in the child (Belsky, 1984). As their mothers have difficulties in interpreting and reacting to the ambiguous emotional signals of their child with ASD, the result may be less parental support for the development of new skills, including regulatory skills (Stansbury & Zimmermann, 1999). However, it seems that it is possible to improve maternal strategies, by means of specific intervention focusing on joint engagement, on joint attention and consequently improve emotion regulation in children with ASD; such interventions could help with the co-regulation of emotions between the two partners (Gulsrud et al., 2009).
In their study, Gulsrud et al. (2009) randomly assigned about 35 toddlers with ASD (with an average mental age of 19 months) and their mothers to both control and joint attention intervention conditions. In the intervention condition, mother-child dyads attended twenty-four ten-minute sessions, organized in ten modules, targeting early joint attention, language skills and joint engagement with the mother, three days a week for eight weeks. Videotape of the children and mothers was used to classify their emotion regulation behaviours using standardized coding, screening for the presence and the absence of any distress episodes. The following aspects of the children's behaviour was coded: "negativity" (in facial and body expressions) and regulation strategies, including symbolic self-soothing, physical self-soothing, repetitive or idiosyncratic behaviours, tension release, avoidance, distraction, maternal orientation, other-directed comfort seeking, and other-directed assistance seeking. The following maternal regulation strategies were coded: prompting/helping, following the child's lead, redirection of attention, active ignoring, reassurance, emotional following, physical comfort, vocal comfort. Moreover, behavioural strategy combinations were applied in order to classify mothers' and children's regulatory behaviours: (a) maternal vocal strategies consisting of the combination of maternal vocal comfort and reassurance; (b) maternal active strategies consisting of the combination of prompting/helping, redirection of attention and physical comfort; (c) children's comfort strategies consisting of physical self-comfort and comfort-seeking; (d) children's physical strategies consisting of tension release, avoidance, and distraction; and (e) children's verbal strategies consisting of cognitive/verbal self-soothing and assistance seeking. Their results showed variability in the intensity of negative expressions and in the number of distress episodes in toddlers with ASD, but almost all displayed an increase of negative arousal during play interactions with their mothers. This observation was interpreted by authors as evidence of profiles of dysregulation. However, these children engaged in a range of emotion regulation strategies, characterized as appropriate active strategies (distraction, avoidance, and tension release) and constructive strategies (orienting to mum, and seeking assistance). Like typical toddlers, they were able to request maternal support and assistance; however, they made less frequent use of sophisticated verbal strategies such as symbolic/verbal self-soothing (which may be impeded by their low expressive language level - less than 20 months). Emotion regulation strategies were used significantly more by toddlers with ASD during episodes of negativity than non-negativity. In addition, mothers of these toddlers with ASD engaged (as also reported for mothers of typically developing toddlers) in a variety of emotion regulation strategies when the child was in distress, from active strategies (redirection, prompting, physical behaviours) to vocal comforting strategies (vocal soothing and reassurance). They continued to use active strategies throughout the intervention more frequently than mothers of typically developing children. Moreover, specific characteristics in the child with ASD and the mother were associated with emotion regulation outcomes. For example, when interacting with their toddlers with behaviour problems, mothers were more stressed and used more active strategies and fewer vocal strategies. These mothers'

ability to redirect attention away from a source of distress for the child and reengage him or her in an ongoing play activity appears to be an important regulatory skill. Concerning the impact of the intervention, this study provides evidence for the effectiveness of an early mother-driven social-communication intervention in decreasing negativity and supporting emotion regulation capabilities in children with ASD. Mothers' improvements in motivational and emotional scaffolding were related to the socialization of emotion regulation in their toddlers with ASD.

These studies showed that it is important to assess and to intervene in co-regulation between children with ASD and those around them, and not only target children's dysregulation.

## 5. The integrative model of regulation in psychological functioning and development in children with ASD and its implications for assessment and intervention

### 5.1 Components of the integrative model

In order to integrate recent relevant models (notably Adrien's and Whitman's theories) and the results of empirical studies of regulation *versus* dysregulation processes, emotion regulation and co-regulation, we propose an integrative model including three levels: (1) micro-functioning, (2) functional abilities *versus* inabilities, and (3) macro-functioning or development (see Fig. 2). These three levels have dynamic and retroactive connections into "streams", and even in a "spiral" in the course of time. They involve different types of assessment and targets for intervention.

The micro-functioning level designates the micro-genetic functioning *versus* dysfunctioning that occurs in very specific contexts of problem solving. It corresponds to the regulation of activity, positive strategies of problem solving, self-regulatory strategies (sustained by executive functions) as well as negative dysregulatory behaviours and neuropsychological dysfunctioning displayed by the child. At this first level, assessment and intervention must focus on the executive functioning, self-regulation strategies, and functional dysregulation in challenging contexts. The examiner must select instruments[25] assessing very specific cognitive functions or strategies, such as self-regulated attention, goal-oriented planning, inhibition of non pertinent elements in tasks, regulation behaviour, etc. At this level, the highlighting of specific dysfunctioning could complement a diagnostic process by focusing on the assessment of specific disorders.

The level of functional abilities versus inabilities relates to abilities mobilized in daily life by the child; his or her social, cognitive, emotional and psychomotor functional abilities[26] and the combination of these abilities help the child to adjust his or her behaviour during life events or to respond to requests from the environment. Lack of ability or inabilities in these

---

[25] The following instruments could be used: the grid for coding self-regulation in problem solving (Nader-Grosbois, 2007); the Regulation Disorders Evaluation Grid, assessing dysregulation (RDEG, Adrien, 1996); and the Behavioral Functional Inventory (BFI, Adrien et al., 1995, 2001b). The neuropsychological instrument NEPSY-II (Korkman, Kirk, & Kemp, 2007), composed of 27 subtests designed for children aged 3 to 12, assesses five functions: attention/executive functions, language, sensorimotor, visuospatial, and memory and learning.

[26] At this level, Nader-Grosbois (2006) suggest that specific relations are constructed between specific abilities in different areas that create "local homology". This neo-Piagetian concept designates the variable intensity of coordination between specific domains (as opposed to Piagetian "general homology").

different areas reduce his or her adjustment to situations. Our definition of this level is founded on an ecological and curriculum-based approach to children. The level includes notably abilities or inabilities in emotion regulation when the child experiences distress, frustration and negative emotions[27] in daily life events. At this second level, assessment[28] and intervention must target abilities in multiple ecological situations.

The level of macro-functioning or development corresponds to a macro-genetic approach to the development profiles of children and to their developmental trajectories in several areas. It could give information about synchrony *versus* asynchrony in development; or in other words, about homogeneity *versus* heterogeneity in developmental profiles. It is possible at this level to identify weaknesses and strengths in domains of development. Our definition of this level is founded on neo-Piagetian conceptions of typical and atypical development. The level enables the developmental stage or developmental age to be identified in cognitive, communicative, psychomotor domains. For assessment, ordinal and multidimensional scales[29] of development, varying depending on the period of development, must be used. The intervention must focus on the emergence of the child's abilities and on the weaknesses in specific domains in order to choose eliciting situations that could improve developmental progression and reduce the heterogeneity of the child's development.

Concerning the connections between these three levels, empirical studies of children with ASD have emphasized:

- positive links between positive self-regulation and functional abilities;
- positive links between positive self-regulation and the developmental level/ homogeneous development;

[27] The parents could complete other-reported scales, such as the Emotion Regulation Checklist (ERC, Shields & Cicchetti, 1997), the Emotional Regulation Rating Scale (ERRS, Carlson & Wang, 2007), or the Emotion Regulation Subscale of the Social Competence Scale (Conduct Problems Prevention Research Group, 1999). Moreover, the examiner could observe the child in a setting inducing emotion regulation in interactive and non-interactive contexts (see studies led by Baurain and Nader-Grosbois, 2011, in press).

[28] For example, the Assessment Evaluation Programming System for infants and children (AEPS, Bricker, 2002), which includes assessment by professionals and parents, and a programme of intervention targeting functional abilities in several domains (social, cognitive, motor, adaptive, communicative) for which training could be given in formal sessions by professionals and in daily life activities by people around the child. Another example: the Vineland Adaptive Behavior Scales-Second Edition (VABS-II, Sparrow et al., 2005) measures multidimensional adaptive behaviour from birth to adulthood: communication, daily living, motor skills and socialization. A Maladaptive Behavior Index is optional. There are four formats: semi-structured interview, expanded interview, parent or caregiver rating form and teacher rating form.

[29] For the sensory-motor period, several neo-Piagetian scales could be used. First, the Infant Psychological Development Scales, IPDS, Uzgiris & Hunt, 1975) or the new version, Evaluation du Développement Cognitif Précoce (EEDCP, Nader-Grosbois, 2009) including seven scales: object permanence, means-end, vocal imitation, gestural imitation, operational causality, spatial relations, and schemes of action. Second, the Early Social Communication Scales (ESCS, Seibert & Hogan, 1982), which uses eight scales to assess three communicative functions (social interaction, joint attention, behaviour regulation) and distinct roles (responding to, initiating and maintaining). Third, the Batterie d'Evaluation du Développement Cognitif et Social (BECS, Adrien, 1996). For the symbolic period, standardized intelligence tests could be applied, but these are difficult to administer to children with ASD. The Snyders-Oomen (SON-R, Tellegen et al., 1998) is a measure of non-verbal intelligence which is easier to administer to children with poor language skills.

- negative links between dysfunctioning in executive function, dysregulation and functional abilities;
- negative links between dysfunctioning in executive function, dysregulation and the developmental levels/homogeneous development;
- positive links between functional abilities and the developmental level.

In other words, the more these children mobilize optimal neuropsychological functions, the more their self-regulatory strategies operate, the more they are able to adjust their functional behaviours in daily life, the more they progress positively in their development and the more their developmental profiles are harmonious, and *vice versa*. Moreover, the more children with ASD display neuropsychological executive dysfunctioning, or dysregulation, the more they present deficits in several self-regulatory strategies, the more they have difficulties in responding adequately to daily life events with efficient functional abilities and with adapting, the less they develop their abilities in several domains of development and the more their developmental profiles are heterogeneous due to the difference in the speed of development in different domains, and *vice versa*.

In order to appraise these inter-connections between the levels in children with ASD, several combinations of instruments could be chosen in an assessment procedure.

Concerning the risk and protective factors that could influence the three levels of functioning and development in children with ASD, on the one hand there are the individual characteristics of the child (gender, age, mental age, type of deficiency, severity of autism, temperament, health, etc.) and on the other hand social environmental factors, including family and parental factors (parents' characteristics, types of scaffolding, other-regulatory strategies, co-regulation, contingency, responsiveness, stress management, etc.) and all components of intervention by professionals. All these factors must be identified in order to adjust the choice of assessment and intervention with respect to children with ASD. In order to illustrate this integrative model of regulation in psychological functioning and development in children with ASD, we represent these components and links between them in Fig. 2.

In a longitudinal approach (see Fig. 3), the components of the three levels of functioning and development, as well as these positive *versus* negative connections between the components of these levels, could be viewed as a dynamic of mutual effects not only into "streams" but also in a "spiral" through time. In other words, specific deficits in the components of the three levels could get worse or decrease in future periods of development; and the intensity of the links between them could fluctuate in individual trajectories, depending in particular on risk and protective endogenous and exogenous factors.

### 5.2 Empirical studies using this integrative model

Nader-Grosbois (2007b) examined dysregulation[30] and self-regulation[31] in 14 boys with ASD (aged from 36 to 92 months; mental age ranged from 10 to 24 months) when they were confronted with a problem-solving set corresponding to assessment situations of different cognitive domains of development (by means of BECS). Their mental age (but not their chronological age) was correlated positively with their self-regulation and negatively with their dysregulation. The severity of autism[32] (mild to severe) was linked negatively to self-

---

[30] Assessed by means of RDEG (Adrien et al., 2001).

[31] A grid of coding of self-regulation and other-regulation (Nader-Grosbois, 2000, 2007) was applied.

[32] Assessed by means of Childhood Autism Rating Scale (CARS-T, Schopler et al., 1986).

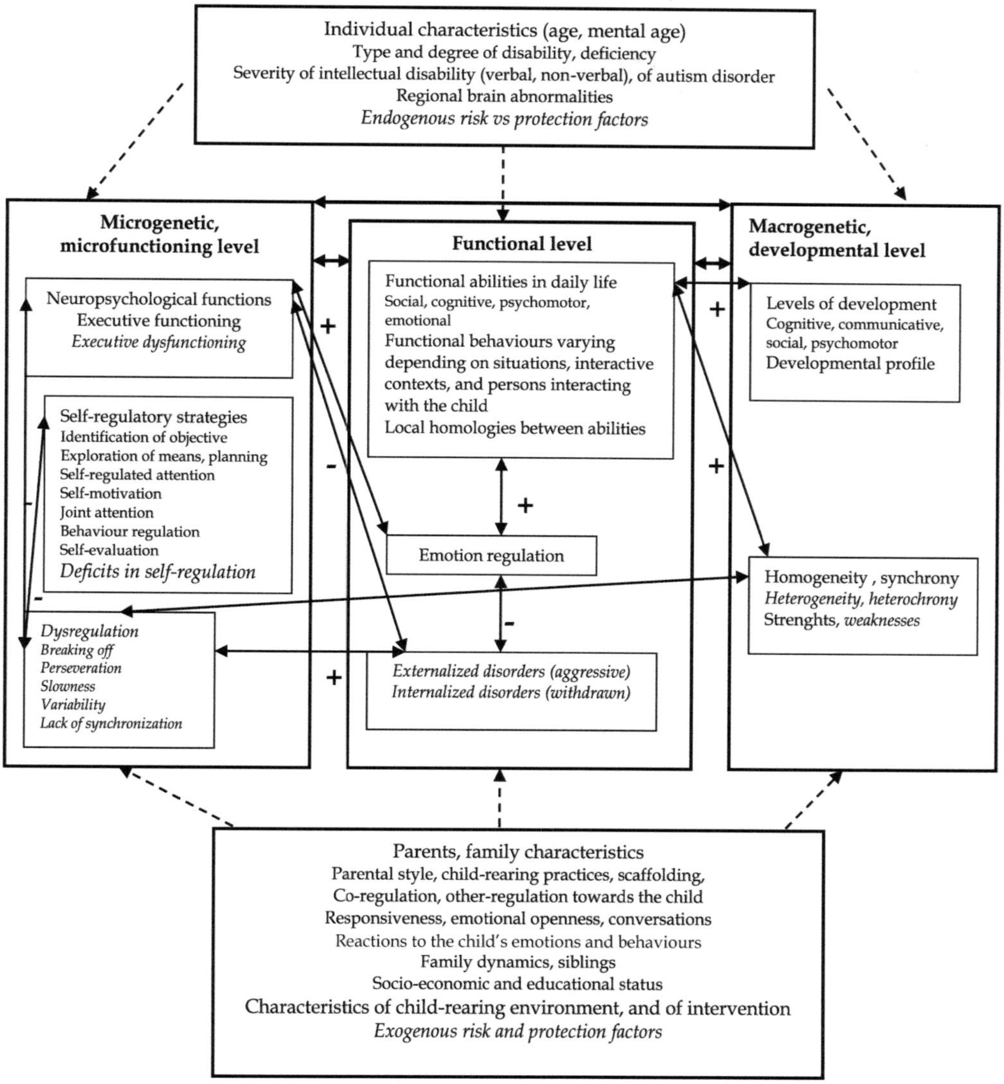


Fig. 2. Integrative model of regulation in the functioning and development of children with ASD

regulation and positively to dysregulation. The self-identification of objective was stronger than other self-regulatory strategies (planning, attention, motivation, evaluation, joint attention, request). Planning in particular was the weakest self-regulatory strategy. The cognitive developmental level was linked positively to overall self-regulation. The positive links between the majority of specific cognitive domains (object permanence, means-end, causality, self-image, symbolic play, schemes of action) and self-regulation varied in significance. Considerable inter-individual variability was observed in the degree of dysregulation and in the type of disorders of regulation. The cognitive developmental level was linked negatively to overall dysregulation. Significant negative links were obtained between specific cognitive domains (object permanence, means-end, self-image, symbolic play) and dysregulation.

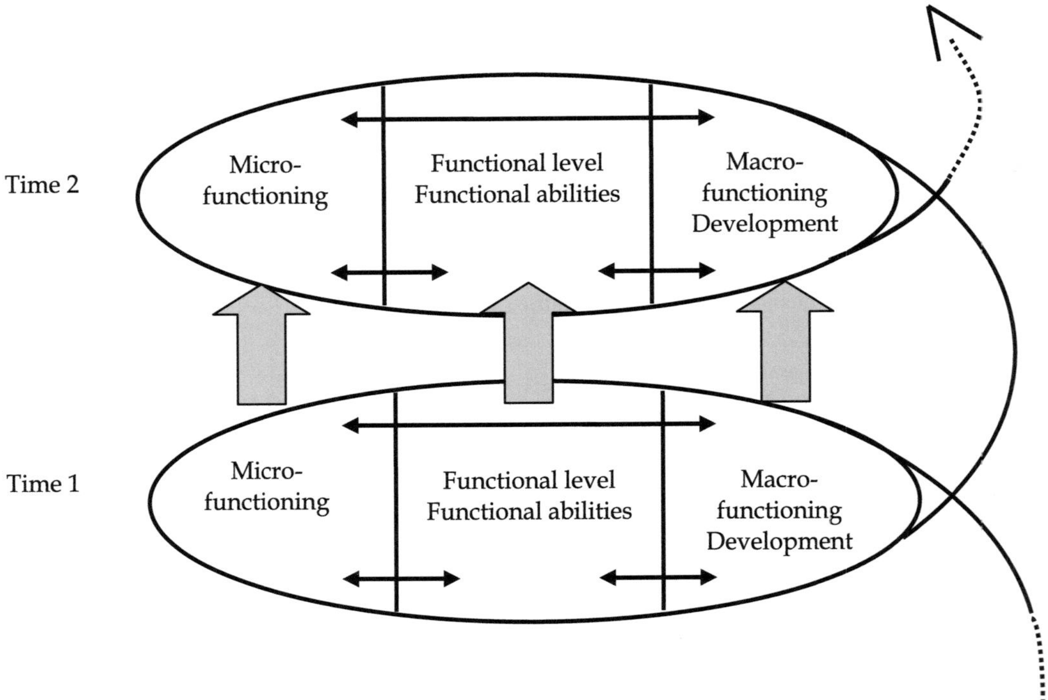


Fig. 3. Integrative, longitudinal "spiral" model of the development of children with ASD

Three comparative studies (Seynhaeve, 2006; Seynhaeve & Nader-Grosbois, 2008a, Seynhaeve et al., 2008b) focused on the impact of neuropsychological dysfunction[33] and of dysregulation[34] in activity on the development of 12 children with ASD matched for developmental age (18 months) with 12 children with intellectual disability (ID).

Seynhaeve (2006) analysed neuropsychological dysfunction in conjunction with cognitive and social development[35] in these both groups. Their results showed higher dysfunction scores in children with ASD than in children with ID. Patterns of neuropsychological dysfunction observed in the two groups presented some similarities concerning their most affected functions, including regulation, association and imitation. Significant negative correlations were found between dysfunction and several developmental scores in both groups, with variability in their patterns of links. These negative links were much more numerous and intense within the ASD group than in the group with ID. Specifically, dysfunction in regulation in the ASD group was negatively linked to overall development and socio-emotional scores, to specific scores in self-image, social interaction, behaviour regulation, joint attention, expressive and comprehensive language and vocal imitation. Within the ASD group, the agglomerate of dysfunctions (regulation, association and imitation) has a strong influence on their speed of development, and particularly on their heterogeneity of development. The more affected these functions are, the greater the overall, socio-cognitive and socio-emotional developmental heterogeneity.

[33] Assessed by means of Behavioral Functional Inventory (BFI, Adrien et al., 1995).

[34] Assessed by means of RDEG (Adrien et al., 2001).

[35] Assessed by means of Batterie d'Evaluation du Développement Cognitif et Social (BECS, Adrien, 1996).

In the same samples, Seynhaeve and Nader-Grosbois (2008a) examined more specifically regulation disorders in activity. Compared with ID children, children with ASD showed more intense and more frequent total dysregulation (as shown by Adrien, 1996; Adrien et al., 2001a; Blanc et al., 2005), dysregulation in maintenance (as shown by Adrien et al., 1995; Adrien et al., 2001a; Martineau et al., 1998) and breaking off as well as slowness dysfunction (as shown by Adrien et al., 2001a). The two groups also showed similarities in displaying greater dysregulation disorders during initiation and maintenance than during achievement of the activity. Dysregulation of activity was negatively linked to development in several domains, but correlations were much more numerous and intense within the ASD group than in the group with ID. Within the ASD group, the mean score for dysregulation as well as the mean scores for each specific disorder (except variability) and of the three times of activity were strongly negatively linked to overall development and, according to the types of regulation disorders, to socio-cognitive and socio-emotional development. The specific developmental domains that are particularly negatively linked to dysregulation are the following: self-image, symbolic play, social interaction, behaviour regulation, joint attention, expressive and comprehensive language and vocal imitation. Moreover, Developmental Quotient on the Brunet-Lézine-Revised scale (BL-R, Josse, 1997) was negatively correlated with the mean score in dysregulation in children with ASD: their cognitive impairments are more severe when dysregulation is more intense.

Seynhaeve, Nader-Grosbois and Dionne (2008b) observed, in the same two groups, the impact of dysregulation on functional abilities in daily life[36]. They also concluded that in both groups total dysregulation was negatively linked to total functional abilities as well as to specific functional abilities in different domains (with and without controlling for chronological age). In the ASD group, as dysregulation decreases, the more functional abilities increase, both overall and in specific domains such as fine motor, cognitive and communicative domains (when not controlling for chronological age) and the social domain (when controlling for chronological age). This study showed that total dysregulation has a differentiated impact in each group: whereas in ASD children, it is linked to weaker communicational and social abilities as well as weaker cognitive or motor abilities, this is not the case in children with ID.

## 6. Perspectives for research

In a paper entitled "The development of emotion regulation and dysregulation: a clinical perspective", Cole, Michel and Teti (1994) encouraged research into these processes in developmental psychopathology. They suggested that they should be studied in children both with and without specific disorders, and in the latter case both at risk and not at risk of them, using a test design assessing various dimensions of emotionality in context, multiple assessments (including observations of children's reactions beyond what they are able to self-report) of their positive and negative emotions, and analyses of their dysregulation patterns. They noted that it is important to focus on the dysregulation process and its links with several dimensions of emotionality: diversity of positive and negative emotions, flexible modulation of their intensity and duration, transitions from one emotion to another, use of social and cultural rules in expression of emotions, reflexion on one's own emotions,

---

[36] Assessed by means of Assessment, Evaluation Programming System for Infants and Children (AEPS, Bricker, 2002) in its "Birth to three" version.

and emotion regulation strategies. They considered that a lack of flexibility in emotional reactions induces dysregulation and a dysregulatory pattern could gradually become stable in the child's development, generating a form of psychopathology. In developmental psychopathology, they pointed out that is important to examine the regulatory role of emotions, how emotion regulation changes over time and under what conditions dysregulation patterns appear in order to detect symptoms of disorders as soon as possible.

In future, we propose that inter-syndrome and inter-disability comparative studies should be conducted to investigate the dynamic between the components of the three levels of functioning and development included in our integrative model, in order to specify with more precision the types of links between them (differentiating bi-directional relations, direct, mediator or moderator effects of some components on others) according to types of psychopathology in children (ASD, with different genetic syndromes, with behaviour disorders)[37]. Moreover, we suggest that future research could combine hierarchical cluster analyses of cases in which regulation disorders are included among the variables for regrouping clinical cases (such as the studies by Adrien, 1996; Seynhaeve & Nader-Grosbois, 2008a) and qualitative case studies (such as the study conducted by Wieder et al., 1999) in order to differentiate diagnosis and individual profiles more precisely; this could have implications for preventive and early intervention, targeting the regulation disorders in particular. Future studies should focus on the design of specific early intervention targeting emotion regulation during interactions and its efficiency; it should also examine the development of higher-order verbal strategies for emotion regulation in children with ASD with a good level of verbal ability (as suggested also by Gulsrud et al., 2010).

## 7. Perspectives for intervention

Early detection of dysfunction in self-regulation or of dysregulation could make it possible to specify which strategies are available to facilitate the acquisition of certain functional or developmental characteristics as well as to prevent the accumulation of dysfunction which could be reflected in the development of children with ASD. A choice of intervention objectives that aims in particular to support self-regulation strategies or to remedy regulation disorders, in various problem-solving situations with objects and/or with persons, could be made, in light of the prior developmental domains.

According to Adrien (2005, pp.10-11)[38], the remediation of functional dysregulation could help the child with ASD to coordinate her or his psychological activities better and consequently to undergo more harmonious development and social integration in his or her social and physical environment. This suggestion is consistent with our integrative model of regulation in the functioning and development of children with ASD. This model can serve as a frame of reference for selecting instruments of assessment according to the goal and the situation of assessment. It effectively permits a coordinated approach to the three levels of

[37] This has been done in studies of children with ASD and with ID conducted by Seynhaeve (2006), Seynhaeve and Nader-Grosbois (2008a) and Adrien and his collaborators.

[38] In the IDDEES programme (Gattegno et al., 2006), an intensive, longitudinal intervention in the ecological environment of young children with ASD aims to improve their regulation in a constant way, in social, interactive, emotional, cognitive activities and learning situations with professionals, in order to promote their development and their social integration.

functioning and development of atypical children for research or intervention purposes, and hence a better understanding of their deficits and their strengths according to the ease or difficulty with which they mobilize their strategies of problem solving or their self-regulation. Intervention could focus purely on the remediation of a dysfunction in the context of specific problem-solving; or coordinate several abilities in distinct areas of daily life; or elicit emerging developmental acquisitions in one or more domains of development by targeting the proximal zone of development; or elicit efficient co-regulation between the child and those around him or her. These types of intervention will have implications at other levels of individual dynamics.

If the intervention aims to improve self-regulation, we offer some suggestions here. As reported in the literature, the type of task, the material, the media (physical, computer) and their familiarity to the children influence their self-regulation and are associated with an inter-situational variability of strengths or weaknesses in self-regulatory strategies (Freund, 1990; Nader-Grosbois, 2007a; Nader-Grosbois & Thomée, 2007; Nader-Grosbois & Lefèvre, 2011). From a Vygotskyan viewpoint (Vygotsky, 1978), various interactive games with adults and with peers and make-believe play (Elias & Berk, 2002, Kraft & Berk, 1998; Vieillevoye & Nader-Grosbois, 2008) between peers are privileged activities which provide an array of opportunities for practising various self-regulatory strategies in cognitive and socio-emotional problem-solving and the use of communicative and language abilities. Such play could consolidate coordination between functional abilities and self-regulatory strategies. In special education, training focusing on executive functions or on self-regulatory strategies (supported by the activation of the prefrontal cortex) in challenging and motivating situations with a varied degree of structure, and training in self-instruction during problem solving (Haelewyck & Nader-Grosbois, 2004; Kraft & Berk, 1998; Winsler et al., 2007), could be efficient at improving self-regulated abilities in children or adolescents with disability, their adjustment to changes and their socio-emotional self-regulation (Nader-Grosbois, 2007). Although some intervention programmes have developed objectives of training sessions focusing on self-regulation, initiatives for young children with ASD are not yet sufficiently supported in early intervention. It seems particularly important to provide training in self-regulation because children, especially those at risk, who begin school with a lack of self-regulation, are less likely to succeed in school and life (Raver & Knitzer, 2002). Pre-school self-regulation levels have stronger links with future school readiness, than with IQ (Blair, 2002) and with cognitive, coping and self-regulatory competence in adolescence (Eigsti et al., 2006).

In addition, if the intervention focuses on the improvement of emotion regulation in children with ASD or another psychopathology (as suggested notably by Cole et al., 1994; Southam-Gerow & Kendall, 2002), here are some guidelines. Some studies have shown the efficiency of programmes promoting the development of socio-emotional development in children with special needs[39] that include training in certain specific strategies, for example, self-control through verbal mediation or self-identification of emotions in order to manage them. Specifically in order to train emotion regulation in children with ASD, on the basis of

[39] Such as "Promoting Alternative Thinking Strategies" (PATHS, Kusché & Greenberg, 1994); the inhibitory control represents a main generative mechanism in the link between PATHS and behavioural outcomes.

a review of the literature and of some recent intervention programmes[40], Nader-Grosbois (2011) gives the following specific guidelines on interventions involving these children through the provision of training in the following skills:

- Identifying their physiological states according to their emotions (respiration, contraction, relaxation of muscles) and to learning to control them;
- Recognizing emotions from various types of stimuli (facial, vocal, gestural, body movements), socio-emotional cues, verbal and non-verbal (attitudes, postures, intonations), giving them meaning and interpreting them in an integrated manner;
- Identifying their emotional states when they are alone and in interactions with others;
- Linking their own emotional states with their own behaviour and that of other persons;
- Distinguishing inappropriate emotional state, inadequate intensity of emotional expression, depending on the circumstances;
- Using language to help modify their emotional states (negative or positive) or the intensity of their expression or of their behaviour;
- Minimizing the negative effect of environmental, social aspects to which they are over-sensitive;
- Discovering efficient emotion regulation strategies (distraction, seeking comfort, modification of emotional valence) when faced with frustrating situations;
- Practicing co-regulation of emotions[41] by means of parental scaffolding or other-regulation likely to support joint attention.

These suggestions could be applied in play or interactive situations (cooperative, competitive, pretend) using various materials (vignettes, videos illustrating social scripts, software) and in daily life.

More generally, Nader-Grosbois (2011) has developed guidelines for intervention from infancy and childhood onwards to improve socio-emotional abilities and social adjustment in children with ASD and other developmental disorders, through the provision of training in:

- precursors of ToM: emotional recognition, using various media (photographs, videos, computer software); face processing; early imitation; joint attention;
- socio-perceptive processing and perceptive integration;
- executive functions and self-regulation strategies;
- social information processing, social knowledge;
- emotional expression, emotion regulation and conventional responses to others' emotions, empathic behaviours in various contexts and towards different persons;

---

[40] In their book "The incredible 5-point Scale: assisting students with autism spectrum disorders in understanding social interactions and controlling their emotional responses", Buron and Curtis (2004) propose a method to help these children and adolescents to understand and control their emotional reactions in daily life events that could provoke inappropriate reactions or behaviour disorders. Macklem (2008) gives a set of guidelines for professionals and parents to reinforce their ability to support the children in regulating their emotions, notably by improving their reactions to the child's negative emotions, their adjustment to the child's temperament, and their exchanges about positive and negative emotions (in critical situations or from examples of scripts); this could facilitate the child's emotion regulation and coping strategies.

[41] According to Gulsrud et al. (2010), as children with ASD are at risk of dysregulation, early mother-child interactions (including joint attention) are an ideal context for socialization of their emotion regulation.

- ToM abilities, such as the understanding of causes and consequences of emotions;
- skills in socio-emotional problem-solving or challenges, social scripts.

## 8. Conclusion

As several authors have drawn attention to the fact that infants and young children diagnosed as presenting ASD display deficits in self-regulation or dysregulation in their activity, and in early emotion regulation, these specificities represent an early risk factor of severe autism and of intense behaviour disorders that need to be detected as soon as possible (Adrien, 2005; Bagnato & Neisworth, 1999; De Gangi et al., 1993, 2000; Gomez & Baird, 2005; Nader-Grosbois, 2007b; Whitman, 2004). It is indispensable to proceed to regular longitudinal assessments in the course of early development and during childhood by focusing on inter- and intra-individual variability, using instruments founded on an integrative model of functioning and development of atypical children and combining various sources of information from professionals and other people around the children (Greenspan & Meisels, 1999).

## 9. References

Adrien, J.-L. (1996). *Autisme du jeune enfant. Développement psychologique et trouble de la régulation.* Paris : Expansion Scientifique Française, Elsevier.

Adrien, J-L. (2005). *Vers un nouveau modèle de psychopathologie de l'autisme.* PsychoMédia, 37-41.

Adrien, J.-L., Martineau, J., Barthélémy, C., Bruneau, N., Garreau, B., & Sauvage, D. (1995). Disorders of regulation of cognitive activity in autistic children. *Journal of Autism and Developmental Disorders, 25*(3), 247-261.

Adrien, J.-L., Rossignol, N., Martineau, J., Roux, S., Couturier, G., & Barthélémy, C. (2001a). Regulation of cognitive activity and early communication development in young autistic, mentally retarded and young normal children. *Developmental Psychobiology, 39*(2), 124-136.

Adrien, J.-L., Roux, S., Couturier, G., Malvy, J., Guerin, P., Debuly, S., et al. (2001b). Towards a new functional assessment of autistic dysfunction in children with developmental disorders: The Behavior Function Inventory. *Autism, 5*(3), 249-264.

Allen, G., & Courchesne, E. (2001). Attention function and dysfunction in autism. *Frontiers in Bioscience, 6,* 105–119.

Argott, P., Buffington Townsend, D., Sturmey, P., & Poulson, C.L. (2008). Increasing the use of empathic statements in the presence of a non-verbal affective stimulus in adolescents with autism. *Research in Autism Spectrum Disorders, 2,* 341–352.

Attwood, A., Frith, U., & Hermelin, B. (1988). The understanding and use of interpersonal gestures by autistic and Down's syndrome children. *Journal of Autism and Developmental Disorders, 18,* 241–257.

Bacon, A.L., Fein, D., Morris, R., Waterhouse, L., & Allen, D. (1998). The responses of autistic children to the distress of others. *Journal of Autism and Developmental Disorders, 28,* 129-142.

Bagnato, S.J., & Neisworth, J.T. (1999). Normative detection of early regulatory disorders and autism: empirical confirmation of EC.-0-3. *Infants and Young Children, 12*(2), 98-106.

Bandura, A.B. (1997). *Self-efficacy: the exercise of control*. New York: W.H. Freeman.

Banerjee, M. (1997). Hidden emotion: Preschoolers' knowledge of appearance-reality and emotion display rules. *Social Cognition, 15*, 107-132.

Baranek, G.T. (1999). Autism during infancy: A retrospective video analysis of sensory-motor and social behaviours at 9–12 months of age. *Journal of Autism and Developmental Disorders, 29*, 213–224.

Baurain, C. & Nader-Grosbois, N. (2009). Evaluation de la régulation émotionnelle et de la résolution de problèmes socio-émotionnels chez des enfants présentant une déficience intellectuelle : études de cas. *Revue Francophone de la Déficience Intellectuelle, 20*, 123-147.

Baurain, C., & Nader-Grosbois, N. (2011). Élaboration et validation d'un dispositif méthodologique pour l'observation de la régulation socio-émotionnelle chez l'enfant. *Enfance, 2*.

Baurain, C., & Nader-Grosbois, N. (in press). Validation of a method of assessment of the socio-emotional regulation in preschoolers. *European Review of Applied Psychology*.

Begeer, S., Koot, H.M., Rieffe, C., Meerum Terwogt, M., & Stegge, H. (2008). Emotional Competence in children with autism. Diagnostic criteria and empirical evidence. *Developmental Review, 28*, 342-369.

Bieberich, A.A., & Morgan, S.B. (2004). Self-regulation and affective expression during play in children with autism or Down syndrome: a short-term longitudinal study. *Journal of Autism and developmental Disorders, 34*(4), 439-448.

Blanc, R., Adrien, J.-L., Roux, S., Barthélémy, C. (2005). Dysregulation of pretend play and symbolic communication in children with autism. *Autism, 9*(3), 229-245.

Blanc, R, Adrien, J.-L, Roux, S, & Barthélémy, C. (2007). Les troubles du jeu symbolique et du développement de la communication chez les enfants autistes : à propos de la dysrégulation de l'activité. In N. Nader-Grosbois (Ed.). *Autorégulation, dysrégulation, régulation* (pp. 150-175). Wavre : Mardaga.

Blanc, R., Tourrette, C., Deletang, N., Roux, S., & Barthélémy, C., & Adrien, J.-L. (2000). Regulation of pretend activity and development of communication in children with autism disorder. *European Review of Applied Psychology, 50*, 369-381.

Boekaerts, M. (1999). Self-regulated learning: where we are today. *International Journal of Educational Research, 31*, 445-457.

Boekaerts, M., Pintrich, P.R., & Zeidner, M. (2000). *Handbook of self-regulation: Theory, research, and applications*. San Diego, CA: Academic Press.

Buron, K.D., & Curtis, M. (2004). *The incredible 5-Point Scale: Assisting students with autism spectrum disorders in understanding social interactions and controlling their emotional responses*. Shawnee Mission, KS: Autism Asperger Publishing.

Bricker, D. (2002). Assessment, evaluation, and programming system for infants and children. Baltimore: Brookes.

Broadhead, P. (2001). Investigating sociability and cooperation in four and five-year olds in reception class settings. *International Journal of Early Years Education, 9*, 23-35.

Bronson, M.B. (2000). *Self-regulation in early childhood. Nature and nurture.* New York: Guilford Press.

Brun, P. (2001). Psychopathologie de l'émotion chez l'enfant : l'importance des données développementales typiques. *Enfance, 53,* 281-291.

Brun, P., & Mellier, D. (2004). Régulation émotionnelle et retard mental : étude chez l'enfant trisomique 21. *Handicap-Revue des Sciences Humaines et Sociales, 101-102,* 19-31.

Brun, P., Nadel, J., & Mattlinger, M.J. (1998). L'hypothèse émotionnelle dans l'autisme. *Psychologie Française, 43,* 147-156.

Calkins, S.D., & Johnson, M.C. (1998a). Toddler regulation of distress to frustrating events: temperamental and maternal correlates. *Infant Behavior and Development, 21,* 379-395.

Calkins, S.D., Smith, C.L., Gill, K.L., & Johnson, M.C. (1998b). Maternal interactive style across contexts: relations to emotional, behavioural, and physiological regulation during toddlerhood. *Social Development, 7,* 350-369.

Campos, J.J., Campos, R.G., & Barrett, K.C. (1989). Emergent themes in the study of emotional development and emotion regulation. *Developmental Psychology, 25*(3), 394-402.

Capps, L., Kasari, C., Yirmiya, N., & Sigman, M. (1993). Parental perception of emotional expressiveness in children with autism. *Journal of Consulting and Clinical Psychology, 61,* 475–484.

Carlson, S.M., & Wang, T.S. (2007). Inhibitory control and emotion regulation in preschool children. *Cognitive Development, 22,* 489-510.

Chang, F., & Burns, B. (2005). Attention in preschoolers: associations with effortful control and motivation. *Child Development, 76,* 247-263.

Charman, T., Swettenham, J., Baron-Cohen, S., Cox, A., Baird, G., & Drew, A. (1997). Infants with autism: An investigation on empathy, pretend play, joint attention, and imitation. *Developmental Psychology, 33,* 781–789.

Charman, T., Swettenham, J., Baron-Cohen, S., Cox, A., Baird, G., & Drew, A. (1998). An experimental investigation of social cognitive abilities in infants with autism: Clinical implications. *Infant Mental Health Journal, 19,* 260–275.

Cole, M.P., Dennis, T.A., Smith-Simon, K.E., & Cohen, L.H. (2009). Preschoolers' emotion regulation strategy understanding: relations with emotion socialization and child self-regulation. *Social Development, 18*(2), 324-352.

Cole, M.P., Martin, S.E., & Dennis, T.A. (2004). Emotion regulation as a scientific construct: methodological challenges and directions for child development research. *Child Development, 75*(2), 317-333.

Cole, P.M., Michel, M.K., & Teti, L.O. (1994). The development of emotion regulation and dysregulation: a clinical perspective. *Monographs of the Society for Research in Child Development, 59*(2-3), 73-100.

Colvert, E., Custance, D., & Swettenham, J. (2002). Rule-based reasoning and theory of mind in autism: a commentary on the work of Zelazo, Jacques, Burack and Frye. *Infant and Child Development, 11,* 197–200.

Contreras, J.M., Kerns, K., Weimer, B.L., Gentzler, A.L., & Tomich, P.L. (2000). Emotion regulation as a mediator of associations between mother-child attachment and peer relationships in middle childhood. *Journal of Family Psychology, 14,* 111-124.

Corbett, B.A., Constantine, L.J., Hendren, R., Rocke, D., & Ozonoff, S. (2009). Examining executive functioning in children with autism spectrum disorder, attention deficit, hyperactivity disorder and typical development. *Psychiatry Research, 166,* 210-222.

Corona, R., Dissanayake, C., Arbelle, S., Wellington, P., & Sigman, M. (1998). Is affect aversive to young children with autism? Behavioral and cardiac responses to experimenter distress. *Child Development, 69,* 1494–1502.

Cuskelly, M., Zhang, A. & Gilmore, L. (1998). The importance of self-regulation in young children with Down syndrome. *International Journal of Disability, Development and Education, 45,* 331-341.

Czapinski, P., & Bryson, S. E. (2003). Reduced facial muscle movements in Autism: Evidence for dysfunction in the neuromuscular pathway? *Brain and Cognition, 51,* 177–179.

Daffe, V. & Nader-Grosbois, N. (2011). Comportements parentaux à l'égard des émotions et des croyances et Théorie de l'esprit chez l'enfant. In N. Nader-Grosbois (Ed.), *Théorie de l'esprit : entre cognition, émotion et adaptation sociale* (pp. 301-321). Bruxelles : De Boeck.

Davidov, M., & Grusec, J.E. (2006). Untangling the links of parental responsiveness to distress and warmth to child outcomes. *Child Development, 77*(1), 44-58.

Dawson, G., Webb, S.J., Carver, L., Panagiotides, H., & McPartland, J. (2004). Young children with autism show atypical brain responses to fearful versus neutral facial expressions of emotion. *Developmental Science, 7,* 340–359.

Dawson, G., Hill, D., Spencer, A., Galpert, L., & Watson, L. (1990b). Affective exchanges between young autistic children and their mothers. *Journal of Abnormal Child Psychology, 18,* 335–345.

DeCooke, P.A., & Brownell, C.A. (1999). Young children's help-seeking in mastery-oriented contexts. *Merrill-Palmer Quarterly, 41*(2), 229-246.

DeGangi, G.A., Porges, S.W., Sickel, R.Z., & Greenspan, S.I. (1993). Four-year follow-up of a sample of regulatory disordered infants. *Infant Mental Health Journal, 14*(4), 330-343.

DeGangi, G.A., Breinbauer, C., Doussard-Roosevelt, J., Porges, S. & Greenspan, S. (2000). Prediction of childhood problems at three years in children experiencing disorders of regulation in infancy. *Infant Mental Health Journal, 21*(3), 156-175.

De La Ossa, J.L., & Gauvain, M. (2001). Joint attention by mothers and children while using plans. *International Journal of Behavioral Development, 25,* 176-183.

Denham, S., Salisch, M.V., Olthof, T., Kochanoff, A., & Caverly, S. (2002). Emotional and social development in childhood. In P.K. Smith & C.H. Hart (Eds.), *Blackwell handbook of childhood social development* (pp. 308-328). Malden, MA: Blackwell Publishing.

Denham, S.A., & Burton, R. (2003). *Social and emotional prevention and intervention programming for preschoolers.* New York: Kluwer-Plenum.

Denham, S.A. (2007). Dealing with feelings: how children negotiate the worlds of emotions and social relationship. *Cognition, Brain, Behavior, 11,* 1-48.

Dennis, T.A. (2006). Emotional self regulation in preschoolers: the interplay of temperamental approach reactivity and control processes. *Developmental Psychology, 42,* 84-97.

Dennis, T.A., & Kelemen, D.A. (2009a). Preschool children's views on emotion regulation: functional associations and implications for social-emotional adjustment. *International Journal of Behavioral Development, 33,* 243-252.

Dennis, T.A. (2007). Interaction between emotion regulation strategies and affective style: implications for trait anxiety versus depressed mood. *Motivation and Emotion, 31,* 200-207.

Dennis, T.A., Malone, M., & Chen, C. (2009b). Emotional face processing and emotion regulation in children: an ERP study. *Developmental Neuropsychology, 34,* 85-102.

Derryberry, D., & Rothbart, M.K. (1988). Arousal, affect, and attention as components of temperament. *Journal of Personality and Social Psychology, 55,* 958-966.

Dissanayake, C., Sigman, M., & Kasari, C. (1996). Long-term stability of individual differences in the emotional responsiveness of children with autism. *Journal of Child Psychology and Psychiatry, 37,* 461–467.

Dodge, K.A., Pettit, G.S., McClaskey, C.L., & Brown, M.M. (1986). Social competence in children. *Monographs of the Society for Research in Child Development, 51*(2, Serial No. 213), 1-85.

Dumas, C., & Lebeau, S. (1998). Le changement représentationnel affectif chez les enfants d'âge préscolaire. *Revue Canadienne de Psychologie Expérimentale, 52*(1), 25-33.

Dumont-Mathieu, T., & Fein, D. (2005). Screening for autism in young children: The modified checklist for autism in toddlers (M-CHAT) and other measures. *Mental Retardation and Developmental Disabilities Research Reviews, 11,* 253–262.

Dunn, J. (2003). Emotional development in early childhood: A social relationship perspective. In R. Davidson, H.H. Goldsmith, & K. Scherer (Eds.), *The handbook of affective science* (pp. 332–346). Oxford, UK: Oxford University Press.

Dyck, M.J., Ferguson, K., & Shochet, I.M. (2001). Do autism spectrum disorders differ from each other and from non spectrum disorders on emotion recognition tests? *European Child and Adolescent Psychiatry, 10,* 105–116.

Eigsti, I.M., Zayas, V., Mischel, W., Shoda, Y., Ayduk, O., Dadlani, M.B., Davidson, M.C., Aber, J.L., & Casey, B.J. (2006). Predicting cognitive control from preschool to late adolescence and young adulthood. *Psychological Science, 17*(6), 478-484.

Eisenberg, N. (2000). Emotion, regulation, and moral development. *Annual Review of Psychology, 51,* 665-697.

Eisenberg, N. (2003). Prosocial behavior, empathy, and sympathy. In M.H. Bornstein, L. Davidson, C.L.M. Keyes, & K.A. Moore (Eds.), *Well-Being: positive development across the life course* (pp.253-265). London: Lawrence Erlbaum Associates, Publishers: London.

Eisenberg, N., & Fabes, R.A. (1990). Empathy: conceptualization, assessment, and relation to prosocial behavior. *Motivation and Emotion, 14,* 131-149.

Eisenberg, N., & Fabes, R.A. (1992). Emotion, regulation, and the development of social competence. In M.S. Clark (Ed.). *Emotion and Social Behavior* (Vol. 14, pp. 119–150). Newbury Park, CA: Sage.

Eisenberg, N., & Fabes, R.A. (1995a). The relation of young children's vicarious emotional responding to social competence, regulation, and emotionality. *Cognition and Emotion, 9,* 203-228.

Eisenberg, N., & Fabes, R.A. (1998a). Prosocial developmental. In W. Damon (Ed.), *Handbook of child psychology 5th Edition: Social, Emotional, and personality development* (pp.701-778). New-York: John Wiley & Sons.

Eisenberg, N., & Miller, P. (1987). The relation of empathy to prosocial and related behaviors. *Psychology Bulletin, 101*, 91-119.

Eisenberg, N., & Morris, A.S. (2001b). The origins and social significance of empathy-related responding. A review of empathy and moral development: implications for caring and justice by M.L. Hoffman. *Social Justice Research, 14*(1), 95-120.

Eisenberg, N., & Mussen, P.H. (1989). The roots of prosocial behavior in children. Cambridge: Cambridge University Press.

Eisenberg, N., Cumberland, A., Spinrad, T.L., Fabes, R.A., Shepard, S.A., Reiser, M., Murphy, B.C., Losoya, S.H., & Guthrie, I.K. (2001a). The relations of regulation and emotionality to children's externalizing and internalizing problem behavior. *Child Development, 72*(4), 1112-1134.

Eisenberg, N., Fabes, R.A., Guthrie, I.K., & Reiser, M. (2000a). Dispositional emotionality and regulation: their role in predicting quality of social functioning. *Journal of Personality and Social Psychology, 78*(1), 136-157.

Eisenberg, N., Fabes, R.A., Karbon, M., Murphy B.C.,Wosinski, M., Plazzi, G.C. & Juhnke, C. (1996a). The relations of children's dispositional prosocial behavior to emotionality, regulation, and social functioning. *Child Development, 67*, 974-992.

Eisenberg, N., Fabes, R.A., Murphy, B., Karbon, M., Maszk, P., Smith, M., O'Boyle, C., & Suh, K. (1994). The relations of emotionality and regulation to dispositional and situational empathy-related responding. *Journal of Personality and social psychology, 66*(4), 776-797.

Eisenberg, N., Fabes, R.A., Murphy, B., Maszk, P., Smith, M., & Karbon, M. (1995b). The role of emotionality and regulation in children's social functioning: a longitudinal study. *Child Development, 66*, 1360-1384.

Eisenberg, N., Fabes, R.A., Murphy, B.C., Karbon, M., Smith, M., & Maszk, P. (1996b). The relations of children's dispositional empathy-related responding to their emotionality, regulation, and social functioning. *Developmental psychology, 32*(2), 195-209.

Eisenberg, N., Fabes, R.A., Shepard, S.A., Murphy, B.C, Guthrie, I.K., Jones, S., Friedman, J., Poulin, R., & Maszk, P. (1997a). Contemporaneous and longitudinal prediction of children's social functioning from regulation and emotionality. *Child Development, 68*, 642-664.

Eisenberg, N., Guthrie, I., Fabes, R., Reiser, M., Murphy, B., Holgren, R., Maszk, P., & Losoya, S. (1997b). The relations of regulation and emotionality to resiliency and competent social functioning in elementary school children. *Child Development, 68*, 295-311.

Eisenberg, N., Guthrie, I.K., Fabes, R.A., Shepard, S.A., Losoya, S., Murphy, B.C., Jones, S., Poulin, R., & Reiser, M. (2000b). Prediction of elementary school children's externalizing problem behaviors from attentional and behavioral regulation and negative emotionality. *Child Development, 71*(5), 1367-1382.

Eisenberg, N., Hofer, C., & Vaughan, J. (2007). *Effortful Control and its Socio-emotional Consequences*. In J.J. Gross (Ed.) *Handbook emotion regulation* (chap.14, pp. 287-306). New York: Guilford Press.

Eisenberg, N., Losoya S., & Guthrie, I.K. (1997c). Social cognition and prosocial development. In S. Hala (Ed.), *The development of social cognition* (pp. 329-363). Hove, East Sussex. Psychology Press.

Eisenberg, N., Shepard, S.A., Fabes, R.A., Murphy, B.C., & Guthrie, I.K. (1998b). Contemporaneous and longitudinal prediction of children's sympathy from dispositional regulation and emotionality. *Developmental Psychology, 34*(5), 910-924.

Ekman, P. (2003). Emotions revealed: recognizing faces and feelings to improve communication and emotional life. New York: Times Books/Henry Holt and Co.

Elias, C.L., & Berk, L.E. (2002). Self-regulation in young children: is there a role for socio-dramatic play ? *Early Childhood Research Quarterly, 17*, 216-238.

Fabes, R.A., Eisenberg, N., Jones, S., Smith, M., Guthrie, I., Poulin, R., Shepard, S., & Friedman, J. (1999). Regulation, emotionality, and preschoolers' socially competent peer interactions. *Child Development, 70*(2), 432-442.

Fantuzzo, J., Sekino, Y., & Cohen, H.L. (2004). An examination of the contributions of interactive peer play to salient classroom competencies for urban head start children. *Psychology in the Schools, 41*, 323-336.

Filipek, P.A., Accardo, P.J., Ashwal, S., Baranek, G.T., Cook, E.H., Jr., Dawson, G., et al. (2000). Practice parameter: Screening and diagnosis of autism: Report of the Quality Standards Subcommittee of the American Academy of Neurology and the Child Neurology Society. *Neurology, 55*, 468–479.

Fisher, N., & Happé, F. (2005). A training study of Theory of Mind and executive function in children with autistic spectrum disorders. *Journal of Autism and Developmental Disorders, 35*(6), 757-771.

Focant, J., Grégoire, J., & Desoete, A. (2006). Goal-setting, planning and control strategies and arithmetical problem solving at grade 5. In M.J. Veenman & A. Desoete (Eds.), *Metacognition in mathematics education* (pp. 51-71). New York: Nova Sciences Publishers.

Freund, L.S. (1990). Maternal regulation of children's problem-solving and its impact on children's performance. *Child Development, 61*, 113-126.

Frye, D., Zelazo, P.D., & Palfai, T. (1995). Theory of mind and rule-based reasoning. *Cognitive Development, 10*, 483–527.

Fujiki, M., Brinton, B., & Clarke, D. (2002). Emotion regulation in children with specific language impairment. *Language, Speech, and Hearing Service in Schools, 33*, 102-111.

Fujiki, M., Spackman, M.P., Brinton, B., & Hall, A. (2004). The relationship of language and emotion regulation skills to reticence in children with specific language impairment. *Journal of Speech, Language, and Hearing Research, 47*, 637-646.

Galyer, K.T., & Evans, I.M. (2001). Pretend play and the development of emotion regulation in preschool children. *Early Child Development and Care, 166*, 93-108.

Garcia-Andres, E., Huertes-Martinez, J.A., Ardura, A., & Fernandez-Alcaraz, C. (2010). Emotional regulation and executive function profiles of functioning related to the social development of children. *Procedia Social and Behavioral Sciences, 5*, 2077-2081.

Gardner, W., & Rogoff, B. (1990). Children's deliberateness of planning according to task circumstances. *Developmental Psychology, 26*, 480-487.

Gattegno, M.-P., Ionescu, S., Malvy, J., & Adrien, J.-L. (1999). Étude préliminaire de la recherche d'un lien spécifique entre les troubles de l'attention conjointe et de la théorie de l'esprit dans l'autisme de l'enfant. *Approche Neuropsychologique des Apprentissages chez l'Enfant, 52*, 41-48.

Gattegno, M.-P., Abenhaim, N., Kremer, A., Castro, Ch., & Adrien, J.-L. (2006). Étude longitudinale du développement cognitif et social d'un enfant autiste bénéficiant du programme IDDEES. *Journal des Thérapies Comportementales et Cognitives, 16*(4), 157-168.

Gauvain, M., & Rogoff, B. (1989). Collaborative problem solving and children's planning skills. *Developmental Psychology, 25*, 139-151.

Gena, A., Krantz, P.J., McClannahan, L.E., & Poulson, C.L. (1996). Training and generalization of affective behaviour displayed by youth with autism. *Journal of Applied Behavior Analysis, 29*, 291–304.

Gepner, B., & Mestre, D. (2002). Brief report: postural reactivity to fast visual motion differentiates autistic from children with Asperger syndrome. *Journal of Autism and Developmental Disorders, 12*, 231-238.

Ghaziuddin, M., & Butler, E. (1998). Clumsiness in autism and Asperger syndrome: A further report. *Journal of Intellectual Disabilities Research, 42*, 43–48.

Gilmore, L., Cuskelly, M., & Hayes A. (2003). Self-regulatory behaviors in children with Down syndrome and typically developing children measured using the Goodman Lock Box. *Research in developmental Disabilities, 24*, 95-108.

Gomot, M., Giard, M.-H., Adrien, J.-L., Barthélémy, C., & Bruneau, N. (2002). Hypersensitivity to acoustic change in children with autism: Electrophysiological evidence of left frontal cortex dysfunctioning. *Psychophysiology, 39*, 577-584.

Gomez, C.R., & Baird, S. (2005). Identifying early indicators for autism in self-regulation difficulties. *Focus on Autism and Other Developmental Disabilities, 20*(2), 106-116.

Gosselin, P. (2005). Le décodage de l'expression faciale des émotions au cours de l'enfance. *Psychologie Canadienne, 46*(3), 126-138.

Gottman, J.M. (1986). The world of coordinated-play: Same and cross-sex friendship in young children. In J.M., Gottman, & J.G., Parker (Eds.), *Conversations of Friends: Speculations on Affective Development* (pp. 139-191). Cambridge: Cambridge University Press.

Grandin, T. (1995). *Thinking in pictures*. New York: Vintage Books.

Gross, J.J. (1998). The emerging field of emotion regulation: an integrative review. *Review of General Psychology, 2*(3), 271-299.

Gross, J.J., & Thompson, R.A. (2007). Emotion regulation: Conceptual foundations. In J.J. Gross (Ed.), *Handbook of emotion regulation* (pp. 3-24). New York, NY: Guilford Press.

Gulsrud, A.C., Jahromi, L.B., & Kasari, C. (2010). The co-regulation of emotions between mothers and their children with autism. *Journal of Autism and Developmental disorders, 40*(2), 227-237.

Guthrie, I.K., Eisenberg, N., Fabes, R.A., Murphy, B.C., Holmgren, R., Mazsk P., & Suh, K. (1997). The relations of regulation and emotionality to children's situational empathy-related responding. *Motivation and emotion, 21*(1), 87-108.

Greenspan, S.I., & Meisels, J. (1999). Toward a new vision for the developmental assessment of infants and young children. In J. Meisels & E. Fenichel (Eds.), *New visions for the developmental assessment of infants and young children* (pp. 11-26). Washington: Zero to Three: National Center for Infants, Toddlers and Families.

Haelewyck M.-C., & Nader-Grosbois, N. (2004). L'autorégulation : une des portes d'entrée vers l'autodétermination des personnes à incapacités intellectuelles? *Revue Francophone de la Déficience Intellectuelle, 15*(2), 173-186.

Hallett, M., Lebiedowska, M.K., Thomas, S.L., Stanhope, S.J., Denckla, M.B., & Rumsey, J. (1993). Locomotion of autistic adults. *Archives of Neurology, 50,* 1304–1308.

Harris, P.L., Johnson, C.N., Hutton, D., Andrews, B., & Cooke, T. (1989). Young children's theory of mind and emotion. *Cognition and Emotion, 3,* 379-400.

Herbé, D., Tremblay, H., & Mallet, P. (2007). La coopération dyadique entre enfants de 5-6 ans: Effets de la complexité cognitive et de l'activité motrice sollicitées pas les situations de résolution de problème. *Enfance, 59,* 393-413.

Hill, E.L. (2004). Executive dysfunction in autism. *Trends in Cognitive Sciences, 8,* 26-32.

Dawson, G., Hill, D., Spencer, A., Galpert, L., & Watson, L. (1990b). Affective exchanges between young autistic children and their mothers. *Journal of Abnormal Child Psychology, 18,* 335–345.

Haynie, D.L., & Lamb, M.E. (1995). Positive and negative facial expressiveness in 7-, 10-, 13-month-old infants. *Infant behaviour and Development, 18*(2), 257-259.

Howes, C., Unger, O., & Matheson, C.C. (1992). *The collaborative construction of pretend: social pretend play functions.* New-York: State University of New York Press.

Huebner, R.A., & Dunn, W. (2001). Introduction and basic concepts. In R. Huebner (Ed.), *Autism: A sensorimotor approach to management* (pp. 61-99). Gaithersburg, MD: Aspen.

Hudry, K., & Slaughter, V. (2009). Agent familiarity and emotional context influence the everyday empathic responding of young children with autism. *Research in Autism Spectrum Disorders, 3,* 74–85.

Hudson, J.A., & Fivush, R. (1991). Planning in the preschool years: the emergence of plans from general event knowledge. *Cognitive Development, 6,* 393-415.

Hudson, J.A., Shapiro, L.R., & Sosa B.B. (1995). Planning in the real world: preschool children's scripts and plans for familiar events. *Child Development, 66,* 984-998.

Hugues, C., Russell, J., & Robbins, T.W. (1994). Evidence for executive dysfunction in autism. *Neuropsychologia, 32*(4), 477-492.

Izard, C.E., & Malatesta, C.Z. (1987). Perspectives on emotional development I: Differential emotions theory of early emotional development. In J.D. Osofsky (Ed.), *Handbook of infant development* (pp. 494–554). New York: Wiley.

Izard, C.E, Fine, S., Schultz, D., Mostow, A., Ackerman, B., & Youngstrom, E. (2001). Emotion knowledge as a predictor of social behavior and academic competence in children at risk. *Psychological Science, 12,* 18-23.

Izard, C.E, Schultz, D., Fine, S.E., Youngstrom, E., & Ackerman, B.P. (2000). Temperament, cognitive ability, emotion knowledge, and adaptive social behavior. *Imagination, Cognition, and Personality, 19*, 305-330.

Jarrold, C. (1997). Pretend play in autism: executive explanations. In J. Russell (Ed.), *Autism as an executive disorder* (pp. 101-140), Oxford, UK : Oxford University Press.

Joseph, R.M., McGrath, L.M., & Tager-Flushberg, H. (2005). Executive dysfunction and its relation to language ability in verbal school-age children with autism. *Developmental Neuropsychology, 27*(3), 361-378.

Josse, D. (1997). *Brunet-Lézine Révisé : Echelle de développement psychomoteur de la première enfance.* Issy-Les-Moulineaux, France: Etablissements d'Applications Psychotechniques.

Kasari, C., Sigman, M., & Yirmiya, N. (1993a). Focused and social attention of autistic-children in interactions with familiar and unfamiliar adults - A comparison of autistic, mentally-retarded, and normal-children. *Development and Psychopathology, 5*, 403–414.

Kasari, C., & Sigman, M. (1996). Expression and understanding of emotion in atypical development : autism and Down syndrome. In M. Lewis & M.W. Sullivan (Eds.), *Emotional development in atypical children* (pp. 109-130). Mahwah, NJ: Lawrence Erlbaum Associates.

Khalfa, S., Bruneau, N., Rogé, B ., Georgieff, N., Veuillet, E., Adrien, J.-L., Barthélémy, C., & Collet, L. (2001). Peripheral auditory asymmetry in infantile autism. *European Journal of Neuroscience, 13*, 628-632.

Konstantareas, M.M., & Stewart, K. (2006). Affect regulation and temperament in children with autism spectrum disorder. *Journal of Autism and Developmental Disorders, 36*, 143–154.

Korkman, M., Kirk, U., & Kemp, S. (2007). *NEPSY-II Review* (2nd edition). San Antonio, TX: Harcourt Assessment.

Kraft, K.C., & Berk, L.E. (1998). Private speech in two preschools: significance of open-ended activities and make-believe play for verbal self-regulation. *Early Childhood Research Quarterly, 13*, 637-658.

Kusché, C.A., & Greenberg, M.T. (1994). *The Paths (Promoting Alternative Thinking Strategies) curriculum.* South Deerfields, MA: Channing-Bete Co.

Lanfaloni, G.A., Baglioni, A., & Tafi, L. (1997). Self-regulation training programs for subjects with intellectual disability and blindness. *Developmental Brain Dysfunctionning, 10*, 231-239.

Lelord, G. (1990). Physiopathologie de l'autisme. Les insuffisances modulatrices cérébrales. *Neuropsychiatrie de l'Enfance et de l'adolescence, 38*(1-2), 43-49.

Lemche, E., Lennertz, I., Orthmann, C., Ari, A., Grote, K., Häfker, J. & Klann-Delius, G. (2003). Emotion regulatory processes in evoked play narratives. *Praxis der Kinderpsychologie und Kinderpsychiatrie, 52*(3), 156-171.

Lengua, L.J. (2002). The contribution of emotionality and self-regulation to the understanding of children's response to multiple risk. *Child Development, 73*(1), 144-161.

Lewis, M., & Sullivan M.W. (1996). *Emotional development in atypical children.* Mahwah, NJ: Lawrence Erlbaum Associates.

Lewis, M., Sullivan, M.W., Stanger, C., & Weiss, M. (1989). Self-Development and Self-Conscious Emotions. *Child development, 60,* 146-156.

Liew, J., Eisenberg, N. & Reiser, M. (2004). Preschoolers' effortful control and negative emotionality, immediate reactions to disappointment, and quality of social functioning. *Journal of Experimental Child Psychology, 89*(4), 298-319.

Lindsey, E.W. & Colwell, M.J. (2003). Preschooler's emotional competence: Links to pretend and physical play. *Child Study Journal, 33,* 39-52.

Loveland, K.A., Tunali-kotoski, B., Pearson, D.A., Brelsford, K.A., Ortegon, J., & Chen, R. (1994). Imitation and expression of facial affect in autism. *Development and Psychopathology, 6,* 433–444.

Luminet, O. (2002). *Psychologie des émotions.* Bruxelles: De Boeck.

Macklem, G.L. (2008). Practitioner's guide to emotion regulation in school-aged children. Manchester: Springer.

Maestro, S., Muratori, F., Cavallaro, M.C., Pecini, C., Cesari, A., Paziente, A., et al. (2005). How young children treat objects and people? An empirical study of the first year of life in autism. *Child Psychiatry & Human Development, 35,* 383–396.

Maestro, S., Muratori, F., Cavallaro, M.C., Pei, F., Stern, D., Golse, B., & Palacio-Espasa, F. (2002). Attentional skills during the first 6 months of age in autistic spectrum disorder. *Journal of the American Academy of Child and Adolescent Psychiatry, 41,* 1239–1245.

Malatesta-Magai, C., Leak, S., Tesman, J., & Shepard, B. (1994). Profiles of emotional development: Individual differences in facial and vocal expression of emotion during the second and third years of life. *International Journal of Behavioral Development, 17,* 239-269.

Martineau, J., Adrien, J.-L., Barthélémy, C., Garreau, B., & Lelord, G. (1998). Association and regulation disorders in infantile autism. *Journal of Psychophysiology, 12,* 275-285.

McEvoy, R.E., Rogers, S.J., & Pennington, B.F. (1993). Executive function and social communication deficits in young autistic children. *Journal of Child Psychology and Psychiatry, 34*(4), 563-578.

McGovern, C.W., & Sigman, M. (2005). Continuity and change from early childhood to adolescence in autism. *Journal of Child Psychology and Psychiatry, 46,* 401–408.

Mellier, D., Brun, P., & Tremblay, H. (2008). *Le langage émotionnel, le comprendre et le parler.* Mont-St-Aignan, France: Publication des universités de Rouen et du Havre.

Mikolajczak, M., Quoidbach, J., Kotsou, I., & Nélis, D. (2009). *Les compétences émotionnelles.* Paris : Dunod.

Mirabile, S.P., Scaramella, L.V., Sohr-Preston, S.L., & Robison, S.D. (2009). Mothers' socialization of emotion regulation: the moderating role of children's negative emotional reactivity. *Child Youth Care Forum, 38,* 19-37.

Mottron, L. (2004). *L'autisme : une autre intelligence.* Bruxelles : Mardaga.

Mundy, P., Sigman, M., & Kasari, C. (1990). A longitudinal study of joint attention and language development in autistic children. *Journal of Autism and Developmental Disorders, 20,* 115–128.

Nadel, J., Croué, S., Mattlinger, M.J., Canet, P., Hudelot, C., Lécuyer, C., & Martini, M. (2000). Do children with autism have expectancies about social behaviour of unfamiliar people? *Autism, 4,* 133-145.

Nader-Grosbois, N. & Day, J. (2011). Emotional Cognition: Theory of Mind and Face Recognition. In J.L. Matson & P. Sturmey (Eds.), *International handbook of autism and pervasive developmental disorders* (chap.9). New York: Springer.

Nader-Grosbois, N. (2006). *Le développement cognitif et communicatif du jeune enfant. Du normal au pathologique*. Bruxelles: DeBoeck.

Nader-Grosbois, N. (2007a). *Régulation, autorégulation, dysrégulation*. Wavre: Mardaga.

Nader-Grosbois, N. (2007b). L'autorégulation et la dysrégulation chez des jeunes enfants à autisme en situation d'évaluation développementale. *Revue Francophone de la Déficience Intellectuelle, 17*, 34-52.

Nader-Grosbois, N. (2009). *Echelles d'Evaluation du Développement Cognitif Précoce (EEDCP) : Manuel illustré d'administration*. Louvain-la-Neuve : Presses Universitaires de Louvain.

Nader-Grosbois, N. (2011). *Théorie de l'esprit : entre cognition, émotion et adaptation sociale*. Bruxelles : De Boeck.

Nader-Grosbois, N., & Lefèvre, N. (2011). Self-regulation and performance in problem-solving using physical materials or computers in children with intellectual disability, *Research in Developmental Disabilities*. doi:10.1016/j.ridd.2011.01.020.

Nader-Grosbois, N., & Thomée, C. (2007). Variabilité de l'autorégulation d'enfants à retard mental en situation de résolution de problème et bénéficiant de l'hétérorégulation parentale. In N. Nader-Grosbois (Ed.), *Régulation, autorégulation, dysrégulation*. (pp. 203-221) Wavre: Mardaga.

Nader-Grosbois, N., Normandeau, S., Ricard, M., & Quintal, G. (2008). Mother's, father's and child self-regulation in learning situation. *European Journal of Psychology of Education, 23*(1), 95-115.

Nader-Grosbois, N., & Vieillevoye, S. (2011). Variability of self-regulatory strategies in children with intellectual disability and typically developing children in pretend play situations. *Journal of Intellectual Disability Research*. doi: 10.1111/j.1365-2788.2011.01443.x

O'Neill, M., & Jones, R.S.P. (1997). Sensory-perceptual abnormalities in autism: A case for more research? *Journal of Autism and Developmental Disorders, 27*, 283–293.

Ornitz, E.M. (1985). Neurophysiology of infantile autism. *Journal of American Academy of Child Psychiatry, 24*, 251-262.

Osterling, J.A., Dawson, G., & Munson, J.A. (2002). Early recognition of 1-year-old infants with autism spectrum disorder versus mental retardation. *Development and Psychopathology, 14*, 239–251.

Ozonoff, S. (1997). Components of executive function in autism and other disorders. In J. Russell (Ed.), *Autism as an executive disorder* (pp. 179-211). Oxford, UK : Oxford University Press.

Ozonoff, S., Pennington, B.F., & Rogers, S.J. (1991). Executive function deficits in high-functioning autistic individuals: Relationship to theory of mind. *Journal of Child Psychology and Psychiatry, 32*(7), 1081-1105.

Palomo, R., Belinchon, M., & Ozonoff, S. (2006). Autism and family home movies: A comprehensive review. *Journal of Developmental and Behavioral Pediatrics, 27*, 59-68.

Paris, B. (2000). Characteristics of autism. In C. Murray-Slutsky, & B. Paris (Eds.), *Exploring the spectrum of autism and pervasive developmental disorders* (pp. 7-23). San Antonio, TX: Therapy Skill Builders.

Parker, J.G., & Asher, S.R. (1987). Peer relations and later personal adjustment: Are low-accepted children at risk? *Psychological Bulletin, 102*(3), 357-389.

Parrila, R.K., Das, J.P., & Dash, U.N. (1996). Development of planning and its relation to other cognitive processes. *Journal of Applied Developmental Psychology, 17*, 597-624.

Pellicano, E. (2007). Links between theory of mind and executive function in young children with autism: clues to developmental primacy. *Development Psychology, 43*, 974-990.

Pellicano, E., Maybery, M., Durkin, K., & Maley, A. (2006). Multiple cognitive capabilities/deficits in children with an autism spectrum disorder: "Weak" central coherence and its relationship to theory of mind and executive control. *Development and Psychopathology, 18*, 77–98.

Perner, J., Lang, B., & Kloo, D. (2002). Theory of mind and self-control: more than a common problem of inhibition. *Child Development, 73*, 752–767.

Perron, M., & Gosselin, P. (2004). Le développement de la simulation des émotions: Une étude de la vraisemblance des expressions faciales produites par les enfants. *Enfance, 2*, 109-125.

Perry, N.E. (1998). Young children's self-regulated learning and contexts that support it. *Journal of Educational Psychology, 90*(4), 715-729.

Phillips, W., Baron-Cohen, S., & Rutter, M. (1992). The role of eye-contact in goal detection: evidence from normal and children with autism or mental handicap. *Development and Psychopathology, 4*(3), 375-383.

Pintrich, P.R. (2000). Multiple goals, multiple pathways: the role of goal orientation in learning and achievement. *Journal of Educational Psychology, 92*, 544-555.

Prevost, R.A., Bronson, M.B., & Casey, M.B. (1995). Planning processes in preschool children. *Journal of Applied Developmental Psychology, 16*, 505-527.

Puustinen, M. (1998). Help-seeking behavior in a problem-solving situation: development of self-regulation. *European Journal of Psychology of education, 13*, 271-282.

Rajendran, G., & Mitchell, P. (2007). Cognitive theories of autism. *Developmental Review, 27*, 224-260.

Raver, C.C., & Knitzer, J. (2002). *Ready to enter: what research tells policymakers about strategies to promote social and emotional school readiness among three- and four-year-old children. Promoting the emotional well-being of children and families Policy Paper*. New-York: National Centre for children in poverty, Mailman School of Public Health, Columbia University.

Receveur, C., Lenoir, P., Desombre, H., Barthelmy, C., & Malvy, J. (2005). Interaction and imitation deficits from infancy to 4 years of age in children with autism: A pilot study based on videotapes. *Autism, 9*, 69–82.

Reddy, V., Williams, E., & Vaughan, A. (2002). Sharing humour and laughter in autism and Down's syndrome. *British Journal of Psychology, 93*, 219–242.

Rieder, S., Perrez, M., Reicherts, M., & Horn, A. (2007). Interpersonal emotion regulation in the family: a review of assessment tools. In A.M. Fontaine & M. Matias (Eds.), *Family, Work and Parenting: international perspectives* (pp. 17-45). Porto: Legis/livpsic.

Rimé, B. (2007). Interpersonal emotion regulation. In J.J. Gross (Ed.), *Handbook of Emotion Regulation* (pp.466-485). New York: Guilford Press.

Roberts, W., & Strayers, J. (1996). Empathy, emotional expressiveness, and prosocial behavior. *Child Development, 67*, 449-470.

Rossignol, N., Adrien, J.-L., Martineau, J., Cochin, S., Barthélémy, C. (1998). Etude préliminaire de la théorie de l'esprit, des troubles de la régulation cognitive et de la fonction d'association dans l'autisme de l'enfant. *Approche Neuropsychologique des Apprentissages chez l'enfant, 4*, 26-31.

Rubin, K.H, Bukowski, W., & Parker, J. (2006). Peer interactions, relationships, and groups. In N. Eisenberg (Ed), *Handbook of child psychology: Social, emotional, and personality development* (6th ed., pp. 571-645). New York: Wiley.

Ruble, L. (2001). Analysis of social interactions as goal-directed behaviors in children with autism. *Journal of Autism and Developmental Disorders, 31*, 471-482.

Russell, J. (1997). How executive disorders can bring about an inadequate 'theory or mind'. In J. Russell (Ed.) *Autism as an executive disorder* (pp. 256-304). Oxford: Oxford University Press.

Russell, J., & Hill, E.L. (2001). Action-monitoring and intention reporting in children with autism. *Journal of Child Psychology and Psychiatry and Allied Disciplines, 42*, 317–328.

Russell, J., Hala, S., & Hill, E. (2003). The automated windows task: the performance of preschool children, children with autism, and children with moderate learning difficulties. *Cognitive Development, 18*, 111–137.

Russell, J., Mauthner, N., Sharpe, S., & Tidswell, T. (1991). The windows task as a measure of strategic deception in preschoolers and autistic subjects. *British Journal of Developmental Psychology, 9*, 331–349.

Rydell, A.-M., Berlin, L., & Boblin, G., (2003). Emotionality, emotion regulation, and adaptation among 5- to 8- year old children. *Emotion, 3*(1), 30-47.

Saarni, C. (1999). *The developement of emotional competence*. New York: Guilford Press.

Sallquist, J.V., Eisenberg, N., Spinrad, T.L., Reiser, M., Hofer, C., Zhou, Q., Liew, J., & Eggum, N. (2009). Positive and negative emotionality: trajectories across six years and relations with social competence. *Emotion, 9*(1), 15-28.

Salovey, P., Hsee, C.K., & Mayer, J.D. (1993). Emotional intelligence and the self-regulation of affect. In D.M. Wegner & J.W. Pennebaker (Eds.), *Handbook of Mental control*. (pp.258-277) Century Psychology series. Prentice Hall: Upper Saddle River.

Scambler, D.J., Hepburn, S., Rutherford, M.D., Wehner, E.A., & Rogers, S.J. (2007). Emotional responsivity in children with autism, children with other developmental disabilities, and children with typical development. *Journal of Autism and Developmental Disorders, 37*, 553–563.

Scaramella, L.V. & Leve, L.D. (2004). Clarifying parent-child reciprocities during early childhood: The early childhood coercion model. *Clinical Child and Family Psychology Review, 7*, 89-107.

Scholnick, E.K. & Friedman, S.L. (1987). The planning construct in the psychological literature. In S.L. Friedman, E.K. Scholnick, & R.R. Cocking, (Eds), *Blueprint for thinking* (pp. 3-38). Cambridge: Cambridge University Press.

Schopler, E., Reichler, R.J., & Rochen-Renner, B. (1986). *The childhood autism rating scale (CARS) for diagnostic screening and classification of autism*. New York: Irvington.

Schultz, D., Izard, C.E., Ackerman, B.P., & Youngstrom, E.A. (2001). Emotion knowledge in economically-disadvantaged children: Self-regulatory antecedents and relations to social maladjustment. *Development and Psychopathology, 13*, 53-67.

Seibert, J.M., & Hogan, A. (1982). *Procedures manual for Early Social-Communication Scales (ESCS)*. Miami, Florida: Mailman Center for Child Development, University of Miami.

Sethi, A., Mischel, W., Aber, J.L., Shoda, Y., & Rodriguez, M.L. (2000). The role of strategic attention deployment in development of self-regulation: predicting preschoolers' delay of gratification from mother-toddler interactions. *Developmental Psychology, 36*(6), 767-777.

Seynhaeve, I., (2006). *Sensorimotor development and neuropsychological dysfunction in young children with autism and with intellectual disabilities*. Ph. D. thesis directed by N. Nader-Grosbois. Louvain-la-Neuve: Catholic University of Louvain.

Seynhaeve, I., & Nader-Grosbois, N. (2008a). Sensorimotor development and dysregulation of activity in young children with autism and with intellectual disabilities. *Research in Autism Spectrum Disorders, 2*(1), 46-59.

Seynhaeve, I., Nader-Grosbois, N., & Dionne C. (2008b). Functional abilities and neuropsychological dysfunctions in young children with autism and with intellectual disabilities. *European Journal of Disability Research, Alter, 2*(3), 230-252.

Shields, A., & Cicchetti, D. (1997). Emotion regulation in school-aged children: The development of a new criterion Q-sort scale. *Developmental Psychology, 33*, 906-916.

Sigman, M.D., Kasari, C., Kwon, J.H., & Yirmiya, N. (1992). Responses to the negative emotions of others by autistic, mentally retarded, and normal children. *Child Development, 63*, 796–807.

Silverman, I.W., & Ippolito, M.F. (1997). Goal-directedness and its relation to inhibitory control among toddlers. *Infant Behaviour and Development, 20*(2), 271-273.

Sissons Joshi, M., & McLean, M. (1994). Indian and English children's understanding of the distinction between real and apparent emotion. *Child Development, 65*, 1372-1384.

Snow, M.E., Hertzig, M.E., & Shapiro, T. (1987). Expression of emotion in young autistic children. *Journal of the American Academy of Child and Adolescent Psychiatry, 26*, 836–838.

Southam-Gerow, M., & Kendall, P. (2002). Emotion regulation and understanding implication for child and psychopathology and therapy. *Clinical Psychological Review, 22*, 189-222.

Sparrow, S., Cicchetti, D., & Balla, D. (2005). *Vineland Adaptive Behavior Scales* (2nd ed.). Minneapolis, MN: Pearson Assessment.

Spinrad, T.L., Eisenberg, N., Cumberland, A., Fabes, R.A., Valiente, C., Shepard, S.A., Reise, M., Losoya, S.H., & Guthrie, I.K. (2006). Relation of emotion-related regulation to children's social competence: a longitudinal study. *Emotion, 6*(3), 498-510.

Spinrad, T.L., Stifter, C.A., Donelan-McCall, N., & Turner, L. (2004). Mothers' regulation strategies in response to toddlers' affect: Links to later emotion self-regulation. *Social Development, 13*, 40–55.

Stahl, L., & Pry, R. (2002). Joint attention and set-shifting in young children with autism. *Autism, 6*(4), 383-396.

Stansbury, K., & Zimmerman, L.K. (1999). Relations among child language skills, maternal socializations of emotion regulation, and child behavior problems. *Child Psychiatry and Human Development, 30,* 121-142.

Stein, N.C., Trabasso, T., & Liwag, M. (1993). The representation and organization of emotional experience: unfolding the emotion episode. In M. Lewis & J.M. Haviland (Eds.), *Handbook of emotions* (pp. 279-300). New York: Guilford Press.

Stipek, D., Recchia, S., & McClintic, S. (1992). Self-evaluation in young children. *Monographs of the Society for Research in Child Development, 57,* 84-87.

St-Laurent, D., & Moss, E. (2002). Le développement de la planification: influence d'une attention conjointe. *Enfance, 4,* 341-361.

Szepkouski, G.M., Gauvain, M., & Carberry, M. (1994). The development of planning skills in children with and without mental retardation. *Journal of Applied Developmental Psychology, 15*(2), 187-206.

Tanguay, P.E. (1990). Early infantile autism: what have we learned in the past fifty years? *Brain Dysfunction, 3,* 197-207.

Tardif, C., Lainé, F., Rodriguez, M., & Gepner, B. (2007). Slowing down presentation of facial movements and vocal sounds enhances facial expression recognition and induces facial-vocal imitation in children with autism. *Journal of Autism and Developmental Disorders, 37,* 1469–1484.

Tellegen, P.J., Winkel, M., Wijnberg-Williams, B.J., & Laros, J.A. (1998). *S.O.N.-R 5.5-17: Snijders-Oomen Nicht-verbaler Intelligenztest.* Lisse: Swets Test Publishers (STP).

Thompson, R.A. (1994). Emotion regulation: A theme in search of definition. In N.A. Fox (Eds.), The development of emotion regulation: Biological and behavior considerations. *Monographs of the Society for Research in Child Development, 59*(2/3), 25-52.

Thompson, R.A., & Meyer, S. (2007). Socialization of emotion regulation in the family. In J.J. Gross (Ed.), *Handbook of emotion regulation* (pp. 249-268). New York: Guilford Press.

Tomanik, S., Harris, G., & Hawkins, J. (2004). The relationship between behaviors exhibited by children with autism and maternal stress. *Journal of Intellectual and Developmental Disability,* 29, 16–26.

Turner, M. (1997). Toward an executive dysfunction account of repetitive behavior. In J. Russell (Ed.), *Autism as an executive disorder* (pp. 57-100). Oxford: Oxford University Press.

Travis, L., Sigman, M., & Ruskin, E. (2001). Links between social understanding and social behavior in verbally able children with autism. *Journal of Autism and Developmental Disorders, 31,* 119–130.

Trevarthen, C. (1989). Les relations entre autisme et le développement socioculturel normal : arguments en faveur d'un trouble primaire de la régulation du développement cognitif par les émotions. In G. Lelord, J.P. Muh, M. Petit, & D. Sauvage (Eds.), *Autismes et troubles du développement global de l'enfant* (pp. 56-80). Paris : Expansion scientifique française.

Uzgiris, I.C., & Hunt, J. McV. (1975) *Assessment in infancy: ordinal scales of psychological development.* Urbana, Illinois: University of Illinois Press.

Vieillevoye, S., & Nader-Grosbois, N. (2008). Self-regulation during pretend play in children with intellectual disability and in normally developing children. *Research in Developmental Disabilities, 29*(3), 256-272.

Volkmar, F.R., & Pauls, D. (2003). Autism. *Lancet, 362,* 1133–1141.

Vygotsky, L.S. (1978). *Mind in society. The development of higher psychological processes.* Cambridge: Harvard University Press.

Walden, T.A., & Smith, M.C. (1997). Emotion Regulation. *Motivation and Emotion, 21*(1), 7-25.

Warreyn, P., Roeyers, H., & De Groote, I. (2005). Early social communicative behaviours of preschoolers with autism spectrum disorder during interaction with their mothers. *Autism, 9,* 342–361.

Welsh, M.C. (1991). Rule guided behaviour and self-monitoring on the Tower of Hanoi disk-transfer task. *Cognitive Development, 6,* 59-76.

Werner, E., Dawson, G., Osterling, J., & Dinno, N. (2000). Brief report: Recognition of autism spectrum disorder before one year of age: A retrospective study based on home videotapes. *Journal of Autism and Developmental Disorders, 30,* 157–162.

Whitman, T. (2004). *The development of autism: a self-regulatory perspective.* New-York: Jessica Kingsley Publishers.

Wieder, S., Kalmanson, B., & Fenichel, E. (1999). Diagnosing regulatory disorders using DC: 0-3: a framework and a case illustration. *Infant and Young Children, 12*(2), 79-89.

Winnykamen, F. (1993). Gestion socio-cognitive du recours à l'aide d'autrui chez l'enfant. *Journal International de Psychologie, 28,* 645-659.

Winsler, A., Manfra, L., & Diaz, R.M. (2007). Should I let them talk? Private speech and task performance among preschool children with and without behaviour problems. *Early Childhood Research Quarterly, 22*(2), 215-231.

Wolters, C.A. (1999). The relation between high school students' motivational regulation and their use of learning strategies, effort and classroom performance. *Learning and Individual Differences, 11,* 281-299.

Wood, H., & Wood, D. (1999). Help seeking, learning and contingent tutoring. *Computers and education, 33,* 153-169.

Yeates, K.O., Dennis, M., Rubin, K.H., Taylor, H.G., Bigler, E.D., Gerhardt, C.A., Stancin, T., & Vannatta, K. (2007). Social outcomes in childhood brain disorder: a heuristic integration of social neuroscience and developmental psychology. *Psychological Bulletin, 133*(3), 535-556.

Yirmiya, N., Kasari, C., Sigman, M., & Mundy, P. (1989). Facial expressions of affect in autistic, mentally retarded and normal children. *Journal of Child Psychology and Psychiatry, 30,* 725–735.

Yirmiya, N., Sigman, M.D., Kasari, C., & Mundy, P. (1992). Empathy and cognition in high-functioning children with autism. *Child Development, 63,* 150-160.

Zelazo, P.D., & Frye, D. (1997). Cognitive complexity and control: a theory of the development of deliberate reasoning and intentional action. In M. Stamenov (Ed.), *Language structure, discourse, and the access to consciousness.* (pp.113-153) Amsterdam & Philadelphia: John Benjamins.

Zelazo, P.D., Burack, J.A., Boseovski, J.J., Jacques, S., & Frye, D. (2001). A cognitive complexity and control framework for the study of autism. In J.A. Burack, T.

Charman, N. Yirmiya, & P.R. Zelazo (Eds.), *The development of autism: Perspectives from theory and research* (pp. 195–217). Mahwah, NJ: Lawrence Erlbaum Associates.

Zelazo, P.D., Jacques, S., Burack, J.A., & Frye, D. (2002). The relation between theory of mind and rule use: evidence from persons with autism-spectrum disorders. *Infant and Child Development, 11*(2), 171–195.

Zeman, J., Cassano, M., Perry-Parrish, C., & Stegall, S. (2006). Emotion regulation in children and adolescents. *Journal of Developmental and Behavioral Pediatrics, 27,* 155–168.

Zilbovicius, M., Boddaert N., Belin P., Poline J.B., Rémy P., Mangin J.F. et al. (2000). Temporal lobe dysfunction in childhood autism. *American Journal of Psychiatry, 157,* 1988-1993.

Zimmerman, B.J. (2000). Attaining Self-Regulation: A social cognitive perspective. In M. Boekaerts, P.R. Pintrich, & M. Zeidner (Eds.), *Handbook of self-regulation: Theory, research, and applications* (pp. 13-41). San Diego, CA: Academic Press.

# 14

# Imitation Therapy for Young Children with Autism

Tiffany Field[1,2], Jacqueline Nadel[3] and Shauna Ezell[2]
[1]*Touch Research Institute, University of Miami Medical School,*
[2]*Fielding Graduate University, Santa Barbara, California,*
[3]*CNRS Centre Emotion, Salpetriere Hospital, Paris,*
[1,2]*USA,*
[3]*France*

## 1. Introduction

This paper reviews the literature on the limitation skills of infants who were later diagnosed with autism and on the enhancing effect of adult imitation on the social behavior of children with autism. Nadel had previously used an adaptation of the still-face paradigm to demonstrate that children with autism showed more expectant behaviors such as looking and touching an adult stranger after being imitated by that stranger. Our studies are then reviewed showing that children with autism respond more to imitative than contingently responsive adults. After repeated imitation sessions the children showed more distal social behaviors (looking, vocalizing) and proximal social behaviors (moving close to and touching adult). In another study children approached more imitative and playful adults. And, children with autism were more imitative with an imitative adult than with their parents. In the final study reviewed the children showed more joint attention behaviors following imitation including referential looking, gaze following and imitation. This literature suggests, then, that children with autism show more social and imitative behavior when they are imitated, highlighting the importance of imitation as an effective therapy for these children.

## 2. Imitation in neonates and young infants

Imitation has been noted as early as the neonatal stage (Field, Greenberg, Woodson, Cohen & Garcia, 1984; Meltzoff & Moore, 1983). In these studies, newborns imitated tongue protrusions (Meltzoff & Moore, 1983) and the basic facial expressions of happy, sad, and surprised (Field et al, 1984). Later at around 3 months reciprocal imitation was noted in the face-to-face interactions between mothers and infants and fathers and infants (Field, 1977). Imitation has also been used as an "interaction coaching technique" to improve or "slow down" the intrusive or over-stimulating behaviors of mothers with their high-risk infants (Field, 1977). Several have suggested that reciprocal imitation and memory for imitation (deferred imitation) are the social bases for empathy and language development (see Meltzoff, 1990 & Nadel, 2006 for reviews).

## 3. Infants later diagnosed with autism rarely showed imitation

Infants who were later diagnosed with autism have shown notably different interaction behaviors (Dawson, Hill, Spencer, Galpert & Watson, 1990). They showed fewer smiles and less frequent eye contact. They were less likely to smile in response to their mother's smile, and their mothers were less likely to smile in response to them. Their pre-verbal behaviors were either delayed or failed to develop including engaging in synchronous imitation (Asendorpf & Baudonniere, 1993; Eckerman & Stein, 1990) and exhibiting deferred imitation (Heimann, Laberg & Nordoen, 2006). Children with autism have rarely shown imitative behavior (Roger & Williams, 2006; Williams, 2008). In one model, early imitation deficits were thought to interfere with social interaction which, in turn, affected language development (Rogers & Pennington, 1991).

## 4. Adult imitation enhances social behavior of children with autism

Several studies have documented the positive effects of adults imitating children in object play situations including non-autistic children (Field, 1977; Lubin and Field, 1981) and children with autism (Dawson and Adams, 1984; Dawson and Galpert, 1990). Typically, the imitation enhanced social responsiveness in the children. Other studies on imitation in children with autism showed that imitative interactions: 1) affected object manipulation (Tiegerman & Primavera, 1981); 2) decreased self-stimulating behaviors (Harris, Handleman & Fong, 1987); and 3) increased gaze behavior (Tiegerman & Primavera, 1984). Each of these studies linked these changes to secondary improvements in interpersonal interaction and affect expression. Others referenced an association between these social behaviors and the development of language (Dawson & Adams, 1984; Nadel, 2006). Studies conducted within the last decade supported these earlier findings (Escalona et al., 2002; Field, Field, Sanders & Nadel, 2001; Heiman, Laberg & Nordoen, 2006; Nadel, Croue, Kervella, Mattlinger, Canet, Hudelot et al., 2000). They demonstrated that children with autism ranging in age from 2 to 11 years improved their eye contact behaviors, increased positive affect, enhanced social responsiveness and decreased perseverative behaviors when an unfamiliar adult imitated them.

Studies by Dawson and Adams (1984) suggested that children with autism and a low level of imitative ability were more socially responsive, showed more eye contact, and played with toys in a less perseverative manner when the experimenter imitated their behavior. The authors suggested that imitation was beneficial to children with lower developmental ages because imitation is a "recognized exchange or connection between two persons and thereby creates a feeling of shared understanding between them" (Dawson & Adams, 1984; Nadel & Peze, 1993). In addition, adult interaction partners have been noted to become more sensitive to their child's cues when they are being imitative (Field, 1977).

## 5. Imitation in the still-face paradigm

Imitation effects on children with autism have also been studied in social play situations such as the adapted version of the still-face paradigm by Nadel and her colleagues (2000). In the original still-face paradigm, designed by Tronick et al, mothers were asked to interact naturally with their infants for 3 minutes, then to sit in a still-face fashion and not move for another 3 minutes, and finally to interact normally for 3 minutes (Tronick, Als, Adamson, Wise & Brazelton, 1978).

In the Nadel et al. (2000) adaptation, children with autism interacted with an unfamiliar adult for four phases, each lasting 3 minutes. In the first phase, the child walked into a room that was furnished with a sofa, a table, chairs and two sets of identical toys. An unfamiliar adult sat on the sofa with a still-face and a body like a statue and did not move for 3 minutes. In the second phase, the stranger imitated everything the child did including the child's autistic-like behaviors, social and toy play behaviors, using toys that were identical to those the child used. The third phase consisted of a second still-face similar to the first one, and the fourth phase was a spontaneous interaction.

Although Nadel et al. (2000) had some concern about the negative effects or at least the potential confusion created by the still-face behavior in contrast to the more social behavior during the imitative segment, they showed that out of the six social behaviors coded (looking at person, positive facial expressions, negative facial expressions, positive social gestures, close proximity, and touching), as many as five occurred more often during the second still-face after the imitative segment compared with the first still-face. These included looking at the adult, negative facial expressions, positive social gestures, close proximity and touching. During that segment the children, according to the Nadel et al. study (2000), displayed significantly more expectant behaviors such as looking at or touching the strangers.

The results of the Nadel et al. (2000) study showed that the children's distal social behaviors (looking and social gestures) and proximal social behaviors (close proximity and touching) occurred significantly more often during the second still-face session than the first still-face session. Thus, the children displayed significantly more expectant behaviors such as looking-at or touching the stranger after the imitation session. The increases in proximity-seeking and touching behaviors were viewed as positive changes because they seemed to indicate attempts on the part of the children to initiate interactions, a rare event for children with autism. It is not clear why the imitative behavior on the part of the adult was so effective, although normal children at the early preschool developmental age have also been noted to be particularly responsive to imitations of their own behaviors (Lubin & Field, 1981).

## 6. Imitation compared with contingently responsive interactions

A shortcoming of the Nadel et al. (2000) study was that it could not be determined whether the imitation per se or simply the interaction being contingently responsive led to their results. Thus, we attempted to replicate the Nadel et al. (2000) study but to compare the effects of the adult being imitative versus simply being contingently responsive in their interaction behavior (Escalona et al., 2000). Using the same paradigm, similarly positive effects of imitation were observed (Escalona, Field, Lundy & Nadel, 2000), this time when imitation sessions were compared with contingently responsive sessions. In this study, twenty children with autism (mean age, 5 years) were recruited for the study from a school for children with autism. The children were randomly assigned to an imitation (N=10) or contingently responsive (N= 10) interaction group based on a stratification table for gender and developmental and chronological age. The sessions consisted of four phases, with each phase lasting 3 minutes. In the first phase, the child walked into a room that was furnished with a sofa, a table, chairs, and two sets of identical toys. An adult was in the room sitting very still like a statue (first still-face condition). In the second phase, the adult either imitated the child or was contingently responsive to the child. In the third phase, the adult sat still again (second still-face condition), and in the fourth phase, the adult engaged in a spontaneous interaction.

The results suggested that during the third phase (the second still-face condition), the children in the imitation group spent less time in gross motor activity and more time being close to the adult and touching the adult, as if attempting to initiate an interaction. The contingency condition appeared to be a more effective way to facilitate a distal social behavior (attention), whereas the imitative condition was a more effective way to facilitate a proximal social behavior (touching). These results highlighted the effectiveness of imitation versus the use of simply contingent responsive behavior.

In at least the two studies just described, increases in social initiation and responsiveness were noted, including increased physical proximity and touching by the children with autism immediately following the imitation by the adult (Escalona et al., 2000; Nadel et al., 2000). The children also showed significantly more negative facial expressions toward the adult during the second still face phase, perhaps suggesting that they may be expressing their disappointment that the adult was no longer imitating them.

In the Escalona et al (2002) study, we randomly assigned children to groups. Thus we controlled for the possibility of imitation merely being a contingently reinforcing response by establishing a control group where half of the twenty subjects were responded to contingently without imitation The results of this study showed that imitation produced a larger effect than merely responding contingently without imitation.

These results also suggest that the child's proximal behaviors may be increased by the adult's imitation and contingent responsivity. Decreased distance from the adult occurred for both groups during the second still-face segment after the imitation and contingently responsive interactions, suggesting that the children were initiating moves toward the adult. Imitation, however, yielded additional improvements, including less motor activity, suggesting that imitation may have made the child more aware of the adult and thus diverted his or her attention from motor activity when the adult stopped imitating the child during the second still-face segment. Although both groups reduced their distance from the adult, the increase in touching the adult by the children was significantly greater for the imitation group and is consistent with data reported in the prototype for this study by Nadel et al. (2000).

According to Nadel et al. (2000), children with autism develop social expectancies during the imitation condition. The children showed these expectancies in both the Nadel et al. (2000) study and the Escalona et al. (2002) study by not only reducing their distance from the adult but also by touching the adult more frequently. They also showed a greater advantage for social interaction relative to the contingent responsivity group by reducing motor activity and vocal stereotypies, as indicated by no decrease in silence. Although the silence category also included no discernible sound, which could also include preverbal vocalizations, this makes this finding difficult to interpret inasmuch as increases in stereotypic speech may be less desirable while increases in other vocalizations may be more desirable, especially if they occur at the same time the children are increasing their attention to an adult.

We suggested in the conclusions of the Escalona et al. (2002) study that a future study might determine the specific ways in which the adult differs during the contingent responsivity and imitation conditions. A larger sample would also enable a comparison between those children who initiated contact by touching the adult after imitation and the other approximately half of the children who did not. The anecdotally reported frequency of social touch aversion in children with autism (Baranek, 1999) highlights the importance of finding interventions such as imitation to enhance the proximity and touch initiations noted in the children with autism in this study. The fact that imitation was more effective in reducing gross motor behavior and increasing the children's social contact behavior (touching) than the contingently responsive interaction highlights the special nature of imitation. It is not only being immediately responsive, as in being contingently responsive, that is important, but it is also responding with the same form of behavior that is effective. The data from these studies as well as those from other studies (Dawson & Adams, 1984; Nadel & Peze, 1993) suggest that imitation by adults may be an effective intervention with young nonverbal children with autism.

## 7. Children with autism display more social behaviors after repeated imitation sessions

In the next study we explored the effects of repeated sessions of imitation (Field et al., 2001). Twenty children were recruited from a school for children with autism to attend three

| | Sessions | | |
|---|---|---|---|
| | 1 | 2 | 3 |
| Stereotypies | 1.6 (2.1) | 1.5 (1.9) | 0.9 (1.7) |
| Inactivity | 19.3[d] (21.2) | 1.7(20.7) | 5.7[c] (19.0) |
| Playing alone | 65.7[a] (67.1) | 54.1 (61.2) | 50.9[a] (60.3) |
| Accepting object | 0.0[d] (0.7) | 3.0 (1.2) | 0.0 (0.9) |
| Playing with object | 60.3[d] (54.9) | 90.6 (62.3) | 80.8[b] (71.5) |
| Looking at adult | 4.5[d] (3.9) | 20.0 (7.8) | 15.7[c] (9.3) |
| Mirror play | 1.0 (2.1) | 6.5 (4.2) | 10.7[a] (5.8) |
| Smiling/laughing | 0.1[d] (0.4)[a] | 8.9 (3.2) | 4.3 (2.7) |
| Vocalizing | 5.0[b] (6.7) | 11.0 (7.2) | 7.3 (5.8) |
| Proximal to adult | 0.7 (0.5) | 0.7 (0.9) | 3.3[b] (1.7) |
| Sitting next to adult | 0.1 (0.4) | 1.0 (0.5) | 7.1[b] (0.8) |
| Touching adult | 0.0 (0.0) | 0.0 (0.0) | 6.2[d] (1.2) |
| Imitation recognition | 0.0[d] (0.0) | 6.8 (0.0) | 7.0[d] (0.0) |
| Reciprocal play | 0.0[d] (0.2)[a] | 6.7 (3.1) | 7.1[d] (3.2)[a] |

Superscripts in column 1 reflect significant differences between sessions 1 and 2. Superscripts in column 3 reflect significant differences between sessions 1 and 3.
[a] $p < 0.05$. [b] $p < 0.01$. [c] $p < 0.005$. [d] $p < 0.001$.

Table 1. Mean percentage time that behaviors occurred during spontaneous play following repeated imitation sessions (contingently responsive play sessions in parentheses). (Adapted from Field et al., 2001).

sessions during which an adult either imitated all of the children's behaviors or simply played with the child. By the second session the children in the imitation group were showing distal social behaviors toward the adult a greater proportion of time including (see table 1): (1) looking; (2) vocalizing; (3) smiling; and (4) engaging in reciprocal play. During the third session, the children in the imitation group spent a greater proportion of time showing proximal social behaviors toward the adult including: (1) being close to the adult; (2) sitting next to the adult; and (3) touching the adult.

These results suggest that both distal and proximal social behaviors may be increased in children with autism by repeated sessions of the adult imitating the child's behaviors. Solitary behaviors including inactivity and playing alone had decreased by the second session and accepting and playing with objects had increased. Distal social behaviors of looking at the adult, smiling and vocalizing toward the adult occurred more often, and reciprocal play and recognizing imitation had also increased by the second session. By the third session the time that proximal social behaviors occurred had increased including mirror play, being close to the adult, sitting next to the adult and touching the adult. Consistent with the suggestions of Dawson and Adams (1984), Nadel and Field (2001) recently reported data showing that only those children with autism who recognized they were being imitated actually increased their social behavior.

Imitation by an adult requires total attentiveness and responsiveness to the child for the child's behaviors to be matched. As in mother–infant interactions featuring imitation (Field, 1977), the adult–child time together becomes more playful and reciprocal. In the better interactions of children with autism (i.e. those where the children approach, are close to and touch the adult more), the adult has been noted to be more playful (Nadel et al., 2007). A larger sample would enable a comparison between those children who approach and touch the adult following imitation and those (approximately half of the children) who do not (Escalona et al., 2002).Those who approach and touch may experience less social touch aversion, frequently reported in children with autism (Baranek, 1999), and have more intimate relationships.

## 8. Children with autism approach more imitative and playful adults

In a subsequent study, the videotapes from the Escalona et al. (2002) study were recoded for children's approach behaviors and for adult behaviors to assess the adult's imitative behavior and to determine what other adult behaviors were associated with the children's approach behaviors (Nadel et al., 2007). The videotapes were first coded for the children's approach behaviors. The children from the high-approach sessions were labeled the high-approach group, and those with low-incidence approach behavior were labeled the low-approach group. The interactions were then coded for the adults' behaviors. Children with autism were selected to be in high-approach and low-approach groups based on a median split of their proximity-seeking behavior with adults (looking at, approaching and touching adults) during videotaped interactions. The same videotapes of those two sets of interactions were then coded and analyzed for the adult partners' behaviors. The adult interaction partner of high approach children showed more looking at the child, smiling at the child, moving toward the child, inviting the child to play, imitating the child in play and being playful (see table 2).

The results suggested that the high-approach group interaction sessions or those in which children with autism showed more approach behaviors were characterized by more interesting behavior in the adults, including more frequent smiling, sound effects, imitative behavior and playfulness. The greater incidence of adult imitative behavior during those high-approach interactions may have been a carryover effect from the imitative phase of the

| Adult Behavior | High approach | Low approach | *t* value | *p* value |
|---|---|---|---|---|
| Looking at child | 52.5 (29.2) | 63.9 (20.8) | 1.01 | N.S. |
| Smiling at child | 11.1 (10.6) | 4.0 (2.4) | -2.81 | 0.001 |
| Moving toward child | 29.7 (24.4) | 21.8 (13.0) | -0.90 | N.S. |
| Relaxed body tone | 72.0 (39.7) | 20.0 (18.5) | -3.73 | 0.001 |
| Adult making sounds | 3.5 (3.2) | 0.0 (0.2) | -3.46 | 0.01 |
| Inviting child to play | 47.6 (29.5) | 28.5 (22.4) | -1.63 | 0.05 |
| Imitating child in play | 3.8 (6.8) | 0.7 (1.8) | -1.44 | 0.05 |
| Being playful | 72.0 (39.7) | 20.4 (18.5) | -3.73 | 0.01 |

Table 2. Mean (standard deviation) percentage of time adult behaviors occurred in high-approach and low-approach interactions. (Adapted from Nadel et al., 2008).

session inasmuch as more of the high-approach interactions occurred following the imitation sessions. More frequent approach behaviors by the child during the spontaneous interactions may relate to the imitative and more playful behavior during those interactions. Consistent with the Nadel *et al.* (2000) suggestion that children with autism can develop social expectancies around socially expressive adults, which then manifest themselves in more approach behaviors such as looking at or touching the adult. The more playful adult may help the child with autism relate to that adult and form more social expectancies, the more playful adult may also be a more interesting playmate and more flexible, allowing the children with autism more freedom to initiate. The child being allowed to initiate seems to be effective in eliciting social contact. A second confound of this study, in addition to the chance finding that more imitation occurred prior to the high-approach sessions, is that more of the high approach sessions featured an adult who was more experienced playing with children with autism. This adult may have learned through interactions with these children that imitation and playfulness are effective behaviors.

Several behavioral techniques have been investigated for increasing imitative behavior in children with autism including discrete trial training, use of stereotypic behaviors to increase play skills, pivotal response training, differential reinforcement of appropriate behavior, *in vivo* modeling and play scripts, video modeling and reciprocal imitation training (Stahmer, Ingersoll, & Carter, 2003). In a study teaching reciprocal imitation skills to young children with autism using a naturalistic behavioral approach, the children with autism increased their imitation skills and generalized these skills to novel environments (Ingersoll & Schreibman, 2006). In addition, the children increased other social-communicative behaviors, including language, pretend play and joint attention.

## 9. Children with autism are more imitative with an imitative adult than their parents

The purposes of our next study were: (1) to determine how much imitative behavior parents show during play interactions with their autistic children as compared to a researcher who was deliberately imitative of the children during a play interaction; and (2) to determine how the more imitative researcher affected the child's social and imitative behavior. Children with autism (mean age = 6 years) were videotaped first interacting with a parent and then with an unfamiliar researcher who imitated the child's behaviors. The researcher showed more imitative and playful behaviors than the parents. In turn, the children showed more imitative behavior when playing with the imitative researcher than with their parents (see table 3 & 4).

| | Interaction | | |
|---|---|---|---|
| | Mother | Researcher | p |
| **Adult** | | | |
| Imitating child | 2.60 (5.33) | 39.33 (14.48) | 0.000 |
| Playful with child | 50.33 (22.28) | 59.67 (15.81) | 0.05 |
| **Child** | | | |
| Smiling at adult | 6.20 (8.10) | 9.27 (10.96) | 0.1 |
| Touching adult | 15.93(23.98) | 5.13 (7.53) | 0.04 |
| Imitating adult | 7.20 (9.17) | 17.33 (16.70) | 0.02 |
| Recognizing being imitated by adult | 1.47 (4.91) | 2.13 (4.47) | 0.25 |

Note: These behaviors are not mutually exclusive nor would they comprise 100% of the individual's interaction behavior.

Table 3. Mean percent time that interaction behaviors occurred in mothers, researchers and children with autism. (Adapted from Field et al., 2010).

| | Interaction | | |
|---|---|---|---|
| | Father | Researcher | p |
| **Adult** | | | |
| Imitating child | .00 (.00) | 39.33 (14.48) | 0.002 |
| Playful with child | 33.40 (13.43) | 59.67 (15.81) | 0.02 |
| **Child** | | | |
| Smiling at adult | 2.80 (2.95) | 9.27 (10.96) | 0.17 |
| Touching adult | 21.40 (32.24) | 5.13 (7.53) | 0.05 |
| Imitating adult | .80 (9.09) | 17.33 (16.70) | 0.05 |
| Recognizing being imitated by adult | .00 (.00) | 2.13 (4.47) | 0.37 |

Note: These behaviors are not mutually exclusive nor would they comprise 100% of the individual's interaction behavior.

Table 4. Mean percent time that interaction behaviors occurred in fathers, researchers and children with autism. (Adapted from Field et al., 2010).

The low levels of imitation among these children with autism (from 7% to 8% time with the parents to 17% time with the researcher) are consistent with the literature suggesting impaired imitation in these children (Malvy et al., 1997; Rogers et al., 2003). Imitation deficits are a risk factor for later development given their relationship to mental age (Roeyers et al., 1998). The children's very infrequent signs of recognizing being imitated in this study may be another risk factor. However, the paradigm used in this study, like that of our other studies (Escalona et al., 2002; Field et al., 2001; Nadel et al., 2000) suggests that

children can display social imitation (Nadel & Peze, 1993), and particularly when an adult is being imitative. This is highlighted by the comparisons between the researcher who was more imitative of the children than the mothers or fathers were. The children, in turn, were more imitative with the more imitative researcher than with their parents.
The reciprocal play and game-like turn-taking during the bouts of imitation could be elicited specifically by the imitative behavior of the adult. Comparisons between sessions that are imitative and those using contingently responsive behavior have suggested that imitative behavior of the adult may be more effective in eliciting imitative behavior of the child (Escalona et al., 2002). The effects of the researcher's more frequent imitative behavior on the imitative behavior of the child, however, were confounded by the researcher also showing more frequent playful behavior. Playful behavior by adults has also been notably effective in eliciting social behavior in children with autism in a recent study (Nadel, Field, Escalona, & Lundy, 2007). The relatively high levels of playful behavior in the parents (33–50% time) and the simultaneously low levels of imitative behavior by the children during play with their parents suggest that the adults' playful behavior is less instrumental than the adults' imitative behavior in eliciting the children's imitative behavior.
These data highlight the effectiveness of adult imitative behavior and suggest that therapists/teachers might model imitative behavior for parents. Since imitation is a process by which most young children learn new skills, the social and cognitive skills of children with autism might also be enhanced by imitation modeling of this kind.

## 10. Imitation and joint attention

A study on imitation and communication involved the recoding of videotapes from the Field et al (2001) study (Field et al., 2001). This included two randomized groups. During the intervention phase, one group of 10 children was imitated by the unfamiliar adult. This constituted the imitation (IM) group. In the other group, the adult interacted in a non-imitative, yet, contingently responsive manner. For this group, the adult was instructed not to imitate the child. Joint attention behaviors were observed in accordance with the definition offered by Carpenter, Pennington, and Rogers (2002). These researchers referred to joint attention as a cluster of behaviors such as referential looking, gaze following, imitation, and gestures such as showing, reaching, and pointing. The young children with autism (4-6 years of age) who were imitated were expected to show a greater percent of time showing joint attention behaviors compared to the children in the group that simply received contingent responsivity, including referential looking, gaze following, imitation, and gestures such as showing, reaching, and pointing sessions.
The percent time the children engaged in joint attention behaviors as demonstrated by referential looking, gaze following, imitation, and gesturing was recorded during two phases of two sessions (during the intervention phase and the spontaneous interaction phase and the first and third sessions). The imitation group showed greater referential looking, gaze following and imitation behaviors (see table 5). Imitating the child's behaviors was significantly related to the increase in percent time the child engaged in three of the four joint attention behaviors by the children including referential looking, gaze following and imitation (see table 6). Adult imitation was not, however, significantly related to the percent time the child spent gesturing.

| Joint Attention Behaviors | | | | |
|---|---|---|---|---|
| | Referential Looking | Gaze Following | Imitation | Gestures |
| Adult Imitates | 30.25 | 67.25 | 24.00 | 23.65 |
| Adult does not imitate | 10.68 | 39.63 | 2.55 | 19.40 |

Table 5. Comparison between groups of the mean percentage time joint behaviors occurred. (Adapted from Ezell & Field, 2011). The groups significantly differ on all behaviors except gestures.

| Joint Attention Behaviors | | | | | |
|---|---|---|---|---|---|
| N=20 | Adult Imitates | Referential Looking | Gaze Following | Child Imitates | Gestures |
| Adult Imitates | - | .567(**) | .466 (*) | .429 (*) | .056 |
| Referential Looking | | - | .409 | .290 | .319 |
| Gaze Following | | | - | .809 (**) | -.036 |
| Child Imitates | | | | - | -.142 |
| Gestures | | | | | - |

Table 6. Correlations between mean percentage time of imitation and joint attention behaviors. (Adapted from Ezell & Field, 2011).

## 11. Summary

This paper reviews the literature on the imitation skills of infants who were later diagnosed with autism and on the enhancing effect of adult imitation on the social behavior of children with autism. Nadel had previously used an adaptation of the still-face paradigm in to demonstrate that children with autism showed more expectant behaviors such as looking and touching an adult stranger after being imitated by that stanger. Our studies are then reviewed showing that children with autism respond more to imitative than contingently responsive adults. After repeated imitation sessions the children showed more distal social behaviors (looking, vocalizing) and proximal social behaviors (moving close to and touching adult). In another study children approached more imitative and playful adults. And, children with autism were more imitative with an imitative adult than with their parents. In the final study reviewed the children showed more joint attention behaviors following imitation including referential looking, gaze following and imitation. This literature suggests, then, that children with autism show more social and imitative behavior when they are imitated, highlighting the importance of imitation as an effective therapy for these children.

## 12. Acknowledgements

We thank the parents and children who participated in these studies and our colleagues for their collaboration. This research was supported by a merit award (MH46586), NIH grants (AT00370 and HD056036) and Senior Research Scientist Awards (MH00331 and AT001585) and a March of Dimes Grant (12-FYO3-48) to Tiffany Field and funding from Johnson & Johnson Pediatric Institute to the Touch Research Institute. Correspondence and requests for reprints should be sent to Tiffany Field, Ph.D., Touch Research Institute, University of Miami School of Medicine, and PO Box 016820, Miami, Florida, 33101. Business phone number (305) 243-6781.

## 13. References

Asendorpf, J. B. & Baudonniere, P.M. (1993). Self-awareness and other-awareness: Mirror self-recognition and synchronic imitation among unfamiliar peers. *Developmental Psychology, 29,* 88-95.

Baranek, G.T. (1999). Autism during infancy: a retrospective video analysis of sensory-motor and social behaviors at 9-12 months of age. *Journal of Autism and Developmental Disorders, 29,* 213-224.

Carpenter, M., Pennington, B. E., & Rogers, S. J. (2002). Interrelations among social-cognitive skills in young children with autism. *Journal of Autism and Developmental Disorders, 32,* 91-106.

Dawson, G. & Adams, A. (1984). Imitation and social responsiveness in autistic children. *Journal of Abnormal Child Psychology, 12,* 209-226.

Dawson, G. & Galpert, L. (1990). Mothers' use of imitative play for facilitating social responsiveness and toy play in young autistic children. *Development and Psychopathology, 2,* 151-162.

Dawson, G., Hill, D., Spencer, A., Galpert, L., & Watson L. (1990). Affective exchanges between young autistic children and their mothers. *Journal of Abnormal Child Psychology, 18,* 335-345.

Eckerman, C.O. & Stein, M.R. (1990).How imitation begets imitation and toddlers' generation of games. *Developmental Psychology, 26,* 370-378.

Escolona, A., Field, T., Lundy, B., & Nadel, J. (2000). Imitation effects on children with autism. *Journal of Autism and Developmental Disorders, 32,* 141-144.

Escalona, A., Field, T., Nadel, J. & Lundy, B. (2002). Imitation effects on children with autism. *The Journal of Autism and Developmental Disorders, 32,* 141-144.

Ezell, S. & Field, T. (2011). Unpublished data.

Field, T. (1977). Effects of early separation, interactive deficits, and experimental manipulations on infant-mother face-to-face interaction. *Child Development, 48,* 763-771.

Field, T., Field, T., Sanders, C. & Nadel, J. (2001). Children with autism display more social behaviors after repeated imitation sessions. *Autism, 5,* 317-323.

Field, T., Greenberg, R., Woodson, R., Cohen, D., & Garcia, R. (1984). A descriptive study of facial expressions during Brazelton neonatal behavior assessments. *Infant Mental Health Journal,* 5, 61-71.

Field, T., Nadel, J., Diego, M., Hernandez-Reif, M., Russo, K., Vchulek, D., et al. (2010). Children with autism are more imitative with an imitative adult than with their parents. *Early Childhood Development & Care, 180,* 513-518.

Harris, S., Handleman, J. S., & Fong, P. L. (1987). Imitation of self-stimulation: Impact on the autistic child's behavior and affect. *Child and Family Behavior Therapy, 9,* 1–21.

Heimann, M., Laberg, K.E., Nordoen, B. (2006).Imitative interaction increases social interest and elicited imitation in non-verbal children with autism. *Infant and Child Development 15,* 297–309.

Ingersoll, B., & Schreibman, L. (2006). Teaching reciprocal imitation skills to young children with autism using a naturalistic behavioral approach: effects on language, pretend play, and joint attention. *Journal of Autism and Developmental Disorders, 36,* 487-505.

Lubin, L. & Field, T. (1981). Imitation during pre-school peer interaction. *International Journal of Behavior Development, 4,* 443-453.

Malvy, J., Rouby, P., Receveur, C., & Sauvage, D. (1997). Natural history of infantile autism (nasography). *Encephale, 23,* 28-33.

Meltzoff, A.N. (1990). Towards a developmental cognitive science. The implications of cross-modal matching and imitation for the development of representation and memory in infancy. *Annals of the New York Academy of Sciences, 608,* 1-31.

Meltzoff, A.N. & Moore, M.K. (1983). Newborn infants imitate adult facial gestures. *Child Development, 54,* 702-709.

Nadel, J. (2006). Does imitation matter to children with autism? In S. Rogers & J. Williams (Eds.), Imitation and the social mind (pp. 118-137). NY: The Guilford Press.

Nadel, J., Croue, S., Kervella, C., Mattlinger, M., Canet, P., Hudelot, C., et al, (2000). Do children with autism have expectations about the social behavior of unfamiliar people. *Autism, 4,* 133-145.

Nadel, J., Field, T., Escolona, A., & Lundy, B. (2007). Children with autism approach more imitative and playful adults. *Early Child Development and Care, 177,* 1-5.

Nadel, J., Martini, M., Escolona, A., Field, T., (2008). Children with autism approach more imitative and playful adults. *Early Child Development Care, 178,* 461-465.

Nadel, J. & Peze, A. (1993). What makes immediate imitation communicative in toddlers and autistic children? In J. Nadel & L. Camaioni (Eds.), *New perspectives in early communicative development.* London, NY: Routledge.

Roeyers, H., Van Oost, P., & Bothuyne, S. (1998). Immediate imitation and joint attention in young children with autism. *Developmental Psychopathology, 10,* 441-450.

Rogers, S.J., Hepburn, S.L., Stackhouse, T., & Wehner, E. (2003). Imitation performance in toddlers with autism and those with other developmental disorders. *Journal of Child Psychology and Psychiatry, 44,* 763-781.

Rogers, S. J., & Pennington, B. F. (1991). A theoretical approach to the deficits in infantile autism. Development and Psychopathology, 3(2), 137–162.

Rogers, S. J., & Williams, J. H. G. (2006). Imitation and the social mind: Autism and typical development. New York, NY: Guilford Press.

Stahmer, A., Ingersoll, B., & Carter, C. (2003). Behavioral approaches to promoting play. *Autism, 7,* 401-413.

Tiegerman, E. & Primavera, L. (1981). Object manipulation: An interactional strategy with autistic children. *Journal of Autism and Developmental Disorders, 11,* 427-438.

Tiegerman, E. & Primavera, L. (1984). Imitating the autistic child: Facilitating communicative gaze behavior. *Journal of Autism and Developmental Disorders, 14,* 27-38.

Tronick, E., Als, H., Adamson, L., Wise, S., & Brazelton, T.B. (1978). The infant's response to entrapment between contradictory messages in face-to-face interaction. *Journal of American Academy of Child Psychiatry, 17,* 1-13.

Williams, J.H.G. (2008). Self-other relations in social development and autism: Multiple roles for mirror neurons and other brain bases. *Autism Research, 1,* 73-90.

# 15

# Interactive Technology: Teaching People with Autism to Recognize Facial Emotions

José C. Miranda, Tiago Fernandes, A. Augusto Sousa
and Verónica C. Orvalho
*Instituto Telecomunicações, Universidade do Porto, Instituto Politécnico da Guarda*
*Portugal*

## 1. Introduction

In daily life, we interact with others by exchanging a huge quantity of information, including our current states of emotions, through facial expressions. Thus, faces are crucial for the recognition and understanding of emotions and for assisting communications and interactions between people. Individuals with autism tend to avoid looking at others' human faces and find it hard to recognize facial expressions and emotions in themselves and in others (Baron Cohen, 1995). This incapacity to read emotions on the human face impairs their ability to communicate with other people (Baron-Cohen et al., 2007).

Previous work has shown that children and adults with Autism Spectrum Disorders (ASD) can improve their emotion recognition skills with computer-based intervention. An increasing number of studies show that computer technologies used in teaching and in therapy are well accepted by individuals with ASD (Golan et al., 2007; Moore et al., 2000; Tanaka et al., 2010). However, most of the current computer-based solutions train patients with ASD using drawings or photographs (Bernard-Opitz et al., 2001; Bolte et al., 2002; Tseng & Do, 2010). When the autistic people try to apply the acquired knowledge to recognize emotions in real life, they are still unable to communicate properly (Golan et al., 2006).

This paper gives an overview of existing methods that have been used for teaching emotion recognition to individuals with autism. We identify some technological limitations that difficult their interpersonal interactions. Lastly, we present our contribution: a different approach to teach autistic people to recognize emotions from facial expression. Our idea is based on real-time facial synthesis of 3D characters. We also suggest a different interaction model to involve the autistic patient more deeply in the process of learning emotions. Creating a solution to solve this problem requires a joint effort from many research fields, such as computer vision, computer graphics, human computer interaction and facial behaviour and emotions.

## 2. Emotions and facial expression

Facial expression should not be confused with emotions. Human emotions are a result of many different factors, like feelings or convictions (Ekman, 1999). Human beings' emotional states might be revealed through a number of different channels, such as emotional voice, pose, gestures, gaze direction and facial expressions. Facial expressions deal with facial

features deformation (purely based on visual information) and emotions are not the only source for facial expression.
In 1971, Ekman and Friesen (Ekman & Friesen, 1971) postulated six primary emotions: happiness, sadness, fear, disgust, surprise and anger. These basic emotions seem to be universal across human ethnicities and cultures. However, not all of researchers agree with this classification. Ortony and Turner (Ortony & Turner, 1990) collated a wide range of research on the identification of basic emotions.
Facial expressions are generated by contractions of facial muscles, which results in temporally deformed facial features such as eye lids, eye brows, nose or lips, often revealed by wrinkles and bulges. These facial movements convey the emotional state of the individual to observers and involve three main concepts: intensity, length and valence.
**Intensity:** subtle expression vs. strong expression. Emotions usually vary in intensity. Strong expressions involve the whole face in large facial movements that can be obvious. Subtle expressions involve small facial movements that often appear only in one region of the face, such as just the brows, eyelids, cheeks, nose or lips. These small movements occur gradually when an emotion begins, when an emotion is repressed, or when an emotion is deliberately masked.
**Length:** micro expression vs. macro expression. Emotions vary in how long they last. A micro expression can be as short as 1/25 to 1/5 of a second. On the other hand, (Ekman & Friesen, 1975) gives the average time for an emotion to unfold to be 2-4 seconds (surprise is the shortest universal emotion). Micro expressions are signs of emotions just emerging, emotions expressed before the person displaying them knows what she is feeling, or emotions the person is trying to conceal.
**Valence:** positive expressions vs. negative expression. Some expressions are termed positive, such as joy. Other expressions are termed negative, such as anger, fear, sad, and disgust. Some expressions are neutral in this spectrum, such as surprise.

### 2.1 Facial expression analysis

In order to analyse and classify facial expressions it is crucial to know the facial signals that imply each facial expression. In this context, it is necessary to accurately describe the *location* of facial features, their *intensity* and their *dynamics* (Fasel & Luettin, 2003). For example, when someone is happy, the implied facial features are: smiling (an open or closed mouth); possible laughter; crows-feet wrinkles at the sides of sparkling eyes; slightly raised eyebrows and head level. Facial expression intensity may be measured by determining either the geometric deformations of facial features or the density of wrinkles appearing in certain face regions. For example the measurement of a smile intensity is conveyed when cheeks and lip corners rise, as well as wrinkle display. Dynamics is related to the timing of a facial expression: not only the nature of the deformation of facial features conveys meaning, but also the relative timing of facial movements and their temporal evolution.
In the past, facial expression analysis was primarily a research subject for psychologists but, in 1978, Suwa et al. (Suwa et al., 1978) presented a preliminary investigation on automatic facial expression analysis from an image sequence. In the nineties, this research area gained great awareness. The reasons for this renewed interest in facial expressions are multiple, but one major motivation is due to the advances in related research areas, such as face detection, face tracking and face recognition, as well as the recent availability of relatively cheap computational power (Fasel & Luettin, 2003).

Most of automatic facial expression analysis approaches (Fasel & Luettin, 2003; Pantic & Rothkrantz, 2000) code facial motion and deformation into visual classes. Facial actions are hereby described by their location and intensity but do not take profit from the temporal component, which is essential in classifying a facial expression. Therefore, a complete description framework would ideally contain all possible perceptible changes that may occur in a face. This is the goal of FACS (Facial Action Coding System) which was developed by (Ekman & Friesen, 1978) and has been considered as a foundation for describing facial expressions. This was designed for human observers to describe changes in the facial expression in terms of observable activation of facial muscles. FACS became a standard used to categorize the physical expressions of emotions, and it was widely adopted by psychologists and animators.

FACS parameterizes facial expressions in terms of Action Units (AU). AUs represent various minimal facial changes, like raising the right eyebrow, and are based on anatomical muscle and bone movements. Along with the definition of various AUs, FACS also provides the rules for AU detection in a face image. By using these rules, it is possible to encode a facial expression that produces the expression. For example, combining the AU1 (Inner Brow Raiser), AU4 (Brow raiser), AU15 (Lip Corner Depressor), and AU23 (Lip Tightened) creates a sad expression (Deng & Noh, 2007).

Despite its popularity, there are some drawbacks of using FACS (Ekman, 1993; Essa et al., 1996; Pelachaud et al., 1994): AUs are purely local patterns while actual facial motion is rarely completely localized; FACS offers spatial motion descriptions but not temporal components. In the temporal domain, co-articulations effects are lost in the FACS system.

The MPEG-4 Facial Animation standard is a direct implementation of FACS and specifies and animates 3D face models by defining a set of Feature Points (FP). The main purpose of the FPs is to provide spatial reference to specific positions on a human face such as major muscles and bones. The MPEG-4 Facial Animation specification was the first facial control parameterization to be standardized into MPEG-4 FBA (Face and Body Animation) (Koenen, 2002; Pandzic & Forchheimer, 2002).

## 3. Autism spectrum disorder background

Autism is a developmental disorder with onset prior to age three and is characterized by cognitive and behavioural difficulties in communication and social interaction (Association, 1994). This psychological illness is characterized by the presence of restricted, repetitive, and stereotyped patterns of behaviour, interests and activities. Autism is part of a range of disorders that include Asperger's Syndrome and other pervasive developmental disorders. These syndromes are jointly referred to as Autism Spectrum Disorders (ASDs).

A fundamental part of these disorders is the failure to recognize emotions in due time (Baron Cohen, 1995). Individuals with autism tend to avoid looking at human faces and find it hard to understand why facial features move in the way that they do. This inability to read emotions on the human face impairs their ability to communicate with other people.

The human face is fundamental in both the expression and communication of emotions, so the majority of studies have focused on the face and tested the recognition of basic emotions (Ekman & Friesen, 1971). Studies assessing recognition of these emotions report inconclusive findings. Some studies report difficulties in recognition of basic emotions from facial expression, voice recordings, and from the matching of stimuli from the two modalities (Deruelle et al., 2004). Other studies have found no such difficulties (Baron-Cohen et al., 1993), and that the deficit only becomes apparent when testing recognition of more "complex" emotions, such as jealousy, embarrassment or pride. These studies have reported that autistic individuals have deficits in complex emotion recognition from photographs of eyes (Baron-Cohen et al., 2001), facial expressions, short voice recordings (Capps et al., 1992), pictures (Bauminger, 2004) and linguistic contextual cues (Happe, 1994).

In contrast to these difficulties, individuals with autism show good and sometimes even superior skills in "systemizing"(Baron-Cohen, 2003). Systemizing is the drive to analyze or build systems, to understand and predict the behaviour of nonagentive events in terms of underlying rules and regularities. Autistic individuals are hyper-attentive to details and prefer predictable rule-based environments, features that are intrinsic to systemizing. In addition, individuals with autism are superior to control on various tasks that involve searching for detail, analyzing and manipulating systems (Shah & Frith, 1993).

Assuming that autistic people possess good systemizing skills, it is possible to explore them to compensate for some of their empathizing difficulties. This might be hard to implement because the socio-emotional world is a context-related open system (Lawson, 2003), often unpredictable and difficult to conceptualize with strict rules. However, if provided with a system of emotions, it is plausible that systemizing skills could be harnessed to help individuals with autism learn to recognize emotions.

### 3.1 Traditional learning tools

Past attempts to teach emotion recognition to adults and children with autism have either focused on the basic emotions (Hadwin et al., 1996), or have been part of social skills training courses, usually run in groups (Barry et al., 2003). These training programs do not focus on systematically teaching emotion recognition, instead, they address other issues, such as speaking, reducing socially inappropriate behaviour, and so forth. In such groups it is difficult to accommodate the individual's specific pace of learning.

Other attempts to teach emotion recognition to individuals with autism have used computer-based solutions (Bernard-Opitz et al., 2001; Bolte et al., 2002; Grynszpan et al., 2005). The use of computer software for individuals with autism has several advantages. First, individuals with autism favour the computerized environment because it is predictable, consistent, and free from social demands, which they may find stressful (Williams et al., 2002). Second, users can work at their own pace and level of understanding (Powell, 1996). Third, lessons can be repeated over and over again, until mastery is achieved (Williams et al., 2002). Fourth, interest and motivation can be maintained through different and individually selected computerized rewards (Moore et al., 2000). Previous studies have found that the use of the computer can help individuals with autism to recognize basic emotions from cartoons and still photographs (Bolte et al., 2002; Tseng & Do, 2010), and to solve problems in illustrated social situations (Bernard-Opitz et al., 2001). However, participants find it hard to generalize their knowledge from learnt material to related tasks (Golan et al., 2006).

A common feature of the computer-based interventions mentioned above is that they use drawings or photographs, rather than more lifelike stimuli, for training. It is possible that the use of more realistic stimuli could improve the knowledge transfer.

### 3.2 Digital media learning tools

Recent approaches to teaching emotion recognition to individuals with ASD use interactive game solutions.

*Mind Reading* (Baron-Cohen et al., 2004) helps children and adults to learn about emotions and their expressions, especially in human faces. It provides an interactive guide and a video library of real people expressing emotions, as well as quizzes and games to check the individual's progress.

*The Transporters* (Baron-Cohen et al., 2007) is an animation series designed to help children with autism to discover the world of emotions. The series involves characters who are mechanical vehicles with human faces, that show emotional expressions in social context.The aim of this project is to attract the children's attention with mechanical motion in order to encourage incidental social learning and increase attention to the face. The evaluation of this project shows that there was greater progress in emotion recognition skills in the autistic children intervention group.

Children with ASD often avoid eye contact with others which prevents them from perceiving and understanding the emotions of others. *FaceSay* is an interactive computer software program that features interactive games that let children with ASD practice recognizing the facial expression of an avatar, or software "puppet". Specifically, this computer game shows these children where to look for facial cues, such as an eye gaze or a facial expression.The study found that children with ASD made significant improvements in their ability to read facial expressions and recognize emotions (Biasini & Hopkins, 2007).

The *Let's Face It! (LFI!)* program is a series of interactive computer games designed to improve the face recognition abilities, including inatention to the eyes (Wolf et al., 2008), and failure to understand faces (Gauthier et al., 2009). This set of games aims reinforce the child's ability to attend to faces, recognize facial expressions and interpret facial cues in a social context. The study of Tanaka (Tanaka et al., 2010) with *LFI!* shows considerable improvements in the face recognition skills of children with autism.

The *SmileMaze* is a face expertise training prototype that teaches children how to recognize and produce facial expressions via a web cam. The program uses state-of-the-art computer techniques in expression recognition and are incorporated into the *LFI!* treatment program. The study of Cockburn (Cockburn et al., 2008) suggest that including real time expressive production into the *LFI!* program is a great benefit to help childrens with ASD to recognize emotions from own facial expression.

The present game solutions indicate that emotion recognition can be improved over a relatively brief training period, when more lifelike stimuli are employed.

### 3.3 Challenges in trainning methodologies

A facial expression is a result of a muscle contraction that produce different facial movements. Assuming these movements as being important in the context of non-verbal communication, it is necessary to ponder methods that include facial motion. Several researchers have claimed that not only the movement itself, but also the timing associated with facial motions are critical parameters in recognizing emotions (Cockburn et al., 2008; Ekman, 1993; Fasel & Luettin, 2003; J. Reilly, 2006).

Nowadays, most methods for teaching facial emotions are based on static photographs of facial expressions. According to the above, those methods present some limitations, as interactive applications to teach emotions recognition.

Another problem that affects the learning process of autistic people is the user interface and interaction model. There is not much research that addresses such an issue, but most of the solutions that have been applied to ASD are based on the traditional style of WIMP interaction (Window, Icon, Menu, Pointing device). This kind of interaction allows the children and adults with autism to input commands using keyboards, mice or touch screens, like the examples presented in previous solutions.

However, it is possible to explore the autistic people's unique learning style: typically, they are much more attracted by the details of a tangible user interface, such as a steering wheel used in a computer game, than by a standard mouse.
Sitdhisanguan et al. (Sitdhisanguan et al., 2007) made a comparative study between the use of both WIMP and tangible user interface. The study shows that autistic childrens' behavior are restricted, by the WIMP interface. Such interaction style could easily lead to boredom. At the same time, autistic children had difficulties in performing point and click actions. Different, when using a tangible user interface, they were more agile in manipulating the interface. The study also concludes that autistic children enjoy technology that supports physical activities.
Most of the computer-based solutions that have been used to help autistic people to learn about emotions aim at a teaching environment. They make use of some of the benefits afforded by computer technology, but are often based on exactly the same concepts as "tried-and-true", lower-tech solutions (Michel, 2004). One could argue that the rather traditional approach of these technologies fails to exploit some of the most novel and interesting properties of computer-based technology.
*Are there ways of extending the use of technology beyond a teaching scenario to help people with autism to look at the human face and learn about emotions?*

## 4. LIFEisGAME: A modular interactive learning system

Based on the review of the findings of past research, we are developing the LIFEisGAME (Learning Facial Emotions Using Serious Games) project, a facial emotion recognition learning system, based on the interaction between humans and 3D avatars. The system, with a game like structure, has a set of activities that will reinforce an understanding of emotions, their causes and consequences, and their associated facial expressions. To define a user interface and a set of interactive activities, a psychotherapy background was necessary.
This project will be based upon a LEGO-like structure. In one hand, we have the possible technologies that can be used, such as motion capture, virtual and augmented reality, digital tables, mobile devices, computers, etc. In the other hand, we have the game concepts, ideas and tasks that must be completed throughout the game. In order to achieve a flexible and expansible platform, it is necessary to consider that the game can be easily adapted to the needs and specifications of the therapists, parents and children. So, both the technology and the game modules will be developed and used as LEGO pieces. For example, imagine that a therapist wants to use the game mode A with a digital table. He will be able of simply choosing the desired module and, if the game is compatible with the digital table, it will be automatically ready for being played. Afterwards, if another therapist wants to play the same game with, for example, motion capture he simply chooses the correct module and the game is auto-reconfigured. The same concept can be used the other way around, i.e., different game modules (LEGO pieces) may fit upon the same technology modules (other LEGO pieces).

### 4.1 Game design

The goal of the game is to help children with ASD recognize emotions through facial expressions. Based on the experiential lerning cycle defined by Kolb (Kolb, 1984), we defined the following pedagogical modes for the game:

1. **Recognize the Expression.** In the first mode, children are encouraged to watch and recognize facial expressions.

2. **Build a Face.** In the second mode, they are encouraged to learn by doing, that is, actively experiment with different possibilities of constructing a desired facial expression.
3. **Become Your Avatar.** In the third mode, children are not only encouraged to recognize and mimic, but also to concretely experience how to make the expression with their own faces.
4. **Live a Story.** Finally, the children are encouraged to generalize or transfer their knowledge of facial expressions to real-life situations, requiring them to understand each emotion.

The four modes differ in their interactivity and engagement. Children will be encouraged to play these modes in a sequential manner, but customizations could be made to allow them to begin with any mode.

**Recognize the Expression.**
In this mode, the player is presented with a sequence of random facial expressions and required to identify a specific (pre-selected) expression from the set. Each session is time-limited, as determined by a therapist, to maximize player attention.
The therapist can create different exercises for facial expression recognition based on the core mechanics embedded in the game. The core mechanics are based on identifying micro and subtle expressions and analyzing the three concepts: intensity, length and valence. Each type of exercise can have different configurable scenarios where the avatar appears with a full face, half face or a mix face:

1. **Full face**: uses all the face to display the expressions. This scenario allows teaching expressions associated to a specific type of avatar.
2. **Half face**: either the upper part or the lower part of the face is hidden. This scenario allows teaching a specific section of an expression.
3. **Mix face**: uses half of the face from one character and the other half of the face from another character. This scenario allows teaching expressions by dissociating them from the type of avatar.

**Build a Face.** This mode asks the player to construct a facial expression on a 3D avatar to match a defined emotion. This mode has two levels. The first level is a free play mode. The player must choose a 3D avatar to play with and an emotion. Then, a drawing area and a 3D model of the chosen avatar will appear. The player must draw on the first area to create a 2D representation of the expression. The system will automatically apply the 2D sketch to the 3D avatar. In this mode, the player can save the expressions that were drawn and create a sequence that can be animated and played. Also, it will be possible to edit these expressions and sequences to create new animations or, for example, change the 3D avatar maintaining the animation sequence. The player can build several models that can be used to produce an animation sequence. The second mode makes use of a webcam to take a picture of the player that may be performing some facial emotion. Then, the player will be able of drawing on the special area, by using the sketching feature, to match the expression of a 3D avatar with the expression from the photo. When the player finishes drawing, the system will calculate the final score of the game based on how close the drawing was to the expression in the photo.
**Become Your Avatar.** The objective of this mode is to improve the children's capabilities of reproducing facial expressions. The player controls a 3D avatar simply by moving his own face. When the player performs a given facial expression, the 3D avatar will mirror its movements. When the game starts, a target expression is presented. The player must

try to achieve this target by performing it with its own face. When the target expression is achieved, the player must hold it for three seconds. This time is used to ensure that the player consciously achieved this expression. This game is divided in three sub-games. The first is a free-play mode in which the 3D avatar simply mirrors the player's expressions; in the second game mode, called "Train an expression" , the player chooses an expression and must achieve it as described above; finally, in the third mode, the player will have to follow the same game mechanics throughout a random sequence of expressions to finish the level.

**Live a Story.** In this mode the player is invited to perform a role in a certain story. The story will unfold until a certain event occurs. At these moments, two things can happen. In the first case, it is expected that the player performs a given facial expression, which will be captured by a camera or motion capture system. For example, we can imagine that at some point in the history, the player can be given a gift. In this situation, it is expected that the player smiles because he was happy. If the expression is not the same as the one that was expected, the story may take a different course. In the case depicted above, the person who gave the player a gift may be sad and the story will have a different ending. In the second case, the player may have to make another type of action, such as choosing an answer from a predefined set of possible answers or performing a physical action such as picking something or doing a movement.

### 4.2 Game technology

The core technology behind our solution is based on the facial synthesis of 3D characters. It strives to solve the synchronization and realism problems, support reusability of facial components, and have an avatar-user interaction model with real time response.

The technology we have developed is capable of not only creating smooth facial deformations in a friendly way, but also making avatars respond to it in real time. It is prepared to reproduce facial animations with cinematographic quality and accepts avatars that range from photorealistic to cartoon. The 3D characters in the game were created by an artist and are intentionally made to be likable and agreeable to children. Therefore, the avatars possess some attractive features such as healthy skin and symmetrical faces. Also, some avatars have child-like traits to appear warmer and more trustworthy for the player (Isbister, 2006).

The technology behind the game mode **Recognize the Expression** is based on keyframe animation. This type of animation is the most commonly used technique in facial animation practice. It consist first on creating different poses and interpolate them to generate animation. We have defined six basic expressions: anger, disgust, fear, happiness, sadness and surprise (Ekman & Friesen, 1971). For each 3D model, an artist custom created these basic expressions.

In the game mode **Build a Face** we aim to develop an interaction model to *draw* facial expressions in an easy and intuitive way, by exploring the emerging domain of interaction usability. Inspired in the way people draw, this interaction model will allow the player to *sketch* smooth facial deformations in a friendly way (Miranda et al., 2010).

The game mode **Become Your Avatar** is based on facial motion capture (MoCap). This technology allows capturing the complex deformations of a human face. The information captured is then mapped to a 3D model and reproduced to animate synthetic characters. Traditional MoCap techniques are based on facial markers. This solution is not suitable for our approach, because is unpleasant and "unnatural" , due to the need of using markers on the face. In order to overcome these problems we sugest using a markerless facial motion capture system based on low cost hardware, like a webcam, to capture the facial features of the player.

In the game mode **Live a Story** we want give the freedom to the player to interact in the digital environment by performing physical actions. These types of actions will be captured by using hardware such as the Wii Remote, Microsoft Kinect or the motion capture system.
The ultimate goal is to allow patients and therapists to create and adapt the contents of each game mode to the patient profile. Creating specific content is expensive, time-consuming and requires highly artistic skills. Thus, the technology presented in this section was designed to allow automatic user content generation.

## 5. Results and discussion

In this article, after describing some emotions and facial expression issues, we reviewed several computer-based solutions that have been used to teach autistic people to recognize facial expressions. The review suggestes that emotion recognition could be improved when systematic methods, with lifelike stimulus, are employed. We then present the basis of a new approach, whose novelty is the interactivity of the process, as opposed to previous methods that use still images and traditional interaction models. We believe that the generalization of the acquired knowledge to real life can be attained with a more natural interaction between the human (patient and/or therapist) and realistic expression 3D avatars. In this approach, we considered that a facial expression plays an important role in the transmission of emotions, so teaching autistic people to recognize emotions requires believable facial animations. However, generating realistic face movements is hard because there are many subtleties to control.
Our approach introduces a novel and sophisticated interaction model that enables patients to learn facial emotions by recognizing and imitating the avatars' movements. It is being developed with a game like structure in a modular way.
We have implemented the first game mode, "Recognize the Expression". Figure 1 shows a young children playing the game and a screenshot of the user interface. The 3D models used in the game were created by an artist.

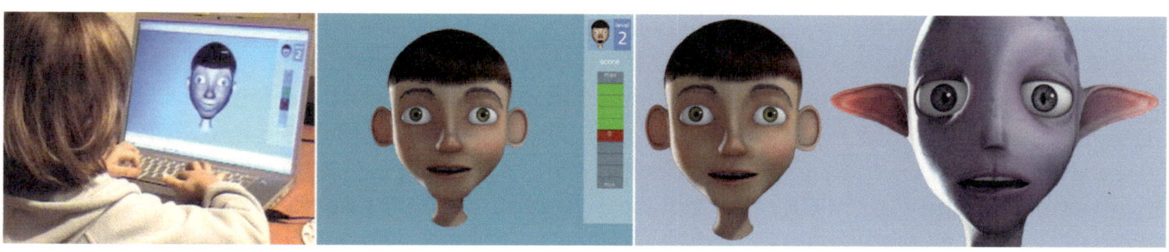

Fig. 1. A young children playing the game (left). User Interface of game mode "Recognize the Expression". Main window with the current expression and left panel that shows the score status, the expression to identify and the difficulty level (middle). Two examples of 3D avatars from the game: a boy and a fantastic creature, all in cartoon style (right).

We are developing a novel sketching control system to draw facial expressions, inspired in the way people draw. The method will be exploited in game mode 2, "Build a face", to speeding up the creation of facial expressions in an easy, natural and intuitive way. Figure 2 shows a screenshot of our sketching system.

### 5.1 Preliminary user study

In order to evaluate our game design, we conducted a user study. Nine participants, seven boys and two girls, ranging from four to eleven years old, with ASDs, participated in the study. Their ASD diagnoses varied. Six were identified as having high-functioning autism

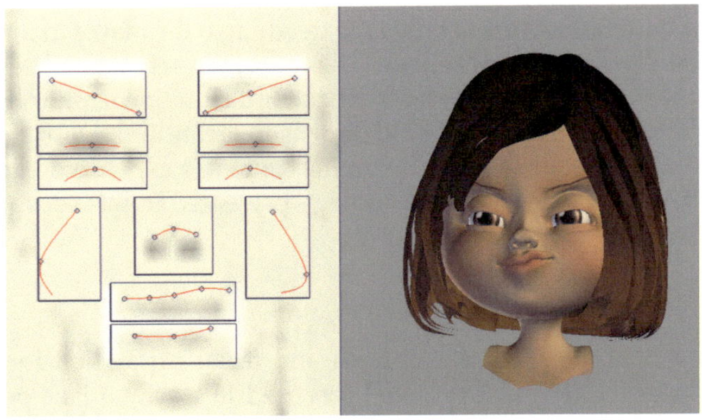

Fig. 2. Sketching System. Drawing area: the boxes represent the canvases where the user can draw the strokes; the background is a 2D image of a generic face (left) ; 3D area: shows a facial expression of the 3D character; the facial expression corresponds to the strokes on the drawing window (right).

or Asperger's syndrome. Two were in the middle of the spectrum. The testing sessions took place at the children's home or cafes designated by the parents. Every child was accompanied by at least one parent, mostly mothers. In the sessions, participants were asked to play two testing versions of the game with only the first game mode, "Recognize the expression", implemented. The first version of the game begins by asking players to select an avatar. After making this selection, the player must choose one of six basic emotions. The available emotions are based on Ekman and Friesen's (Ekman & Friesen, 1971) six primary and cross-cultural emotions. After choosing the emotion, the player must recognize and correctly identify the emotion on the avatar, which randomly cycles through facial expressions representing the six emotions. Players also select from three levels of difficulty. The second version of the game differs in that players are given the option to play additional modes where particular facial features, such as the eyes or mouth, may be covered on the avatar. Participants were instructed to play as long as they wanted. After ending play, the children were interviewed about what they liked and disliked about the game and how we could make the game more enjoyable. The parents were also interviewed with similar questions. In situations where the children did not wish to talk, we only interviewed the parents. The game play sessions were video recorded, and the interviews were audio recorded. The testing results suggest that overall, the children responded favorably to the game. When selecting avatars, all of the male participants preferred to play with the young-boy avatar, while the girls expressed a preference for the young-girl avatar. The majority of male participants requested to play with the alien-like avatar. Several parents discussed the importance of game context. They expressed an interest in a game that included storylines involving social scenarios. In terms of feedback, all of the participants enjoyed the auditory feedback; however, several children deliberately made wrong selections because they preferred the wrong-answer feedback. This suggests that the game design should allow for customization, including the ability to turn off or adjust colors and sounds, or provide a less engaging wrong-answer response. Additionally, in the testing version of the game, players had to choose the correct facial expression of an emotion, which is selected, in the current game design, from a series of images. One issue we observed was that children selected the correct answer by matching rather than by recognizing the expression. In order to reinforce learning and avoid matching, the correct answer image should be changed to text or represented by a different face.

Changing the correct answer image not only has the ability to reinforce a player's learning, but also enhance a player's ability to generalize the expression to other faces.

### 5.2 Future work

One future extension of our interaction model includes tangible user interfaces. In this context, several studies can be done to implement an interface where users interact in the digital environment with real objects in a natural way. We believe this kind of physical interaction will involve autistic patients more deeply in the emotions learning process and, consequently, improve their interaction with other people.
We will attempt to develop a set of facial synthesis algorithms and a classification method for facial emotion analysis. The classification method, in an extended way to the FACS system, will be used to analyze which facial movements, produced by the 3D character, correspond to the rules that define the different facial expressions.
We will perform future user studies to validate the game design and the usability enabled by the methodologies we are developing.

### 5.3 Acknowledgements

The authors would like to thank Cristina Queirós for her valuable feedback on the psychology of emotion recognition and Pamela Davis for feedback on the design of facial expressions. We would also like to thank Yan Zhang for her contribution on the user study. This work is partially supported by Instituto de Telecomunicações, Fundação para a Ciência e Tecnologia (SFRH/BD/46588/2008) and the UT Austin | Portugal Program CoLab grant (FCT) UTA-Est/MAI/0009/2009.

## 6. References

Association, A. P. (1994). *DSM-IV diagnostic and statistical manual of mental disorders (4th Edn.)*, Washington DC: American Psychiatric Association.

Baron Cohen, S. (1995). *Mindblindness: An essay on autism and theory of mind.*, MIT Press/Bradford Books.

Baron-Cohen, S. (2003). The essential difference: Men, women and the extreme male brain, London: Penguin.

Baron-Cohen, S., Golan, O., Chapman, E. & Granader, Y. (2007). Transported into a world of emotion, *The Psychologist* (20(2)): 76–77.

Baron-Cohen, S., Golan, O., Wheelwright, S. & Hill, J. J. (2004). *Mind reading: The interactive guide to emotions*, Jessica Kingsley Limited, London.

Baron-Cohen, S., Spitz, A. & Cross, P. (1993). Can children with autism recognize surprise?, *Cognition and Emotion* (7): 507–516.

Baron-Cohen, S., Wheelwright, S., Spong, A., Scahill, V. L. & Lawson, J. (2001). Are intuitive physics and intuitive psychology independent? a test with children with asperger syndrome, *Journal of Developmental and Learning Disorders* (5): 47–78.

Barry, T. D., Klinger, L. G., Lee, J. M., Palardy, N., Gilmore, T. & Bodin, S. D. (2003). Examining the effectiveness of an outpatient clinic-based social skills group for high-functioning children with autism, *Journal of Autism and Developmental Disorders* (33): 685–701.

Bauminger, N. (2004). The expression and understanding of jealousy in children with autism, *Development and Psychopathology* (6(1)): 157–177.

Bernard-Opitz, V., Sriram, N. & Nakhoda-Sapuan, S. (2001). Enhancing social problem solving in children with autism and normal children through computer-assisted instruction, *Journal of Autism and Developmental Disorders* (31): 377–398.

Biasini, F. & Hopkins, M. (2007). Demonstration and evaluation of avatar assistant: Encouraging social development in children with autism spectrum disorders, *University of Alabama at Birmingham* .

Bolte, S., Feineis-Matthews, S., Leber, S., Dierks, T., Hubl, D. & Poustka, F. (2002). The development and evaluation of a computer-based program to test and to teach the recognition of facial affect, *International Journal of Circumpolar Health* (61(Suppl. 2)): 61–68.

Capps, L., Yirmiya, N. & Sigman, M. (1992). Understanding of simple and complex emotions in non-retarded children with autism, *Journal of Child Psychology and Psychiatry* (33): 1169–1182.

Cockburn, J., Bartlett, M., Tanaka, J., Movellan, J., Pierce, M. & Schultz, R. (2008). Smilemaze: A tutoring system in real-time facial expression perception and production in children with autism spectrum disorder, *Proceedings from the IEEE International Conference on Automatic Face & Gesture Recognition, 978-986.* .

Deng, Z. & Noh, J. (2007). *Computer Facial Animation: A Survey. Data-Driven 3D Facial Animation*, Springer London.

Deruelle, C., Rondan, C., Gepner, B. & Tardif, C. (2004). Spatial frequency and face processing in children with autism and asperger syndrome, *Journal of Autism and Developmental Disorders* (34(2)): 199–210.

Ekman, P. (1993). Facial expression and emotion, *American Psychologist* (48(4)): 384–392.

Ekman, P. (1999). Basic emotions, *Handbook of Cognition and Emotion* .

Ekman, P. & Friesen, W. (1971). Constants across cultures in the face and emotion, *Journal of Personality and Social Psychology* (17(2)): 124–129.

Ekman, P. & Friesen, W. (1975). *Unmasking the face: a guide to recognizing emotions from facial clues*, Prentice-Hall, Inc., Englewood Cliffs, New Jersey.

Ekman, P. & Friesen, W. (1978). Facial action coding system, *Consulting Psychologist Press* .

Essa, I., Basu, S., Darrell, T. & Pentland, A. (1996). Modeling, tracking and interactive animation of faces and heads using input from video, *Computer Animation* 0: 68.

Fasel, B. & Luettin, J. (2003). Automatic facial expression analysis: a survey, *PATTERN RECOGNITION* 36(1): 259–275.

Gauthier, I., Klaiman, C. & Schultz, R. T. (2009). Face composite effects reveal abnormal face processing in autism spectrum disorders, *Vision Research* 49(4): 470 – 478.
URL: *http://www.sciencedirect.com/science/article/B6T0W-4VF4YN3-2/2/0881cd9f173bb7a062f971e5d1cf3a6b*

Golan, O., Baron-Cohen, S., Chapman, E. & Granader, Y. (2007). Facilitating emotional understanding and face processing in young children with autism spectrum conditions, using animations of vehicles with faces, *Paper presented at the International Meeting for Autism Research (IMFAR)* .

Golan, O., Baron-Cohen, S., Wheelwright, S. & Hill, J. J. (2006). Systemizing empathy: Teaching adults with asperger syndrome and high functioning autism to recognize complex emotions using interactive multimedia, *Development and Psychopathology* (18): 589–615.

Grynszpan, O., Martin, J.-C. & Nadel, J. (2005). Human computer interfaces for autism: assessing the influence of task assignment and output modalities, *CHI '05 extended*

*abstracts on Human factors in computing systems*, CHI EA '05, ACM, New York, NY, USA, pp. 1419–1422.
URL: *http://doi.acm.org/10.1145/1056808.1056931*

Hadwin, J., Baron-Cohen, S., Howlin, P. & Hill, K. (1996). Can we teach children with autism to understand emotions, belief, or pretence?, *Development and Psychopathology* (8): 345–365.

Happe, F. G. (1994). An advanced test of theory of mind: Understanding of story charactersÕ thoughts and feelings by able autistic, mentally handicapped, and normal children and adults, *Journal of Autism and Developmental Disorders* (24): 129–154.

Isbister, K. (2006). *Better Game Characters by Design: A Psychological Approach*, Morgan Kaufmann.

J. Reilly, J. Ghent, J. M. (2006). Investigating the dynamics of facial expression, *Proceedings of the International Symposium on Visual Computing*.

Koenen, R. (2002). Overview of the mpeg-4 standard. http://www.cselt.it/mpeg/standards/mpeg-4/mpeg-4.htm.

Kolb, D. (1984). *Experiential Learning: Experience as the Source of Learning and Development*, Englewood Cliffs, NJ.

Lawson, J. (2003). Depth accessibility difficulties: An alternative conceptualisation of autism spectrum conditions, *Journal for the Theory of Social Behaviour* (33): 189–202.

Michel, P. (2004). The use of technology in the study, diagnosis and treatment of autism., *Final term paper for CSC350: Autism and Associated Development Disorders.* .

Miranda, J., Blanco, X., Sousa, A., Gutierrez, D., Orvalho, J. & Orvalho, V. (2010). Painting on canvas: a facial sketching control system, *ACM SIGGRAPH/Eurographics Symposium on Computer Animation*.

Moore, D., McGrath, P. & Thorpe, J. (2000). Computer-aided learning for people with autism - a framework for research and development, *Innovations in Education and Training International* (37): 218–228.

Ortony, A. & Turner, T. J. (1990). What's basic about basic emotions?, *Psychological Review* (97): 315–331.

Pandzic, I. . S. & Forchheimer, R. (2002). *The origins of the mpeg-4 facial animation standard. In MPEG-4 Facial Animation, The Standrad, Implementation and Application.*, John Wiley & Sons Ltd.

Pantic, M. & Rothkrantz, L. (2000). Automatic analysis of facial expressions: The state of the art, *IEEE TRANSACTIONS ON PATTERN ANALYSIS AND MACHINE INTELLIGENCE* 22(12): 1424–1445.

Pelachaud, C., Badler, N. & Viaud, M. (1994). Final report to nsf of the standards for facial animation workshop, *Technical Report, National Science Foundation* .

Powell, S. (1996). The use of computers in teaching people with autism, *National Autistic Society Conference* pp. 128–132.

Shah, A. & Frith, U. (1993). Why do autistic individuals show superior performance on the block design task?, *Journal of Child Psychology and Psychiatry and Allied Disciplines* (34): 1351–1364.

Sitdhisanguan, K., Dechaboon, A., Chotikakamthorn, N. & Out, P. (2007). Comparative study of WIMP and tangible user interfaces in training shape matching skill for autistic children, *TENCON 2007 - 2007 IEEE REGION 10 CONFERENCE, VOLS 1-3*, pp. 660–663.

Suwa, M., Sugie, N. & Fujimora, K. (1978). A preliminary note on pattern recognition of human emotional expression, *Proceedings of the 4th International Joint Conference on Pattern Recognition*, pp. 408–410.

Tanaka, J. W., Wolf, J. M., Klaiman, C., Koenig, K., Cockburn, J., Herlihy, L., Brown, C., Stahl, S., Kaiser, M. D. & Schultz, R. T. (2010). Using computerized games to teach face recognition skills to children with autism spectrum disorder: the letŠs face it! program, *Journal of Child Psychology and Psychiatry* 51(8): 944–952. URL: *http://dx.doi.org/10.1111/j.1469-7610.2010.02258.x*

Tseng, R.-Y. & Do, E. Y.-L. (2010). Facial expression wonderland (few): a novel design prototype of information and computer technology (ict) for children with autism spectrum disorder (asd), *Proceedings of the 1st ACM International Health Informatics Symposium*, IHI '10, ACM, New York, NY, USA, pp. 464–468. URL: *http://doi.acm.org/10.1145/1882992.1883064*

Williams, C., Wright, B., Callaghan, G. & Coughlan, B. (2002). Do children with autism learn to read more readily by computer assisted instruction or traditional book methods? a pilot study, *Autism* (6(1)): 71–91.

Wolf, J. M., Tanaka, J. W., Klaiman, C., Cockburn, J., Herlihy, L., Brown, C., South, M., McPartland, J., Kaiser, M. D., Phillips, R. & Schultz, R. T. (2008). Specific impairment of face-processing abilities in children with autism spectrum disorder using the let's face it! skills battery, *Autism Research* 1(6): 329–340. URL: *http://dx.doi.org/10.1002/aur.56*

# 16

# Promoting Peer Interaction

Barbro Bruce and Kristina Hansson
*Malmö University and Lund University*
*Sweden*

## 1. Introduction

Positive experience from peer interaction is a key to language as well as cognitive and social development. On the other hand language skills, i.e. the ability to understand and make oneself understood, is a prerequisite for gaining access to peer interaction. Social status in peer relations is crucial for self esteem. In peer interaction identity and awareness of self - both positive and negative - emerge and develop.

Problems with peer interaction and peer communication can occur both as a core symptom and as a secondary consequence in several developmental diagnoses during childhood. Such problems are often secondary in for example specific speech- and/or language impairment and developmental language disorder, while they are part of the core problems in for example autism spectrum disorders. For children with problems in language and communication, this scenario entails a risk for marginalization and exclusion in peer play. This is particularly problematic, since these children need more, rather than less, experiences from peer interaction to support their development of language and communication skills. It is therefore important to indentify intervention models that address peer interaction and peer communication.

Peer interaction is something that children commonly manage by themselves already at an early age, and therefore are supposed to manage without too much involvement from adults. As soon as an adult is involved, it is per definition no longer primarily a peer interaction. This turns out to be a dilemma both for parents and professionals working with children with problems of language and communication. What seems so easy and natural in typically developing children is something that for children with problems is so hard to enhance, promote and compensate for in professional intervention. Therefore models for intervention need to take their point of departure in spontaneously occurring interaction between peers, and aim to increase and optimize such interactions. Such interactive experiences from familiar and meaningful contexts enhance flexible and generalized use of communication skills (Landa, 2007).

In this chapter we discuss factors to take into account when promoting peer interaction in children with communication problems, based on our studies of children with specific language impairment (SLI) in interaction with different types of peers. We begin by giving a background picture of the importance of positive experience from practicing peer interaction for the development of language and communication skills. After that we present some risk scenarios for children with problems in language and communication. We then describe the methodology and the results from our research addressing the question of how interaction between children with SLI and peers with typical language development can be enhanced and promoted. The main focus is on contextual influence and how systematic variation of contextual factors can be used as an intervention model. The issue is how children with language and communication problems can get enough support and scaffolding as well as challenges, in order to develop their language and communication skills. Our intention has been to focus on how the main results from our research can be interpreted and generalized to a wider spectrum of children with language and communication problems.

## 2. Background

### 2.1 Peer interaction

Language and communication skills emerge and develop in social interactions before they can be used as strategies in individual learning. From the Vygotskian perspective follows the picture of social communication being a joint venture characterized by reciprocity and co-construction, in which both partners rely on each other and are mutually dependent in shaping each other's context (Linell, 2009).

Another main idea relies on the assumption that contextual factors are highly relevant for the emergence of social communication skills (Linell, 2009). Contextual factors or conditions, for example the situation and the partner that you are interacting with, seem to govern the extent to which you manage and succeed in social language skills.This is true from both a perspective of possibilities and a perspective of constraints in communication skills (e.g., Perkins, 2007). It is particularly true for children with serious problems with language and communication, who are in great need of support and scaffolding from their interactional partner. The more severe problems the child has, the more s/he will rely on the support that the conversational partner can offer.

Furthermore, depending on the type and extension of communication problems, it is reasonable to assume that the child will develop more or less functional coping strategies. From this perspective, communication skill is both a goal in language development, and a coping strategy to manage verbal interaction. Therefore it is important to identify conditions that enhance, promote and motivate the child to develop his/her communication skill. Earlier studies have pointed out that the way the conversational partner acts will affect how the child with language problems contributes to the dialogue (Nettelbladt et al., 2001). On the other hand, the interactional as well as the linguistic behavior of the child with language and communication problems will affect the way the conversational partner acts (Conti-Ramsden & Dykins, 1991). This mutual influence opens up for possibilities, as well as for risk scenarios for the child with language and communication problems. If the conversational partner offers scaffolding, coherence in the dialogue may be promoted, while too much scaffolding may lead to dependence. There is a risk for the child to become too dependent on adults to scaffold and interpret what s/he is saying. This might preserve a dependence of support, and the child may avoid and then miss more challenging situations, which could promote development towards more independence.

Another argument why peer interaction is important is that everybody contributes to his/her own language input. The more verbally active a child is the more language input s/he receives from his/her interactional partner in reactions, answers, new questions and comments. The importance of peer interaction in play cannot be overemphasized; it is a prerequisite for further development. Play situations are characterized by a reciprocal focus, a high level of activity with dynamic exchanges, not limited to "joint attention" but also entail "joint action". Since they are frequently and regularly occurring in everyday situations generalization is promoted (Landa, 2007, p. 22).

> Transactional, developmental, and social-pragmatic approaches view language learning as a co-created process shared by child and other. Perhaps the most distinguishing features of the transactional/developmental approaches pertain to the emphasis on reciprocal, affective, self-regulatory, relationship-building, and discovery processes. Through interactions with others, such as joint action routines, shared experiences and meanings are developed. (Landa, 2007, p. 22)

Peer interaction starts early, already at a pre-verbal developmental age, and can be regarded as a prerequisite as well as a predictor of language development. For example, the ability to participate in games and routines has been shown to significantly predict language production in a longer perspective (4-5 years) in children with autism spectrum disorders (Bopp & Mirenda, 2010). Furthermore, peer interaction can be viewed as a platform for sharing of experiences and co-learning in adopting others' perspectives, which is essential for both social and cognitive development (Williams, 2007). One important quality in peer interaction is to be able to take other's perspectives, to mentalize, which is essential in social interaction. Social communication in peer interaction entails opportunities to practice listening and language comprehension, a prerequisite for responsiveness, as well as expressing oneself, a prerequisite for assertiveness. Reading other people's minds as well as asserting oneself with body posture, gestures, eye movements can be seen as precursors of interactive skills (Halliday, 1975; Tomasello, 2008).

## 2.2 Communication problems in children

Regardless of specified diagnosis, children with constraints in language and communication and/or neuropsychiatric functioning, e.g. autism spectrum disorder (ASD), attention deficit/hyperactivity disorder (ADHD), conduct disorder, all have problems with communication. In some cases the core problem primarily affects structural language, but also has consequences for the use of language, since these children may have reduced speech intelligibility, which makes it hard for other children to understand what they are saying. In other cases the primary problem is the use of language in social contexts, i.e. a pragmatic language problem. However, the relationship between structural language skills and functional language in social communication has not been found to be straightforward (Bonifacio et al., 2007). This means that problems with peer interaction have to be addressed separately, and it cannot be taken for granted that they disappear as language structure develops.

Communication problems can also occur in combination with other problems often referred to as co-morbidity. It is well known that there is an overlap - or sharing of symptoms - across disorders identified during childhood (Gillberg, 2010). Some of the most commonly occurring symptoms that elicit concern in parents, pediatricians and teachers already at an early age involve language, communication and social relations. The symptoms can also be found in the fields of behavior, activity, attention, and motor coordination as well as mood (Gillberg, 2010). Such commonly occurring problems have been shown to persist over time, sometimes with changes in manifestations. Therefore, according to Gillberg (2010), children with any of those symptoms manifested at an early age, need a general neurodevelopmental clinical examination with a broad focus (ESSENCE: Early Symptomatic Syndromes Eliciting Neurodevelopmental Clinical Examination, Gillberg, 2010). Another example of overlap or co-occurrence was found by Gilmour et al. (2004), who identified pragmatic language problems, i.e. problems with social communication, in two-thirds of children diagnosed with conduct disorders. As suggested by Gilmour et al. (2004), co-occurrence of symptoms may also have implications for intervention, e.g. by ameliorating social and communicative skills, disruptive behavior is likely to decrease.

A further characteristic is instability in diagnoses involving language and communication problems. For example, diagnoses such as developmental language disorder and specific language impairment (SLI), have both been shown to be unstable over time. Children diagnosed with developmental language disorder at an early age may have symptoms characteristic of autism spectrum disorder at a later age (Norbury & Bishop, 2002; Bishop & Norbury, 2002; Bishop et al., 2008; Mouridsen & Hauschild, 2009). For these reasons it is wise to address a wide perspective of diagnoses involving language and communication in assessment as well as in planning intervention for children with such problems.

### 2.3 Peer interaction in children with communication problems

All children with language and communication problems share a common core problem or risk, namely to be ignored and marginalized by peers and to have trouble in gaining access to social interactions with peers. As a consequence they miss valuable social experience and language input as well as practice of language skills (Corsaro, 1979; Craig & Washington, 1993; Brinton & Fujiki, 1999; 2005; Horowitz, 2005). According to Ladd (1984) peer relationship difficulties can be manifested in at least three ways: "peer isolation/withdrawal, lack of popularity (including peer neglect and rejection) and friendlessness" (Ladd, 1984, p.326). However, these manifestations of peer relationship difficulties may be regarded as secondary, i.e. consequences that originate from different underlying problems, either related to a core problem of the child him/herself, or to contextual factors.

Regardless of specific diagnosis, all children with problems with social interaction and communication have a "moment 22" dilemma in common: first, social communication skills are stimulated and enhanced in peer interactions, and second, social communication skills are required to gain access to peer interaction. The consequences of such a dilemma can be understood through the following: in peer interaction each participant creates and sets the limits for his/her own language input and learning. The more responsive and assertive a child is in relation to others, the easier it will be for others to respond, comment, and thereby prolong and deepen the conversation. If there is a risk for not being involved in spontaneous peer interactions, e.g. as is the case for children with language and communication impairments, the problems of marginalization and exclusion will increase as the child falls further behind. Children with language problems seem to find it easier to communicate with adults, in particular with professionals, probably because they scaffold and give support in a systematic way. This has been shown in studies which have found that adults are preferred as conversational partners (Rice et al., 1991). However, the dependence on rich support from adults can also develop into a lack of interactional independence and turn into a constraining factor as the child becomes older.

### 2.4 Intervention targeting peer interaction and communication skills

It is difficult to promote interaction between children with communication problems and typically developing peers with didactic means in direct intervention. As soon as an adult - parent or professional - enters a moment of peer interaction, it is per definition no longer interaction between peers. In the opposite scenario - if we do nothing - children with communication problems will get marginalized and thereby miss even more valuable experience of peer interaction and may get caught in a vicious circle.

Given that peer interaction is hard to promote with direct and didactic means, peer-mediated social skills training aiming at improving communication skills is an attractive alternative. For example, Chung et al. (2007) showed that peer-mediated training was effective in order to improve communication skills in young children with high-functioning autism, although they claim that "there is a tremendous need to develop an effective social skills training manual for teachers, parents, and paraprofessionals" (Chung et al., 2007, p. 435). There are two possibilities when choosing a peer-mediated intervention: either to try to increase the social interaction skills of children with communication problems, or to train typically developing children to interact with peers with communication problems. According to Pollard (1998) the last alternative, focusing on the typically developing peers, seems to be the most common approach targeting preschool children with autism.

Sometimes the intervention is a placement in a preschool (Language Acquisition Preschool; Rice & Hadley, 1995) or school language unit. Such models are based on the assumption that a placement in a smaller group of children with teachers specialized in the field of language and communication, is beneficial in itself. However, there are different set-ups of language preschools and language units. Some models are based on the assumption that children with language and communication problems develop optimally in interaction with peers representing a similar language developmental stage, and moreover also having problems with their language development. Such a segregated group only consists of children with language and communication problems. Other models are based on the assumption that children with language impairment will develop most optimally in mixed groups, where they can interact with peers who offer them both support and challenge. In such an integrated model, children with language and communication disorders are mixed with typically developing children.

First of all the intervention must fit the needs of the child, and be functional in relation to the social needs of the child (Johnston, 1985). Furthermore, the intervention should result in an increase of social experience and be "ecologically valid" as defined by Ladd (1984 p. 331), that is, "relevant to the types of tasks children must perform in the peer group". This means that research on different models of intervention must be performed in situations where peer interaction typically occurs; otherwise the outcome may not be representative and difficult to generalize. Wang et al. (2011), compared the effectiveness of peer-mediated and video-modeling social interventions for children with autism spectrum disorders, and found both methods to be equally effective. The age of the child predicted the effect significantly: the younger the child at the time for intervention, the better. For this reason, intervention that promotes peer interaction at an early age is often more effective given that it works proactively in aiming at minimizing the risk for marginalization and exclusion. Furthermore, early intervention is motivated by the fact that communication disorders often appear early and affect several aspects of development, not just language and communication

> Communication intervention for children with autism will envelop many aspects of development, including social engagement, social reciprocity, joint attention, imitation, play, vocal-manual coordination, language, flexible communicative contingencies, and social communicative abilities. (Landa, 2007, p. 22).

The more language skills are used, the more robust and accessible they become. It is therefore important to enhance and encourage peer interaction. The intervention model must generate many occasions for practice, in order to obtain change and to facilitate generalization to other contexts and to make the acquired skills permanent and stable over time. Therefore it is important to identify contexts that are natural and regularly occurring and that do not require special arrangements. McConkey et al. (2010) recommend an intervention model based on structured communication offered in the children's homes by family members for preschoolers with autism spectrum disorders.

We do not have enough knowledge about how to implement learning outcome from individual training to spontaneous peer interactions, or about how to optimize the conditions for social communication. Most intervention models target structural aspects of language rather than functional language in social contexts. Since children with communication problems often have problems to generalize from one context to the other, functional/social language skills have to be consciously targeted by professionals in natural contexts without "taking over" the responsibility of the interaction.

Leaf et al. (2009) evaluated the effectiveness of a special intervention aiming to increase social skills and pro-social behavior in children diagnosed with autism. The intervention, called "Teaching interaction procedure", was based on reinforcement and priming in targeting four social behaviors: 1. conversation, 2. play, 3. emotional skills and 4. choosing the same friend throughout the day. Leaf et al. (2009) found that the teaching package was effective, but since the study involved only three children during a period of just two months, the question of generalization still remains.

Intervention models must thus include the question of generalization over time and over situations, and not be restricted to what has been didactically practiced within an intervention session. They should take their point of departure in underlying contextual conditions, e.g. by facilitating for children with communication problems to meet and be involved in joint actions with their peers.

## 3. A study of children with specific language impairment interacting with different peers

One of the aims of our research on children with SLI is to study co-construction and reciprocity in interaction between children with language impairment and typically developing peers. The main focus is not on the individual participants in verbal interaction, but on the dynamics, dominance, and coherence conditions in the dialogues as wholes. The following is an overview of the results reported in Bruce et al. (2010), which we use to discuss from a wider perspective of relevance for all children with communication problems.

### 3.1 The participating children

Thirty children with Swedish as their first language were engaged in the studies. Ten (five girls and five boys) had a diagnosis of specific language impairment (SLI) and 20 were children with typical language development. Of these, ten (three girls and seven boys) were of similar chronological age as the children with SLI, and ten (five girls and five boys) were on a similar stage of language development. Apart from the requirements with respect to age and language stage, the typically developing peers also had to belong to the usual playmates of the children with SLI. The children in the SLI group were aged 3;9-5;0, the age similar peers 3;8-5;1, and the language similar peers were aged 2;11-3;10. All children had normal hearing and non-verbal cognitive ability. The pre-testing included assessment of phonology, grammatical production and sentence comprehension. The children in the SLI group had significant problems with grammar in language production, whereas only one of them had significant problems with sentence comprehension. They all also had problems with output phonology. The children in the other two groups performed within age expectations. The age similar group scored significantly higher than the other two groups on grammar and phonological production, whereas there was no difference between the SLI and language similar group.

### 3.2 Material and analyses

15 minutes of interaction between each child with SLI and each of their peers was video- and audiotape-recorded. A set of small toys was used in all the dialogues. Altogether, the data consist of 10 dialogues.

The dialogues were transcribed orthographically and coded with respect to how each turn linked backwards to earlier turns, "response properties" and how they carried the conversation forward, "initiation properties" (Bruce et al., 2010, Linell et al., 1988). The typical response properties are linking up with focal (as opposed to peripheral) aspects of the partner's (as opposed to with the speaker's own) immediately (as opposed to earlier) preceding turn. Initiation properties contribute new information and can be either statements, which are non-soliciting, or questions/directives, which are explicitly soliciting a response. Most turns have both response and initiation properties. Turns with only response properties are minimal responses and turns with only initiation properties are turns that introduce new topics. Utterances that are not intended or treated as contributions to the ongoing dialogue, for example self-talk or utterances directed to someone else in the room are not treated as turns, and were coded as non-contributing utterances. For a more detailed description of the method for analysis, initiative-response analysis(IR-analysis), see Bruce et al. (2010), Hansson et al. (2000) and Linell et al. (1988).

The different turn codings are scored on a scale from 1 to 6 according to their strength, where solicitation and non-focal, non-local and self-linking get a higher score than non-soliciting and focal, local other-linking turns. Using this scoring, a mean "strength" of the contributions in the dialogue can be computed, an "IR-index", which is a measure of the dominance conditions and dynamics of the dialogue. A dialogue with a high IR-index (> 3) is a dynamic dialogue which is likely to cover different topics and to contain many questions/directives. In a dialogue with a lower IR-index (< 3) the participants are likely to stick to the same topic and to contribute new information in statements rather than asking questions. The IR-index is computed for the dialogue as a whole, as well as for each individual participant. The difference between the IR-index of the two participants is the IR-difference and reflects the general dominance conditions within the dialogue.

The coding of response and initiation properties was also used to obtain more specific variables to characterize the dialogues. *Responsiveness* is the proportion of turns that link to the focal aspects of the partner's immediately preceding turn and also has initiation properties. *Topic shift* is the proportion of turns introducing a new topic. *Self-linking* is the proportion of turns where the speaker links up with his/her own earlier turn. We also computed the proportion of *non-contributing utterances*. The focus was on the dialogues as wholes, but in order to assess the mutual influence within the dialogues individual values were also computed for each participant.

## 4. Peer interaction; similarities, differences and correlations

### 4.1 Coherence

An important characteristic of a well-functioning dialogue is coherence, that is, that the participants adhere to the topic at hand, and contribute to topic continuation by contributing new information for the partner to respond to. One important aspect of coherence is responsiveness when comparing the two types of dialogues. Responsiveness tended to be higher in the dialogues with age similar peers compared to the dialogues with language similar peers. From another perspective, coherence, or rather lack of coherence, is also reflected in the frequency of topic shifts and self-linkings as well as in the proportion of non-contributing utterances. All these variables tended to be lower in the dialogues with age similar peers than with language similar peers and the differences between the two types of dialogues were significant. The different aspects of coherence in the two types of dialogues at time I are illustrated in Figure 1.

In the individual contributions of the children with SLI, the overall pattern was the same, i.e. their turns contributed to higher coherence with the age similar peer than with the language similar peer, although very few of the differences were significant.

### 4.2 Assertiveness

The IR-indexes in the two types of dialogues were around 3 (mostly slightly below 3), which is expected from a spontaneous conversation between equals. Looking at the IR-difference, the children with SLI were likely to be dominated by their age similar peer (see Figure 2). The IR-difference was negative from the perspective of the child with SLI in nine out of ten dialogues with age similar peer. The children with SLI had a higher IR-index with language similar peers than with age similar peers. The child with SLI had a negative value for IR-difference in five dialogues and a positive value in five dialogues with language similar peers.

### 4.3 Mutual influence

Mutual influence was explored through correlation analyses between the participants' individual values for the different variables. The responsiveness of the conversational partner was positively associated with the responsiveness of the child with SLI, and negatively with topic shift, as well as percentage of non-contributing utterances in the child with SLI. This illustrates how important scaffolding and challenges from the conversational partner are for the development of communication skills. All of the results reported are confirmed and strengthened in an ongoing follow-up study with the same participants, using the same method. Most differences between the two types of dialogues seem to remain and the differences between the two types of dialogues are mirrored in the comparison between the first and second occasion (Bruce et al., manuscript).

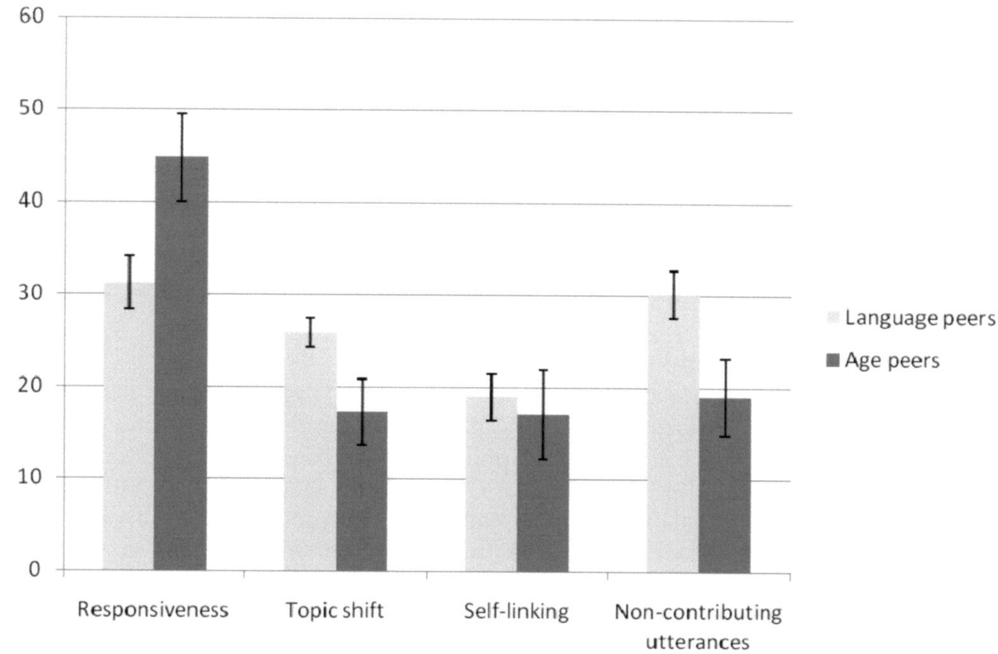


Fig. 1. Mean percentages and standard error of the mean for the measures of coherence, i.e. responsiveness, topic shift, self-linking, and non-contributing utterances in the two types of dialogues as wholes.

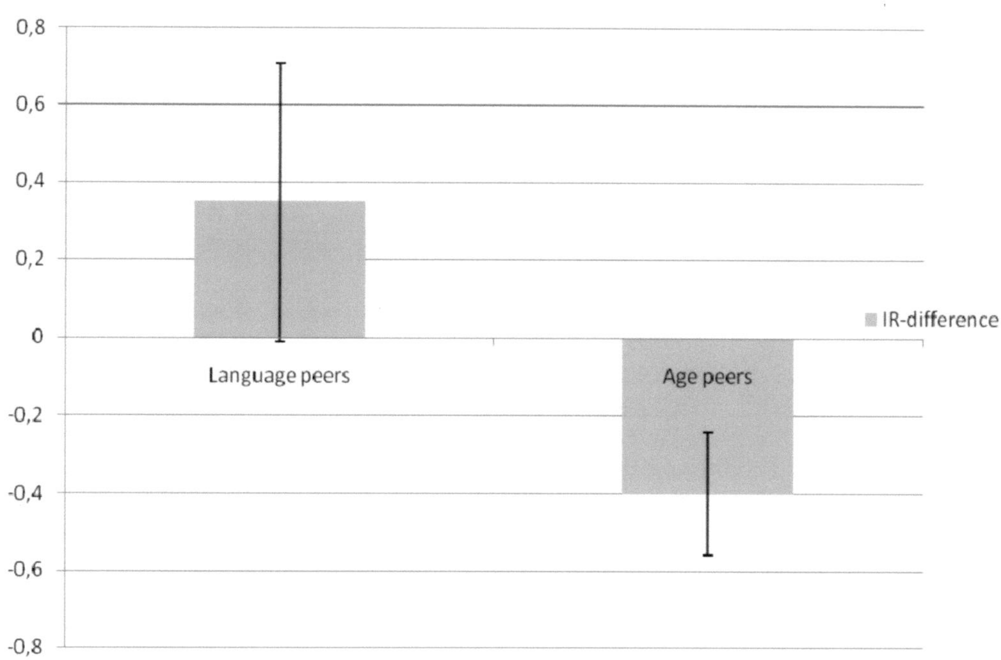


Fig. 2. The IR-difference, i.e. the difference in "strength" between the participants in the two types of dialogues.

## 5. Discussion

We will use these results to discuss how interaction between the larger group of children with language and communication problems, including children with ASD and typically developing peers, can be promoted. Our focus is on what is going on in different peer interactions, and particularly on the contextual conditions for peer interaction to be initiated as well as maintained, and from this identify relevant implications for intervention. Children with severe communication problems, in particular children with ASD, are also in great need of direct training programs performed and supervised by professionals, but this might be complemented by efforts to promote peer interaction.

### 5.1 Early proactive intervention

Promotion of interaction between peers of different age and language developmental stage can be made with an ambition to work proactively using indirect intervention methods. Early proactive intervention could focus on optimizing the contextual conditions for peer interaction to occur. All children, in particular children with language and communication problems, need qualitatively as well as quantitatively rich input as well as experiences of practicing their communication skills. The more children will be able to engage in conversations, the more reactions, answers and comments they will get back as responses. Early proactive intervention aims at preventing the risk of communication problems to grow permanent and at decreasing the risk of negative consequences, e.g. bullying and marginalization. Experience from early social interactions, that have been systematically varied and tailored to the abilities and needs of the child seems to promote the emergence of social communication skills (Landa, 2007). Such an association is derived from the discovered principle of an experience-dependent neuroplasticity of the brain, and generates implications for intervention (Landa, 2007). The main idea of our work was to "break ground" for initiating and maintaining peer interactions in children with communication problems. This was performed by selecting a specific conversational partner and vary qualities of the conversational partner, such as age and level of language development. Using this strategy in a systematic way might lessen the risk for marginalization of children with language and communication problems. Making children meet and take part in joint actions and reciprocal interactions will increase their experience of participation, which is a prerequisite for communication. This kind of indirect intervention, often called incidental or naturalistic intervention model takes its point of departure in spontaneously emerging situations in everyday life. However, to be able to promote such valuable situations in everyday life requires awareness of how important peer interactions are, and how interaction with peers can be initiated, and sustained (Bygdeson-Larsson, 2005).

We sort our findings and reflections under the main headings *support*, *challenges*, and *mutual influence*. These aspects represent aspects that are essential for all children in order to develop language and communication skills. Furthermore, they highlight the importance of contextual factors such as the preconditions for peer interactions to occur, as well as different qualities in different types of peer interactions. Peers representing different age and language developmental stage offer different proportions of these aspects, but there is scaffolding as well as challenges in all. Interactions with typically developing peers of similar age - *age similar interactions* – mainly seem to promote coherence, while interactions with peers representing similar language development - *language similar interactions* – mainly offer challenges and chances to "grow" from the perspective of a child with vulnerability in language and communication.

### 5.2 Support and scaffolding

Responsiveness makes the dialogue progress in a coherent and cohesive way. Topic shifts, self-linking, and non-contributing turns have the opposite effect, i.e. they fragmentize the interaction. Dialogues with age similar peers, compared to those with language similar peers, are characterized by significantly higher responsiveness, which contributes to coherence and the creation of mutually shared meanings. Listening and responding to the interactional partner, generates more coherent dialogues with respect to topic continuation. The ability to listen and respond to each other develops with increased age, maturity, but particularly with augmented experiences of interaction. As the child becomes older, s/he will be less dependent on scaffolding from the conversational partner to keep the topic and maintain the interaction. Coherent, cohesive and well-structured conversations have also been shown to have a scaffolding effect on language development (Bruce et al., 2010; Van Balkom & Verhoven, 2004).

At the same time as responsiveness is promoted in interaction with an age similar peer, fragmenting aspects (topic shift, self-linking and non contributing turns) diminishes (see Figure 1). The age similar peer is more responsive, maybe because of his/her more developed expressive language. On the other hand, in interactions with a less language developed and less experienced partner, the occurrence of fragmenting characteristics will increase. Taking part in such less scaffolding dialogues also adds important experience to conversational skills that the child needs in order to develop into an independent conversational partner. This maturation of conversational skill is indicated by a tendency for fragmentaione to decrease with increased age. All these considerations reflect the influence of contextual factors and are important to be aware of when planning intervention for children with communication problems.

### 5.3 Challenge and assertiveness

There is a risk for the child with communication problems to be dominated by his/her conversational partner, particularly in interactions with typically developing children of similar age. We saw evidence of this in our study. This indicates that it is hard to outgrow the role as being a less assertive conversational partner in peer interaction, see Figure 2. The challenge for the child with communication problems is different in the two types of dialogues. With the age similar peer, the challenge is to be assertive in spite of comparatively lower communicative skills. With the language similar peer the challenge is to take more responsibility for the interaction because the conversational partner does not offer scaffolding. The interaction with language similar peers is likely to be more symmetrical. However, these interactions might also be characterized by less coherence as reflected in more topic shifts, more self-linkings and non-contributing turns. Not unexpectedly, the follow up indicates that verbal interactional skills seem to increase with age and experiences, as shown by an increase of responsiveness, and a decrease of fragmenting features, like topic shifts, self-linking and non-contributing turns.

Dialogues involving older children with more developed language tend to be less dynamic than dialogues involving younger and less experienced children. From the perspective of the child with communication problems, the interactional patterns that reflect conditions of dominance, may be negative in dialogues with more language competent peers. In interactions with language similar peers, the pattern is likely to be more equal or symmetrical. It seems that with a younger peer on a similar language level, a child with language and communication problems will be more likely to take the lead and to take more of the responsibility in the interaction. This may be gained from experience of interactions with age similar peers, where the child with communication problems is offered more scaffolding. This can be carried over to the dialogue with a peer of the same language developmental stage, in which the child with communication problems takes more responsibility for the interaction. The difference between the two contexts is illustrated in Figure 3, showing the possible combinations of assertiveness and responsiveness. Dialogues with a peer of the same age as the child with communication problems tend to be high in responsiveness and low in assertiveness, while the opposite pattern is likely to be seen in dialogues with a peer representing the same language developmental stage as the child with communication problems. The idea of illustrating different combinations of assertiveness and responsiveness in a graph comes from Fey (1986), who used a cross-table representing presence or absence of these qualities. However, the main point of our figure also representing assertiveness and responsiveness is that such interactional behaviours are fluctuating and contextually dependent - not stable characteristics of an individual.

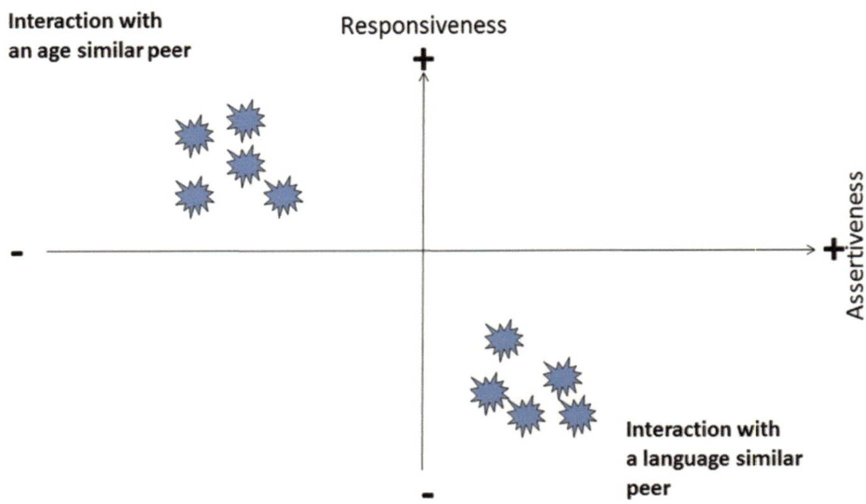


Fig. 3. Possible pattern in interactions between a child with problems with language and communication and typically developing peers of similar age or similar language development.

### 5.4 Mutual and contextual influence

Conversational partners constitute each other's context and influence each other "for better or for worse" in co-constructing their conversations. Such a mutual influence has been studied primarily in dialogues between adults and children (Conti-Ramsden & Dykins, 1991; Nettelbladt et al., 2001). As seen in Bruce et al. (2010), our research indicates that this also is true for peer interactions with conversational partners representing different age and stage of language development.

The most influential variable seems to be responsiveness in the conversational partner, which is positively associated with both the features of coherence, i.e. responsiveness, and the features of fragmentization, e.g. topic shift, self-linking and non-contributing turns in the contributions of the child with communication problems. This reflects the importance of support as well as challenge from the conversational partner. However, there are both pros and cons with all peer relations. Therefore it is important to try to identify what different conversational partners can offer in terms of support as well as challenge. Interaction with different conversational partners offers different proportions of scaffolding as well as challenges. Furthermore, the proportions and distributions of these aspects continuously vary during ongoing interactions because of a mutual influence between the interactional partners. What is important is that children with constraints of communication skills should not be left alone to manage initiation in peer play by themselves since this puts them at risk to be ignored. One way to avoid this scenario and to help them "over the threshold" is by introducing them to one - deliberately selected - peer at a time, with an adult still within reach although not actively participating. It is important to bear in mind that a need of scaffolding can easily turn into dependency and a feeling of "helplessness". At the same time the proportion of challenge will decrease. Furthermore, it is reasonable to believe that there is a transfer from one peer relation to another, for example if a child with communication problems acquires support from his/her interactional partner in one peer relation, s/he might be better able to offer scaffolding in another peer relation, where s/he feels relatively more competent. The mutual influence reveals that context plays an important role for the emergence of conversational ability, which the child cannot acquire without interacting with others. It is therefore important to promote and enhance peer interaction in children with some kind of language and/or communication problem.

### 5.5 Implications

An important and challenging question is how to apply the findings of relevance for peer interaction between children with communication problems and typically developing peers, and furthermore, how already attained goals can be maintained and generalized. Increased awareness of the importance of peer interaction in professionals and methods for systematic variation of contextual factors, such as group size, mix of children representing different age and stage of language development, introduction of one peer at a time, are some ideas. Bygdeson-Larsson (2005) used a model to facilitate professional awareness of social interaction between the children at preschool, with a program called "Educational Process Reflection", which was shown to "bring a shift of the teacher's perception of children, and enhanced inter-subjectivity in communication" (Bygdeson-Larsson, 2005, p.161). The model was introduced in Swedish pre-school practice and highlighted democratic values of interaction and play processes. The outcome was enhanced inter-subjectivity in communication, which in turn resulted in more interaction experiences. All these suggestions aim to offer support, scaffolding as well as challenges in order to foster independence and an increased status of children at risk.

## 6. Conclusions

Our conclusion is that different contextual conditions offer different kinds of support and present different types of challenges for children with problems of language and communication. Interaction with age similar typically developing peers are more supportive and can serve as "good models", while interaction with younger, language similar peers challenges the child to take a more active and assertive role. Children may take different roles in verbal interaction depending on how much support/scaffolding the conversational partner can offer. Communication - skills as well as problems - is strongly contextually dependent, and varies with general factors like purpose, number of persons involved and their relations, as well as with the characteristics of the conversational partners, like age, language skills and interests. The solution might be to design optimal contextual conditions for peer interaction to occur by deliberately choosing one conversational partner at a time. Contextual factors can be controlled for and systematically altered, but in order to make conscious adaptations and tailoring, we must know more about how, and to what extent different contextual factors influence peer communication.

## 7. Acknowledgements

This work was supported by the Swedish Council for Working Life and Social Research, grants No. 2001-2048 and 2007-0235.

## 8. References

Bishop, D.V.M. & Norbury, C. (2002). Exploring the borderlands of autistic disorder and specific language impairment: a study using standardized diagnostic instruments. *Journal of Child Psychology and Psychiatry,* 43, 917-929.

Bishop, D.V.M, Whitehouse, A., Watt, H. & Line, E. (2008). Autism and diagnostic substitution: evidence from a study of adults with a history of developmental language disorder. *Developmental Medicine and Child Neurology,* 50, 341-345.

Bonifacio, S., Girolametto, L., Bulligan, M., Callegari, M., Vignola, S. & Zocconi, E. (2007). Assertive and responsive conversational skills of Italian-speaking late talkers. *International Journal of Language and Communication Disorders,* 42, 607–623.

Bopp, K. & Mirenda, T. (2010). Prelinguistic predictors of language development in children with autism spectrum disorders over four–five years. *Journal of Child language.* doi:10.1017/S0305000910000140

Brinton, B. & Fujiki, M. (1999). Social interactional behaviors of children with specific language impairment. *Topics in Language Disorders,* 19, 49-69.

Brinton, B. & Fujiki, M. (2005). Social competence in children with language impairment: making connections. *Seminars in Speech and Language,* 26, 151-59.

Bruce, B., Hansson, K. & Nettelbladt, U. (2010). Assertiveness, responsiveness, and reciprocity in verbal interaction: Dialogues between children with SLI and peers with typical language development. *First Language,* 30, 493-507.

Bruce, B., Nettelbladt, U. & Hansson, K. (manuscript). Children with SLI interacting with age similar and language similar peers. A follow-up study.

Bygdeson-Larsson, K. (2005). Giving Voice to the Swedish Pre-school Child: Inclusion through Educational Process Reflection. *Child Care in Practice,* 11:2, 161/177.

Chung, K.-M., Reavis, S., Mosconi, M., Drewry, J., Matthews, T. & Tassé, M. J. (2007). Peer-mediated social skills training program for young children with high-functioning autism. *Research in Developmental Disabilities* 28, 423–436.

Corsaro, W.A. (1979). We're friends, right? Children's use of access rituals in a nursery school. *Language in Society,* 8, 315-336.

Conti-Ramsden, G., & Dykins, J. (1991). Mother-child interactions with language-impaired children and their siblings. *British Journal of Disorders of Communication,* 26, 337-354.

Craig, H. & Washington, J. (1993). Access behaviors of children with specific language impairment. *Journal of Speech and Hearing Research,* 36, 322-37.

Fey, M. (1986). *Language intervention with young children.* San Diego: College-Hill, Press.

Gillberg, C. (2010). The ESSENCE in child psychiatry: Early symptomatic syndromes eliciting neurodevelopmental clinical examinations. *Research in Developmental Disabilities* 31, 1543-1551.

Gilmour, J., Hill, B., Place, M. & Skuse, D.H. (2004). Social communication deficits in conduct disorder: a clinical and community survey. *Journal of Child Psychology and Psychiatry* 45:5, 967–978.

Halliday, M. (1975). *Learning how to mean – explorations in the development of language.* London: Edward Arnold.

Hansson, K., & Nettelbladt, U. & Nilholm, C. (2000). Contextual influence on the language production of children with speech/language impairment. *International Journal of Language & Communication Disorders,* 35, 31-47.

Horowitz, L. (2005). *Conflict resolution and development of communication competence in preschool boys with language impairment.* Doctoral thesis. Stockholm University.

Johnston, J. (1985). Fit, focus and functionality: an essay on early language intervention. *Child Language Teaching and Therapy,* 1, 125-134.

Ladd, G. (1984). Social skill training with children: issues in research and practice. *Clinical Psychology Review,* 4, 317-337.

Landa, R. (2007). Early communication development and intervention for children with autism. *Mental retardation and developmental disabilities research reviews,* 13, 16-25.

Leaf, J., Taubman, M., Bloomfield, S., Palos-Rafuse, L., Leaf, R., McEachin, J. & Oppenheim, M. (2009). Increasing social skills and pro-social behavior for three children diagnosed with autism through the use of a teaching package. *Research in Autism Spectrum Disorders,* 3, 275–289.

Linell, P., Gustavsson, L. & Juvonen, P. (1988). 'Interactional dominance in dyadic communication: A presentation of initiative-response analysis'. *Linguistics,* 26, 415-42.

Linell, P. (2009). *Rethinking language, mind and world dialogically. Interactional and contextual themes of human sense-making.* Charlotte, NC: Information Age Publishing.

McConkey, R., Truesdale-Kennedy, M., Crawford, H., McGreevy, E., Reavey, M. & Cassidy, A. (2010). Preschoolers with autism spectrum disorders: evaluating the impact of a home-based intervention to promote their communication. *Early Child Development and Care,* Vol. 180:3, 299–315.

Mouridsen, S.E. & Hauschild, K.-M. (2009). A longitudinal study of autism spectrum disorders in individuals diagnosed with a developmental language disorder as children. *Child: care, health and development,* 35:5, 691–697.

Nettelbladt, U., Hansson, K. & Nilholm, C. (2001). Why ask questions? Contextual effects on the grammatical structure in the language production of children with SLI. *Child Language Teaching and Therapy,* 17, 89-106.

Norbury, C. & Bishop, D.V.M. (2002). Inferential processing and story recall in children with communication problems: A comparison of specific language impairment, pragmatic language impairment and high-functioning autism. *International Journal of Language Disorders,* 37, 227-251.

Perkins, M. (2007). *Pragmatic Impairment.* Cambridge University Press, Cambridge.

Pollard, N. (1998). Development of Social Interaction Skills in Preschool Children with Autism: A Review of the Literature. *Child & Family Behavior Therapy*, 20: 2, 1-16.

Rice, M. & Hadley, P. (1995). Language outcomes of the language-focused curriculum. In: M. Rice & K. Wilcox (Eds.). *Building a language-focused curriculum for the preschool classroom* (pp. 155–169). Baltimore, MD: Paul H. Brookes.

Rice, M., Sell, M. & Hadley, P. (1991). Social interactions of speech- and language-impaired children. *Journal of Speech and Hearing Research*, 34, 1299-1307.

Tomasello, M. (2008). *Origins of Human Communication.* Cambridge, Mass.:The MIT Press.

van Balkom, H. & Verhoven, L. (2004). Pragmatic disability in children with specific language impairments. In: L. Verhoven and H.v. Balkom (Eds.), *Classification of developmental language disorders. Theoretical Issues and clinical implications*, pp. 283-305. Mahwah, New Jersey: Lawrence Erlbaum Associates.

Wang, S.-Y. & Cui, Y. & Parrila, R. (2011). Examining the effectiveness of peer-mediated and video-modeling social skills interventions for children with autism spectrum disorders. *Research in Autism Spectrum Disorders*, 5, 562-569.

Williams, P. (2007). Children teaching children. *Early Child Development and Care*, 177:1, 43–70.

# 17

# Augmentative and Alternative Communication Intervention for Children with Autism Spectrum Disorders

Gunilla Thunberg
*DART – centre for AAC and Assistive Technology, Sahlgrenska University Hospital, Sweden*

## 1. Introduction

The main purpose of this chapter is to present the field of augmentative and alternative communication (AAC) intervention, its application to children with autism spectrum disorders (ASD), and what we know of the effects so far.

## 2. Communication in children with autism spectrum disorders

### 2.1 Difficulties with communication and language as part of the spectrum

Major advances have been made over the two past decades in understanding the social-communication difficulties of children with ASD, resulting in greater emphasis on early social-communication features in the diagnostic criteria (Wetherby, 2006). The second of the three main criteria for autism in both diagnostic systems (DSM-IV and ICD-10) specifically concern communication, while the first concerns impairment in social interaction, which involves body communication to a great extent (table 1). Most parents of children with autism first begin to be concerned that something is not quite right in their child's development because of early delays or regressions in the development of speech (Short & Schopler, 1988). Problems with communication, in terms of both understanding and expression, are often said to be one of the main causes of the severe behaviour problems that are common among persons with severe autism and mental retardation (Carr et al., 1997). The lack of meaningful, spontaneous speech by age five has been associated with poor adult outcomes (Billstedt, 2007; Billstedt, Gillberg, & Gillberg, 2005; Howlin, Goode, Hutton, & Rutter, 2004; Shea & Mesibov, 2005). Certainly, communication and communication problems are at the heart of what ASD is all about.

Although all persons diagnosed with autism have problems with communication, their type and degree vary a lot and the work of identifying different subgroups has just begun. It has been estimated that between one-third (Bryson, 1996) and one-half (Bryson, Clark, & Smith, 1988) of children and adults with autism have no speech. However, recent research results indicate that the proportion of non-speaking children with ASD is much smaller, approximately 14% to 20%, among those who received very early intervention (Lord, Risi, & Pickles, 2004).

Two phenotypes of speaking children with ASD were identified by Tager-Flusberg and Joseph (2003): children with normal linguistic abilities (phonological skills, vocabulary, syntax, and morphology) and children with impaired language that is similar to the phenotype found in specific language impairment. Another potential subgroup may experience verbal dyspraxia or dyspraxia of speech (Rogers, 2006; Tager-Flusberg, Paul, & Lord, 2005; Wetherby, Prizant, & Schuler, 2000). Voluntary motor control is disturbed in children with dyspraxia, which also affects their ability to imitate. The new research on the role of the 'mirror neurons' in the parietal and frontal lobes may provide some answers on the relationships between motor control and imitation but also on the possible link with the development of intersubjectivity (Rogers, 2006).

In spite of the heterogeneity of language abilities in children with ASD, social-communication or pragmatic impairments are universal across all ages and ability levels (Tager-Flusberg, Joseph, & Folstein, 2001). According to Wetherby (2006), the social-communication deficits in children with ASD can be organized into two major areas: (1) the capacity for joint attention and (2) the capacity for symbol use. Since joint attention emerges before words, this deficit may be more fundamental and a number of longitudinal studies provide evidence of a relationship between joint attention and language outcomes (Charman et al., 2003; Mundy, Sigman, & Kasari, 1990). According to Wetherby (2006, p. 11), 'deficits in initiating and responding to joint attention have a cascading effect on language development since language learning occurs within the context of the modelling by the caregiver of words that refer to objects and words that are jointly regarded'. Wetherby (2006) states that deficits in imitation and observational learning are other main causes of the problems with symbol use experienced by children with ASD. Learning shared meanings, imitating and using conventional behaviours, and being able to decontextualize meaning from the context constitute the symbolic deficits in children with ASD (Wetherby, Prizant, & Schuler, 2000).

### 2.2 Development of communication and language in children with ASD

Because autism is usually not diagnosed until age three or four, there is relatively little information about language in very young children with autism (Tager-Flusberg et al., 2005). Retrospective studies using parent reports and/or videotapes collected during infancy, together with studies of children considered likely to develop autism, show severely delayed language acquisition with respect to both receptive and expressive skills (Dahlgren & Gillberg, 1989; Osterling & Dawson, 1994; Watson et al., 2007). Another typical phenomenon described by 25% of parents of children with ASD is language loss after initially developing some words (Chawarska et al., 2007; Kurita, 1985). Lord, Schulman, and DiLavore (2004) found that this language regression is unique to autism and does not occur in other children with developmental delays. Chawarska et al. (2007) hypothesize that these early-acquired speech-like productions are lost by children with ASD because the link between these expressions and a network of symbolic communication fails. There is significant variability in the rate at which language progresses among children with ASD who do acquire speech.

The few longitudinal studies of language acquisition in children with ASD suggest that progress within each domain of language follows similar pathways as it does in typically developing children (Lord et al., 2004; Tager-Flusberg et al., 2005). However, the speech of children with ASD is also characterized by some typical deviations. One of the most salient aspects is the occurrence of echolalia, which can be either immediate or delayed. Although some echolalia seems to be self-stimulating, both types of echolalia can serve communicative purposes for the speaker (Tager-Flusberg et al., 2005). At an early stage of language development, this may be the only way in which the child can actually produce speech. Tager-Flusberg et al. (1990) found that, over the course of development, echolalia rapidly declined for all the children with ASD and Down's syndrome in their study. Another prominent feature of language in children with ASD is general problems with deixis, which are most often manifested as pronoun confusion (Tager-Flusberg et al., 2005). Features such as vocal quality, intonation and stress patterns often result in problems for persons with ASD, although there is a lack of research in this field. Taken together, the findings suggest that the difficulties are due not only to problems in social intent but also to problems affecting a more basic aspect of vocalization (Tager-Flusberg et al., 2005).

Less research attention has focused on the comprehension skills of individuals with ASD although deviations in response to language and comprehension have been found to be strong indicators of ASD (Dahlgren & Gillberg, 1989; Lord, 1995). According to Tager-Flusberg et al., it seems that ASD children 'not only may have limited ability to integrate linguistic input with real-world knowledge but also may lack knowledge about social events used by normally developing children to buttress emerging language skills and to acquire increasingly advanced linguistic structures' (Tager-Flusberg et al., 2005, p. 350).

The pragmatic aspects of language have been studied in numerous ways. Children with autism share important similarities across different language levels (Tager-Flusberg et al., 2005). The speech acts that are missing or rarely used in the conversations of children with autism often concern social, rather than regulatory, uses of language (Wetherby, 1986). Ghaziuddin and Gerstein (1996) suggested that people with Asperger syndrome do not engage much in turn-taking and may talk too much. Ramberg, Ehlers, Nydén, Johansson, and Gillberg (1996) found that children with ASD were impaired in taking turns during dyadic conversations. Tager-Flusberg and Anderson (1991) found that children with autism had difficulty dealing with new information and produced more noncontingent utterances. A higher proportion of initiations rather than responses was found in a study by Bishop, Hartley, and Weir (1994). Tager-Flusberg et al. (2005) suggest that there is a basic difficulty in establishing and maintaining reciprocity in conversation - that is, in the ability to engage in mutual, co-operative social dialogue. Although the basic intention to communicate often exists, the person with autism has impaired skill in participating in communicative activities involving joint reference or shared topics (Tager-Flusberg et al., 2005, p. 354).

## 3. Augmentative and Alternative Communication (AAC) for individuals with ASD

### 3.1 Which children are in need of AAC intervention?

As stated above, many individuals with ASD never develop functional speech, while those who do still have problems with language and communication to different degrees, in different situations and during different periods in their life. 'The need for a range of augmentative strategies to enhance the communication skills of children with autism is evident given the severity and pervasiveness of their speech and language deficiencies' (Howlin, 2006, p. 237).

Augmentative and Alternative Communication is the term used since the 1980s for the field, which encompasses research, clinical and educational practice. The American Speech-Language-Hearing Association (ASHA) defines AAC as 'attempts to study and when necessary compensate for temporary or permanent impairments, activity limitations, and participation restrictions of persons with severe disorders of speech-language production and/or comprehension, including spoken and written modes of communication (ASHA, 2005, p. 1).

AAC should be thought of as a system with four primary components: symbols, aids, strategies and techniques (ASHA, 2005, pp. 1–2). Symbols of various kinds can be included in an AAC system: graphic, auditory, gestural, and textured or tactile symbols, which may be unaided (such as signs, gestures or facial expressions) or aided (such as real objects, pictures, line drawings, or orthography). Aids refer to electronic or non-electronic objects that are used to transmit or receive messages, and techniques to the ways in which messages can be transmitted. Finally, strategy refers to the ways in which messages can be conveyed most effectively with respect to, for instance, timing, grammatical formulation or communication rate (Beukelman & Mirenda, 2005). According to Beukelman and Mirenda (2005), the ultimate goal of an AAC intervention is to enable an individual to efficiently and effectively engage in a variety of interactions and participate in the activities of their choice.

Von Tetzchner and Martinsen (2000) have defined three different groups of individuals who need AAC: (1) the expressive language group, characterized by a gap between their understanding of other people's speech and their ability to express themselves through spoken language. The difficulties of this group are persistent and they need an AAC system that can be used permanently. (2) The supportive language group needs an AAC system at certain periods of their life or in certain situations and is divided into two subgroups in this respect: the developmental group and the situational group. For the developmental group, the AAC is often a step towards the development of speech. The situational group is made up of individuals who have learned to speak, but who have difficulty in making themselves understood, most often with people who do not know them well. (3) Finally, the alternative language group consists of individuals who will need their alternative language form for the rest of their lives. Intervention comprises both comprehension and production and the communication partners will also need to use the AAC mode. Von Tetzchner and Martinsen (2000) specifically mention children with autism as belonging to the third group. This is often true of children with autism and intellectual disabilities and definitely of those who do not develop speech. Probably the majority of children diagnosed within the autism spectrum who develop speech fall within the supportive language group, often due to their persistent problems with the comprehension of speech and language. Some rare individuals with ASD might fit better into the expressive language group in that they only communicate through alphabet boards or speech-generating devices (SGDs) but have a comparatively good understanding of speech.

### 3.2 AAC and autism in a historical perspective

#### 3.2.1 Manual sign communication

Historically, the first studies describing AAC techniques being used for persons with autism appeared in the 1970s; they reported on the use of sign language to improve communication (Howlin, 2006). These studies appeared at the same time as the unsatisfactory results of spoken-language-training programmes were being published. Studies by, for example, Lovaas et al. (1973) and Howlin (1989) reported little change after many hours of intensive treatment, and the results were particularly poor for the children whose comprehension and vocal skills were most impaired (Howlin, 2006). Initially, most signing programmes were built on formal sign language systems, but it became evident that these were often too complex and abstract, and so specially adapted systems were developed and implemented.

Sign-based programmes spread rapidly in schools for children with autism in many countries. This was also the case in Sweden, where the positive research results obtained by Johansson (1981), who used methods primarily involving sign communication for children with Down syndrome, influenced the communication programmes in most clinics and schools.

### 3.2.2 The shift to visual-graphic AAC

During the 1980's and 1990's a shift was seen within AAC practice for children with ASD. Use of manual sign communication decreased in favour of increased use of photos, pictures, and symbols alone or in combination with speech output on dedicated devices or computers. Mirenda and Erickson (2000) explain that the shift away from the use of signing to visual-graphic communication occurred as a result of research findings in three main areas: imitation, iconicity, and intelligibility. In addition to the evidence of a generalized imitation deficit in autism, there were also studies showing that some children with ASD had extremely poor sign imitation skills (Yoder & Layton, 1988) due to difficulties with motor planning, control and execution (Seal & Bonvillian, 1997). With respect to iconicity manual signing was thought to be too an abstract system for individuals on the autism spectrum, having easier to use and understand symbols with more resemblance to their referents. Problems with intelligibility refers to the fact that manual signs are not so easy to interpret for communication partners not so familiar with the child and/or the system of manual signing. According to Howlin (2006), the shift from the use of manual signs to visual methods was also due to the fact that visual methods had proven to be effective in enhancing general skill acquisition, mainly within the TEACCH programme (Treatment of Education of Autistic and related Communication-handicapped CHildren; Schopler, Reichler, & Lansing, 1980) developed during the 1970s. A variety of symbol systems were also developed, beginning with Blissymbolics (Bliss, 1965; Blissymbolics Communication International, 2011) and Rebus (Widgit Software, 2002; Woodcock, Clark, & Davies, 1968), followed by Pictogram (Maharaj, 1980) and Picture Communication Symbols (Mayer-Johnson, 1981). The improvements in computer technology made these symbol sets easily available in the form of practical software packages. The development of digital cameras during the 1990s also increased the possibility of including personal photos in AAC systems, which, according to clinical reports, seemed to increase motivation and facilitate understanding of pictures, particularly for individuals with ASD (Danielsson & Jönsson, 2001).
There are, however, also reports of problems in teaching symbols to children with ASD, mainly in teaching them to use the pictures spontaneously and for communicative functions other than requesting (Howlin, 2006). It was precisely these problems that led Bondy and Frost (1994) to develop the method called Picture Exchange Communication System (PECS). PECS is a systematic approach to communication training specifically developed for children with autism. The elements that make PECS different from other visual-graphic techniques are the use of the concrete hand-to-hand exchange of the picture and also the highly prescriptive user manual with its six levels to follow in sequence.

### 3.2.3 Speech output technologies and computer assisted instruction

Historically, the use of speech output technologies (i.e the use of dedicated and/or mainstraeam products, mainly computer applications, where it is possible to use synthetic

or digitized speech) for individuals with ASD has not been a matter of course (Schlosser & Blischak, 2001). Computer technology was introduced into educational settings for children with autism late, not only in North America, but also in Sweden. Three Swedish surveys done at the end of the 1990s (Eklöf Wicksell, 1998; Olsson, 1998; Thunberg, 2000) clearly revealed that the number of computers used at school and/or supplied by the county councils as personal communication aids was remarkably low compared to the situation for individuals with communication impairments with other causes than autism.
In Sweden, professionals feared that people with ASD would become even more aloof if they were encouraged to sit in front of a computer screen. Concerning speech-generating devices (SGDs i.e communication aids with speech out), a common view was that they would only stimulate echolalia in children with ASD, and that there would be too much noise in the classroom. By the end of the 1990s, scepticism had decreased. This was probably due to reports of some studies of successful computer-assisted instruction (CAI) carried out in Sweden. By using the interactive multimedia software Delta Messages, Heimann, Nelson, Tjus, and Gillberg (1995) showed that a group of 11 children with autism were able to make significant gains in reading, phonological awareness, verbal behaviour, and motivation. Another study within this project showed that 13 children with autism, regardless of the initial cognitive and language level, increased their reading skills and reading speed following the use of CAI (Tjus, Heimann, & Nelson, 1998). The interaction between the children and their teachers was also studied during the CAI sessions. It was suggested that the intervention promoted an increase in verbal expressions and enjoyment for the participating children, and specifically for the children with autism compared to the other children who were also included in the project. The children's verbal expressions were more relevant at the end of the study period, and this was most marked for the children at low language levels. Concerning the teachers' behaviour, it was seen that they tended to use more physical directives towards children with a low language level while the children with higher language levels received more praise (Tjus et al., 1998).

## 4. Evidence-based practice and AAC

The term evidence-based used as a prefix and a denominator of interventions and methods comes from medicine. The term evidence based means that the choices of interventions and assessments are based on a research of scientific literature and not only professional experience or previous practice. Within the field of AAC a discussion was started during the end of the 90's and in 2003 the book "The Efficacy of Augmentative and Alternative Communication. Towards Evidence-based Practice » was published (Schlosser, 2003). Editor and also author of many chapters of this book, was Ralph W. Schlosser, professor at NorthEastern University, USA. His work has been of great importance, partly because he is spreading knowledge about evidence-based practise (EBP) and due to the many thorough compilations of research that he has done but also in demonstrating the problems and shortcomings using EBP in relation to the field of AAC. One of these problems concerns the use of the RCT as the golden standard, as RCT studies are almost non-existent within the AAC field. There are many reasons to this but the main ones are that (1) children with communicative disabilities are so heterogenous and (2) that randomization is extremely difficult to put through due to ethical reasons. Schlosser has therefore suggested an alternative evidence hierarchy placing the meta-analysis on top (2003; Schlosser & Raghavendra, 2004). Schlosser and other prominent AAC-researchers recommend the use of well-controlled single-subject research designs that can form the base for systematic meta-analyses.

## 5. The evidence-base for AAC intervention directed to children with autism

### 5.1 Which mode and method of AAC is best for children with autism?

#### 5.1.1 Studies of manual sign communication for children with autism

The evaluative research on sign communication for individuals with ASD is limited. In a review article, Goldstein (2002) identified ten studies involving sign communication for children with ASD that met experimental requirements. The findings varied and mostly focused on the number of signs learned rather than functional aspects. The results suggested that sign teaching may be more effective at increasing communication in children with ASD than the teaching of spoken language.

In the results of a meta-analysis of AAC intervention outcomes for children with autism done by Wendt, Schlosser, and Lloyd (2004), 11 single-subject studies met the inclusion criteria. It was suggested that manual signs constitute a viable communication option based on a particular effectiveness measure, the Percentage of Nonoverlapping Data (PND), that is, the percentage of data points during intervention that exceeded the highest data point during baseline. The PND value for nine of the ten multiple baseline design studies was 90% to 100%; for the remaining one, it was 70% to 90%. None of these studies were published after the 1980s, which might reflect the gradual change in AAC intervention for persons with autism, as it became more focused on visual-graphic communication. Von Tetzchner and Martinsen (2000), though, report on a Norwegian survey of 64 children and adolescents with ASD in which it was seen that progress in terms of quality of language was seen only in those individuals who had been given systematic manual sign teaching. Von Tetzchner and Martinsen (2000, p. 82) criticized the fact that manual signing interventions were being abandoned and stated that 'this limits the variety of strategies that are applied and hence opportunities for learning for individuals with autism.

In a Swedish review of early intervention for children with communicative disabilities no new studies (i.e. published during the last ten years) other than review articles, involved manual sign communication alone. However, two very interesting studies comparing Picture Exchange Communication System (PECS) and manual signing were found. In the first of these it was seen that manual signing resulted in more eye-contact and vocalizations than did PECS (Anderson, 2002). However, PECS was learned faster than signing and the individuals initiated more using PECS. PECS was also better generalized to other situations (Anderson, 2002). Better generalization was also found in the other comparative study by Chambers & Rehfeldt (2003). One interesting review that reports manual signing being used within the frame of positive behaviour support is written by Bopp, Brown & Mirenda (2004). This review primarily focuses on the role of the speech-language pathologist in the delivery of positive behavior support and concludes that all 6 individuals in the survey who were trained to use signs as an alternative to the challenging behavior made progress (Bopp et.al., 2004).

#### 5.1.2 Studies of graphic symbol use for children with autism

Experimental research is also fairly limited within the area of visual-graphic AAC for children with ASD except for an increased number of studies in the last couple of years being done on PECS (reported below). In two review articles, Mirenda (2001, 2003) reports ten studies where non-electronic communication boards were used. According to Mirenda, the participants in these studies were usually taught to request desired objects or activities, and given appropriate opportunities and instruction many children, adolescents and adults across the range of ability can learn to use aided techniques communication for functional communication (2003, p. 205). In the previously mentioned article on the role of speech language pathologists and use of AAC in providing Positive Behavior Support, it was revealed that those studies that made use of visual schedules to enhance understanding could show that the individuals could learn to use these quickly and decrease their amount of challenging behaviours (Bopp, Brown & Mirenda, 2004).

There is now more evidence available to support the effectiveness of PECS. Preston and Carter in 2009, published a comprehensive review, also including a meta-analysis of some studies. Building on the results of altogether 456 individuals the authors concluded that PECS is an effective intervention for children with ASD as well as for children having communication problems due to other causes. PECS give children with no or limited functional communication a way of expressing themselves, Positive effects with respect to interaction and challenging behaviours were also seen in many studies. The children's use of speech also was stimulated but these effects were more limited and not so well studied. Preston and Carter points out that it is the first three steps in the PECS method that are known to be effective since almost no research has been done on the last three steps supporting different communicative functions and syntactic development.

In the studies that compare PECS with other interventions it was seen that children seemed to learn PECS faster than manual signing. In a study that compared PECS to an intervention where parents learned how to use responsive strategies and milieu teaching (RPMT) some interesting results were seen (Yoder & Stone, 2006). PECS seemed to stimulate the communication development more for those children who had poor joint attention skills. The children who had difficulties manipulating objects gained more using RPMT (Yoder & Stone, 2006). There is some evidence suggesting that children who use ecolalic speech develop speech better and faster using PECS than children who don't (Ganz, Simpson & Corbin-Newsome, 2008). In a study of PECS-training in a school setting it was concluded that it seems to be of great importance to provide continuous support and guidance to the staff to maintain the positive communication effects gained after training in and introduction of PECS (Howlin, Gordon, Pasco, Wade & Charman, 2007).

The last few years it has been more common to stress the importance of providing children with ASD with a continuous support for understanding language. This could be done using manual signing but also through pointing to pictures or graphic symbols while speaking. This method was first introduced in the 1980's by Goosens and was namned Aided Language Stimulation, shortened ALS or today ALgS (1989). The method has been used increasingly since then within the AAC field and other researchers and interventionists has adjusted the method somewhat and named it Aided Language Modeling or ALM (Drager, 2009), Natural Aided Language or NAL (Cafiero, 2005), Point-talking (Jonsson, Kristoffersson, Ferm & Thunberg, 2011) and used on a speech-generating device, System for Augmenting Language or SAL (Romski & Sevcik, 1986; Romski et.al., 2010). Many studies of graphic AAC intervention make use these methods, but few have tried to evaluate the specific effects of this intervention part. A newly published study by Romski et. al.(2010), however excluding children with ASD, show that SAL combined with training of AAC-use is en effective method to stimulate development of speech and language (2010). Compared to direct training of speech and language competencies it was proven even more effective.

According to a review by Drager (2009) on ALM for children with ASD "we have preliminary evidence that changing adults' behavior through aided modeling interventions can be effective for children with ASD" (p. 118). Drager hypothesize that it is the combination of the following that makes the different methods of aided modeling interventions effective: 1) implementation during opportunities that arise out of natural contexts and 2) presentation of both verbal and aided symbol augmented input to expand vocabulary.

### 5.1.3 Studies of the use of speech-generating devices for children with ASD

Speech-generating devices (SGDs), also referred to as VOCAs (Voice Output Communication Aids) in the literature, are portable electronic devices that produce synthetic or digitized speech output. Pictures or text of any kind can be used to represent the messages on the display. SGDs were first used in the 1980s and since then a range of models have been developed, from very simple ones with a single message, to advanced models in which large - theoretically infinite - vocabularies can be used. The latter are typically software-based and most also have pre-programmed applications available, free or for sale, that are designed to meet the needs of users at different language levels and ages. Unfortunately, with very few exceptions, they are only available in English. Improvements in computer technology in recent years have changed the relationship between low- and high-technology-based pictorial systems with respect to access and portability. SGDs, apart from the simplest models, used to be problematic to access and transport for people with communication problems who were not wheelchair-bound, while a communication book of some sort was often easier to carry around. A communication book can still be small and handy, but today it is more limited than commercial handheld computers and smartphones. The latter can contain large vocabularies with speech output and at the same time allow more advanced users to take and store photos, record messages, make phone calls and send symbol-based text messages. The development of improved speech output software has also resulted in computers becoming far more effective means of communication (Howlin, 2006).
A potential advantage with SGDs is the ability to facilitate natural personal interactions and socialization by virtue of the speech output they provide (Mirenda, 2003). A study that reports on these variables was done by Schepis, Reid, Behrmann, and Sutton in 1998. The four children in this study, all of whom were three to five years old and diagnosed with autism, were given access to an SGD; through naturalistic teaching procedures, they learned to make requests, answer questions, and make social comments during natural play and/or a snack routine at their preschool. There was also an increase in classroom staff members' communicative interactions with the children. The authors speculated that this increase might be due to the recent training, but that it might also be due to the new ease of understanding the children's SGD communication. This study was done on children at a prelinguistic level, using SGDs in a school setting; the same is true of almost all of the research done in the field of SGD intervention for children (and adolescents) with ASD.
In the series of studies by Sigafoos and colleagues (2001, 2003, 2004a, 2004b, 2004c, 2005), different aspects of SGD intervention were studied. In their 2001 article, Sigafoos and Drasgow used a case study to demonstrate the need for individuals with severe communication impairments to have access to different modes of AAC to use in different situations and settings and with different communications partners. The participant in this

study demonstrated rapid acquisition and conditional use of manual signing and an SGD. The boy always chose to use the SGD when it was present, but when it was absent, he used his corresponding manual sign to communicate. It was speculated that the SGD was visually more salient and that it was a more efficient response because it appeared to require less effort to use. In this case, contrary to other clinical reports, the boy used only his own speech together with manual signing, and not an SGD. Sigafoos et al. (2003) studied the specific role of speech output. Following the acquisition of the ability to request preferred objects using an SGD, rates of requesting and vocalization across speech output conditions (on and off) were compared. No major differences were found and the authors suggested that access to preferred objects, rather than the effect of the speech output, was the critical variable in maintaining the use of SGDs. One of the three children began to speak single words during the intervention, suggesting that SGD intervention may facilitate speech in some cases. In the next study, Sigafoos et al. (2004b) reported on an intervention to teach students to locate their AAC device or SGD, when it was not accessible. After an initial period of teaching the students to request access to preferred objects, a least-to-most prompting procedure was implemented to teach them to locate their device. The intervention proved effective in all three adolescents who participated in the study. The students were also taught to turn the device on. The speech output seemed to provide an important source of feedback the participants needed to master this skill. Sigafoos et al. (2004a) investigated whether two students at a prelinguistic level could learn to use an SGD to repair communicative breakdowns. The intervention was effective and the participants also began to use the SGDs to initiate requests even when communication breakdowns had not occurred.

Romski and Sevcik (1996), are the only researchers reporting a longitudinal study. Two individuals with autism were included in the investigation of the System of Augmenting Language (SAL). The individuals with ASD in the study both belonged to the group of participants who achieved the best success. Although the rest of the group were not diagnosed with ASD, it should be mentioned that Romski and Sevcik suggested that factors related to speech comprehension and representational skills seemed to distinguish the advanced from the beginning achievers in their group of 11 participants (Romski & Sevcik, 1996).

#### 5.1.4 Answer to the question of best AAC-approach

The answer to this question is that there is no clear answer, or at least no answer depicting one AAC-mode as better than the others. The three main methods being manual signing, graphic AAC including PECS and graphic AAC used together with speech output seem all to be effective in promoting communication and development of speech and language. There have also been very few attempts to compare the relative effectiveness of these approaches. In a systematic review of the research done on manual signs and graphic symbols used in ASD the author comes to the conclusion that the research base is not large enough to reliably inform clinical decision making (Wendt, 2008). He states that "Individuals with ASD constitute a very heterogeneous group; evidence is emerging to indicate that the selection of an AAC approach must be made relative to specific task demands and individual characteristics, rather than on the basis of general predictive and prescriptive indicators." However, Wendt in his review summarizes the advantages and disadvantages of manual and graphic AAC according to the information in table 1:

| Approach | + Advantages | - Disadvantages |
|---|---|---|
| Graphic symbols | + Visual learning often intact and good in ASD<br><br>+ Less demand on memory<br><br>+ Easy to understand for partners<br><br>+ Easier to prompt | - Visual discrimination skills<br><br>- Low rate of communication<br><br>- Problems with access, must be carried<br><br>- Turntaking more difficult<br><br>- Grammatical and/or semantic relations more diffifult to transmit<br><br>- Access to good technologies, tools and knowledge to produce symbol material and apps |
| Manual signing | + Always accessible<br><br>+ Possible to develop to a full and rich language system<br><br>+ More natural, transient and easy to fit into human interaction, including eye contact | partners must be able to produce and understand signs<br><br>problems with executive functions and motor impairment such as dyspraxia, motor planning problems, memory and mobilization may prevent acquisition and use |

Table 1. Disadvantages (-) and advantages (+) with manual and graphic AAC (Wendt, 2008).

A study by Sigafoos et al. (2009) compared the use of Picture Exchange and SGD for an adolescent boy with Down Syndrome and an autistic disorder. The conclusion was that the two systems were equally viable modes of communication.

Instead several studies, especially the more recently published, seem to arrive to the same recommendations in their discussion and conclusions, namely that the use of combined modes, multimodal AAC, seems to work best for children with communication difficulties (Branson & Demchak, 2009; Mirenda & Beukelman, 2005). Communication is multimodal in nature and the use of different modes to different extents depending on the situation, topic and the partner, is inherent. So in a way it's given and not surprising that the same must apply to children with disabilities. Different modes support and complement each other. For example, there is strong evidence that pictures are better learned when they are presented together with speech ouput (Schlosser & Sigafoos, 2006). Wendt in his review of manual and graphic AAC suggests that "Given the high training demands placed on communication partners by manual signs and their relatively high fine motor (hand) requirements, manual signs might best be included as one component of a multimodal communication system that also includes graphic symbols, SGDs, and individuals extant communication modalities (e.g., gestures, vocalizations, facial expressions)." (2008).

### 5.2 Does AAC hinder or facilitate development of speech?

Whether AAC hinders or facilitates the development of speech is a very important question. In spite of the multimodal nature of human communication it seems to be an innate force in humans and parents to promote use of speech. As soon as the prelinguistic child starts to use spoken words these are responded to and reinforced by the parent to a greater extent than other signals such as gestures (Volterra, Caselli, Capirci & Pizzuto, 2004). Since speech seems to be on the parental agenda it's important to discuss speech development and AAC with parents, even in if it's not brought up (Jonsson, Kristoffersson, Ferm & Thunberg, 2011). Unfortunately we don't yet have so much evidence when it comes to effects on the use of AAC on speech development. There are several studies that report effects on speech development but almost all of them as a side effect since most AAC interventions have the goal to improve communication, not specifically oral language (Beukelman & Mirenda, 2005). A high-quality review done by Millar, Light & Schlosser (2006) on the effects reported on speech in AAC-studies included several individuals with autism. It was concluded that AAC interventions do not appear to have a negative effect on speech production. One of the authors of this review article updated the search only including individuals with ASD (Millar, 2008). The result of the earlier review was again confirmed and it was seen that most of the existing research suggests that AAC may enhance speech development in individuals with ASD. It was also seen that a variety of instruction methods used in the interventions seemed to trigger speech, for example the use of time delay (Millar, 2008).

### 5.3 When can you start to use AAC – are there any necessary prerequisites that must be met?

The question of when you should start an AAC intervention has also been a matter of discussion, and partly connected to the above mentioned wish and hope in parents to train and/or wait for speech. Earlier, during the 1980's and 1990's, it was also common among professionals within AAC-teams and other professionals to regard certain skills as necessary prerequisites for a successful AAC-introduction. Among these were the capacity to interpret pictures/symbols, good seating, a means of pointing/indicating, understanding of language.

During the last ten years there has been a change in thinking and what is said now is that it never can be too early to start a communication intervention, and that AAC is an important tool (Branson & Demchak; 2009, Sigafoos, Drasgow & Schlosser, 2003). Both researchers and clinicians often work according to the insights and theories of typical development of language and communication: namely that a child has to be exposed to language long before he/she is expected to understand or use it him/herself (Drager, 2009). The mere thought of only using spoken words to a little child that we know he or she can understand is ridiculous. We immediately realize this is impossible - but still that is how we have done with respect to AAC, specifically graphic AAC with or without speech output. When it comes to SGDs some practitioners might well have stated that a SGD was too advanced for the child whilst he or she still used a lot of spoken language to the child.

Today, most researchers and AAC specialists hold that the very early and multimodal start of AAC is the only ethical one; we have to provide all the help that we can; With respect to iconicity manual signing was thought to be too an abstract system for individuals on the autism spectrum having easier to use and understand symbols with more resemblance to their referents. Problems with intelligibility refers to the fact that manual signs are not so easy to interpret for communication partners not so familiar with the child and/or manual signs. We can't know in beforehand what modes or methods that are going to work best in the future for the child, in a given situation and with a certain communication partner (Branson & Demchak; 2009, Sigafoos, Drasgow & Schlosser, 2003). If any prerequisites are needed these are connected to the communication partner, not the child. A basic knowledge in communication and the use of responsive strategies probably is needed to make AAC work in daily interactions (Thunberg, Ahlsén & Dahlgren Sandberg, 2007, Iacono, 1999).

### 5.4 What to consider to make AAC work in daily interaction?

During my more than 20 years working as an AAC specialist I have seen just too many examples of AAC systems not being used. It is important to ask oneself if it might be that it is not working to use technologies (be they low- or high-) in human interaction? It probably is very difficult and demanding but as a specialist I also have seen some really good examples when everything works beautifully.

I have also had the opportunity to try AAC myself – in my own home and reality. About a year after my second child was born I realized that he had problems with communication, since he did not show any interest in speech. At the age of three when he finally was given his diagnosis of autism and we landed as a family, I had the energy to start up AAC intervention in my own home. We used a multimodal intervention: manual signs, picture boards, visual schedules, SGDs and computers. And it worked! In my son's case it was the SGD that really helped him to crack the code of language: after hundreds and hundreds of activations of his messages on the SGD he realized what spoken words were all about. During a year he used this beautiful mix of all communication modes and began to speak more and more – the computer and SGD maybe being the best teachers: so patient and so consequent.

This experience led me into research and my doctoral studies. During a year I video-taped four families communicating with or without an SGDs in different activities using SAL (Thunberg, 2007). It was seen that the access to the device improved communication in most activities, which was very positive. Observing all the tapes I also realized that the families would have needed more knowledge in communication and responsive strategies. It was very common to observe that the parents used a dominant communication style characterized by directives. Knowing the families so well I could see that the results with respect to interaction would probably have been much better had I given the families a better basic knowledge in communication and strategies to use.

This led me to my ongoing projects: one about parental education (AKKtiv) and one about creating communicative environments in schools for children with ASD. Common for both these projects is that the introduction of AAC is preceeded by education and training in the use of responsive strategies (Jonsson, Kristoffersson, Ferm & Thunberg, 2011). Our results so far are very positive and goes along the line of other research that also point out the

importance of providing basic knowledge in communication and responsive strategies before introducing AAC (Iacono, 1999).
Another important factor to make AAC work is that the people involved, the network, have been part of the AAC process and in decision-making (Granlund, Björck-Åkesson, Wilder & Ylvén, 2008, Goldbart & Marshall, 2007). No matter what fancy AAC-systems a specialist team can provide - if the significant persons surrounding a child are not involved and feel insecure or resistant - this system won't have a chance to work due to the transitional nature of communication. In the planning of an AAC solution the energy therefore are best spent on assessing environmental factors and the social network rather than the more traditional structural/functional factors. This assessment is also important for identifying the communicative interactional needs that helps identifying the topics and vocabulary that will be meaningful to use for the child. And this factor is also one predicting a positive outcome of an AAC intervention.

## 6. Conclusion

The field of AAC is a fairly new field of knowledge that has gradually grown as there is a growing interest in functional communication and in ensuring the communicative rights of individuals with disability. There has also been an explosion of available communication technologies and methods that can support and improve communication for individuals with autism. We have probably and hopefully only seen the dawn of these new options. It is also possible to see that we are moving from using one technique or approach at the time to working with multimodal techniques or approaches were different tools and methods combined with an understanding of communication and use of interactional strategies build a total system of communication.
The research base with respect to AAC used by children with autism has grown in recent years. This research mostly consists of singe-subject-design studies and case studies, with very few controlled group studies being done. On the other hand there are some well-done meta-analyses published that compile results from singe-subject research studies. Due to the difficulties of conducting RCT studies within the field of AAC-intervention the meta-anlyses are important and can be seen as the golden standard.
In conclusion, meta-analyses and other studies show that AAC-interventions are cost-effective and give fast results and tend to stimulate speech development. The best results seem to be reached when the social network surrounding a child is given support and resources to be able to use responsive strategies and provide communication opportunities and direct training using AAC in natural daily interactions. AAC intervention should be started as soon as communication difficulties are displayed or suspected since AAC promotes communication, language and speech. AAC-intervention has also been proved to effectively decrease challenging behaviors. There is today no mode of AAC that is known to be better than any other. Instead multimodal approaches seem to be the most effective. However, graphic AAC seem to be acquired at a faster rate and also easier to generalize to other situations. PECS has been proved to be an effective AAC method, specifically at early stages of communication and with respect to the first three phases of the method.

## 7. Acknowledgment

Parts of chapter two and three was first published in the author's thesis (Thunberg, 2007).

## 8. References

American Psychiatric Association. (1994). *Diagnostic and statistical manual of mental disorders* (4th ed.). Washington, DC: Author.

American Speech-Language-Hearing Association. (2005). Roles and responsibilities of speech-language pathologists with respect to augmentative and alternative communication: Position Statement. Rockland, MD: Author.

Anderson, A.E. (2002). *Augmentative communication and autism : A comparison of sign language and the Picture Exchange Communication System*. Doctoral dissertation, University of California at Santa Barbara, 2001. *Dissertation Abstracts International : Section B : The Sciences and Engineering*, 62, 4269.

Beukelman, D. R., & Mirenda, P. (2005). *Augmentative and alternative communication* (3rd ed.). Baltimore, MD: Paul H. Brookes Publishing.

Billstedt, E. (2007). *Children with autism grow up: Use of the DISCO (Diagnostic Interview for Social and COmmunication disorders) in population cohorts*. Göteborg: Göteborg University.

Billstedt, E., Gillberg, I. C., & Gillberg, C. (2005). Autism after adolescence: Population-based 13-22-year follow-up study of 120 individuals with autism diagnosed in childhood. *Journal of Autism and Developmental Disorders*, 35, 351–360.

Bishop, D., Hartley, J., & Weir, F. (1994). Why and when do some language-impaired children seem talkative? A study of initiation in conversation of children with semantic-pragmatic disorders. *Journal of Autism and Developmental Disorders*, 24, 177–197.

Bliss, C. (1965). Semantography. Sidney: Semantography Publications.

Blissymbolics Communication International. (2011). Retrieved April 2011, from http://www.blissymbolics.org.

Bondy, A., & Frost, L. (1994). The Picture Exchange Communication System. Focus on Autistic Behavior, 9, 1–19.

Bopp, K., Brown, K. & Mirenda, P. (2004). Speech-Language Pathologists' Roles in the Delivery of Positive Behaviour Support for Individuals With Developmental Disabilities. *American Journal of Speech-Language Pathology, vol 13,* 5-19

Bryson, S. (1996). Brief report: Epidemiology of autism. *Journal of Autism and Developmental Disorders*, 26, 165–167.

Bryson, S., Clark, B. S., & Smith, T. M. (1988). First report of a Canadian epidemiological study of autistic syndromes. *Journal of Child Psychology and Psychiatry*, 29, 433–445.

Cafiero, J. M. (2005). *Meaningful Exchanges for People with Autism*, Bethesda, MD: Woodbine House.

Carr, E. G., Levin, L., McConnachie, G., Carlson, J. I., Kemp, D. C., & Smith, C. E. (1997). *Communication-based intervention for problem behavior*. Baltimore, MD: Paul H. Brookes Publishing.

Chambers, M., & Rehfeldt, R. A. (2003). Assessing the acquisition and generalization of two mand forms with adults with severe developmental disabilities, *Research in Developmental Disabilities*, 24, 265-280.

Charman, T., Baron-Cohen, S., Swettenham, J., Baird, G., Drew, A., & Cox, A. (2003). Predicting language outcome in infants with autism and pervasive developmental disorder. *International Journal of Language and Communication Disorders*, 38, 265–285.

Chawarska, K., Paul, R., Klin, A., Hannigen, S., Dichtel, L. E., & Volkmar, F. (2007). Parental recognition of developmental problems in toddlers with autism spectrum disorders. *Journal of Autism and Developmental Disorders*, 37, 62–72.

Dahlgren, S. O., & Gillberg, C. (1989). Symptoms in the first two years of life: A preliminary population study of infantile autism. *European Archives of Psychiatric and Neurological Science*, 283, 169–174.

Danielsson, H., & Jönsson, B. (2001). Pictures as language. *Paper presented at the International Conference on Language and Visualisation,* Stockholm.

Dawson, G., & Osterling, J. (1997). Early intervention in autism. In M. J. Guralnick (Ed.), *The effectiveness of early intervention* (pp. 307-326). Baltimore, MD: Paul H. Brookes Publishing.

Drager, K. (2009). Aided modeling interventions for children with autism spectrum disorders who require AAC. *Perspectives on Augmentative and Alternative Communication.* 114-120.

Eklöf Wicksell, G. (1998). *Kartläggning av förskrivning av datorbaserade hjälpmedel sett ur skolperspektivet [A survey of prescription of computerized aids from a school perspective].* Stockholm: Swedish Handicap Institute.

Fombonne, E. (2005). Epidemiological studies of pervasive developmental disorders. In F. Volkmar, R. Paul, A. Klin & D. Cohen (Eds.), *Handbook of autism and pervasive developmental disorders* (Vol. 1, pp. 42–69). Hoboken, NJ: John Wiley & Sons.

Freeman, B. J. (1997). Guidelines for evaluating intervention programs for children with autism. *Journal of Autism and Developmental Disorders*, 27(6), 641-651.

Ganz, J. B., & Simpson, R. L. (2004). Effects on communicative requesting and social development of the Picture Exchange Communication System in children with characteristics of autism. *Journal of Autism and Developmental Disorders*, 34, 395–409.

Ghaziuddin, M., & Gerstein, L. (1996). Pedantic speaking style differentiates Asperger syndrome from high-functioning autism. *Journal of Autism and Developmental Disorders*, 26, 585–595.

Goldstein, H. (2002). Communication intervention for children with autism: A review of treatment efficacy. *Journal of Autism and Developmental Disorders*, 32, 373–396.

Goossens, C. (1989). Aided communication intervention before assessment: a case study of a child with cerebral palsy. *Augmentative and Alternative Communication, 5,* 14-26.

Granlund, M., Björck-Åkesson, E., Wilder, J., & Ylvén, R. (2008). AAC interventions for children in a family environment: Implementing evidence in practice. *Augmentative and Alternative Communication, 24,* 207-219.

Heimann, M., Nelson, K., Tjus, T., & Gillberg, C. (1995). Increasing reading and communication skills in children with autism through an interactive multimedia computer program. *Journal of Autism and Developmental Disorders*, 25, 459–480.

Howlin, P. (1989). Changing approaches to communication training with autistic children. *British Journal of Disorders of Communication*, 24, 151–168.

Howlin, P. (2006). Augmentative and alternative communication systems for children with autism. InT. Charman & W. Stone (Eds.), *Social and communication development in autism spectrum disorders* (pp. 236–266). New York: The Guildford Press.

Howlin, P., Goode, S., Hutton, J., & Rutter, M. (2004). Adult outcomes for children with autism. *Journal of Child Psychology and Psychiatry*, 45, 212–229.

Howlin P., Gordon K., Pasco G, Wade a., Charman T. (2007). The effectiveness of Picture Exchange Communication System (PECS) training for teachers of children with autism: a pragmatic, group randomised controlled trial.

Iacono, T., (1999). Language Intervention in Early Childhood. International journal of Disability, Development and Education, 46, 383-420.

Johansson, I. (1981). Språk- och talutveckling hos barn med downs syndrom [Development of language and speech in children with Downs syndrome]. Umeå: Department of Linguistics.

Jonsson, A., Kristoffersson, L., Ferm, U., & Thunberg, G. (2011). The ComAlong communication boards: Parents' use and experiences of aided language stimulation. Forthcoming in *Augmentative and Alternative Communication.*

Kurita, H. (1985). Infantile autism with speech loss before the age of 30 months. *Journal of the American Academy of Child Psychiatry*, 24, 191–196.

Lord, C. (1995). Follow-up of two-year olds referred for possible autism. *Journal of Child Psychology and Psychiatry*, 36, 1365–1382.

Lord, C., Risi, S., & Pickles. (2004). *Trajectory of language development in autism spectrum disorders.* In R. M & S. Warren (Eds.), Developmental language disorders: From phenotypes to etiologies (pp. 7–29). Mahwah, NJ: Lawrence Erlbaum.

Lord, C., Schulman, C., & DiLavore, P. (2004). Regression and word loss in autistic spectrum disorders. *Journal of Child Psychology and Psychiatry*, 45, 936–955.

Lovaas, O. I., Koegel, R. L., Simmons, J. Q., & Long, J. S. (1973). Some generalization and follow-up measures on autistic children in behaviour therapy. *Journal of Applied Behavior Analysis*, 6, 131–166.

Maharaj, S. (1980). *Pictogram ideogram communication.* Regina, SK: The George Reed Foundation for the Handicapped.

Marshall, J., Goldbart, J. (2007) 'Communication is everything I think.' Parenting a child who needs Augmentative and Alternative Communication (AAC)', *International Journal of Language & Communication Disorders*, 43: 1, 77 -98.

Mayer-Johnson, R. (1981). *The picture communication symbols book.* Solana Beach, CA: Mayer-Johnson Co.

Millar, D. C. (2008). Effects of AAC on the natural development speech development of individuals with autism spectrum disorders. In P. Mirenda & T. Iacono (Eds), *Autism Spectrum Disorders and AAC* (pp. 171-192). Baltimore : Paul H. Brookes Publishing.

Mirenda, P. (2001). Autism, augmentative communication, and assistive technology: What do we really know? *Focus on Autism and Other Developmental Disabilities*, 16, 141–151.

Mirenda, P. (2003). Toward functional augmentative and alternative communication for students with autism: Manual signs, graphic symbols, and voice output communication aids. Language, Speech, and Hearing Services in Schools, 34, 203–216.

Mirenda, P., & Erickson, K. A. (2000). Augmentative communication and literacy. In B. M. Prizant & A. M. Wetherby (Eds.), *Autism spectrum disorders: A transactional developmental perspective* (pp. 369–394). Baltimore, MD: Paul H. Brookes Publishing.

Mundy, P., Sigman, M., & Kasari, C. (1990). A longitudinal study of joint attention and language development in autistic children. *Journal of Speech and Hearing Research*, 38, 157–167.

Olsson, G. (1998). *Kartläggning av förskrivning av datorbaserade hjälpmedel [Survey of prescription of computerized aids*]. Stockholm: Swedish Handicap Institute.

Osterling, J., & Dawson, G. (1994). Early recognition of children with autism: A study of first birthday home videotapes. *Journal of Autism and Developmental Disorders*, 24, 247–258.

Preston, D. & Carter, M. (2009). A Review of the Efficacy of the Picture Exchange Communication System Intervention. *Journal of Autism and Developmental Disorders (2009) 39:1471-1486*

Ramberg, C., Ehlers, S., Nydén, A., Johansson, M., & Gillberg, C. (1996). Language and pragmatic functions in school-age children on the autism spectrum. *European Journal of Disorders of Communication*, 31, 387–413.

Rogers, S. (2006). Evidence-based interventions for language development in young children with autism. In T. Charman & W. Stone (Eds.), *Social and communication development in autism spectrum disorders* (pp. 143–179). New York: The Guildford Press.

Romski, M. A., & Sevcik, R. A. (1996). *Breaking the speech barrier: Language development through augmented means.* Baltimore, MD: Paul H. Brookes Publishing.

Romski, M. A., & Sevcik, R. A., Adamson, L. B., Cheslock, M., Smith, A., Barker, R. M., & Bakeman, R. (2010). Randomized comparison of augmented and nonaugmented language interventions for toddlers with developmental delays and their parents. *Journal of Speech, Language and Hearing Research*, 53, 350-364.

Schepis, M. M., Reid, D. H., Behrmann, M. M., & Sutton, K. A. (1998). Increasing communicative interactions of young children with autism using voice output communication aids and naturalistic teaching. *Journal of Applied Behavior Analysis*, 31, 561–578.

Schlosser, R. W. (2003a). Roles of speech output in augmentative and alternative communication: Narrative review. *Augmentative and Alternative Communication*, 19(1), 5-27.

Schlosser, R. W. (2003b). *The Efficacy of Augmentative and Alternative Communication: Towards Evidence-Based Practice. Baltimore*: Paul Brookes.

Schlosser, R. W., & Blischak, D. M. (2001). Is there a role for speech output in interventions for persons with autism. *Focus on Autism and Other Developmental Disabilities*, 16, 170–176.

Schlosser, R. W., Raghavendra, P. (2004). Evidence-Based Practice in Augmentative and Alternative Communication. *Augmentative and Alternative Communication, 20,* 1-21.

Schopler, E., Reichler, R., & Lansing, M. (1980*). Teaching strategies for parents and professionals.* Austin, TX: PRO-ED Inc.

Seal, B. C., & Bonvillian, J. D. (1997). Sign language and motor functioning in students with autistic disorders. *Journal of Autism and Developmental Disorders*, 27, 437–466.

Shea, V., & Mesibov, G. (2005). Adolescents and adults with autism. In F. Volkmar, R. Paul, A. Klin & D. Cohen (Eds.*), Handbook of autism and pervasive developmental disorders* (pp. 288–311). Hoboken, NJ: John Wiley & Sons.

Short, C., & Schopler, E. (1988). Factors relating to age of onset in autism. Journal of Autism and Developmental Disorders, 18, 207–216.

Sigafoos, J., Didden, R., & O'Reilly, M. (2003). Effects of speech output on maintenance of requesting and frequency of vocalizations in three children with developmental disabilities. *Augmentative and Alternative Communication*, 19, 37–47.

Sigafoos, J., & Drasgow, E. (2001). Conditional use of aided and unaided AAC. *Focus on Autism and Other Developmental Disabilities*, 16, 152–161.

Sigafoos, J., Drasgow, E., Halle, J. W., O'Reilly, M., Seely-York, S., Edrisinha, C., et al. (2004a). Teaching VOCA use as a communicative repair strategy. *Journal of Autism and Developmental Disorders*, 34, 411–422.

Sigafoos, J., Drasgow, E., & Schlosser, R. (2003). Strategies for Beginning Communicators. I Schlosser (Red.), *Efficacy in Augmentative and Alternative communication* (pp. 323-346). Amsterdam: Academic Press.

Sigafoos, J., O'Reilly, M., Ganz, J. B., Lancioni, G. E., & Schlosser, R. W. (2005). Supporting self-determination in AAC interventions by assessing preference for communication devices. *Technology and Disability*, 17, 143–153.

Sigafoos, J., O'Reilly, M., Seely-York, S., & Edrisinha, C. (2004b). Teaching students with developmental disabilities to locate their AAC-device. *Research in Developmental Disabilities*, 25, 371–383.

Sigafoos, J., O'Reilly, M., Seely-York, S., Weru, J., Son, S. H., Green, V. A., et al. (2004c). Transferring AAC intervention to the home. *Disability and Rehabilitation*, 26, 1330–1334.

Sigafoos, J., Green, V., Payne, D., Son, S., O'Reilly, M., & Lancioni, G. E. (2009). A comparison of picture exchange and speech-generating devices : acquisition, preference, and effects on social interaction. *Augmentative and Alternative Communication*, 25, 99-109.

Tager-Flusberg, H., & Anderson, M. (1991). The development of contingent discourse ability in autistic children. *Journal of Child Psychology and Psychiatry*, 32, 1123–1134.

Tager-Flusberg, H., & Joseph, R. M. (2003). Identifying neurocognitive phenotypes in autism. *Philosophical Transactions of the Royal Society of London, Series B: Biological Sciences*, 358, 303–314.

Tager-Flusberg, H., Joseph, R., & Folstein, S. (2001). Current directions in research on autism. *Mental Retardation and Developmental Disabilities Research Reviews*, 7, 21–29.

Tager-Flusberg, H., Paul, R., & Lord, C. (2005). Language and communication in autism. In F. Volkmar, R. Paul, A. Klin & D. Cohen (Eds.), *Handbook of autism and pervasive developmental disorders* (Vol. 1, pp. 335–364). Hoboken, NJ: John Wiley & Sons.

Thunberg, G. (2000). *Konsekvenser av IT-insatser för personer med autism [Consequences of IT-based interventions to individuals with autism]*. Stockholm: Swedish Handicap Institute.

Thunberg, G. (2007). Using speech-generating devices at home. A study of children with autism spectrum disorders at different stages of communication development. *Gothenburg Monographs in Linguistics* 34. Göteborg, Sweden: Göteborg University.

Thunberg, G., Ahlsén, E., & Dahlgren Sandberg, A. (2007) Autistic Spectrum Disorders and Speech-Generating Devices - Communication in Different Activities at Home. *Clinical Linguistics and Phonetics*, 21, 457-479.

Tjus, T., Heimann, M., & Nelson, K. (1998). Gains in literacy through the use of a specially developed multimedia research strategy: Positive findings from 13 children with autism. *Autism: International Journal of Research and Practice*, 2, 139–156.

Volterra, V., Caselli, C., Capirci, O., & Pizzuto, E. (2004). *Gesture and the emergence and development of language.* Rome: Unpublished manuscript.

von Tetzchner, S., & Martinsen, H. (2000). *Introduction to augmentative and alternative communication.* London: Whurr Publishers.

Watson, L. R., Baranek, G. T., Crais, E. R., Reznick, S. J., Dykstra, J., & Perryman, T. (2007). The first year inventory: Retrospective parent responses to a questionnaire designed to identify one-year olds at risk for autism. *Journal of Autism and Developmental Disorders,* 37, 49–61.

Wendt, O. (2008). Research on the use of manual signs and graphic symbols in autism spectrum disorders A systematic review. In P. Mirenda & T. Iacono (Eds), *Autism Spectrum Disorders and AAC* (pp. 83-139). Baltimore : Paul H. Brookes Publishing.

Wendt, O., Schlosser, R. W., & Lloyd, L. (2004). A meta-analysis of AAC intervention outcomes in children with autism. *Paper presented at the 11th biennial conference of the International Society for Augmentative and Alternative Communication,* Natal, Brazil.

Wetherby, A. M. (1986). Ontogeny of communicative functions in autism. *Journal of Autism and Developmental Disorders,* 16, 295–316.

Wetherby, A. M. (2006). Understanding and measuring social communication in children with autism spectrum disorders. In T. Charman & W. Stone (Eds.*), Social and communication development in autism spectrum disorders* (pp. 3–34). New York: The Guildford Press.

Wetherby, A. M., Prizant, B. M., & Schuler, A. L. (2000). Understanding the nature of communication and language impairments. In A. M. Wetherby & B. M. Prizant (Eds.), *Autism spectrum disorders: A transactional developmental perspective* (pp. 109–141). Baltimore, MD: Paul H. Brookes Publishing.

Widgit Software. (2002). *Widgit rebus symbol set.* Retrieved March 2007 from www.widgit.com/products/wws2000/about_symbols/WWS2000Widgit-Rebus.htm.

Woodcock, R., Clark, C., & Davies, S. (1968). *Peabody rebus reading program.* Circle Pines, MN: AGS Publishing.

Yoder, P. J., & Layton, T. L. (1988). Speech following sign language training in autistic children with minimal verbal language. *Journal of Autism and Developmental Disorders,* 18, 217–230.

Yoder, P. & Stone, W. L. (2006). A Randomized Comparison of the Effect of Two Prelinguistic Communication Interventions on the Acquisition of Spoken Communication in Preschoolers With ASD. *Journal of Speech, Language and Hearing Research, August 2006, Vol. 49, pp. 698-771.*

# 18

# Mobile Communication and Learning Applications for Autistic People

Rodríguez-Fórtiz M.J, Fernández-López A and Rodríguez M.L
*ETSIIT. CITIC-UGR. University of Granada.*
*Spain*

## 1. Introduction

People with autism can experience limitations in their intellectual functions, in their interpersonal development, in their adaptive behaviour and thinking, and in the language they use (verbal and non verbal, in both semantic and pragmatic aspects). In order to improve their functioning and achieve wellbeing on an emotional and physiological level, they need forms of support that are centred on the person, and based on an analysis of their particular needs.
Just like anybody else, they should have the opportunity to take part in family life, in school, in a job, and in their community in general. Sources of support and opportunities to participate must be offered as early as possible and must continue for their entire livesand be adapted to match the evolution of the individual. Professionals, families and the rest of society must be involved in the process.
Technologies can help autistic people and their social environment particularly in the sphere of education and communication. Thanks to the personal adaptation and use of specific technology in their daily lives, we are observing that people with autism can be helped to relate better to others, to learn, and to feel better in themselves.
The use of mobile devices also offers the possibility of using applications that help the user to communicate in different environments and places. These devices also allow families, educators and professionals to intervene in the educational process. Their portability also enables users to perform learning activities any time, anywhere. In addition, the connectivity between mobile devices is very useful in performing communication and learning activities in a group setting, helping the integration of the user in their social environment.
We are working on two projects that take advantage of these possibilities. The first is the Sc@ut Project (Rodriguez et al., 2009) (Sc@ut, 2011), for designing adapted communicators, which runs on computers, Pocket PCs and Nintendo DS. The second is Picaa (Fernandez et al, 2009) (Picaa, 2011), a platform for creating adaptable and collaborative didactic activities via the iPhone, iPod touch and iPad devices.
In this paper we present the main characteristics of these devices and our experiences of their use, highlighting the benefits observed amongst the population using them.

## 2. Related works

In the context of interactive environments such as learning and teaching, several tools have been developed, for example:

- VTech (Vtech, 2011) has commercialized multiple products that combine entertaining electronic formats and engaging content that help children learn. However, these products are not targeted at children with special needs.
- JClic (JClick, 2011) is an environment that allows the creation of individual activities, but it only runs on desktop computers.
- Hot Potatoes (Hot Potatoes, 2011), a suite to create interactive multiple-choice, short-answer, jumbled-sentence, crossword, matching/ordering and gap-fill exercises for the World Wide Web.
- In (Schelhowe, 2009) a mobile application is presented, designed for people with special needs who exhibit a mild to severe level of mental disability. It is focused on fostering the learning process directly within the context of use, with a flexible learning speed and a fixed structure. A server is used to feed clients´ mobiles with learning materials that are adapted to the learner profile. A customization and decision engine is used to fulfil this objective. User profiles are provided by the application but they are not configurable. The teacher does not intervene in their creation and they cannot be modified.
- Some learning applications have been developed for the iPhone OS system, such as iWriteWords (iwritewords, 2011). This teaches children handwriting while they play an entertaining game. Meanwhile Proloquo2Go (proloquo, 2011) is a product that provides a communication solution for people who have speaking difficulties. These applications are designed for individual use only and they are not configurable.

None of these systems proposes an adaptive approach that takes into account professional directives in an educational context and user-specific needs, and nor do they provide mobility capabilities together with functionalities for cooperative work.

**In the following sections we present two of our products that are being used by autistic people for communication and learning.**

## 3. Communication - the Sc@ut project

Language is the main medium for communication and information. It is an instrument to structure thinking, and to regulate the personality and social behaviour. Language allows us to express what is inside. Lack of communication can impoverish a person as it can make them come across as unfriendly, provoking anomalous behaviours that affect their social relationships and their life in general.

Augmentative and alternative communication systems (AAC) (Mirenda, 2003) help people with the above mentioned problems to communicate, and enable them to be trained in social abilities. When making interventions relating to language, the use of total communication (Schlesinger, 1986) is a good choice. Total communication includes the use of images (pictograms, photos, or drawings), sounds (words or sentences), written language and gestures during the communication process. All of these media provide alternative forms of support to people with cognitive problems, such as autistic people, because they help the individual communicate with others (Schaeffer et al, 1980).

In the next section we describe Sc@ut, the tool that we have developed to provide AAC, with total communication. Its main advantages over other systems are that it is adaptable to the user at interface and content levels, and that it can run in mobile devices.

### 3.1 Sc@ut - description

Sc@ut consists of two applications: the *communicator* and the *generator* of communicators.
A communicator is an electronic device for supporting augmentative and alternative communication. The Sc@ut *communicator* shows a structure of templates with images, similar to a communication board made with paper. Images can be pictograms, photos or drawings, which represent objects that the user can ask for, actions that can be carried out or things that the user wants to say (feelings or opinions, for instance) (Figure 1). When an image is selected, an associated sound, previously stored, is heard. This sound, which can be a word or a sentence, represents reinforcement for the user and allows people who listen to it to know what the user wants. Moreover, our communicator provides links between templates. Visiting a new template is possible from a previous one, when a specific image is selected in it. This navigation between templates allows the construction of structured sentences, or the classification of actions and elements.

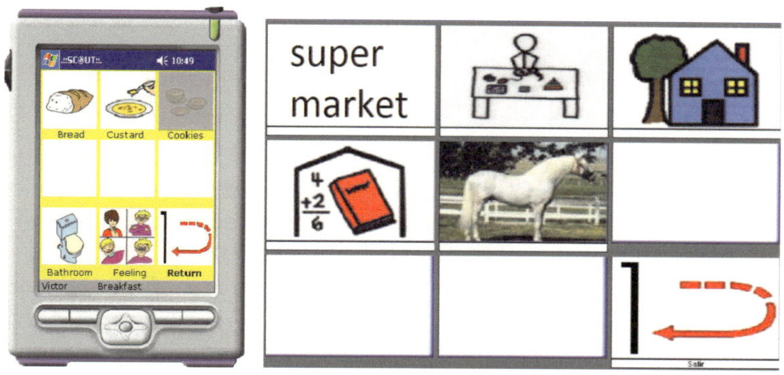


Fig. 1. The Sc@ut Communicator

An animated pictogram can be also shown when an image is selected. We have used this property to support total communication, presenting an animated character that performs a gesture, showing the text and sound associated (Figure 2) . We have drawn 2,200 animated pictograms (aumentativa, 2011) from the gesture language of Benson-Schaeffer. The vocabulary of this language has been designed to be used by people with cognitive impairment as an alternative language with which to communicate.
As Figure 2 shows, Sc@ut provides a version for the NintendoDS portable game console. The arrival of the Nintendo DS game console in the market was presented as an interesting possibility, offering several advantages over other devices:

- Feedback: Two screens (one of them touch) allowing more possibilities of interaction.
- Multimedia: Being a gaming device, it offers tremendous multimedia capabilities (sound, video, graphics).
- Battery life: Approximately 11 hours.
- Robustness: A device intended to be used by children (bumps and scratches on the screen).
- Motivation: Commercial games can also be used in addition, or as a reward for the child.

Thanks to the new possibilities that this offers it is possible to introduce new functionality in the communicator, taking full advantage of Nintendo DS features, such as new concepts based on visual and auditory stimulation, in addition, of course, to its work as a communicator. Being a two-screen device, the top screen can be used to provide feedback. Thus animations can be shown without losing the context of the action, presenting the cause and the effect of the action together. This helps to identify the sound and image with the concept, and therefore promotes learning.

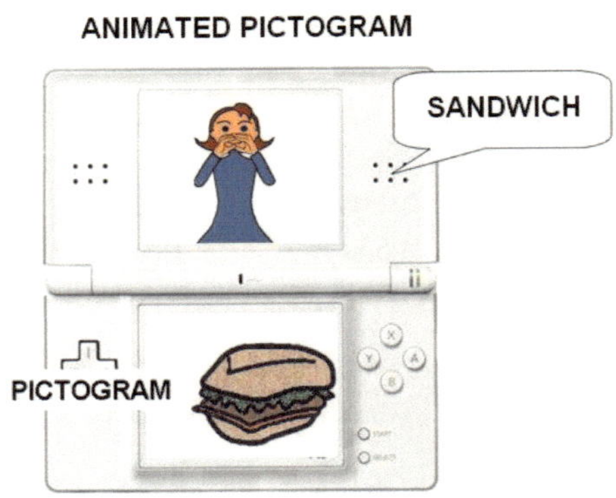


Fig. 2. Total Communication with Sc@ut in Nintendo DS.

The second tool provided by Sc@ut is the *generator*. It is used by educators and families to create and modify communicators, which are adapted to the needs, capabilities, interests, abilities and evolution of users. The generator allows the user profile and the templates for each user to be specified (Figure 3). For example, it offers the possibility of indicating the order in which the images of a template can be selected, and the time during which an image is shown, avoiding the selection of another one. In addition, it allows an agenda and a timetable of actions for each day of the week to be designed, thus helping users to know what can they do and to organize their time.

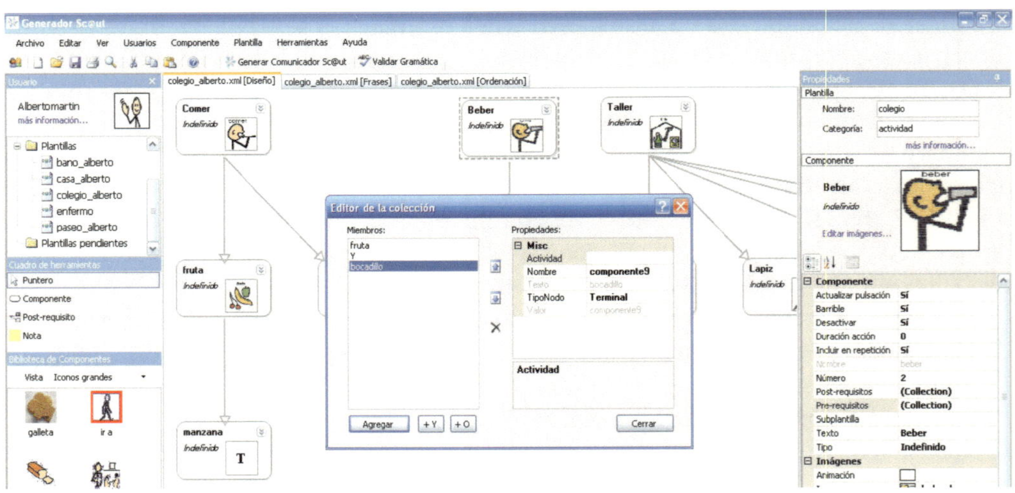


Fig. 3. The Sc@ut generator.

### 3.2 Sc@ut - experience of use

We have been working on this project since 2006. Sc@ut has been used under controlled conditions by approximately 100 handicapped people, mainly with autism, from the South of Spain (Andalusia), at educational centres and schools, but also at occupational units for adults. The duration of the interventions varied from six months to one year, depending on the population and teachers.

The overall objective of our studies had been to show the benefits of using Sc@ut amongst people with severe problems of language and communication and of differing ages, for which we propose the following study hypotheses:

H1: The use of Sc@ut by autistic adults and school-age students improves communication, language development and learning.

H2: Improving communication leads to the reduction of disruptive and challenging behaviour.

H3: Sc@ut supports total communication, helping teachers to adapt and customize the content and structure of the communicators.

In addition, we also propose the following objectives:

- To give support to teachers and families who use these tools at any time.
- To collect user feedback and improve the tool and its usability to make it more flexible and adaptable to the difficulties that people with alternative communication needs may have.
- To promote the University's commitment to society.

The intervention process was performed in the following stages:

1. Definition of hypotheses to be validated in the project.
2. Presentation of the project to address the participating institutions and professionals.
3. Training of professionals involved in the systems of augmentative and alternative communication, the use of ICTs, in particular the Sc@ut program. Providing them information on the process to be followed in the study and the materials to be used.
4. Evaluation and selection of candidate students participating in the intervention. In selecting students we consider their communication needs and their scope for interaction according to their cognitive and motor limitations. Their experience with alternative augmentative communication systems is also taken into account. In addition, we identify the communicative behaviours of users that can be improved with communication support.
5. Implementation – intervention with Sc@ut as a communication system:
   - Performing a pre-test amongst all participants.
   - For each student, choosing the device to use, from among all those available, according to which one will be best suited to his/her needs.
   - Selecting pictograms, photographs, sounds, videos, scenarios and animations of sign language gestures.
   - For each student, designing his/her personal communicator: the user profile for the presentation of content and interaction, templates, and the agenda.
   - Use of the communicator by the student two or three times weekly for approximately forty-five minutes each time. The professionals can make adjustments and modifications to the communicator during the intervention to adapt to the progress and responses from the student.
   - Involving tutors and family to generalize what they learned in other settings.
   - The development team visits the users to interview the professionals and families, and observe the use of programs.
6. Evaluation of results from the pre-test, undertaking the post-test, distributing questionnaires to gather the opinions of the professionals concerned, and video recording in some cases. This allows the validity of the hypotheses to be checked.

7. Modification of software to fix bugs detected and incorporate participants´ suggestions for improvement and feedback from questionnaires and observations made during the visits of the development team for monitoring.
8. Creation of a website providing free download of the software. Dissemination via conferences, training courses and journals.

### 3.3 Sc@ut benefits

All of the autistic people that participated in the study had specific communicative limitations. At best, they only spoke single words, which could only be understood by their parents and close relatives. Not all had this form of expression, making it very difficult to understand them. Some of them used gestures (three or four at most), while others simply looked to the interlocutor in the hope they would guess their needs. Several students presented disruptive behaviour, for instance they appeared to be in despair because they felt misunderstood, and this led them to cry, scream, throw a tantrum and self-harm or, in extreme cases, assault their classmates or adults responsible for their care. They commonly presented a lack of communication, and visible isolation.
We performed the statistical studies in real situations with a degree of quasi-experimental control as we left many variables (staff, facilities, schedules, illnesses, absenteeism, etc.) without control. For the purpose of testing assumptions, we used nonparametric tests, in particular, the Mann-Whitney U test and the Wald-Wolfowitz test. The number of individuals involved in a first study, only for autistic students, was 22. The second study involves 67 students (80% with autism). We used observation questionnaires as the Exam of the existing abilities of communication, the Communication interview and a Scale of evaluation of the communicative pattern in deficient subjects. Observing the values obtained by the tests in the control and experimental groups, in both experiments, we conclude that the degree of significance is high. It implies that intervention is effective, concluding that Sc@ut helps students in several of the aspects suggested by Baumgart (Baumgart, 1990):

- Decreased disruptive behaviours: Some students worked specifically to display communication options to prevent such conduct, and others exhibited less disruptive behaviour simply because of feeling better understood and increased personal satisfaction.
- Improved oral language through auditory and visual reinforcement and systematic work: For those individuals with opportunities to develop oral language, Sc@ut represents a useful speech tool when phrases or words constructed with the communicator are repeated. Some individuals even learn to anticipate particular components, after confirming that the device tells them what they already know. The verbal label associated with the concepts is useful for helping students to read, being a tool of learning and reinforcement.
- Helps solve communication issues: The student can access a wide range of templates to be used in different scenarios to express needs, feelings and ideas. In some individuals, the templates have been used to train in social skills and respond to daily situations.
- Reduced level of anxiety, which affects daily living and learning. In particular, the improved communication calms the user, and their level of anxiety caused by misunderstanding of the social environment is brought down to more acceptable levels.
- Increasing the impulse to communicate: Once they feel confident that they will be understood, some individuals begin to take the lead on communication and participation, which was unthinkable before the intervention.

- Learning and consolidation of gestural vocabulary, increasing the use of gestures for communication: This implies that the student has internalized the gesture as a means of communication, making it independent of any external communication device and promoting spontaneity. We think the use of characters with these signs is more stimulating and encourages users to imitate them. Despite the use of sign language, users must continue with the device to communicate with people who do not understand his/her gestures.
- Improved communication between peers and teachers, thus promoting integration and standardization in their social environment.

We have also proved that Sc@ut helps teachers and family, concluding the following:

- The generator helps the professional to make a personalized intervention, allowing them to adapt templates, the number and size of pictograms, photographs and images and sounds, animations, etc. It also facilitates the modification of the communicators when the student progresses.
- Improved coordination between professionals and family. In many cases, this improvement is thanks to the interest shown by the student, which led to his or her speech therapist communicating with their tutors and parents to share the experience with them.
- The familiarity of the supporting devices, and the low cost and free devices of the computer program have also encouraged some families to use Sc@ut in their homes.
- Professionals from occupational centres and day-stay units are grateful for the initial training that was given in augmentative and alternative communication and the use of ICTs for education. In general, they are specialists in specific fields (such as ceramics, graphic arts, textiles, etc.) but not in AAC.
- With regard to interventions using pictograms with signs, the professionals value their utility in teaching the total communication model to the students.

Table 1 summarises the contributions of Sc@ut.

| Users | Characteristic to be improved | Contribution |
|---|---|---|
| Autistic People | Disruptive behaviours | Decreases |
| | Oral language | Improves |
| | Solve communication issues | Helps |
| | Level of anxiety | Reduces |
| | Impulse to communicate | Increases |
| | Gestures vocabulary | Improves learning and consolidation |
| | Communication between peers and teachers | Improved |
| Education professionals and families | Personalised intervention | Adaptation of learning contents, methodology and evaluation |
| | Devices and software | Low cost or free |
| | Training | Helps professionals use the tools |
| | Coordination between professionals and family | Participation of all, generalized use of AACs |
| | Total communication | Helps in the intervention |

Table 1. Observed benefits of the use of Sc@ut

Sc@ut has been developed for the Linux platform, thanks to a project funded by the Consorcio Fernando de los Ríos, Spain. The usability of the generator tool has also been improved.

## 4. Learning - Picaa

Learning to read, write, make calculations and solve problems is the basis for living an autonomous life and for being integrated both at work and in daily life.

Education of people with cognitive impairments, including those with autism, must begin as early as possible. People with autism require ongoing intervention that has to be systematic and based on personal motivation. The person has to work on each task in accordance with their skills, bearing in mind that their personal work rhythm and learning style may differ from those of others. Therefore, individualization of the learning process is necessary. However, at the same time, the students must learn to interact with others. Cooperative learning in a classroom setting prepares them to perform daily activities and to integrate in their social environment.

Cooperative learning (Johnson et al, 2000) is a pedagogical method that applies some of the ideas from social constructivism, a psycho-pedagogical paradigm based on the theories of Vigotsky and Piaget. Cooperative learning requires students to work together on a common task. It promotes the personal growth processes, developing the potential of each individual to learn by himself or with others in different situations. Therefore, it is very useful for students with cognitive impairments. The teacher intervenes to create activities and to assign group learning tasks, manages time and resources, and monitors whether the students and groups are working well (Smith, 1996). The main contributions that the cooperative relationship can offer the students with autism are (Barkley, 2005): teachers and classmates can act as role models to imitate; opportunities to do, to say and to feel; team and personal auto-regulation; observing different perspectives from a same subject; constant positive reinforcement; and development of cognitive, social and affective abilities.

The use of technology allows the learning content and user interaction to be adapted, helping the teachers to design personalized learning activities that can be carried out in a group setting. The tactile interaction on mobile devices, which includes learning activities with multimedia content, stimulates the students, gains their attention and reinforces their learning. Picaa, a learning mobile platform for teachers and students which provides an adaptive and cooperative learning tool, works to this particular objective.

### 4.1 Picaa - description

Picaa integrates, in a single application running on a mobile device, features that allows children and educators to interact with different elements, according to the actions they will carry out and the educational approach.

Its main objective is to facilitate the user's curricular adaptation by the educator. Learning activities and content must be sufficiently flexible to adapt to the characteristics of each user and integrate the personal data of their inner world, respecting their own particular work rhythm. Activities must be also modified by educators according to user progress or changes in his or her environment. The content, structure and user interface of the applications can be adapted depending on such requirements in order to achieve accessible applications. This is very useful because there are many differences between the interests and learning needs of autistic children, therefore the personalization of learning activities is essential in class.

The Picaa platform allows four kinds of activities to be defined that cover the basic learning tasks. The kinds of activities designed are:

- Exploration: sequencing of screens to navigate across a hypermedia system. This allows simple communicators, agendas or stories to be created. Images, sounds and animations are presented. (Figure 4).
- Association: assignation of elements to sets. This provides a basis for memory exercises, calculation, discrimination and categorization. (Figure 5.a).
- Puzzle: includes pieces with different shapes and numbers. (Figure 5.b).
- Sort: consists of items that the student must put in the correct sequence. This activity can be performed with graphics or text. (Figure 5.c).

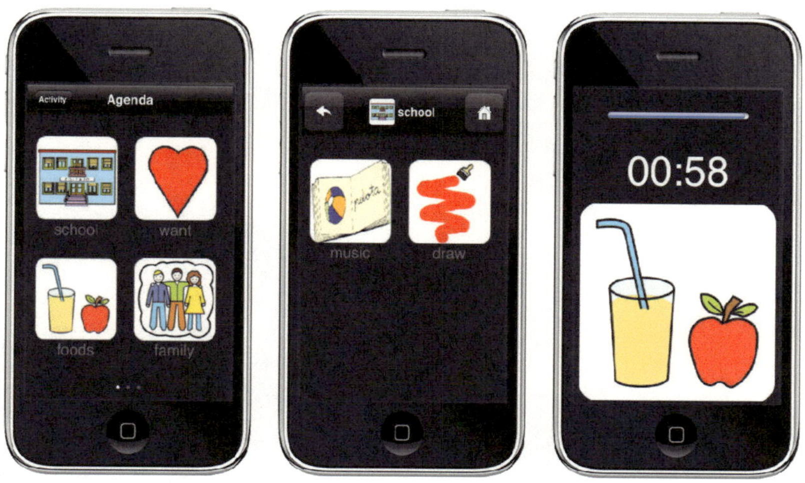


Fig. 4. Exploration activity in iPod touch.

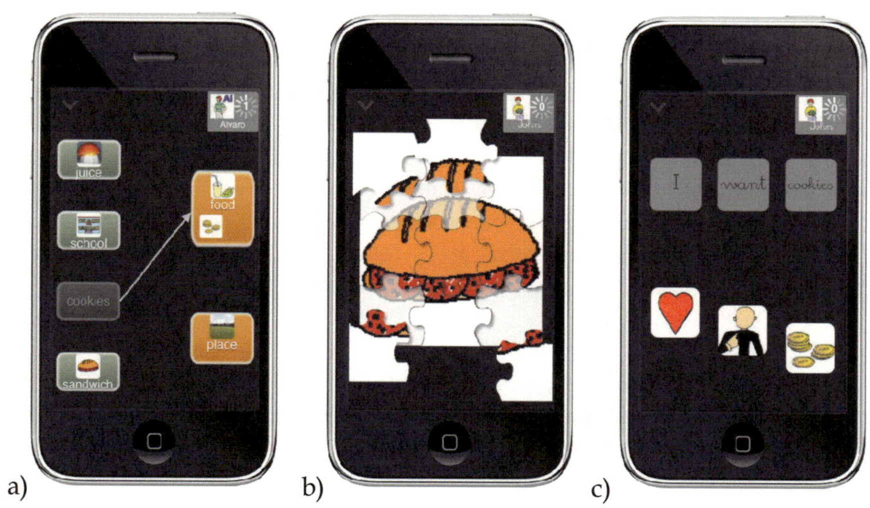


Fig. 5. a)Association, b)Puzzle and c)Sort activities.

These activities are aimed at developing the following skills and abilities:

- Perception and visual and auditory discrimination.
- Acquisition and expansion of vocabulary and understanding of meaning.
- Development of memory.
- Improvement of phonetics, syntax and pragmatics of language.
- Working hand-eye coordination (fine motor).
- Examining assumptions, conclusions and interpretations.
- Learning cause and effect.
- Generalization of concepts.
- Coordination.
- Managing notions of space/time.
- Development of attitudes such as responsibility, cooperation and collaboration.
- Development of skills for handling numbers and their applications.
- Learning strategies for soling simple problems.

The application is available for three types of devices: the iPhone smartphone, the iPod touch device and the iPad tablet (Figure 6).

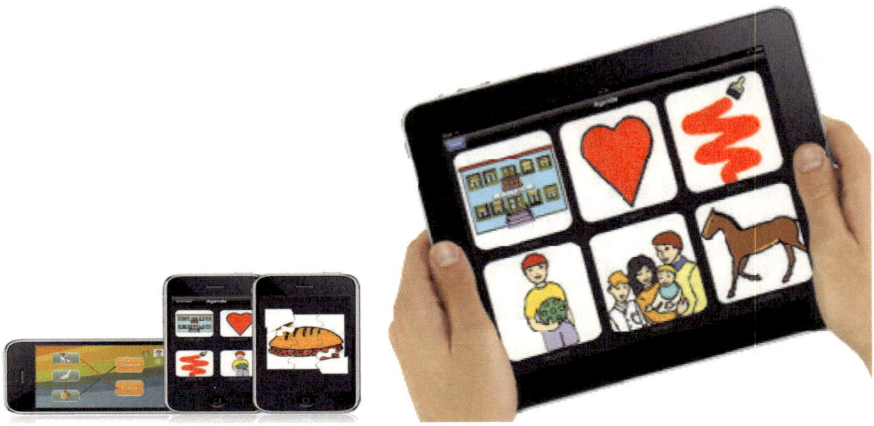

Fig. 6. iPod touch device and iPad tablet running *Picaa* activities.

Picaa, as with Sc@ut, differentiates between two kinds of use. As we have seen, the students can perform activities, but, the educators can also use it to define user profiles, design the activities and plan a daily agenda (Figure 7). The educator can configure aspects of the activities relative to their content and presentation, for instance: number of components or concepts to be taught, screen composition, screen position (rotation or not), multimedia used to represent the components, difficulty level (goals of the exercise, working out the punctuation), reinforcements and help to the users. Figure 7 shows how to design one of the exercises and the personal agenda.

Additionally, the educator can configure some of the rules to be considered when working in a group context. For instance, the order to be followed when selecting components and the information that the users can see about the interaction performed by other users when they work in a group (number of participants, orderly turns, punctuation, etc.).

### 4.2 Picaa - experience of use

We began to develop Picaa in 2009. It is available for free, in both English and Spanish, at the online store App Store where it has been downloaded by over 4,000 users worldwide.

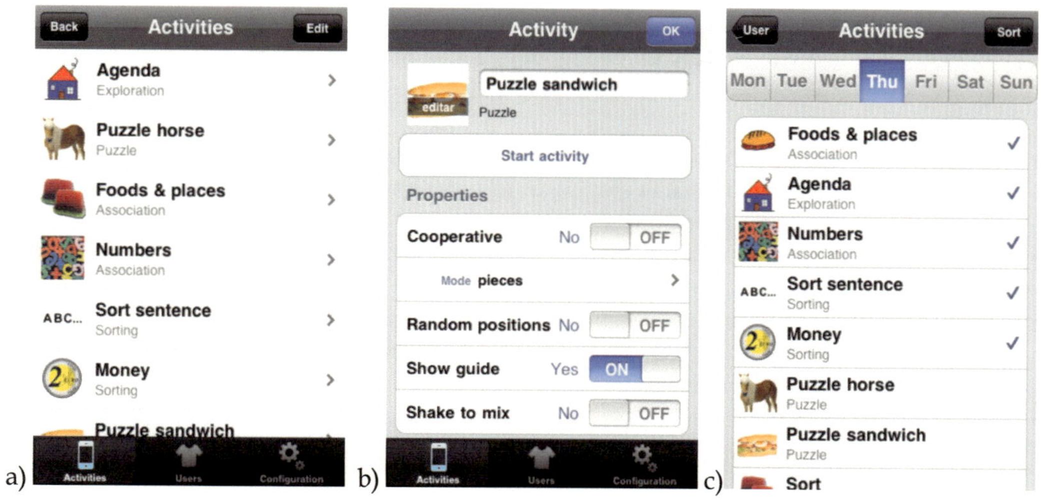


Fig. 7. Picaa for the Educator: a)list of activities, b)activity design and c)agenda.

To include the educators and students in the development and validation process, we performed a pilot project during a school term. The overall objective of Picaa was to serve as a support tool for people with learning disabilities and poor communication, for which we propose the following hypotheses:

- H1. The use of Picaa in school improves communication, and facilitates learning and the development of language.
- H2. The integration of the tool on a completely mobile platform system favours adaptation by professionals, families and students.

Some 13 autistic children with ages ranging from 4 to 12 and their teachers participated in the pilot project at several schools from the Andalusia and Murcia regions of Spain. Picaa was mainly used for the following purposes:

- Communicative use of exploration activities, as an AAC tool.
- Planning and anticipating circumstances through images based on what is going to happen.
- Teaching specific topics from curricular areas by designing specific activities.
- Working on reading and language comprehension.
- Agenda.
- Bits of Intelligence.

The intervention process was performed following the same stages as applied in the Sc@ut pilot.

### 4.3 Picaa benefits

The participation of students and educators in the development process has been very useful because the resulting feedback and suggestions have allowed improvements to be made to the user interface, the tool to be more accessible and usable, and the functionality of the program to be more complete and versatile. Table 2 summarizes the main benefits.

The initial evaluation of teachers is very positive and highlights benefits both for themselves and for their students. We now summarize the main views expressed in the questionnaires that have permitted us to validate the initial hypotheses:

- They consider the tool to be simple and easy to use, highlighting the key advantage as being the capacity to both work on the device and make changes more quickly. Thanks to its design and tactile interaction it is intuitive even for people with little knowledge of IT.
- The multimedia resources used in activities are integrated into the device itself. Using them is easy because the use of electronic resources means that no scissors, glue, paper, photocopying, recording, etc are required, and that the tool can be reused.
- Students have the opportunity of performing activities that were not previously accessible to them, because both the interface and the content can be adapted.
- The students can perform the tasks anywhere, thanks to the mobility of the system. This allows their families to intervene in the educative process and facilitates their communication with the school environment.
- The use of electronic devices with multimedia content becomes more stimulating and attractive to students than traditional resources and in some cases may even be the only alternative for students with sensory limitations.

| Users | Characteristic to be improved | Contribution |
|---|---|---|
| Autistic People | Disruptive behaviours | Decreases |
| | Learning content | Adapted content, multimedia and learning activities more stimulating and attractive for students |
| | Communication between peers and with teachers | Improved |
| Education professionals and families | Personalized intervention | Adaptation of learning content, methodology and evaluation |
| | Devices and software | Low cost or free. Design-use-modifications in the same device. |
| | Training | Not necessary for all, ease of use |
| | Coordination between professionals and family | Participation of all, can be used in any location |
| | Total communication | Helps in the intervention |

Table 2. Observed Benefits of the use of Picaa

## 5. Conclusion

Mobile devices can be used to provide customized and integrated support for people with autism. We have designed two applications: Sc@ut for AAC and Picaa for Learning. Both of these can be configured by educators to enable users to follow their own work rhythm, and also integrate with peers, educators and family.

The transfer of our experiences of these applications is easy considering that the software is free and available via the Internet. The devices are inexpensive, readily available and in many cases already present in homes and schools. Our recommendations for transfer are to follow a systematic approach to intervention and to promote widespread use by education professionals and families.

Regarding to the creation of software for people with special needs, we recommend a user-centred design, based on the participation of end users in the specification, design and evaluation of prototypes. In this sense, pilot studies are essential to validate the benefits, detect errors and draw on new suggestions from users to improve the programs and deliver quality products.
As a working group, our assessment is positive and also highlighted the importance of the involvement of the University in applied projects, which may benefit disadvantaged sectors of society.

## 6. Acknowledgment

This research is funded by the Spanish Government's Ministry of Science and Innovation, via the projects TIN2008-05995/TSI.
The pictograms of the examples have been granted by the Divertic Association (http://www.divertic.org) and CATEDU (http://catedu.es/arasaac/) under Creative Commons license.

## 7. References

Aumentativa. Animated Pictograms with gestures from Benson-Schaeffer. http://www.aumentativa.net/signos.php

Barkley, E. F., Cross, K.P. & Major C.H. (2005). *Collaborative Learning Techniques*. John Wiley, San Francisco

Clic Zone: Resources and information about Clic. http://clic.xtec.cat/es/index.htm

Click. http://clic.xtec.cat/en/index.htm

Fernández, A., Rodríguez-Fórtiz, M. J. & Noguera, M. (2009). Designing and Supporting Cooperative and Ubiquitous Learning Systems for People with Special Needs. OTM 2009 Workshops. *Lecture Notes in Computer Science* 5872, pp:423-432, Springer, Berlin

Hot Potatoes suite. http://hotpot.uvic.ca/

iWriteWords handwriting game. http://www.ptgdi.com/gdiplus/iWriteWords/

Johnson, D.W. & Johnson, R.T. (2000). Stanne. M.B.: Cooperative Learning Methods: a Meta-analysis. Available from: http://www.clcrc.com/pages/cl-methods.html

Mirenda, P. (2003). Toward functional augmentative and alternative communication for students with autism: manual signs, graphic symbols, and voice output communication aids. *Language Speech and Hearing Services in Schools, 34*, 203-216.

Picaa platform. http://scaut.ugr.es/picaa

Proloquo2go communication system. http://www.proloquo2go.com/

Rodríguez-Fórtiz, M. J., González, J. L., Fernández, A., Entrena, M., Hornos, M. J., Pérez, A., Carrillo, A. & Barragán, L. (2009). "Sc@ut: Developing Adapted Communicators for Special Education". *Procedia - Social and Behavioral Sciences*, 1 (1), pp. 1348-1352. Elsevier.

Schaeffer, B., Musil,A. & Y Kollinzas, G. (1980). *Total communication. A signed speech program for nonverbal children*, Illinois, Research Press.

Schelhowe, H & Zare, S. (2009). *Intelligent Mobile Interactions: A Learning System for Mentally Disabled People (IMLIS)*. In C. Stephanidis Ed. Universal Access in HCI. Part 1. Lecture Notes in Computer Science 5614. pp: 412-421. Springer Verlag.

Schlesinger, H. (1986). *Total communication in perspective.* In D.M. Luterman (Ed.), Deafness in Perspective .pp. 87–116. College-Hill Press: San Diego, CA.

Sc@ut Project. http://scaut.ugr.es

Smith, K.A. (1996) *Cooperative Learning: Making "Group Work" Work. New Directions for Teaching and Learning*. Jossey-Bass, San Francisco

V-Tech. http://www.vtech.com/

# 19

# Autism and the Built Environment

Pilar Arnaiz Sánchez[1], Francisco Segado Vázquez[2]
and Laureano Albaladejo Serrano[2]
[1]*Universidad de Murcia*
[2]*Universidad Politécnica de Cartagena*
*Spain*

## 1. Introduction

Heidegger (2001) ended his essay entitled "Building, dwelling, thinking", with an exhortation to *"build out of dwelling, and think for the sake of dwelling"*. Many definitions have been given for Architecture throughout history, but it is (or at least it should be) clear that its centre, its aim, its main objective, is the act of dwelling. This is the reason why Norberg-Schultz (1980) affirms that, in order to research and better know architectonic space, it is necessary to understand what he names *"existential space"*, i.e., that concept of space that permits an individual to construct a stable image of what is around him, and, at the same time, makes him belong to a society and a culture.

The need of a space that can be lived, inhabited, or dwelled in underlies an architect's work (even if it is consciously or not) in order for a building to become true architecture. It's this existential experience of space that grants it the sense of place and not of a mere abstraction. As Montaner i Martorell (2002) has stated, *"Space has an ideal, theoretical, generic and undefined condition, while place has a concrete, empirical, existential, articulated character, defined down to its details"*.

The perception, the understanding, and, thus, the appropriation[1] each person makes of the environment around him is different. However, there is a number of factors (for instance biological, social, cultural, psychological ones, among others) which are common to the vast majority of inhabitants –*users*, if we wanted to use a colder word– that allow us to assert that, even within this diversity, the built environment will be apprehended, used and dwelled in in a certain way, or, in the worst case, with slight deviations from the way it has been planned to be.

Also, it is well known that, since a few decades ago, architecture practice is carried out having in mind that there are individuals with different types and degrees of disabilities (mainly visual, hearing and motoric impairments), and architects plan and design (whether convinced –this is the most common situation– or just impelled by regulations) spaces so that these can be also inhabited by those people. We speak then about *accessibility*, but, in fact, this word has come to convey a mostly physical concept: *accessibility* is, therefore, a way to grant people with disabilities physical access to building or spaces, what, ultimately, allows them to inhabit those spaces.

---

[1] In the very etymological sense of the word: the action of making something one's own

There are, however, many other impairments or disabilities that are not so "visible", and that are, usually, ignored in this task of making the environment accessible. In this sense, Smith (2009) states that, in the design process of buildings (or streets, cities and interiors) almost exclusively two paradigms come into play: that of the client and that of the architect. That is, it is these two agents' vision of reality, of how things –spaces, communications, spatial connections, ...– work and are perceived, what actually shapes the built environment around us. What is more, this is usually accomplished with the assumption that this environment is just a container or a mere scenario in which certain activities or functions are carried out, forgetting the active role it can –and does– play.

On the contrary, for people with particular cognitive or sensory impairments –which are *"less visible"* as Smith puts it–, among which individuals with autism can be found, this assumption about how spaces will be perceived and dwelled in is far from correct: due to their impairments, they are forced to make an effort, enormous at times, to get to grasp and understand the environment around them. When that struggle takes place, because of their difficulty in processing the information they receive through their senses, a number of elements –music too loud in a supermarket or mall, or just the accumulation of placards, symbols or neon signs, to cite two examples– can become a barrier, somehow *jamming* the understanding of the environment, and, in turn, originate frustration and strange behaviour (gestures, verbal utterances, weird movements...). Smith points out that, in the eyes of a casual observer being at that precise time in that precise space, the whole situation would be perceived simply as an inappropriate behaviour in a given situation, while, actually, it has been the imbalance between the environment and an individual's ability to adapt to it, to apprehend it, what has triggered the seemingly bad behaviour.

So the surroundings, the built environment, has to be considered an important factor that greatly influences –directly and indirectly– individuals with *"less visible"* impairments. As architect John Jenkins states, in reference to the design of educational spaces for children with autism –though we consider his affirmation can be applied to individuals of any age and to any type of building–, says:

> "Mainstream children are probably more 'able to cope' with badly designed spaces than an autistic child would be. So the responsibility to create a 'good' environment is brought into sharp relief" (as cited in Scott, 2009, p. 41).

If, in a broad sense, constant reflection on the relationship between the individual and the space around him, between an individual and his (built) environment, is important for the architectural discipline, the particularization of this reflection in the inhabitant with autism can become a significative contribution not only to the architectural field itself –since Architecture, like other Arts and disciplines such as Philosophy, grows when it's rethought–, but also to the understanding of the way people with autism confront spaces and environments, and, what is more important, to the achievement of a greater well-being for them, as well as to the social consideration of their needs and the difficulties they find in their daily life.

## 2. Autism

Although it is probably not necessary for the reader of this chapter to be given a definition or description of autism, we believe it is important here to recall some key concepts and highlight some points that are relevant to the process of designing spaces for people with autism. Also, this will allow us to explicitly declare what we will understand for *autism* when referring to spaces designed for autism or simply designed with individuals with autism in mind [2]. It is well known that the definitions of the autistic disorder, its etiologic accounts, the nosologic considerations, and even, of course, the *treatments*, have been suffering modifications along time, obviously in tune with progress made on research being done on autism from such different –if complementary– fields as Medicine, Psychology, Psychiatry, Pedagogy or even Philosophy. But, again, it is important to know what characteristics are –or can be– present in individuals with autism so that we can determine what attributes must a built environment have to facilitate its apprehension by them. This will, also, lead to achieve other goals, which lay beyond –but in many ways depend on– the architectural discipline itself, such as aiding the learning process, promoting autonomy, facilitating socialization, ensuring independence or even, from a wider point of view, preserving the dignity of individuals with autism.

### 2.1 General concept

Without any doubt, autism is one of the most fascinating disorders Medicine and Psychology have confronted. In Riviere's words,

> "is autistic that person to whom other people become opaque and unpredictable, that person who lives like absent –mentally absent– towards people present, and whose conduct these latter feel incompetent to rule by means of communication". (as cited in Escobar Solano, Caravaca Cantabella, Herrero Navarro & Verdejo Bolonio, 2008)

This isolation or loneliness is one of the most enigmatic characteristics of autism. In fact, when Austrian-born American psychiatrist Kanner (1943) first describes the autistic disorder, he considers that its pathognomonic sign is the inability to communicate with other people, what leads to an *"extreme autistic aloneness"*. In this very first description, Kanner specifies a number of aspects common to the children he has studied, which we can briefly enumerate as follows:

1. Inability to relate to other people, at least in an ordinary way
2. Extreme autistic aloneness, that seemingly isolates the child from the outer world
3. Apparent resistance to being embraced or lifted
4. Impairments in language, which can include mutism, pronoun reversal, echolalia or idiosyncratic utterances, among others
5. In some cases, an excellent rote memory
6. Preference for certain specific foods, since early age
7. Fear of intense noises
8. Obsessive desire for repetition and insistence on sameness
9. Limited variety of spontaneous activities (like normal play)
10. Strange motoric stereotypies, as spinning or balancing
11. Normal physical appearance
12. Onset during the first three years of life

[2] We discuss further on in this chapter the differences between designing buildings and spaces which are specific for people with autism and others that, not being specific, are to be used by them and, thus, must be thought and planned bearing in mind their needs.

Several months later, in 1944, Austrian Hans Asperger, without previous knowledge of Kanner's work, published an article entitled "'Autistic psychopathy' in childhood" (see Asperger, 1991), where he studied the cases of several children whose main disorder was the limitation of their social relationships. According to Escobar Solano et al. (2008), and even thought the contrary has been affirmed, the cases described by Asperger correspond to the same symptoms as those depicted by Kanner, although the former covered a wider condition range, from severe neurological damage to children with almost normal development.

### 2.2 Brief history of the concept of autism

Along the years after the appearance of Kanner's and Asperger's article, and due to the spread of psychoanalytical theories, and even though Kanner himself pointed to a probable biological origin, it was considered that a psychodynamic etiology was in the root of the autistic disorder, i.e., that it was elicited by emotional causes. This lead to blame progenitors and to speak about cold mothers or uncaring fathers. Within this line of thought, assertions were made such as that the cause of autism was the desire of the parents that the child did not exist (Bettelheim, 2001). The psychoanalytical therapies that were used aimed at restoring emotional wounds and rebuilding supposedly broken affections. This type of psychodynamic treatment, in many current researchers' opinion, has not contributed too much[3](see, for instance, Escobar Solano et al., 2008; Wing, 1968).

From the mid 1960s and until, approximately, the middle of the 1980s, autism started to be considered due to a neurological origin, and thus conceptualized as a cognitive "disarrangement", instead of an affective one (Escobar Solano et al., 2008). Autism began to be researched in a further methodical and rigorous way, so as to try to understand its communication and language alteration, as well as associated social relationship impairments, resistance to change, etc. (for instance, Rutter & Schopler, 1984; Wing & Gould, 1979).

Since that stage, and thanks to those advances in research, autism has come to be considered as a development disorder. Hence, it is included among the Pervasive Developmental Disorders (PDDs), which, aside from autistic disorder[4], comprises others such as Asperger syndrome, Rett syndrome, childhood disintegrative disorder and PPD-not otherwise specified (or PDD-NOS). More recently it has been realized that it is often hard to set clear boundaries among these disorders, but, in fact, there is a continuum within which three main areas are –in some degree– affected. These three are communication –verbal and non-verbal, as impairments are not constrained to heard and spoken language–, social reciprocity and imagination [5]. That is the reason why the expression Autistic Spectrum Disorders (ASD) became the usual name of what we know, generally speaking, as autism. In fact, as it is well known, future fifth edition of *Diagnostic and Statistical Manual of Mental Disorders* (DSM-5) by American Psychiatric Association (APA), expected by next year (2013), contemplates this naming [6].

---

[3] Aside from the distress and suffering this kind of assertions may have put on parents, the current literature renders these therapies –advocated, for instance, by Bettelheim (2001) or Tustin (1996)– obsolete and superceded by more recent research and praxis.

[4] Which would correspond to Kanner's or *classic* autism.

[5] The term *'imagination'* here must be understood in its widest sense: the ability to mentally view or think of things that are not really present at a given moment –or even that don't exist at all. The impairment in imagination entails, for instance, the lack of symbolic play, imaginative behaviours, and the existence of repetitive interests and activities.

[6] See http://www.dsm5.org/ProposedRevisions/Pages/proposedrevision.aspx?rid=94.

### 2.3 Current accounts

Since Kanner's publication, many theories have tried to account for the behaviour and development observed in people with autism. The aim is not only to find a clear etiology (whether it considers one only cause or combination of different factors, or a range of different causes that lead to the same cerebral injuries, and, therefore, the same symptoms), but also to try to explain the cognitive, emotional or sensory processes carried out by individuals with autism. We will summarize now three of these theories that can be considered to be the most influencing ones in recent times.

#### 2.3.1 Theory of mind

Postulated by Baron-Cohen, Leslie & Frith (1985), this account considers that people with autism lack a "Theory of Mind", i.e., that they are incapable of assigning mental states (emotions, thoughts, etc.) to other people. The well-known Sally-Anne experiment showed that a majority of children with autism failed the test due to their inability to understand that Sally has a particular state of mind (she is unaware of the fact that Anne has moved the marble) which is independent of that of the own child's one. On the contrary, children in the control groups (one of them made of of *normal* children and a second one comprising children with Down syndrome, with mental ages that were even inferior to those of the autistic group), passed the test with no great difficulty.
This absence of a Theory of Mind (or *blindness* to other people's mental states) would explain, to a great extent, social impairments observed in people with ASD: social world seems chaotic to them, verbal messages are interpreted in a literal manner, and they do not find it easy to participate in a normal social interaction, since, while it is taking place, it is crucial that each agent or interlocutor be able to understand the fact that the other has a concrete state of mind (he knows something, is thinking about something, feels in a particular way, etc.). It would also account for the usual observation that the child with autism treats people "like objects", since he is not able to recognize a mind in them. It could also mean a lack of self-consciousness (Frith & Happe, 1999).

#### 2.3.2 Theory of central coherence

According to Frith (2006), people with autism would present an impairment of the cerebral mechanism that confers coherence to the wide range of stimuli we receive. Central coherence would allow us, in usual conditions, to assign a meaning to a given stimulus, by means of extracting information from its context. As people with autism would lack this ability to integrate information coming from outside –and even that which is stored, taken from past experiences–, they will not apprehend its meaning or, if they come to grasp it, this meaning will not be readjusted when in new contexts. Consequently, this theory would also explain the ability, at times amazing, that some individuals with autism have to focus on details, whereas they remain unable to integrate the different parts in a meaningful whole [7]. "Weak" central coherence, as Frith names it, would also account for issues as literal understanding of verbal messages –since they are interpreted out of their context–, something that, in turn, occasionally prevents them from discerning irony, metaphorical senses or mere jokes.

[7] Bogdashina (2005) talks about *gestalt* perception, meaning the act of grasping all the details in a single –sensory– image. The term *gestalt*, then, tries to refer to a holistic perception, but not, as it may seem, to the integration of all the details in a whole.

### 2.3.3 Theory of executive functions

Executive functions are certain mental and cognitive processes such as attention, concentration, planning, etc., used to achieve an objective that has been previously chosen. According to this theory, people with autism lack control –or at least enough control– over these executive functions, an impairment that would limit their ability to carry out things like task switching or focusing their attention on different things –on a given stimulus or on another one, at will–, in order to complete a planned goal. Therefore, this impairment would also be the origin of stereotypied and repetitive behaviours, which would not be correctly governed by an *executive or supervisory* system (Frith, 2006, p. 31).

## 3. Design criteria: literature review

In this section we will expound –and at times discuss– a number of design criteria, extracted from the scarce existent literature on this matter, that can be applied to the built environment in order to facilitate its apprehension –and appropiation– by people with ASD.

One of the first publications regarding this matter –which should be considered a pioneering work– is that of Richer & Nicoll (1971). Through a combination of a careful design of a playroom space and its fixtures and some guidelines for the caring staff, the authors aimed to achieve two main goals:

1. Reduction of frustration and arousal.
   - By subdividing space in smaller areas, overstimulation and an excessive number of social interactions are avoided. Also, the design provided a *retreat box* in which the child could calm down.
   - Space for activities such as climbing, rolling, sliding, etc. was provided. When children are involved in this kind of games, they are less likely to become overaroused, and this, in turn, facilitates social interactions.
   - Stereotypies were not stopped by any means. On the contrary, toys which could easily be played with in repetitive movements were included in the playroom.
2. Reduction of *flight behaviours*, i.e., all those actions a child with autism carries out to avoid social interactions (moving away, retreating, looking away, etc.), and, simultaneously, facilitation of approaches.
   - Structures and fixtures were robust and firmly anchored, so that there was no need to interrupt the children's games with safety warnings or instructions.
   - Areas were provided in which the children could demand two types of social interaction: a close tactile contact, and a *rough and tumble* play.
   - In some areas, as in what they called the *activity house*, physical boundaries somehow *force* social interaction, but these will be rewarding, since they are framed in a rewarding activity.

It is important to recall that this was not a design-only intervention, but also some guidelines were given to staff about how the playroom was to be used, and what their attitudes should be. The main concern was to avoid approaching the children as much as possible, unless it was the children themselves who were demanding these approaches. Even looking at the children was considered a form of approaching them, unless they seemed motivated enough to begin an interaction. As a result of this intervention on the physical environment, as well as the application of these guidelines, the children with autism developed an increased number of social interactions, and, at the same time, were less involved in their stereotypies.

Let us highligh some of the design criteria used by Richer & Nicoll (1971), some of which we find in other authors, too, later in this chapter:

- Subdivision of spaces, cutting off one from another, in a certain way. Mostafa (2008) also carries out a *spatial sequence compartmentalization* in her intervention in a classroom space.
- Safety and robustness of elements, furniture, or fixtures.
- Minimize intrusion of carers as much as possible, leaving the children free to play, jump, slide, roll, interact, how and when they feel the need to.
- Inclusion of a *retreat box.*
- Use of elements and materials that are durable (although the authors themselves comment on two failures in their design: the PVC cover of some foam rubber objects turned out to be not bite-proof, and a water fountain was installed incorrectly, what led to floods, and ultimately, had to be removed).
- Controlled sensory stimulation in the different subspaces, ranging from no-stimulus (retreat box) to highly stimulating areas such as the activity house or the so-called *stimulus wall.*
- Use of light dimmers, to allow staff to create different atmospheres when needed.

Khare & Mullick (2008; 2009) have been carrying out a research by means of which they aim to obtain a series of conclusions that can be applied to so-called *Universal Design*, particularly in educational spaces. It is important to recall here what this expression refers to: Universal Design (sometimes abbreviated UD) is a paradigm –not exclusively architectural, but indeed applicable to this discipline– which aims at designing objects –buildings, interiors and urban spaces, etc., in our case– in such a way that they can be used by the largest possible number of people, regardless of their particular conditions.
This study by Khare & Mullick has been divided in six phases, summarized below:

1. Establishing users' needs
2. Laying down environment considerations for autism
3. Definition of design parameters
4. Assessment of the selected design paramenters
5. Preparation of design criteria or recommendations
6. Selection of principles applicable to Universal Design

It is remarkable that this research process and methodology have been designed so that the design suggestions can be assessed later, and, thus, their validity can be verified. Even though the conclusions have not been published yet, we believe it is important to highlight the design parameters –we would better say they are objectives to be accomplished by means of, or with the help of, design– the authors choose –and later assess– as the most beneficial to children with ASD (Khare & Mullick, 2008):

1. Physical structure: organize environment with clear visual and physical boundaries. These will help to create a definite context for each activity in association with a given space.
2. Maximize visual structure: organize visual environment by means of concrete visual cues. This would comprise aspects as colour coding, numbers, signs, labels, etc.

3. Provide visual instructions: indicate the sequence of steps to be followed when performing certain activities –in the spaces where these are carried out– by means of not only written guidance, but also images, pictures, visual schedules, etc.
4. Opportunities for community participation: pupils should be involved in everyday social activities.
5. Opportunities for parent participation: involve parents in school activities, thus aiding to address pupils' educational needs.
6. Opportunities for inclusion: provide an environment for children with autism that allows them to interact with their peers.
7. Maximize future independence: create an environment in which the child can learn everyday life skills, as well as vocational ones, that allow them to be independent in the future.
8. Generous spatial standards: these will help children with autism to face social demands, since they are rather wary about their personal space (see note 11 on page10).
9. Provision of withdrawal spaces[8]: quiet areas in which pupils with autism can retire to avoid or mitigate the stress they can feel in certain moments, when they are in spaces where socially demanding situations may occur.
10. Maximize safety: minimize risks derived from pupils' own conditions, including, in many cases, the misperception of dangers.
11. Maximize comprehension: clear arrangement of spaces, direct routes between them, neat zoning, use of simple forms, and uncluttered interiors help children with autism to perceive –and to apprehend– their school environment.
12. Maximize accessibility[9]: impairments in movement coordination and balance, epilepsy, restricted attention span, and other difficulties demand that the building be physically accessible.
13. Provide assistance: there should be space enough to help a pupil with autism in doing their learning activities, or in the toilet or the dining room, etc.
14. Maximize durability and minimize maintenance costs: equipment, furnishing, fixtures, fittings, and materials and systems in general should be durable –especially taking into account possible aggressions and misuse by pupils– and require little and inexpensive maintenance.
15. Minimize sensory distractions: environments should not present elements that can become visual, auditive, tactile, etc., distractions –other than the ones specifically and strategically set out for this precise objective –as stated in next point.
16. Facilitate sensory integration[10]: include multisensory stimuli within the environment, providing opportunities to roll, jump, spin, as well as vibrations, music, visual experiences, etc.
17. Provide flexibility: environment has to be flexible enough to accommodate a wide range of functional skills and different teaching paradigms.

[8] Mostafa (2008) talks about *haven* spaces.
[9] In this case restrictedly understood as easy *physical* access (see above, page 1)
[10] Davis & Dubie (2004), for instance, also face sensory integration

18. Allow monitoring for assessment and planning: it is necessary to control or monitor pupils with the lesser degree of distraction and intrusion, in order to assess them, grant their safety and plan activities, teaching strategies, etc.

It could be argued that some of the criteria enumerated above –if not most of them– may not seem specific to pupils with autism. And it would be true to a certain degree, but the fact it is that in that particular case, those parameters become not only adequate –as they would surely be be when talking about individuals without ASD– but essential, and therefore they have to be emphasized and carefully taken into account.

Another interesting contribution Khare & Mullick (2009) make is the use of evaluation tools to assess the presence of different design criteria in the environment, as well as to measure the performance of children with autism. Their research shows that a high score when evaluating the environment from this point of view was related to a high performance result for children with autism in a given educational setting.

Humphreys (2008) sketches a variety of criteria to be considered when designing buildings for people with ASD. He refers to some clearly architectural concepts that the designer should include in his creations. Thus, he suggests seeking:

- Calm, order and simplicity:
  As a example, he mentions a school designed by him and located in Newcastle, United Kingdom, in which younger and older pupils are separated and use each of two units adjacent to a shared piece which holds common services, administration, departments, etc. Each units has a courtyard shaped in an golden spiral which becomes a permanent visual reference along the circulation spaces in the building. Furthermore, the sense of calm and simplicity is not limited to the way in which the plan and sections have been designed, but also applies to the use of materials. At this point Humphreys refers to medieval cistercian cloisters, where the same material is used for every element –pillars, floors, walls, etc.–, and suggests that, doing so, i.e., selecting a limited palette of materials, finishings, textures or colours, the same sense of calm we can find in those places can be achieved.
- Minimal details and materials:
  Aside from the above mentioned sense of order, this strategy can minimize the visual distraction excessive detailing brings. Any unnecessary detail should be avoided, altogether with hard edges. Reducing the background visual stimulation to a minimum allows carers and teachers to introduce the precise degree of stimulation according to each child's needs. Also, it is a good idea to consistently define heights of elements such as doors, handles, light switches and others.
- Proportion: With this idea Humphreys brings us back to ancient proportional systems, to Vitruvius, to classical Greek architecture, to the Parthenon's golden proportion, or to the use of Fibonacci series. To sum up, the author suggests trying to confer harmonious proportions on buildings and spaces designed for people with autism.
- Natural light:
  Humphreys advocates an extensive use of natural light, but warns against some possible errors: dazzling sun entrance, deep shadows or excessive contrasts, patterned or rhythmic shadow-light sequences, etc., may produce visual overstimulation. Sandblasted –or otherwise similarly treated– glass generates a convenient diffuse and homogeneous illumination out from natural light. Also, the precise design and placing of windows determines the way natural light spreads out in a given space. Skylights, too, or, even better, clerestory windows, can help getting this kind of diffuse lighting.

- Proxemics[11]:
  Proximity relationships in people with autism may be different to the usual ones. That is the reason we can speak about *particular proxemics* in individuals with ASD, meaning they may need more space for social relationships, and this has to be taken into account in the design process –including classrooms, corridors, halls, dining-rooms, etc.
- Containment:
  This concept refers to the need to monitor children with ASD, but, simultaneously, to the opportunity for them to wander –whenever their schedules and tasks allow them to. To accomplish this goal, the crucial point is to create a safe place where a child with ASD can walk freely. Humphreys exhorts us to look back into history and nature, zen courtyards or natural forms that can provide a convenient degree of containment. He also suggests designing exterior walls that are not obtrusive nor unpleasant.
- Observation:
  As noted before, this will fulfil the need of supervision, but avoiding, at the same time, excessive intrusion in the child's activities or interactions.
- Acoustics:
  People with ASD often have to make an enormous effort to differentiate sounds, and are more sensitive than other people to noises. The acoustic properties[12] of materials and constructive elements and systems must be taken into account.

To sum up, the most interesting aspect in Humphrey's work is the use of architectural concepts that convey beneficial outcomes for children with autism. In other words, certain intrinsic characteristics or qualities of a given architectural space can –and will–, if wisely employed, have a positive effect on children –or adults– with ASD.
An magnificient report entitled "Advancing full spectrum housing" (Ahrentzen & Steele, 2009) must be considered as one of the most in-depth studies on the matter we are discussing up to date. It summarizes previous research which analysed a number of residential settings, including different type of buildings –independent detached and attached houses, clusters of attached homes with common spaces, single-room occupancy units...–, different situations of dwelling –with or without family, with selected friends or agency chosen room-mates–, mixed or exclusionary residential complexes, and different types of care and support situations. The study and, therefore, the report, focuses on adults with ASD and on housing buildings, as the title shows. Several main design goals applicable to residential buildings for people with ASD were worked out, and are enumerated below:

1. Ensure safety and security
2. Maximize familiarity, stability and clarity
3. Minimize sensory overload
4. Allow opportunities to control social interaction and privacy
5. Provide independence and choice opportunities
6. Foster health and wellness

[11] Proxemics is the study of the spatial relationships –and, thus, of the amount of space laid– between individuals in different kinds of social and personal situations.
[12] Impact, air and flank transmission, reverberation, noise reduction coefficient or acoustic absorption, to name just a few

7. Improve own dignity
8. Ensure durability
9. Achieve affordability
10. Ensure accessibility and support

To achieve these objectives, the report presents many design criteria or recommendations relative to different aspects of a residential project, as its location, its plan layout, exterior spaces, living and community rooms, kitchens, halls, stairs, ramps, bedrooms, sensory –Snoezelen– rooms, bathrooms, laundry rooms, and also deals with aspects such as technology, visual cues, ventilation, lighting, materials, acoustics, appliances and fixtures. The list of suggestions for each of these sections is comprehensive and detailed. What is more, within each section, each recommendation has been correlated to one of the aforementioned design goals –although some of the suggestions might be considered to be related to more than one of those objectives–. Also, it is to be noted that some of the recommendations provided are not really specific for people with autism, but quality standards that could be employed in any building. However, it is clear that this quality must be more firmly ensured when the inhabitant is an individual with ASD.

Another greatly interesting article is that written by Vogel (2008). Although it specifically focuses on classroom design, the ideas presented can be, as the author herself states, extrapolated to other environments people with ASD have to cope with. In addition, Vogel –without dismissing them– goes beyond considerations about sensory, material or textural issues, or even about spaces layout and conditioning. Again, as was the case of Humphrey's work, some architectural qualities are brought out. According to Vogel, these are, summarized, the qualities a built environment for people with autism must have:

1. Flexible/Adaptable
2. Non-threatening
3. Non-distracting
4. Predictable
5. Controllable
6. Sensory-Motor attuned
7. Safe
8. Non-institutional

In relation to the first characteristics of space enumerated above, it could be argued if this might go against the resistance to change people with autism show. However, in many occasions changes in the use of space are necessary, and a given space may be used in different ways along time –even along a day–. Flexibility, therefore, when correctly understood and wisely introduced in design, would allow use transitions to be made without distorting space, i.e., without abrupt modifications that might alter children with ASD.

Especially relevant are Vogel's thoughts about the need to design spaces which are *legible* –readable– and *'imageable'* –qualities that render them predictable–, since these terms remind us of Kevin Lynch's book "The image of the city" (Lynch, 1998). We will recall now the idea of appropriation and apprehension of the built environment we mentioned in our introduction: the space, the environment, must be read and imagined –i.e., converted to a mental image–, before such a process of appropriation takes place. It is, in fact, the process by means of which a *space* becomes a *place*, and therefore stops being what French anthropologist Marc Augé names a *non-place* (Augé, 1993).

British architect Christopher Beaver has published on several occasions (Beaver, 2003; 2006; 2010) about the creation of architectural environments suitable for people with ASD. In particular, he explains certain strategies put into play in the development of a residential-educational centre projected by himself, and suggests them as valid approaches for other type of design projects involving users with autism. These strategies can be summarized as follows:

- Corridors were designed in such a way that they are not any longer mere spaces dedicated to circulate, but can be used, for instance, as playrooms. This, in turn, discharges some other spaces, as the living room, so that they can remain reserved for quieter activities. Also, this approach permits this space's appropriation by the children.
- Ample spaces, to allow the development of the children's activities without excessive proximity.
- Beaver designs two curved walls, that seemingly result in a more pleasant aspect. The building assessment carried out some time after it was put into use (Whitehurst, 2007) –which is one of the few evaluations of this type existent in the literature– states that these curved surfaces are liked by children and that, occasionally, they help them circulate, since children actually walk in contact with them.
- Acoustics are taken into account, avoiding too polished materials, for instance. As Beaver says, sometimes it is difficult to combine this aspect with the need to clean the flooring –soft materials like carpet can be useful to absorb noise, but the downside is that they are harder to clean than shinier ones, whose acoustic behaviour can be problematic.
- Safety is important when designing showers and toilets, and therefore pipes must not remain exposed, and fittings must be firmly fixed –otherwise they could be pulled out of their place. It is also necessary to provide enough common showers and toilets because incontinence is not a rare problem in some children with autism.
- Beaver recommends underfloor heating or radiant ceiling panels, and cross-ventilation, preferably from bottom to top, by means of two windows placed in opposite walls. In common areas he suggests the use of passive ventilation.
- Windows may be a safety problem, and hence Beaver's advice on placing mechanisms to restrict their opening. Also, he suggests that the windows can be locked from the interior. Glazing should be made out of safety glass –both on the exterior and the interior sides–. Another interesting possibility is the opportunity to place blinds inside double glazings.
- Regarding lighting fixtures, Beaver remarks that they have to be resistant even to abuse, but their lines should not imprint on the building and its spaces a sense of institution. They could be even hidden to sight, thus achieving indirect and diffuse illumination. Specifically reminds us to avoid traditional fluorescent lamps, as people with ASD might be greatly sensitive to the flickering produced by them, even though other people will never notice it. A good option which lighting industry offers us is the use of dimmers to control different illumination scenarios, each of which will generate a different ambience.
- It is also important to provide "quiet rooms" where a child having a tantrum –or simply experiencing too much stress, due to sensory overload, for example– can calm. This also helps to prevent the undesirable behaviour to expand to other children, as those conducts sometimes have a 'contagious' quality. Beaver does not seem to treat these spaces as

"haven" spaces, as Khare & Mullick (2008; 2009) and Mostafa (2008) do, but they can be also used as such: places where children –or adults– with ASD can retire to and where they may resort to the stereotypies that help them get calmed.

- It is also advisable to provide sensory rooms and gardens, which generate visual, auditive, tactile or olfactory stimuli.
- Colour palette should be adequately chosen, in order to create environments that provide a warm but not overstimulating amtmosphere.

Beaver also points out an important subject: the contrast between the measured, pleasant and protective environment we –hopefully– achieve for the individual with autism and other contexts and spaces in which he will have to manage when away from that precise building, which will not be, probably, so *autism-friendly*, i.e., will not conveniently accommodate their particular needs and impairments. We will quote his thoughts on this matter, since we believe this reflection is absolutely pertinent:

> "But where do we draw the line between environments that prepare the individual for the outside world and the protected environment of the purpose designed building? This is a difficult one for me as I am not a policy maker; I respond to a client's brief. But I do see a dilemma for organisations that seek to provide the ideal autism-friendly building for their children (or adults) who then go out into the world only to find that it is a noisy and confusing place with many dangers for which they are not prepared. The low functioning individual will no doubt find this less of a problem as he/she will more likely be in care for life. It is the individual who lives in both worlds that may have more difficulty. Designers must be aware of this and try to find the right balance for the particular user group that will inhabit his/her building."(Beaver, 2010)

Finally, we will refer to an article written by Ian Scott (2009), who analyses British regulations on inclusive schools in the light of the particular needs of children with ASD. He also reviews Humphreys' work cited above (see page 9 onward). From these two starting points, and out of his professional experience, he extracts several requirements –again mostly focused on educational spaces– which are listed below:

1. To create an ordered and comprehensible spatial structure
2. To generate a mix of small and large spaces
3. Provide the user with more control over environmental conditions
4. To accommodate different teaching strategies for pupils with autism
5. To achieve a balance between safety and independence
6. To reduce and simplify detailing
7. To grant the user active participation in the brief building and design process
8. To appropriately use technology to aid the learning experience of pupils with autism
9. To provide adequate technical specification

However, maybe the most interesting respect in Scott's article is the analysis –based on the requirements he has established beforehand– of four schools: New Struan, in Alloa, Scotland; Netley Primary School ASD Unit, in Camden LA, London; Whitton School ASD Unit, in Twickenham, Richmond LA; and Mossbrook Special Primary School, in Norton, Sheffield. Highly valuable are, too, some comments made by the designers of those buildings, as well as by several representatives of the schools, whom the author interviewed [13]. For instance, Jim Taylor, the headteacher at Struan School, in reference to the need of withdrawal spaces that are not excluded from the spatial fabric of the building, says:

> "At one point the architects had proposed a withdrawal room or 'snoozelin', where a child could withdraw and calm down if things got too much. We rejected that as we felt that would have been a failing in itself. We wanted the children to have the opportunity to withdraw, but still remain within the social fabric of the school and the building allows for that." (Scott, 2009, p. 38)

Or Sarah Wigglesworth, designer of Mossbrook Special Primary School, who reflects on the necesary balance between the need of boundaries and their sense of confinement:

> "Typically it seems a large part of the agenda in relation to designing for autism seems to be about ensuring the children can remain within boundaries with which they are familiar. There are two sides to that in that we understand how the limits of a human environment can provide security and be very comforting, but at worst it could reflect confinement. We wanted to create a balance with something that could be 'outward oriented' and engage the world beyond the classroom, whilst at the same time making the kids feel secure. On a philosophical level you can see architecture as a vessel that gathers the world into it-self and this building certainly does that in lots of ways." (Scott, 2009, p. 49)

Scott's article is, in sum, an outstanding example of the extremely scarce studies of several buildings analysing their adaptation to the concrete needs of people with ASD.

## 4. Synopsis of design criteria

In this section we will outline several responses that architectural design may –by means of project and design mechanisms– give to the needs of people with autism. Whilst it may not be an exhaustive compilation, we will group these strategies according to different impairments that may be aided by them, for the purpose of systematising our discourse.

### 4.1 Imagination

Resistance to changes and a limited ability to imagine are, as has been stated above, two of the most common symptoms present on individuals with ASD. These characteristics lead to difficulties or extreme nervousness when switching tasks or even when walking from a given space to another. The main issue is that they may be unable to imagine, i.e., to elaborate a mental image, what lays behind a door or a wall, even if they know the room they are entering. In their school or home environments this issue is usually faced up to through *anticipation* of activities that are to be held soon, and avoiding or mitigating, as much as possible, unexpected changes in scheduled tasks and routines.

From the architectural design point of view, the inability to construct a mental image of the environment, as well as to integrate parts in a whole, can be addressed by providing the building with a clear structure, along with elements[14] that endow it with certain order and unity, in such a way that it becomes easily readable, predictable, *imaginable*.

[13] See also one of these comments by John Jenkins, quoted on page 2

[14] For instance, Southerington (2007) uses a handrail that runs along walls in all the spaces of the building she designs, thus providing an element to achieve a degree of visual consistency.

With regard to transitions between spaces, anxiety may be reduced, for instance, with the help of colour coding of doors –showing the use of the spaces behind them– pictograms or even actual pictures that anticipate what we are about to find, or with a decidedly architectural strategy such as creating intermediate transitional *threshold spaces* where the necessary anticipation can be achieved (see, for instance Scott, 2009, p. 42).

### 4.2 Communication

Impairments in verbal and non-verbal communication, in conjunction with difficulties in information processing, make it essential

> "to remove certain psychological 'barriers' and to adapt the environment with cues that [...] are characterized by being concrete and easily perceivable (versus subtle), simple, i.e., comprising few elements (versus complex) and permanent (versus temporary)".(Tamarit et al., 1990)

An individual with ASD usually needs visual support to communication, and often pictograms, pictures of objects and people, among other aids, are used. The built environment should be able to accommodate these forms of communication, planning their right location and integration. As stated above, coding elements with colours, for instance, can also help communication.
It is also of cardinal importance that the visual background be as neutral as possible. An effort must be put on decluttering the environment, removing superfluous elements, minimizing detailing and employing reduced non-vivid chromatic ranges.

### 4.3 Social interaction

Impairments in social interaction are, by definition –although in different degrees– present in individuals with ASD. That is the reason why the different educative strategies aim at aiding in this dimension. Therefore, it will be necessary to provide spaces to allow and even favour those interactions, but bearing in mind that individuals with ASD may present peculiar proxemics (see above, page 10), thus needing ample spaces in which such interchanges can take place. A proper combination of large spaces and small ones –in which one can, at will, interact closer to each other– is advisable.
Furthermore, in some situations an individual with autism may feel overcome by a social demanding situation –he might find himself impelled to participate in different interactions, even in several at the same time– and thus needs a space where to retire in search of greater intimacy, or just a simpler interaction –fewer people, or more familiar ones–.

### 4.4 Sensory difficulties

Difficulties in the reception or processing of sensory stimuli is also a frequent symptom of ASD. These impairments may take the form of visual, auditory, vestibular, olfactory, proprioceptive or tactile hypersensitivity –or hyposensitivity at times–. Multichannel perception –sounds that elicit images or smells, for instance–. Consideration towards this issue will lead us to carefully select colours –not excessively contrasting, saturated or bright–; textures and patterns –again avoiding high contrasts–, acoustic properties of the different materials and constructive elements, lighting –trying to achieve a diffuse, preferably natural, illumination, and remembering to avoid fluorescent tubes, as its flickering and buzzing can alter an individual with auditory or visual hypersensitivity; fixtures; heat, ventilation and air conditioning –reducing gradients of temperature and limiting noises and vibrations–; etc.

Yet another possible sensory dysfunction is that of pain sensation. For instance, a child –or an adult– with autism may suffer from severe burns if he washes his hands or has a shower with water at high temperature, as he will not pull away. To avoid this type of problems, thermostatic taps can be used, or, at least, the temperature water reaches must be conveniently adjusted. Other elements should also be designed and materials and finishings should be selected in such a way that no one –especially someone insensitive to pain– may not suffer from any accidental injuries.
Aside from these considerations, it is interesting to remember that multisensory stimulation rooms –also called *Snoezelen* rooms– allow people with autism to 'attune' their sensory perception, –whether mitigating or arising them, in cases of hyposensitivity–, and also to reduce anxiety at given moments.

### 4.5 Behaviour and safety

Behavioural problems are, too, frequent in cases of ASD. Aggressive conduct may arise, and, therefore, elements present in the built environment must be designed and chosen bearing in mind the possibility of eventual abuses. In particular, bathroom equipment, lighting fixtures and mechanisms, hardware, banisters, wall and floor tiles, etc., must be well anchored.

## 5. Conclusions

We have shown that the literature on built environments and their relation to people with ASD and their needs is scarce, in spite of the enormous amount of research on autism that has been carried out in recent years. This interest responds to an important increase in diagnosed cases, due to which prevalence studies show ratios well above the estimations of 1 to 3 cases in 10,000 children that were worked out in last century's early 90s –and even lower before–. It has been stated recently that the proportion reaches one child with autism in 110 births (Center for Disease Control and Prevention, 2009). It is obvious that the rise in prevalence ratios does not correspond to a real increment in the number of cases –at least not exclusively–, but also to the expansion of the very concept of autism and its diagnostic criteria, and to improvements in educational and health services that permits for an earlier diagnosis, altogether with a higher degree of awareness on autism (Ahrentzen & Steele, 2009). In spite of that, those ratios bring up the fact that people with autism constitute a wide population group, that require attention and services from society. The disciplinary field of Architecture should move in this direction, too. Within a few decades architects and urban planners have become aware of the need to design without the so-called 'architectural barriers' which limit access and mobility for people with —physical– disabilities. However, within this concept of barrier there has been no place for those elements that limit the use of our environment for individuals with cognitive or mental disabilities. We, thus, need to learn that, as Baumers & Heylighen (2009; 2010) state, these people perceive space in a unique, different style: with the "eyes of the mind".
It is mandatory to advance in research on this matter, with further analyses and assessments of architectural realisations that have been designed and built for people with autism, and of the adaptation to these users' needs. Innovative and imaginative design solutions should be pointed out by this research, as well as failures and errors.
In spite of the fact that it is difficult –i.e., costly– to produce interventions in the built environment, even when scales are small, examples as Magda Mostafa's work (2008) show that they are possible and that, when systematically carried out and assessed, they can provide

us with useful information about how, and to what extent, these realisations improve the experience people with ASD have in their environment.
We will finish this chapter quoting Spanish architect Luis Fernández-Galiano. His words may help other architects and designers –actually, any agent involved in designing and planning buildings– to grasp what their role should be, and especially what challenges are to be faced when shaping environments for people with autism:

> ´´Dwelling is a difficult job. As the trade of living, that of dwelling requires continuous learning and attention, demands a meticulous and systematic effort, and involves an inordinate investment of time and energy. It is therefore surprising to verify the naturalness with which the majority of us get to execute the complicated rituals of habitable space. As happens with languaje, expertise is achieved with habit, that rules and domesticates gestures and voices through everyday reiteration of movements and words. Well, this exhausting and habitual trade has in the architect an obstacle or an ally" (as cited in Oyarzun, 2005).

## 6. References

Ahrentzen, S. & Steele, K. (2009). Advancing full spectrum housing, *Technical report*, Arizona Board of Regents, Phoenix, USA.

Asperger, H. (1991). Autistic psychopathy in childhood, *in* U. Frith (ed.), *Autism and Asperger syndrome*, Cambridge University Press, Cambridge, p. 37.

Augé, M. (1993). *Los no lugares, espacios del anonimato : antropología sobre modernidad*, Gedisa, Barcelona.

Baron-Cohen, S., Leslie, A. & Frith, U. (1985). Does the autistic child have a "theory of mind"?, *Cognition* 21(1): 37–46.

Baumers, S. & Heylighen, A. (2009). The eyes of the mind. architecture and mental disability, *Engaging Artifacts*, Oslo.

Baumers, S. & Heylighen, A. (2010). Harnessing different dimensions of space: The built environment in auti-biographies, *in* P. Langdon, P. J. Clarkson & P. Robinson (eds), *Designing Inclusive Interactions: Inclusive Interactions Between People and Products in Their Contexts of Use*, Springer-Verlag, London, UK, pp. 13–23.

Beaver, C. (2003). Breaking the mould, *Communication* 37(3): 40.

Beaver, C. (2006). Designing environments for children and adults with ASD, Cape Town.

Beaver, C. (2010). Autism-friendly environments, *The autism file* (34): 82–85.

Bettelheim, B. (2001). *La fortaleza vacía: Autismo infantil y el nacimiento del yo*, number 29 in *Saberes Cotidianos*, Paidós, Barcelona.

Bogdashina, O. (2005). *Communication issues in autism and Asperger syndrome: do we speak the same language?*, Jessica Kingsley Publishers.

Center for Disease Control and Prevention (2009). Prevalence of Autism Spectrum Disorders. Autism and Developmental Disabilities Monitoring Network, United States, 2006, *MMWR* 58(SS-10): 1–20.

Davis, K. & Dubie, M. (2004). Sensory integration: Tips to consider, *The Reporter* 9(3): 3–8.

Escobar Solano, M., Caravaca Cantabella, M., Herrero Navarro, J. & Verdejo Bolonio, M. (2008). Necesidades educativas especiales del alumnado con trastornos del espectro autista., Atención a la diversidad: materiales para la formación del profesorado, Consejería de Educación, Formación y Empleo de la Región de Murcia. Centro de Profesores y Recursos de Cieza, Murcia.

Frith, U. (2006). *Autismo: hacia una explicación del enigma*, Alianza Editorial, Madrid.

Frith, U. & Happe, F. (1999). Theory of mind and Self-Consciousness: what is it like to be autistic?, *Mind and Language* 14(1): 82–89.

Heidegger, M. (2001). *Conferencias y artículos*, Ediciones del Serbal, Barcelona.

Humphreys, S. (2008). Architecture and autism.
URL: *http://www.auctores.be/auctores_bestanden/UDDA%2003102008%20S%20Humphreys.pdf*

Kanner, L. (1943). Autistic disturbances of affective contact, *Nervous child* 2(2): 217–230.

Khare, R. & Mullick, A. (2008). Educational spaces for children with autism: design development process, *CIB W 084 Proceedings, Building Comfortable and Liveable Environment for All*, Atlanta, USA, pp. 66–75.

Khare, R. & Mullick, A. (2009). Incorporating the behavioral dimension in designing inclusive learning environment for autism, *International Journal of Architectural Research* 3(3): 45–64.

Lynch, K. (1998). *La imagen de la ciudad*, Gustavo Gili, Barcelona.

Montaner i Martorell, J. (2002). *La modernidad superada : arquitectura, arte y pensamiento del siglo XX*, Gustavo Gili, Barcelona.

Mostafa, M. (2008). An an architecture for autism: Concepts of design intervention for the autistic user, *International Journal of Architectural Research* 2(1): 189–211.

Oyarzun, D. (2005). *Arquitectura y discapacidad. Centro de atención integral para niños autistas.*, Proyecto de título, Universidad de Chile, Santiago de Chile.

Richer, J. M. & Nicoll, S. (1971). A playroom for autistic children, and its companion therapy project, *British Journal of Mental Subnormality* 17(33): 132–143.

Rutter, M. & Schopler, E. (eds) (1984). *Autismo. Reevaluación de los conceptos y el tratamiento*, Alhambra Universidad, Alhambra, Madrid.

Scott, I. (2009). Designing learning spaces for children on the autism spectrum, *Good Autism Practice* 10(1): 36–51.

Smith, D. (2009). Spatial design as a facilitator for people with less visible impairments, *Australasian Medical Journal* 1(13): 220–227.

Southerington, E. A. (2007). *Specialized Environments: Perceptual Experience as Generator of Form*, Master project, Cincinnati, USA.

Tamarit, J., de Dios, J., Domínguez, S. & Escribano, L. (1990). Proyecto de estructuración ambiental en el aula de niños autistas, *Technical report*, Consejería de Educación de la Comunidad Autónoma de Madrid y Dirección General de Renovación Pedagógica del Ministerio de Educación y Ciencia, Madrid.

Tustin, F. (1996). *Estados autísticos en los niños*, number 109 in *Psicología Psiquiatría Psicoterapia*, Paidós, Barcelona.

Vogel, C. L. (2008). Classroom design for living and learning with autism, *Autism Asperger's Digest* .

Whitehurst, T. (2007). Evaluation of features specific to an ASD designed living accommodation, *Technical report*, Sunfield Research Institute.

Wing, J. (1968). Review of Bettelheim: "The empty fortress", *British Journal of Psychiatry* 114: 788–791.

Wing, L. & Gould, J. (1979). Severe impairments of social interaction and associated abnormalities in children: epidemiology and classification, *Journal of autism and developmental disorders* 9(1): 11–29.

# 20

# Quality of Life and Physical Well-Being in People with ASDs

Carmen Nieto[1] and Rosa Ventoso[2]
[1]*Department of Psicología Básica, Autónoma University of Madrid*
[2]*Asociación de Padres de Personas con Autismo (APNA)*
*Spain*

## 1. Introduction

The term Quality of Life (QoL) started to be used in relation to disability in the 1980s. Persons with disabilities have the right to a good quality living. In the 1990s it became a goal to be achieved, verified and measured. The next step was mandatory: if progress is to be made towards achieving QoL for people, then it is necessary to specify what QoL is. In 2002 Schalock and Verdugo published 12 basic principles for conceptualising, measuring and implementing it. They defined a multidimensional concept that is influenced by personal and environmental factors, and their interaction, and is improved with self-determination, resources, life purpose and a sense of belonging. They translated their multidimensional proposal into eight dimensions: emotional well-being, interpersonal relations, material well-being, personal development, physical well-being, self-determination, social inclusion and rights. The importance of the concept of QoL lies in the fact that it provides: a conceptual framework from the individual's perspective; 2) a guide to action; 3) a criterion for assessing both strategies and results. QoL becomes the goal to be reached for the person, the organisations, the politicians and the funders concerned. It is a guarantee with regard to objectives, procedures and quality outcomes.

To improve an individual's QoL we must focus on their point of view, their needs and their context. The QoL model helps us, in the first place, to know where to look. We have eight dimensions, but might there not exist a hierarchical structure among them? Kreuger et al., (2008) conducted a study to identify the priority needs of persons with severe intellectual disabilities. One of their findings was that the physical well-being dimension is of crucial importance for these persons. Chou et al., (2007) carried out a study in Taiwan in which they assessed the QoL of adults with intellectual disabilities. They found that of the eight dimensions in the model put forward by Schalock & Verdugo (2002), the one singled out as most important was the physical well-being dimension.

The eight dimensions of QoL are inter-related and it is likely that improving one will result in an improvement in one or more others. Of course, the converse is also true. This is particularly evident in regard to the physical well-being dimension. Physical well-being and emotional well-being are closely related. Indeed, in populations with communication difficulties, one of the ways pain or physical discomfort may be manifested is through displays of anxiety, increased motility, crying and even tantrums with acts of aggression and/or self-aggression (Nieto et al., 2008). Physical well-being becomes a key item for generating the motivation that leads individuals to set themselves goals to do with social interaction, personal development and so on. Moreover, in general, physical discomfort will affect the other dimensions. This is how the results of the studies by Kreuger et al., (2008) and Chou et al., (2007) can be interpreted. Perhaps it is not quite accurate to say that physical well-being is what contributes most to individuals' QoL, but it does seem that lack of it has an extremely deleterious effect on the other dimensions. In short, actions aimed at ensuring a healthy state must be a priority objective of persons, organisations, politicians and funders.

## 2. What is the health of persons with Autism Spectrum Disorders like?

Autism spectrum disorders (ASDs) are heterogeneous and multifactorial neurodevelopmental disorders. They are neurobiological disorders for which genetic aspects appear to have a decisive influence in interaction with environmental factors (Sigman et al., 2006). This complex interaction shows up clearly in studies of monozygotic and dizygotic twins in which the concordance ratio between the former is 88%, whereas between the latter it is 31% (Rosenber et al., 2009). It is possible to speak of a syndrome in which there is a phenotype with common underlying general features caused by different biological mechanisms (Coleman & Betancur, 2005). There is no specific local problem in the brain; rather, various neuronal systems are probably affected (Akshoomoff et al., 2002; Schultz & Robins, 2005), especially those involved in regulating neuronal connections during development (Minshew et al., 2005); or underconnectivity (Just et al., 2004; Cassanova, 2006; Dosenbach et al., 2010).
Autism spectrum disorders are associated with different biological conditions. Epilepsy is one of the most frequent comorbid disorders of autism (Canitano, 2007; Tuk et al., 2009) and it is even mentioned in The Diagnostic and Statistical Manual of Mental Disorders Fourth Edition [DSM-IV] (1994), although it is not included as a diagnostic criterion. There is a high degree of variability in respect of its prevalence. According to Tuchman & Rapin (2002), about 30% of persons with autism develop epilepsy as adults. The risk of epilepsy varies also depending on the subtype of autistic spectrum. The lowest prevalence (4%) is associated with Asperger syndrome (Cederlund & Gillberg, 2004) and the highest (77%) with childhood disintegrative disorder (Mouridsen et al., 1999). Amit et al., (2008) found that the risk of epilepsy increases as a function of two factors: intellectual disability and female gender.
Gastrointestinal problems are also frequent in this population (Nikolov et al., 2009). Buie, et al., (2010) carried out a wide-ranging study from which they concluded that the prevalence and best treatment of these conditions are still incompletely understood. A key problem is the difficulty this population has in recognising and characterising gastrointestinal dysfunction because of their communication difficulties. Many parents report improved behaviour following medical or nutritional intervention. In this connection, some studies have reported improvements associated with changes in diet (Knivsberg et al., 2002). The high frequency of gastrointestinal problems in persons with autism has made this the focus of a number of studies investigating the aetiology of the disorder. Cassanova (2008) looked for connections between gastrointestinal symptoms and failures in neuronal architecture, in particular, minicolumnar disturbance. Kimberly et al., (2009) carried out a comprehensive review of studies investigating the association between autism and viral infections (Rubella, *Toxoplasma gondii*, Varicella, etc.), neuroimmune studies (including gastrointestinal factors)

and the role of vaccines. It is important to point out that so far no data have been found to support a possible causal relation between the triple viral vaccine and the appearance of autism, and this hypothesis has been ruled out on the basis of strong scientific evidence (D´Souza et al., 2006; Rutter, 2005).

Another crucial aspect of the health of persons with ASDs is the high proportion that are treated with psychotropic medication. There are no medicines that improve the core disorders of autism, but treatments are often prescribed with the aim of alleviating certain symptoms such as aggression, self-injury behaviours, stereotypes and hyperactivity (Hollander et al., 2003). Aman et al., (1995) found that 30% of children with ASDs were using some psychotropic medication. Green et al. (1996) conducted an internet survey of 552 parents of persons with autism in which 52% reported habitually administering psychotropic medication. Recently, Mandell et al., (2011) investigated a sample of 60,641 children with ASDs in the USA. In their sample, 56% were treated with at least one psychotropic medication, 20% of whom were prescribed three or more medications at the same time. The use of these drugs was common even in children aged 0 to 2 years (18%) and 3 to 5 years (32%). Neuroleptic drugs were the most common (31%), followed by antidepressants (25%) and stimulants (22%). In their conclusions they stress that the effects of these treatments on development are not yet known and argue the need to assess the risks, benefits, and costs of the use of this type of medication. Fuentes et al. (2008) develop PHARMAUTISME TR, a protocol to administrate psychotropic medication to people with mental disabilities and ASDs. This protocol is followed in Gipuzkoa, País Vasco (Spain) and the use of these drugs in this population is less than 30%.

There are also other problems commonly found in persons with ASDs that can have negative repercussions on their health and need to be taken into consideration. These include issues to do with the lack of a balanced diet due to food selectivity (Ventoso, 2000) or overeating; difficulties in maintaining suitable hygiene habits, especially oral and dental hygiene (Shapira et al., 1989; Dias et al., 2010); sleeping problems (Berthier et al., 1992; Polimeni et al., 2005; Allik et al., 2006); the lack of physical exercise, with prolonged stress and anxiety (White et al., 2009; Green & Ben- Sasson, 2010) and the difficulty of foreseeing and controlling risks.

Lastly, there is another fact showing that the health of persons with ASDs is worse, or more threatened, than that of other people, namely the mortality ratio data. The different studies conducted on this (Shavelle & Strauss, 1998; Shavelle et al., 2001; Mouridsen et al., 2008; Gillberg et al., 2010) have revealed that persons with autism have a shorter life expectancy than the rest of the population and a higher mortality ratio. High mortality ratios have been reported for circulatory disorders (2.3) and cancer (1.9), which leads to the formulation of the hypothesis that the higher mortality from these causes may be due to late diagnosis of the disease as a consequence of the communication difficulties present in persons with autism. Recently, Gillberg et al., (2010) have published the results of a longitudinal study which was completed in 2008. It was carried out in Sweden with a sample of 120 persons with ASDs born between 1962 and 1984 who were followed up between the ages of 13 and 22. They report that the main causes of death were associated with medical disorders and accidents. They also found that the mortality ratio was higher in women.

As can be seen, persons with ASDs are at greater risk than the population with typical development of suffering various problems affecting their health. In addition, they are at a disadvantage in recognising and expressing their discomfort, and in allowing themselves to be examined. It is common for persons with ASDs, even when they possess language (about

50% of them fail to develop spoken language), not to report on their internal state. So on many occasions we lack information on their psychological and/or physical condition. In addition, they may have difficulty identifying pain and discomfort as a result of altered sensory thresholds, so it is quite possible that they are unable to locate the source or nature of the discomfort (Boghashina, 2003; Ventoso & Osorio, 1997). They are people who do not usually ask for help or consolation consistently when they are in discomfort or suffer pain. Pain is often manifested in behaviour problems, irritability, etc. Relatives and clinical professionals formulate successive hypotheses about the cause of such behaviour and it is not always easy to find the real connection between cause and effect. On some occasions an extreme situation -such as a very high temperature, the discovery of major physical lesions that have become quite evident- provide the key to explaining –a posteriori- serious behaviour disorders that have been going on for years (Nieto et al., 2008). Medical professionals are faced with people coming to their clinics who do not use any means of communication to describe their symptoms, define them incompletely or even deny them, and who, moreover, do not allow an adequate examination to be performed, which means the practitioner tends to act on the basis of trial and error. To this must be added the fact that not all health care environments have sufficient information and training on the treatment and adaptations necessary to optimise examinations (Carbone et al., 2010; Merino et al., 2010).

Taking these factors into account, it is essential for health care education programmes to be implemented that are clear, simple and well-defined, and also demonstrate their effectiveness. The QoL model becomes a guide guaranteeing quality practice.

## 3. Towards an integral health plan for persons with ASDs

The integral health plan put forward here comprises 12 aspects that have a direct connection with, and may have an influence on, physical well-being and, inseparably, on emotional well-being. Some of these factors depend on, or are more directly related to, the person with ASDs and require specific teaching programmes to be run for particular groups or individuals, according to their needs and level of competence. Others focus on the contexts and it is these that need to improve their knowledge and put in place specific assessment and monitoring systems, and action protocols.

The 12 dimensions of the integral health plan constitute, on the one hand, a proposal for 12 different programmes to be carried out and, on the other, offer a schema or basic outline for drawing up health assessment protocols that will help to determine needs, enable intervention goals to be set and serve as a monitoring tool. They provide information that helps to carry out specific intervention programmes for persons with ASDs depending on their particular disorders within the spectrum.

To help with these proposals, the main contents referred to in each of them are described briefly below

### 3.1 Disease prevention and treatment

The “physical” health problems of persons with ASDs may be no different from those of the rest of the population. However, the health care they receive may be different and of inferior quality due to the difficulty some of these persons have, especially in childhood, in allowing adequate examinations to be performed. That is why carrying out programmes designed to get persons with ASDs used to examinations and their contexts by employing specific strategies, such as a routine maintained over time and providing information beforehand using analogous material (photographs or drawings), has proved to be useful (Nieto et al., 2008). Gradual, ongoing habituation from infancy prevents many health care problems, especially in persons with more pronounced disorders within the autism spectrum.

Another component of this prevention dimension is the advisability of carrying out regular "general" health check-ups (primary health care normally performed by general practitioners) and dental check-ups, especially in persons with more pronounced disorders. A regular check-up (for instance, every two months) enables the habituation learning to be maintained and also makes it possible to detect complaints in their initial stages and treat them appropriately and simply (Nieto et al., 2008). For example, a person with ASDs with serious communication limitations, even though they possess language, may, just like anyone else, have a wax blockage in their ear. The manifestations may be the expected lack of attention, in which case there is a considerable likelihood of this being misinterpreted. But it is also not infrequent for the discomfort to be manifested through maladjusted, even self-harming, behaviours that can lead to interventions far removed from what is really needed and, among other negative consequences, aggravate the original health problem. Routine, regular check-ups do not imply excessive "medicalisation" of this population and may have enormous personal and social benefits.

In high-functioning persons who may experience anxiety or rejection when being medically examined, anticipating and explaining such situations using Carol Gray's (1994, 2010) social stories technique may be of great help.

### 3.2 Medication

The aspects to do with the medication dimension are diverse. On the one hand, as happens with the rest of the population, many children may reject the administration of drugs via the different routes and in the different formats. It is important to assess the child's acceptance of the medication formats and administration routes to plan the intervention. Again, employing teaching procedures that include routine, successive approximations and prior visual information about what the child is expected to do and the consequences it will have for their well-being, is extremely useful.

In the case of high-functioning adults, it is advisable to review their ability to follow autonomous administration guidelines. If necessary, specific programmes can be carried out that include a scientific explanation of the effect of the drug and the need to use it at the appropriate times and in the appropriate amounts, the use of external reminding systems such as reminders in watches or diaries.

### 3.3 Food

Food problems are common in persons with ASDs in childhood and some authors have even suggested them as a diagnostic indicator (Ahearn et al., 2001). They appear with various manifestations, but usually present with food hyperselectivity as a common feature, the child accepting only limited ranges of food and completely refusing to eat or even try any others (Field et al., 2003; Martins et al., 2008). Some children display from the very earliest months of life problems in ingesting the necessary amounts, but the most common problem arises when the time comes to change the type of food from milk to baby food and then to introduce solids. Some children will only eat if they are offered a particular type of food, flavour or presentation. Various factors can affect this, one of which is the possible existence of gastrointestinal disorders such as gastro-oesophageal reflux and other digestive problems (Lightdale et al., 2001; Fombonne & Chakrabarti, 2001; Horvath & Perman, 2002) that lead to the refusal of food. The presence of sensory disorders is also common. These tend to be specially pronounced and serious in the early years of development (Williams, 1996). It is likely that some children with autism have a basic sensory disorder problem affecting taste, smell, touch, sight, sensitivity to temperature, etc. (Field et al., 2003) so they find certain foods unpleasant or even unbearable, whereas others, with strong and strange tastes are among their favourites. In addition, changing flavours, smells and sensations, or even simply the visual stimulation conditions of the plate, cutlery, etc. may present a challenge for the cognitive system of a child with ASDs. Mental inflexibility is a central characteristic of autistic processing (DSM-IV-TR; Ozonoff, 1995; Ozonoff et al., 1991; Rivière, 1997) and may manifest itself in the absolute rejection of anything new to do with food. Parents and teachers generally fail to understand the reason for this rejection and often the only way they find to deal with this is by forcing the child to eat so that, by a classical conditioning process, the child comes to associate the intake of new food or the entire stimulation complex of the eating situation with a negative emotional state which the child rejects. Persisting in forcing the child to eat reinforces the association between negative emotion and feeding situations so that some children cry at the simple sight of food or an attempt to give them a little piece of food unleashes a strong temper tantrum.

The food programmes try to break this negative conditioning gently but firmly and gradually, and must be carried out in a personalised way bearing in mind the children's sensory characteristics and their previous history of routines during feeding. Ventoso's (2000) programme proposes a change of attitude in the people in charge of feeding and suggests they take into account various general considerations: turning meals into a pleasant and peaceful time, which requires the adult to display serenity and firmness at all times; associating food only with eating; creating and performing every day a meal ritual shaped by the adult, forcing slightly without entering into a "battle" with the child; requiring the child to eat a small pre-established amount.

The programme includes a number of steps to be followed to make the changeover from minced food to solid food:

- Collect information from the family about foods, the ways of taking them, cutlery preferences, bibs, etc.
- Create a routine and keep the physical conditions constant;
- Finish the meal with a highly gratifying situation such as playing an interactive game, letting the child see a favourite advertising brochure, etc., in other words an activity that is highly desired by the child;
- Begin the new programme in a different context from the usual one;
- Begin with a small amount of the food the child likes best offered in a small spoon. Insist in multiple tries with the utmost tranquillity and strategies of successive approximations plus reinforcement for each one;
- Gradually increase the amount of food accepted;
- Choose a totally new situation for offering new foods;
- Introduce new flavours by choosing a food of similar flavour to the child's favourite and the same texture and temperature;
- When moving from purés to solid foods, change textures, for example, extremely gradually and carefully, introducing a small spoonful of food in a slightly different form into the food in the form the child accepts.

She also recommends some methodological principles that should be adhered to: provide visual information beforehand about what the child is going to eat by showing it to them; present only an amount that one is certain the child is going to eat; always give the child's favourite dessert and do not change it at the beginning; prevent the child from getting wet or dirty and clean them gently and immediately if this does happen; do not mix different foods; do not offer a new spoonful until the child has swallowed the previous one; make sure the food is at the ideal temperature for the child; etc.

Other specific problems, such as the child's leaving the food in their mouth without swallowing it, swallowing without chewing, not accepting new foods, etc., require special adjustments.

At the opposite extreme, some persons with ASDs overeat and lack the comprehension and communication mechanisms that would make it possible to explain to them the reason why it is not good to eat all they want.

Strategies involving feeding at set times to a strict, but fairly frequent, routine -five meals a day- are a good idea. It is important for mealtimes to be set and be known in advance by the individual (Schopler et al., 1995). It is useful to include large amounts of dietary fibre in the food, especially at breakfast and tea time. It is important for persons who are overweight or have nutrition problems due to the limited variety of their food intake to be supervised by a doctor who is an expert in nutrition who can make suggestions about diet and monitor their evolution (Volkmar & Wiesner, 2004).

High-functioning persons with food problems may benefit from diet education programmes that include an intellectual explanation of the food pyramid, the need for a balanced diet and suggested examples of diets.

### 3.4 Physical exercise and posture control

It is obvious that physical exercise and posture control are two fundamental aspects to be looked after, especially in adults, just as in the rest of the population. However, the high incidence of mortality due to circulatory disorders in persons with ASDs (Shavelle et al., 2001) makes it advisable to pay particular attention to this.

Moderately intense physical exercise is a useful tool in reducing stress. Doing moderately intense routine physical exercise is advisable. Individual sports such as swimming, skating, using exercise machines in a gym, trekking, etc., are particularly suitable. With low-medium functioning persons, visual or physical signs can be used to help them understand when an activity begins and ends, e.g. by means of warning devices, route signs in open spaces or indicators showing the number of times an exercise has to be done, eg passing a counter or washer from one container to another after every go (Peeters, 1997).

A much neglected aspect in this population is care in maintaining a suitable posture. There is no information on the effects this may have, but the existence of discomfort must be obvious. It is important, especially in adult care homes, that residents are helped to maintain appropriate postures and are provided with appropriately adapted furniture where necessary. Care and supervision by physiotherapists may also be highly advisable.

### 3.5 Hygiene

Persons with ASDs fairly often lack an understanding of the need for hygiene and its benefits. Nevertheless, most of them have adequate hygiene habits or allow suitable hygiene procedures to be performed; many of them even avoid dirt and try to take their clothes off if they do get dirty. In children, oral and dental health problems are often associated with deficient hygiene (Shapira et al., 1989; Dias et al., 2010). The mouth is a specially sensitive area in which sensory disorders can occur as a result of the brush, the toothpaste or the brushing action. To deal with this, programmes have been carried out to teach carers how to perform hygiene. These teaching programmes often employ a behavioural methodology known as backward chaining supplemented by visual information: drawings of the mouth with the number of times the teeth have to be brushed or numbers to be counted while using an electric toothbrush. Using an electric toothbrush may benefit some children, but it is aversive to others, so an individual assessment is needed. The taste and strength of the toothpaste are aspects that can help or hinder teeth cleaning.

Hand hygiene requires special care due to its implications for health. Hygiene programmes must include the need for the person to wash their hands after going to the toilet, always before handling food or after handling any substance that may be harmful. Here too visual information plus routine are two suitable complementary procedures. Action guides with analogous images are extremely useful, but an intellectual explanation using illustrations of the health consequences may also be of great help to many children and adults with autism with poor communication and comprehension ability.

Cutting nails and hair, especially in the case of children, are two other activities for which special programmes are commonly needed. Adults require special attention to be given to their feet, as they may have discomfort that causes them a great deal of pain. Procedures based on routine, successive approximations, contingent reinforcement and visual anticipation, in the same way as in the medical examination habituation programme, are extremely useful.

### 3.6 Sleep

Sleep problems are quite common in persons with autism and are of various kinds. Generally they include difficulty in getting to sleep, waking up during the night, sleeping for only a short time and waking up very early (Honomichl et al., 2002; Wiggs & Stores, 2004). In general, persons with ASDs appear to sleep for a shorter total time than control groups (Elia et al., 2000). Complicated rituals or strange behaviours for going to bed or getting back to sleep are common and force parents to go to bed with their children or perform complicated rituals to keep them asleep (eg having to leave one of the parents' arms on the child's body or let the child sleep while holding a lock of their mother's hair in their hand). There is a strong association between sleep problems and family stress (Schreck et al., 2004) and although a direct empirical relation between sleep problems and state of health in person's with ASDs has not been established, it is an aspect requiring assessment and intervention.

In some cases drug treatment can alleviate this problem (Filipek, 2005), but intervention via specific programmes is necessary. In such programmes the following kinds of strategies are useful: having the person do moderate physical exercise every day a few hours before going to bed, trying to keep excitement levels low as it gets near bedtime, creating rituals keeping to strict times, ensuring the stimulus conditions (bedroom temperature, weight of bedclothes, etc.) are optimum for the child in question depending on their sensory profile, and, of course, depriving the child of sleep during the day and keeping social attention and stimuli to a minimum if the child wakes up during the night (Durand, 1998).

| |
|---|
| PREVENTION AND TREATMENT OF ILLNESS |
| • Allow examination and use of medication by family members at home<br>• Become habituated to health care contexts and allow standard medical examinations (by paediatrician and dentist)<br>• Allow special medical examinations: medical tests |
| MEDICATION |
| • Accept taking medication when necessary<br>• Take medication autonomously |
| FOOD |
| • Take solid and varied foods<br>• Take an adequate amount of food |
| PHYSICAL EXERCISE AND POSTURE CONTROL |
| • Do regular physical exercise<br>• Maintain suitable postures in different situations |
| HYGIENE |
| • Perform appropriate oral and dental hygiene every day<br>• Maintain hygiene habits: shower and rinse off soap, wash hands before handling food, hygiene after using the toilet<br>• Cut nails, hair, etc. or allow them to be cut |
| SLEEP |
| • Suitable sleep habits: bedtime, appropriate length of sleep, appropriate strategies for getting to sleep at the right time, etc |
| HEALTH COMMUNICATION |
| • Recognise and express physical discomfort and pain<br>• Give and receive information in medical contexts |
| KNOWLEDGE ABOUT HEALTH AND THE HEALTH CARE CONTEXT |
| • Know and name parts of the body<br>• Know the meaning of the specific terms for illnesses, the course of an illness, etc.<br>• Get to know health care contexts: vocabulary and action guides<br>• Be independent in health care contexts |
| RELAXATION |
| • Have strategies for managing stress<br>• Keep healthy life habits to reduce stress |
| SEX EDUCATION |
| • Know the anatomy and appropriate vocabulary<br>• Know and use suitable ways of releasing sexual tension |
| INFORMATION TO HEALTH CARE CONTEXTS |
| • Have general information about ASDs<br>• Know the characteristics of the communication limitations and possible sensory peculiarities. Adapt the environment and forms of treatment. Use alternative information and communication systems<br>• Possess information on the associated biological conditions and the need for assessment using agreed protocols<br>• Possess up-to-date knowledge on the limits and benefits of psychotropic medication and its effects. |
| HEALTH ACTION AND MONITORING PROTOCOLS |
| • Draw up and periodically apply state-of-health assessment and recording protocols<br>• Protocols for periodical general and dental health check-ups<br>• Draw up protocols to ensure continuity between educational, social and health care services |

Table 1. Integral Health Plan: Summary of the dimensions involved

### 3.7 Health communication

Communication difficulties are one of the basic criteria in diagnosing ASDs (DSM-IV). Programmes to improve communication by means of language or alternative systems are a priority and a central component of intervention. Prizant & Wetherby (2005) have pointed out that limited social communication is directly related to the appearance of behaviour problems. Many problematic behaviours, such as self-injury, tantrums, aggression, preservative use of speech, and so forth may be the only means by which an individual with ASD can exert social control. With such behaviours they may achieve certain goals, such as putting an end to unwanted situations, ensuring physical contact or attention, and initiating or regulating social interaction (Carr et al., 1994). But these maladapted behaviours may be the insidious manifestation of physical discomfort (Buie et al., 2010). It is difficult for persons with ASDs to convey pain and discomfort for various reasons: in the first place, they may not find it easy to identify or locate the sensation precisely due to sensory disorders and a lack of basic body awareness; in addition, their communication is clearly limited, which means they do not engage in spontaneous expressive behaviours or requests for help; and lastly, they often have limited vocabulary -whatever the code they employ- with which to describe specific ailments. In view of this, an important aim of health programmes is helping to express internal states, especially pain and discomfort, is.

A programme designed to help express pain may begin by teaching the person to understand what is happening to them and to express it simply by means of drawings when it is happening. There are situations in which pain is easy to detect: a fall, a cut finger, a grazed foot. At such a time it is appropriate to make a simple drawing of the situation and show it to the child so they can see it and at the same time understand that afterwards they will be helped to share the drawing and show it to people they are familiar with who can console and help them. Ventoso & Osorio (1997) suggest making one or two sketches, entitled "Important", in red describing what has happened that can be shared by showing them to others and saying the appropriate words (eg "knee hurts") if the child has spoken language.

This incidental intervention strategy may be backed up by a broader programme for the expression of sensations. Fun situations can be designed for children to learn, at particular times as part of the regular school activities in the area of communication, to express, by means of spoken language or any other alternative system, sensations, such as "my x itches", "y cold", "z hot", etc., that do not refer directly to pain, but develop the ability to express frequently "what is happening" in their body precisely and accurately. At the same time, it may be useful to have a panel visible or handy by way of a dictionary with drawings depicting common bodily sensations or pains -"head hurts", "tummy ache", "want sick", "hungry", "thirsty"- so that when something happens to them they have a better chance to express it. Stick-on graphics that can be detached by the child and handed to an adult provide enhanced possibilities for communication (Frost & Bondy, 1994).

It is sometimes necessary to explain to high-functioning persons, especially during childhood, the difficulty of identifying sensations and naming them. It is a good idea to help them to recognise the internal parts of the body by providing them with some knowledge of anatomy while explaining the need to ask for help to make things better. Using the social stories format devised by Carol Gray (1994, 2010) can also help a great deal in understanding why it is necessary to express ailments, what consequences this can have and how to react to discomfort.

### 3.8 Knowledge about health and the health care context

As part of the school curriculum dealing with knowledge of the environment, it is extremely important for children with ASDs to be given information allowing them to:
Learn and name parts of the body.

- Learn the meaning of the particular terms for illnesses, the course of diseases, etc.
- Be aware of health care contexts: the different places, vocabulary and guides to action in each one.
- Be independent in health care contexts.

To achieve this, it is proposed to create a special image-based book dealing with these subjects. The format of double fold-out images that the child can match up while someone shows them and explains them to her or him may help the child gain a better understanding and make the knowledge stick (*Autismo Sevilla*, 2010).

This "Health Knowledge" book can be for general use, but personalised for particular children. For example, if a particular child often has diarrhoea, it will be useful to include a page explaining what diarrhoea is, what it implies, what to do about it and when it finishes. As already indicated, the presentation format should be simple, realistic drawings.

The section on health care contexts might cover learning what a health centre or hospital is like, getting to know the rooms and specialities, staff names and material, and brief descriptions of what doctors, nurses and patients do. Naturally, the level at which this is dealt with must be adapted to the different capacities and developmental ages. It is important to back up the theoretical lessons with actual visits to the places to give the child simple experiences in them in accordance with fundamental educational principles (routine, visual anticipation and the possibility of repeating the experience several times in a similar fashion).

Higher-functioning persons can be given more ambitious targets, such as making an appointment, keeping a calendar of visits to doctors, etc., but achieving this also requires teaching with clearly programmed goals and structured and repeated learning opportunities.

### 3.9 Relaxation

Many high-functioning persons with ASDs report that, because of their sensory disorders – hypo- or hypersensitivity- they sometimes feel exposed to excessive stimulation that overwhelms them (Grandin, 1992; Williams, 1994). Some of them may feel panic, for example, if they experience certain noises, touch, certain smells or combinations of stimuli they find too much for them.

On the other hand, limited communication competences, the constant need to adapt to social demands and rules they don't understand, the perception of being different and limited social relations may cause persons who are less affected by such disorders to experience high levels of anxiety and stress and considerably diminish their emotional and physical well-being (Arick, et al, 2005). Each person must be assessed individually to detect the possible stressful stimuli or situations.

There are many strategies for preventing or reducing anxiety and stress in everyday life. One of the most useful is providing a routine with analogous visual information in advance about the activities to be performed and how to carry them out (Mesibov et al., 2005), and especially giving information beforehand when major changes in routine are going to be made. Two other important strategies are having the adult look out for subtle signs of discomfort and doing work on expressive communication.

Arick et al. (2005) made some concrete proposals for reducing stress in high-functioning children in a school setting: identifying one person as a reference and support figure to whom they can turn whenever they need to and who routinely makes sure to ask them how they are, as many persons with ASDs may have difficulty in recognising and expressing their fears and anxieties; making agreed plans for temporary "escape" from the classroom when they cannot stand the stress; combining, in daily life, more demanding activities of limited duration with others more to the child's liking and with a positive value, and allowing "time-outs" in between activities to do relaxing activities, such as wandering around the classroom for a little while, going into another room to be alone for a few minutes or playing with an anti-stress ball.

Other strategies that work for some people with ASDs are routinely doing physical exercise (Grandin, 1992) and occupational therapy focusing on sensory integration (Myles et al., 2000). Harrington et al., (1991), and Baron et al., (2007) have devised programmes of special relaxation techniques for persons with ASDs. They have also produced visual supports to help them detect when they are starting to get nervous and which techniques to use to relax. It seems especially important to teach self-detection systems and immediate calming strategies that can be used by even low-functioning persons. So, for example, when an adult detects signs of anxiety in a child, they can gently guide the child to the bathroom to wet their face, if water has previously proved to relax them. After having done this on several occasions, steps can be taken to offer an alternative communication system with the image of a bathroom that the child can learn to pick up and hand to the adult.

Some organisations (eg *Autismo Burgos* in Spain) regularly employ a jacuzzi and hydrotherapy to reduce anxiety and stress levels.

### 3.10 Sex education

Sexual tension and the limitations on getting to know appropriate ways of relieving it are frequently a cause of discomfort and can give rise to behaviour problems in persons with ASDs. In persons with intellectual disability these are commonly associated with not being able to find any way of releasing sexual tension, the presence of autosexual behaviours without respecting the social environment, seeking release with inappropriate objects and failing to perform appropriate hygiene measures (Ruble & Dalrymple, 1993; Van Bourgondien et al. 1997). With high-performing persons the difficulties are of another kind and are usually associated with the need to have sexual relations with persons of the opposite sex, but not knowing how to achieve this or what to do if they succeed, which may cause confusion, sadness and frustration.

Sex education must begin in childhood, ensuring that the basic principles of privacy are respected. Particular objects can be used to associate moments of sexual release with a specific private place, such as the bedroom, at a particular time of the day and in comfortable conditions. Explanations employing drawings representing where and where not to engage in such behaviour are also of help. On occasions putting on tight-fitting clothes, combined with an offer of an incompatible activity limits the possibility of touching the genitals in inappropriate places and at inappropriate times. It is essential to teach hygiene routines. To do this, the person can be given visual guides to the steps involved by placing the materials to be used in order (eg wet wipes, clean clothes, etc.) or doing the same with drawings.

Sex education programmes for persons with a sufficient level of understanding usually include information on parts of the body and the correct vocabulary for private parts, genital hygiene, the concept of privacy and the appropriate degrees of intimacy with strangers, sporadic acquaintances, regular acquaintances, sporadic dates, friends, boy/girlfriend, wife/husband, family, etc., adjustment of the intensity of the relationship depending on the context, masturbation, sexual relations with other people, emotions to do with sexual relations and the ways to express them, and any other issues particular persons need to clear up (Koller, 2000; Shea & Gordon, 1984; Aizpuru et al., 1998)

### 3.11 Information for health care contexts

In spite of its being presented as just another dimension of the integral health plan, the information given to health care contexts and adaptation of these contexts constitute an enormous programme in themselves because of their possible scope, but also because of the major positive repercussions such a programme can have on persons with ASDs.

In order for them to attend appropriately to persons with ASDs, healthcare professionals working in primary health care and the different specialities should have the following simple but accurate information:

- General information on persons with ASDs. Their behavioural and psychological traits which explain the need to be understood and cared for in a special way.
- Information on the biological conditions commonly associated with ASDs, such as epilepsy and the type of ailments the literature reports as being frequent, such as gastrointestinal disorders and allergies, and the need for assessment in accordance with agreed protocols.
- Detailed knowledge of the communicative limitations of persons with ASDs even though they may be able to speak, possible sensory disorders (hypo- or hypersensitivity), anxiety linked to lack of knowledge and the possible anomalous ways of expressing discomfort, making an accurate diagnosis difficult.
- Appropriate adaptations to the environment and ways of treatment. Use of alternative systems to provide information and facilitate communication.
- Up-to-date knowledge of the limits and benefits of psychotropic medication and its effects.
- Periodically updated expert knowledge for professionals in key specialities for ASDs: neurology, psychiatry, electrophysiology, genetics, digestive system, allergology.

These information programmes can be carried out in very different ways: campaigns with talks, the issuing of brochures, the appointment of volunteer professionals to spread the information, etc. Whatever the form in which the information is conveyed, it is advisable for it to be brief, clear and attractive, for the health care professionals to play an important part, for the information to be regularly updated, and for support to be provided

### 3.12 Health action and monitoring protocols

The last dimension concerns the necessary collection of data and the ways of keeping and sharing important health data (always respecting the relevant privacy laws) to ensure continuity and appropriate care, and the need for suitable prevention and care protocols. The following proposals are made in this connection:

- In both the educational and health care contexts, draw up questionnaires for the initial gathering of health data: present and past illnesses, tests performed, sensory disorders, ways of manifesting discomfort, behaviour during medical examinations, etc. as well as all the possible information resulting from the proposed integral plan.

- A protocol for the ongoing inclusion of health data: check-ups and tests and their results, and especially records of medication and its effects (in educational and health care contexts).
- Simple protocols for "fixed" routine periodical general health and dentistry check-ups, eg every two months. Less frequent routine physiotherapy, eyesight and foot health check-ups, eg once a year.
- Specific protocols for attending to persons with ASDs in various settings: at the health centre, at hospital, in accident and emergency, etc. setting out simply the person's needs and how to respond to them.
- Protocols to ensure continuity between social, health care and educational services.

In this area it is important for there to be agreement among all the institutions involved, for all the professionals to be convinced of the need for such measures, and for the possibility of easily introducing small adaptations into other protocols that are already being used, for example, with persons with disabilities.

## 4. Conclusion

The quantity and complexity of factors that can influence the health of a person with ASDs make it advisable to specially monitor and look after this dimension of QoL through comprehensive health care programmes (Volkmar & Wiesner, 2004).

We know that persons with ASDs can be very different from each other in regard to their degree of competence on various dimensions. Their health needs may therefore also be very different, but the highest-functioning persons may need special monitoring and care when it comes to certain aspects of their physical health (Belinchón, Hernández and Sotillo, 2008). That is why for a long time many organisations dedicated to caring for persons with ASDs have been running programmes dealing with different aspects of health care (e.g. Fuentes, 2010; Alvárez et al., 2007; Autismo Burgos, 2010; GAUTENA; Asociación de Padres de Personas con Autismo [APNA]; Autimo Sevilla; Autismo Galicia) and guides for good practices and action protocols have been published (e.g. The National Autistic Society; Merino et al., 2010)

The integral health plan presented here is based on an assessment of the health care context and the treatment it dispenses to persons with ASDs. It has been designed on the basis of the characteristics of persons with ASDs and what they need to ensure they have a healthy life. This action plan seeks to provide a framework that will serve as a guide so that those involved will know where to look, and offer guidelines on how to act with regard to the initial assessment, the intervention strategies and the final assessment recording the results obtained.

The physical health dimension deserves to be accorded the importance that belongs to it. For a long time the mistaken belief was held that, unlike people with other types of disability, persons with ASDs enjoyed good health. Some recent studies with the families of high-functioning persons with ASDs have verified that this mistaken belief about the latters' general good state of health still exists (Belinchón et al., 2008). The health problems associated with this condition, the difficulties persons with ASDs have in identifying and communicating health problems, and allowing themselves to be examined, and the still scant information and training health care personnel have about these disorders produce an interaction of factors that diminishes these persons' QoL and life expectancy.

## 5. References

Ahearn, W. H., Castine, T., Nault, K., & Green, G. (2001). An assessment of food acceptance in children with autism or pervasive developmental disorder-not otherwise specified. *Journal of Autism and Developmental Disorders,* Vol., 31, pp. 505–512, ISSN 0162-3257

Aizpuru, O., Perez, I., García, T., Garcia, F., & Santaya, M.P. (1998). Desarrollo Afectivo Sexual, In: *AETAPI,* http://www.aetapi.org/materiales.htm

Akshoomoff, N., Pierce, K. & Courchesne, E. (2002). The neurobiological basis of autism from a developmental perspective. *Development and Psychopathology,* Vol.14, No.3, pp. 613-634, ISSN 0954-5794

Allik, H., Larsson, J.O. & Smedje, H. (2006). Sleep patterns of school-age children with Asperger syndrome or high-functioning autism, *Journal of Autism and Developmental Disorders,* Vol. 36, No.5, pp.585-95 ISSN 0162-3257

Alvárez, R. Lobatón, S. & Rojano, M. A. (2007) *Las personas con autismo en el ámbito sanitario. Una guía para profesionales de la salud, familiares y personas con TEA.* Federación Autismo Andalucía: www.autismoandalucia.org

Aman, M.G., Van Bourgondien, M.E., Wolford, P.L., & Sarphare, G. (1995). Psychotropic and multi-convulsant drugs in subjects with autism: Prevalence and patterns of use. *Journal of American Academy of Child and Adolescent Psychology,* Vol. 34, No.12, pp. 1672 -1681 ISSN 0890-8567

American Psychiatric Association (1994). *Diagnostic and Statistical Manual of Mental Disorders,* American Psychiatric Association, ISBN: 0890420254 Washington, DC, USA.

Amit, C., Gourfinkel-Ann, I., Bouzamondon, A., Tordjman, S., Baulac, M., Lechat, P., Mottron, L. & Cohen, D. (2008) Epilepsy in Autism is Associated with Intellectual Disability and Gender: Evidence from a Meta-Analysis. *Biological Psychiatry,* Vol., 64, pp. 577-582, ISSN 0006-3223

Arick, J.R., Krug, D.A., Fullerton, A., Loos, L. & Falco, R. (2005). School-based Programs, In: *Handbook of autism and pervasive developmental disorders* (3rd Edition), F. Volkmar, R. Paul, A. Klin & D.J. Cohen (Eds.),1003-1028, J. Wiley, ISBN 0471716987, New Jersey, USA

Asociación de Padres de Personas con Autismo www.apna.es

Autismo Burgos www.autismoburgos.org

Autismo Galicia www.autismogalicia.orgAutismo Burgos (2010). *Desarrollo del bienestar físico dentro del modelo de calidad de vida".* Accésit al Premio de Buenas Prácticas "Ángel Rivière". AETAPI. 18-20 de noviembre de 2010, Zaragoza, Spain

Autismo Sevilla www.autismosevilla.org/

Baron, M.G., Groden, J., Groden, G. & Lipsitt, L.P. (2006). *Stress and Coping in Autism,* Oxford University Press, ISBN 9780195182262, New York, USA

Belinchón, M., Hernández, J. M. & Sotillo, M. (2008). *Personas con Síndrome de Asperger. Funcionamiento, detección y necesidades,* CPA-CAE-FESPAU-ONCE, ISBN 978-84-96913-20-2, Madrid, Spain

Berthier, M.L., Santamaría, J., Encabo, H. & Tolosa, E.S. (1992) Recurrent hipersomnia into adolescent males with Asperger's syndrome. *Journal of the American Academy of Child & Adolescent Psychiatry,* Vol. 31, pp. 735-738, ISSN 0890-8567

Boghashina O. (2003) *Sensory perceptual issues in autism and Asperger syndrome,* Jessica Kingsley Pubishers, ISBN 978-1-84310-166-6, London, UK

Bondy, A. & Frost, L. (1994) The Picture-Exchange Communication System. *Focus on Autistic Behaviour*, Vol. 9, pp. 1-19, ISSN 0887-1566

Buie T, Campbell DB, Fuchs GJ 3rd, Furuta GT, Levy J, Vandewater J, Whitaker AH, Atkins D, Bauman ML, Beaudet AL, Carr EG, Gershon MD, Hyman SL, Jirapinyo P, Jyonouchi H, Kooros K, Kushak R, Levitt P, Levy SE, Lewis JD, Murray KF, Natowicz MR, Sabra A, Wershil BK, Weston SC, Zeltzer L & Winter H. (2010) Evaluation, diagnosis, and treatment of gastrointestinal disorders in individuals with ASDs: a consensus report. *Pediatrics*, Vol. 125, Suppl. 1, pp. S1-18, ISSN 0210-5721

Canitano, R. (2007). Epilepsy in autism spectrum disorders, *European Child and Adolescent Psychiatry*, Vol. 16, pp. 61–66. ISSN 1018-8827

Carbone, P., S., Behl, D., D., Azor, V., Murphy, N.A. (2010) The medical Home for Children with Autism Spectrum Disorders: Parent and Pediatrician Perspectives. *Journal of Autism and Developmental Disorders*, Vol. 40, pp. 317-324, ISSN 0162-3257

Carr, E.G., Levin, L., McConnachie, G., Carlson, J.I., Kemp, D.C., & Smith, C.E. (1994). *Communication-based intervention for problem behavior. A user's guide for producing positive change*, Paul H. Brookes, ISBN 1-55766 -159-6, Baltimore, USA

Cassanova, M.F. (2006) Neuropathological and Genetic Findings in Autism: The Significance of a Putative Minicolumnopathy, *Neuroscientist*, Vol. 12, No. 5, pp. 435-41, ISSN 03064522

Cassanova. M.F. (2008) The Minicolumnopathy of Autism: A link between migraine and gastrointestinal symptoms. *Medical Hypotheses*, Vol. 70, pp. 73-80, ISSN 0306-9877

Chou, Y.C., Schalock, R.L.,Tzou, L.C., Lin, L.C., Chang, A.L., Lee, W.P. & Chang, S. C.(2007). Quality of life of adults with intellectual disabilities who live with families in Taiwan. *Journal of Intellectual Disabilities Research*, Vol. 51, pp. 875-883, ISSN 0964-2633

Cederlund, M. & Gillberg, C. (2004). One hundred males with Asperger syndrome: a clinical study of background and associated factors. *Developmental Medicine and Child Neurology*, Vol. 46, pp. 652-660, ISSN 0012-1622

Coleman, M. & Betancur, C. (2005). Introduction. In: *The neurology of Autism*, M. Coleman (Ed.), 3-39, Oxford University Press, ISBN 0-19-518222-7, New York, USA

Dias, G. G., Prado, E.F.B., Vadasz, E. & y Siquiera, J.T.T. (2010) Evaluation of the efficacy of a dental plaque control program in autistic patients. *Journal of Autism and Developmental Disorders*, Vol. 40, No. 6, pp. 704-708, ISSN 0162-3257

Dosenbach, N.U., Nardos, B., Cohen, A.L., Fair, D.A, Power, J.D. & Church J.A.(2010) Prediction of individual brain maturity using fMRI, *Science*, Vol. 329, pp. 1358–1361, ISSN 0036-8075

D´Souza, Y., Fombonne, E. & Ward, B. (2006). No Evidence of Persisting Measles Virus in Peripheral Blood Mononuclear Cells from Children with Autism Spectrum Disorder, *Pediatrics*, Vol. 118, No. 4, pp.1664-1675, ISSN 0210-5721

Durand, V.M. (1998). *Sleep better! A guide to improving sleep for children with special needs*, Brookes Publishing ISBN 1-55766-315-7, Baltimore, MD, USA

Field, D., Garland, M., & Williams, K. (2003). Correlates of specific childhood feeding problems. *Journal of Paediatric Child Health*, Vol. 39, pp. 299-304, ISSN 1034-4810

Filipek, P., A. (2005) Medical Aspects of Autism. In: *Handbook of Autism and Pervasive Developmental Disorders. Volume one: Diagnosis, Development, Neurobiology and*

*Behavior (3rd Edition)* F. Wolkmar, R. Paul, A. Klin & D. Cohen (Eds.), 534-578, John Wiley & Sons, ISBN: 0-471-71696-0, New Yersey, USA

Fombonne, E. & Chakrabarti, S. (2001) No evidence for a new variant of measles-mumps-rubella-induced autism. *Pediatrics, Vol.* 108, No. 4, pp. E58, ISSN 0210-5721

Fuentes, J. (2010). Nuestro deber: el derecho a la salud de las personas con autismo. In: XV *Congreso Nacional de profesionales del autismo. AETAPI.* 18-20 de noviembre de 2010, Zaragoza, Spain

Fuentes, J., Gallano, I., Isasa, I., Cundín, M. & Martin, A. (2008). *Pharmautisme TR.* KZ Lankidetza - SPRI del Gobierno Vasco, www.pharmautisme.org

GAUTENA www.gautena.org

Gillberg, C. Billstedt, E., Sundh, V. & Gillberg, I. C. (2010) Mortality in autism: a prospective longitudinal community-based study. *Journal of Autism and Developmental Disorders,* Vol. 40, pp. 352-357, ISSN 0162-3257

Grandin, T. (1992). An inside view of autism. In: *High functioning individuals with autism,* E. Schopler y G. Mesibov (Eds.), 105-126, Plenum Press, ISBN 0-306-44064-4, New York, USA

Gray, C. (1994). *Comics strip conversations and social stories.* Future Horizons, ISBN 1- 885477-22- 8, Arlington, TX, USA

Gray, C. (2010). *The New Social Story Book.* Future Horizons, ISBN 978-1-935274-05-6, Arlington, TX, USA

Green, S. & Ben- Sasson, A. (2010). Anxiety Disorders and sensory over-resposivity in children with Autism Spectrum Disorders: Is there a causal relationship? *Journal of Autism and Developmental Disorders,* Vol. 40, No. 12, pp. 1495-1504, ISSN 0162-3257

Green, V.A., Pituch, K.A., Itchon, J., Choi, A., O'Reilly, M, & Sigafoos, J. (2006). Internet survey of treatments used by parents of children with autism. *Research in Developmental Disabilities,* Vol. 27, pp. 70-84, ISSN 0891-4222.

Harrington, B. & Samdperil, D.L., (Producers). Groden, G. & Groden, J. (Directors) (1991). *Breaking the barriers II* (Videotape), Groden Center, Providence, RI, USA

Hollander E., Phillips A. & Yeh. C. (2003). Targeted treatments for symptom domains in child and adolescent autism. *Lancet,* Vol. 362, No.,9385, pp. 732-734, ISSN 0140-6736

Honomichl, R.D., Goodlin-Jones, B.L., Burnham, M.M., Gaylor, E.E., & Anders, T.F. (2002). Sleep patterns of children with pervasive developmental disorders. *Journal of Autism and Developmental Disorders,* Vol. 32, pp. 553-561, ISSN 0162-3257

Horvath & Perman, 2002 Autism and gastrointestinal symptoms. *Current Gastroenterology Reports,* Vol. 4, No. 3, pp. 251-258, ISSN 1522- 8037

Just, M.A., Cherkassky, V.L., Keller, T.A. & Minshew, N.J. (2004) Cortical activation and synchronization during sentence comprehension in high-functioning autism: evidence of underconnectivity. *Brain,* Vol. 127, pp. 1811-1821, ISSN 0006-8950

Knivsberg, A-M., Reichelt, K. L., Hoien, T., & Nodland, M. (2002). A randomised, controlled study of dietary intervention in autistic syndromes. *Nutritional Neuroscience,* Vol. 5, pp. 251-261, ISSN 1476-8305

Koller, R. (2000). Sexuality and adolescents with autism. *Sexuality and Disability,* Vol. 18, No. 2, pp.125-135, ISSN 0146-1044

Kreuder, L., van Exel, J & Nieboer, A. (2008) Needs of Persons with Severe Intellectual Disabilities: a Q-Methological Study of Clients with Severe Behavioural Disorders and Severe Intellectual Disabilities. *Journal of Applied Reseacher in Intellectual Disabilities,* Vol. 21, pp. 466-476, ISSN 1468-3148

Lightdale, J.R., Siegel, B. & Heyman, M.B. (2001). Gastrointestinal symptoms in autistic children. *Clinical Perspectives in Gastroenterology,* Vol. 1, pp. 56-58, ISSN 1098-8351

Mandell, D. S., Morales, K. H., Marcus, S.C., Stahmer, A.C., Doshi,J., & Plsky, D.E. (2008) Psychotropic Medication Use Among Medicaid-Enrolled Children with Autism Spectrum Disorders, *Pediatrics,* Vol.121, No. 3, pp. E441-e448, ISSN 0210-5721

Martins, Y., Young, R., L., Robson, D., C., (2008). Feeding and Eating Behaviors in Children with Autism and Typically Developing Children. *Journal of Autism and Developmental Disorders,* Vol. 38, pp. 1878-1887, ISSN 0162-3257

Merino, M., García, M.J., Martínez, M., Olivar, J.S., Arnáiz, J., De la Iglesia, M., Hortigüela, V., Nieto, M., García, Ch., Esteban, N. (2010). El acceso a la prestación de asistencia sanitaria de las personas con TEA: un problema sin resolver. *Siglo 0.* Vol. 41, pp. 66-77, ISSN 0210-1696

Minchew, N.J., Sweeney, J.A., Bauman, M.L., & Webb, S.J. (2005). Neurological aspects of autism. In: *Handbook of Autism and Pervasive Developmental Disorders.*(3RD Edition), F. Wolkmar, R. Paul, A. Klin & D. Cohen (Eds.), 473-514, John Wiley & Sons, ISBN 0-471-71696-0, New Yersey, USA

Mouridsen S.E., Brønnum-Hansen H., Rich, B. & Isager T., (2008). Mortality and causes of death in Autism Spectrum Disorders: an update. *Autism: The International Journal of Research & Practice,* Vol. 12, pp. 403-414, ISSN 1362-3613

Mouridsen, S. E., Rich, B., & Isager, T. (1999). Psychiatric morbidity in disintegrative psychosis and infantile autism: A long-term follow-up study. *Psychopathology,* 32, 177-183 ISSN 0254-4962

Myles, B. S., Cook, K. T., Miller, N. E., Rinner, L., & Robbins, L. (2000). *Asperger Syndrome and sensory issues: Practical solutions for making sense of the world.* Autism Asperger Publishing Company. ISBN 0967251478

Nikolov, R., N., Bears, K.E., Lettinga, J., Erickson, C., Rodowski, M., Aman, M.G., McCraken, J.T., McDougle, C. J., Tierney, E., Vitiello, B., Arold, L. E. Shah, B., Posey, D. J., Ritz, L., Scabill, L. (2009). Gastrointestinal Symptoms in a Sample of Children with Pervasive Developmental Disorders. *Journal of Autism and Developmental Disorders,* Vol. 39 pp.405-413 ISSN 0162-3257

Nieto, C., Ventoso, R., Covaleda, A., Andériz, D. & de Oro, E. (2008) Programa de educación sanitaria para personas con Trastornos de Espectro Autista. *Anales de Pediatría,* Vol. 68, pp.149-157, ISSN 1695-4033

Ozonoff, S. (1995). Executive functions in autism. In: *Learning and Cognition in Autism,* E. Schopler & G. Mesibov, (Eds), 199-215, ISBN 0- 306-44871- 8, Plenum Press, New York:USA

Ozonoff, S., Pennington, B.F. & Rogers,S.J.(1991). Executive function deficits in high-functioning autistic individuals: relationship to theory of mind. *Journal of Child Psychology and Psychiatry,* Vol. 32, No.7, pp. 1081-1105, ISSN 0021-9630

Peeters, T (1997). *Autism: From Theoretical Understanding to Educational Intervention.* Whurr publishers, ISBN 90- 5240 -230- 2, London, UK

Polimeni, M., Richsdale, A. & Francis, A. (2005). A survey of sleep problems in autism, Asperger's disorder and typically developing children. *Journal of Intellectual Disability,* Vol. 49, No. 4, 260-268 ISSN 0964-2633

Prizant, B.M. & Wetherby, A. M. (2005). *Critical issues in enhancing communication abilities for persons with autism spectrum disorders.* In: Handbook of autism and pervasive developmental disorders (3rd Edition), F. Volkmar, A. Klin & Paul, R. (Eds.), 925-946, Wiley, ISBN 0471532428,Hoboken, NJ

Rivière, A. (1997). *Tratamiento y Definición del espectro autista II: Anticipación, flexibilidad y capacidades simbólicas.* In: El Tratamiento del Autismo: Nuevas Perspectivas, A. Rivière & J. Martos (Comp.), 107-160, APNA, ISBN 84-88986-70-X, Madrid, Spain

Rosenberg, R.E., Law, J.K., Yenokyan, G., McGready, J., Kaufmann, W.E. & Law, P.A. (2009) Characteristics and concordance of autism spectrum disorders among 277 twin pairs. *Archives of Pediatrics and Adolescent Medicine* Vol. 163, pp. 907–914, ISSN 1072-4710

Ruble, L.A. & Dalrymple, N.J. (1993). Social/sexual awareness of person's with autism: A parental perspective. Archives of Sexual Behavior, Vol. 22, No.,3, pp. 229-240, ISSN 1573-2800

Rutter M. (2005) Incidence of autism spectrum disorders: changes over time and their meaning. Acta Paediatrica, Vol. 94, No.1, pp. 2-15, ISSN 0803-5253

Stigler, K.A., Sweeten, T.L., Posey, .DJ. & McDougle CJ. (2009) Autism and immune factors: a comprehensive review. *Research in Autism Spectrum Disorders,* Vol. 3, No. 4, pp.840-860, ISSN 1750-9467

Schopler, E., Mesibov, G. & Hearsey, K. (1995). Structures teaching in the Teacch System. In: *Learning and Cognition in Autism,* E. Schopler & G. Mesibov (Eds), 243-267, Plenum Press, ISBN 0- 306-44871- 8, New York, USA

Schultz, R.T. & Robins, D.L. (2005). Functional neuroimaging studies of autism spectrum disorders. In: *Handbook of autism and pervasive developmental disorders* (3rd Edition), F. Volkmar, R. Paul, A. Klin & D.J. Cohen (Eds.),515-533, J. Wiley, ISBN 0471716987, New Jersey, USA

Schreck, K. A., Mulick, J. A., & Smith, A. F. (2004). Sleep problems as possible predictors of intensified symptoms of autism. *Research in Developmental Disabilities,* Vol. 25, pp. 57-66, ISSN 0891-4222

Shalock, R.L. & Verdugo, M.A. (2002). Handbook on Quality of Life for Human Service Practioners. American Association on Mental Retardation, ISBN 0-940898-77-2, Washington, DC, USA

Shapira, J., Mann, J., Tamari, I., Mester, R., Knobler, H., Yoeli, Y. & Newbrun, E. (1989). Oral health status and dental needs of an autistic population of children and young adults. Special Care Dentistry, Vol. 9, No. 2, pp. 38-41, ISSN 0275-1879

Shavelle, R.M. & Strauss, D.J. (1998). Comparative mortality of persons with autism in California, 1980-1996. *Journal of Insurance Medicine,* Vol. 30, pp. 220-225, ISSN 0743-6661

Shavelle, R.M., Strauss, D.J. & Pickett, J. (2001). Causes of death in autism. *Journal of Autism and Developmental Disorders,* Vol. 31, pp. 569-576, ISSN 0162-3257

Shea, V. & Gordon, B. (1984) *Growing up: A social and Sexual education picture book for young people,* Chapel Hill-NC, ISBN 9780563516385, North Carolina, USA

Sigman, M., Spence, S.J., & Wang A.T. (2006). Autism from developmental and neuropsychological perspectives. *Annual Review of Clinical Psychology,* Vol. 2, pp. 327-55, ISSN 1548-5943

The National Autistic Society http://www.autism.org.uk/en-gb/working-with/health.aspx

Tuchman, R.F. & Rapin, I. (2002). Epilepsy in autism. *Lancet Neurology*, Vol. 1, pp. 352-358 ISSN 1474-4422

Turk, J., Bax, M., Williams, C., Amin, P., Eriksson, M. & Gillberg, C. (2009). "Autism spectrum disorder in children with and without epilepsy: impact on social functioning and communication. Acta Paediatrica, Vol. 98, pp. 675–681, ISSN 0803-5253

Van Bourgondien, M.E., Reichle, N.C., & Palmer, A. (1997). Sexual behaviour in adults with autism. *Journal of Autism and Developmental Disorders*,Vol. 27, No.2, pp. 113-125, ISSN 0162-3257

Ventoso, R. (2000) Los problemas de alimentación en niños pequeños con autismo. Breve guía. In A. Rivière & J. Martos (Comp.), 153-172, APNA, ISBN84-607-0261-8, Madrid, Spain

Ventoso, R. & Osorio, I. (1997) El empleo de materiales analógicos como organizadores del sentido en personas autistas. In: El Tratamiento del Autismo: Nuevas Perspectivas, A. Rivière & J. Martos (Comp.), 565-588, APNA, ISBN 84-88986-70-X, Madrid, Spain

Volkmar, F.R. & Wiesner, L.A. (2004). *Healthcare for Children on the Autism Spectrum. A Guide to Medical, Nutritional, and Behavioral Issues*. Woodbine House, ISBN: 0933149972, Bethesda, MD

Wiggs, L., & Stores, G. (2004). Sleep patterns and sleep disorders in children with autistic spectrum disorders: Insights using parent report and actigraphy. *Developmental Medicine and Child Neurology*, Vol. 46, No. 6, pp. 372-380.

Williams, D. (1996) *Autism: An Inside-Out Approach*. Jessica Kingsley, ISBN 1853023876, London, UK

White, S., Oswald, D., Ollendick, T., & Scahill, L. (2009). Anxiety in children and adolescents with Autism Spectrum Disorders. *Clinical Psychology Review*, Vol. 29, No. 3, pp. 216–229, ISSN 0272-7358